AF700649

# Writing and Defending Your IME Report
## The Comprehensive Guide

**Steven Babitsky, Esq.**
**James J. Mangraviti, Jr., Esq.**
**J. Mark Melhorn, MD**

**SEAK, Inc.**
**Falmouth, Massachusetts**

*Writing and Defending Your IME Report: The Comprehensive Guide*
Copyright © 2004 by SEAK, Inc.
ISBN: 1-892904-24-1

All rights reserved. Printed in the United States of America. This book is for informational purposes only. It is not intended to constitute legal advice. An attorney or other appropriate source should be consulted if necessary.

No part of this work may be reproduced in any manner whatsoever or by any electronic or mechanical means, including information on retrieval and storage systems, without permission in writing from the publisher, except by a reviewer who may quote brief passages in a review. For information, send a written request for permission to SEAK, Inc., P.O. Box 729, Falmouth, MA 02541. 508-457-1111.

# CONTENTS

# Acknowledgments

The authors wish to acknowledge the following persons whose assistance in the production of this book was invaluable: Christopher R. Brigham, MD; Charles N. Brooks, MD; Lorne K. Direnfeld, MD; Anthony J. Dorto, MD; Thomas S. Eagan, MD; Preston B. Fitzgerald, Sr., DC; Stephen F. Freifeld, MD; Kathy Lamson; Kurt V. Miller, MD; Dee Netzel; Jerome H. Poliacoff, PhD; James Robinson, MD, PhD; Paul S. Sandhu, MD; Dorothy Sims, Esq.; Matthew Shafner, Esq.; and Nathan Zasler, MD.

# Related Products by SEAK, Inc.

TEXTS
*The Comprehensive IME System*
*How to Excel During Depositions*
*The Comprehensive Forensic Services Manual*
*Cross-Examination: The Comprehensive Guide for Experts*
*The Successful Physician Negotiator*

SEMINARS
*IME Summit*
*How to Be a Successful Independent Medical Examiner*
*Medical Witness Summit*
*How to Be an Effective Medical Witness*
*Expert Report Writing Workshop*
*Testifying Skills Workshop*
*Advanced Cross-Examination Workshop*
*SEAK Law School for Physicians ™*
*Malpractice Survival Training for Physicians*
*How to Be a Successful Independent Medical Examiner*
*SEAK Negotiating Skills for Physicians ™*
*SEAK Business School for Physicians ™*
*National Expert Witness and Litigation Seminar*

AUDIOTAPE PROGRAMS
*How to Be a Successful Independent Medical Examiner*
*Achieving Success as a Medical Witness*
*Marketing Your Forensic Practice*
*Law School for Experts*

VIDEOTAPES
*Symptom Magnification, Malingering, and Deception*
*How to Perform an Excellent Independent Medical Examination*
*How to Be an Effective Medical Witness*
*The Expert Medical Deposition: How to Be an Effective and Ethical Witness*

DIRECTORIES
*SEAK, Inc. National Directory of Independent Medical Examiners™*
*SEAK, Inc. National Directory of Medical Experts™*
*SEAK, Inc. National Directory of Physician's Counsel*

For more information call SEAK at 508/457-1111. Inquiries may also be addressed to SEAK, Inc. at P.O. Box 729, Falmouth, MA 02541. Fax 508/540-8304; e-mail address: seakinc@aol.com; Internet address: http://www.seak.com

# About the Authors

**Steven Babitsky, Esq.,** is the President of SEAK, Inc. He was a workers' compensation trial attorney for twenty years and is the former managing partner of the firm Kistin, Babitsky, Latimer & Beitman. He is the founder of the National Organization of Social Security Claimants' Representatives, the co-founder of the American Board of Independent Medical Examiners, and the creator of the AMA *Guides* Newsletter. Mr. Babitsky is the co-author of the texts *Understanding the AMA Guides in Workers' Compensation, Litigating Stress Cases in Workers' Compensation, Cross-Examination: The Comprehensive Guide for Experts, Writing and Defending Your Expert Report: The Step-by-Step Guide with Models, How to Excel During Cross-Examination: Techniques for Experts That Work, The Comprehensive Forensic Services Manual: The Essential Resources for All Experts,* and *How to Excel During Depositions: Techniques for Experts That Work.* Attorney Babitsky is the co-developer of the "How to Be an Effective Medical Witness" seminar, the seminar leader for the National Expert Witness and Litigation Seminar and the annual IME Summit, and the scriptwriter for the videos "How to Be an Effective Medical Witness" and "The Expert Medical Deposition: How to Be an Effective and Ethical Witness." Mr. Babitsky is the co-producer of the videotapes "How to Use the AMA *Guides,* Fourth Edition." He trains hundreds of physicians every year.

**James J. Mangraviti, Jr., Esq.,** has trained hundreds of physicians across the United States and Canada. He is a former trial lawyer with experience in defense and plaintiff personal injury law and insurance law. He currently serves as Vice President and General Counsel of SEAK, Inc. Mr. Mangraviti received his BA degree in mathematics *summa cum laude* from Boston College and his JD degree *cum laude* from Boston College Law School. His publications include the texts *SEAK Law School for Physicians, Law School for the Safety and Health Professional, The Independent Medical Examination Report: A Step-by-Step Guide with Models, The Successful Physician Negotiator: How to Get What You Deserve, Understanding the AMA Guides in Workers' Compensation, Litigating Stress Cases in Workers' Compensation, Cross-Examination: The Comprehensive Guide for Experts, Writing and Defending Your Expert Report: The Step-by-Step Guide with Models, How to Excel During Cross-Examination: Techniques for Experts That Work, The Comprehensive Forensic Services Manual: The Essential Resources for All Experts,* and *How to Excel During Depositions: Techniques for Experts That Work.* He trains hundreds of physicians each year.

**J. Mark Melhorn, MD, FAAOS, FAADEP, FACS,** is an occupational orthopaedic physician who specializes in the hands and upper extremities. He received his BS from McPherson College and his MD from the University of Kansas. Dr. Melhorn is board certified in orthopedic surgery with added qualifications in surgery of the hand. In addition to his practice of orthopaedics at The Hand Center in Wichita, Kansas, Dr. Melhorn is a Clinical Assistant Professor, Section of Orthopaedics, Department of Surgery, University of Kansas School of Medicine–Wichita. He has authored over 150 articles, chapters, and publications about his research of workplace injuries and illnesses; return-to-work options; impairment and disability;

and prevention of musculoskeletal pain in the workplace. He has lectured extensively to physicians, employers, insurers, administrators, and legislators on industrial, musculoskeletal, upper extremity disorders, and prevention of musculoskeletal pain (MSD) in the workplace. He is currently the Chairman for the American Academy of Orthopaedic Surgeons' continuing education course on "Occupational Orthopaedics and Workers' Compensation: A Multidisciplinary Perspective." Dr. Melhorn serves on the Committee for Occupational Health and for Continuing Medical Education for the American Academy of Orthopaedic Surgeons, on the Industrial Injuries and Prevention Committee for the American Society for Surgery of the Hand, on the Return to Work Committee for the American College of Occupational and Environmental Medicine, and is a Musculoskeletal Chapter Reviewer for the American Medical Association's fifth edition of the *Guides to the Evaluation of Permanent Impairment*. Dr. Melhorn is also a previous member of the Ergonomic Committee for the American College of Occupational and Environmental Medicine, he serves as faculty and 2004 co-chairperson for the American Academy of Disability Evaluating Physicians' Annual Continuing Education Meeting, and is past president of the Kansas Orthopedic Society.

# Preface

Over the past several years, we have traveled across the United States and trained thousands of physicians in law, in testifying skills, and in how to be more effective and ethical expert witnesses. We try to make our training as realistic as possible. One technique we use to do this involves cross-examining physicians with redacted versions of actual IME reports used in closed cases.

We have, unfortunately, found far too many poorly written IME reports. These reports needlessly open up the examiner to devastating cross-examination. This work has been written to be a comprehensive text to assist examiners in writing high-quality IME reports and in defending their IME reports during cross-examination.

There are innumerable ways to draft high-quality, defensible IME reports. Perhaps the best place to start is by looking at some other well-written reports. Chapter 18 provides examples of some of the better reports that we have come across. The reader can get good ideas on formatting, style, and content from these reports. A highly defensible IME report can then be drafted by following the advice contained in the chapters of this work, which are summarized in Chapter 1 and explained in detail in Chapters 2 through 17.

As in our previous works, we get directly to the point, use numerous examples, and make this an easy-to-use reference. The examples show why the report's language was effective or why it was problematic, the consequences thereof, and how the language could have been easily improved. We have also listened to our clients and have dedicated entire chapters to how to defeat the cross-examining attorney's tactics and how to answer the most difficult trick questions dealing with IMEs. For the first time, we have also added a "Defending the Report As Written" section to almost all of the examples. This is in response to our clients' request for our advice as to how difficult cross-examination questions might be answered. Your feedback is always welcome.

Steven Babitsky, Esq.
James J. Mangraviti, Jr., Esq.

SEAK, Inc.
P.O. Box 729
Falmouth, MA 02541
Phone: (508) 457-1111
Fax: (508) 540-8304
www.seak.com

# Chapter 1 Introduction and Executive Summary

## 1.1 Introduction

IME reports should be well written. Examiners should also be prepared to defend their reports from counsel's tricks and tactics during cross-examination. Examiners who wish to prepare well-written, defensible IME reports and want to defend their reports during cross-examination should carefully consider the advice contained in this book.

The importance of a well-drafted and defensible IME report cannot be overstated. The IME report will likely be an important component of a disputed legal claim. A poorly written report will reflect badly on the examiner who wrote it and may result in injustices in the underlying litigation. On the other hand, a well-written report can serve as an offensive weapon during cross-examination and will increase the demand for the examiner's expertise.

## 1.2 Answer Only the Questions Asked

Examiners should only answer the questions posed by the referring client. These questions should be answered truthfully, without giving any benefit of the doubt to the referring client. Examiners should not opine on other areas. If there is any doubt regarding what issues the client would like addressed, these should be cleared up with a quick phone call to the referral source.

**Example 1.21: Questions to be answered**

*Report States:*

> I appreciate the opportunity of seeing Mrs. Weiss for an Independent Medical Examination. I do not have a letter identifying the questions relating to this, but I suspect I have been asked to determine the current medical status.

*Resulting Cross-examination:*

**Q.** Doctor, you didn't know what you were doing when you examined Mrs. Weiss for an IME, correct?

**A.** I am a board certified orthopedic surgeon, so I clearly know what I am doing.

**Q.** You would agree that an IME could be set up to determine any number of issues?

**A.** Yes.

**Q.** What are the typical issues you are asked to deal with in an IME?

**A.** Causation, prognosis, maximum medical improvement, permanent impairment, work capacity, appropriateness of care, diagnosis, and current medical status.

**Q.** Did you know which one of these eight issues you were supposed to be dealing with and examining for?

**A.** Not precisely.
**Q.** In fact, you state right in your IME report, "I do not have a letter identifying questions relating to this, but I suspect I have been asked to determine the current medical status," isn't that correct?
**A.** Yes.
**Q.** So you took a guess about the purpose and performed an exam based on a suspicion?
**A.** An educated guess.
**Q.** So you really didn't know what you were doing when you did this IME, correct?

**Comment:** IME physicians need a clear understanding of the issues and why the IME is being requested so that they can properly address the issues in their reports. Doing an IME report based on an educated guess or suspicion is ill-advised. When there is ambiguity as to the issues to be addressed, the IME physician should clarify the purpose of the exam before proceeding.

> I did not have a letter identifying the issues to be addressed. I called the insurer and determined that the purpose of the exam was to determine the examinee's current medical status.

**Defending the Report As Written:** The IME physician can use his experience when a clear cover letter does not accompany the referral.

**Q.** Doctor, you didn't know what you were doing when you examined Mrs. Weiss for an IME, correct?
**A.** I received all of the medical records for the examinee without a cover letter. I was unable to get a hold of the insurer, so I performed a current medical status exam, which I learned the next day was what was intended. I am prepared to discuss my medical findings after you stop insulting me. I assume you are reluctant to do so when this is what you are asking me about.

**Example 1.22: Superfluous causation opinion**
*Report States:*

> He is also complaining of low back pain. No medical records are available regarding his back. His back problems may be secondary to favoring his right leg during the recovery phase from his right knee surgery.

*Resulting Cross-examination:*
**Q.** Doctor, you stated in your IME report that the examinee's right knee injury was causally related to his injury at work?
**A.** Yes, I did.
**Q.** You then expressed the further opinion that, "His back problems may be secondary to favoring his right leg during the recovery phase from his right knee surgery," correct?
**A.** Yes, that's my opinion.
**Q.** Do you hold your opinion about the cause of the back problems to a reasonable degree of medical certainty?
**A.** Yes, I do.

**Q.** Thank you, Doctor.

**Comment:** When an IME physician is asked to evaluate causation and work capacity arising out of a knee injury, that is what he should do. In the above example, the IME physician "volunteered his opinion" about a back injury. By volunteering this opinion and then agreeing that it was held to a reasonable degree of medical certainty, he may have created substantial problems for the insurer who requested the IME for the right knee. This passing comment could cost the insurer thousands of dollars and result in substantial litigation.

**Defending the Report As Written:** When an IME physician suspects that opposing counsel is trying to use him to make his case, the physician need not cooperate. He needs to tell the truth, but he can do so in an artful manner.

**Q.** Do you hold your opinion about the cause of the back problems to a reasonable degree of medical certainty?
**A.** No. That's why I said "maybe." I had no medical records for his back and didn't perform an examination of his back. I cannot express an opinion one way or the other on that issue.

## 1.3 Just Say "No"

A crucial trait of quality independent medical examiners is the ability and willingness to say "no" to the referring client. Saying "no" is the best way to deal with many potential problems that can arise in IMEs, including:

- being asked to opine on areas outside of the examiner's true area of expertise,
- being asked to opine without being provided with crucial records and documents,
- being asked to take a history from an examinee who does not speak English without being provided with a translator,
- being asked to work for referral sources that edit or perform "quality control" on reports and then attach the examiner's electronic signature,
- being pressured by the referral source to come to a certain conclusion, and
- being asked to evaluate a patient whom the examiner has treated in the past.

**Example 1.31: Prior medical treatment of examinee**
*Report States:*

Interestingly, initially I saw the examinee for purposes of treatment two years ago.

*Resulting Cross-examination:*
**Q.** Doctor, the examinee is a patient of yours, correct?
**A.** Former patient.

**Q.** As such, you have or had a patient/treating physician confidential relationship?
**A.** As I said in my IME report, "I saw the examinee for purposes of treatment two years ago." So I had a patient/treating physician confidential relationship with him.
**Q.** You breached this confidential relationship during this IME process, did you not?
**A.** Absolutely not. This IME is two years after I treated him. One has nothing to do with the other.
**Q.** Do you not use the confidential information you garnered while treating him to paint him as a liar in your IME report?
**A.** That's not true and is an outrageous accusation.
**Q.** Do you not say on page 2 of your IME report, "I saw the examinee on 6/4/2000 for purposes of treatment. At that time, the examinee told me that his low back pain started at work on 2/2/2000 when he was lifting cartons of copy paper while employed at Smithe Office Supplies. Today the examinee denied any occupational back injury while working for Smithe Office Supplies."

**Comment:** Physicians who have previously treated a patient should not perform an IME exam on that same patient at a later time. In addition to the confidentiality issue evidenced in the above example, issues of prior treatment, appropriateness of care, rendering of future medical treatment, and billing provide too many potential conflicts. IME physicians are better served by informing the requesting party that due to a potential conflict of interest they will not be willing to perform the IME.

**Defending the Report As Written:** When confronted with prior treatment of an examinee, the IME physician can make the best of a difficult situation.

**Q.** As such, you have or had a patient/treating physician confidential relationship?
**A.** Yes. That is why prior to performing the IME, I made full disclosure to the requesting party and the examinee and his counsel. All parties signed a letter indicating they were aware of the past treatment, that they consented to the IME, and that they consented to me releasing the past records of the examinee in my possession. If someone wanted to object to the IME, they should have done so before I issued my IME report with its findings, not afterwards, Counsel.

## 1.4 Background Information and Transmittal Letters

Examiners should expect the reader to focus extra attention on the beginning of the IME report. This is only natural. To make the beginning of reports effective and defensible, the authors recommend the following.

- Document identifying information, such as the name of the examinee, the date of the evaluation, the date of the injury, the file number, and the referral source in an easy-to-read, professional-looking format.
- Include an "Executive Summary" or "Summary of Diagnoses" at

the beginning of lengthy reports.

- Avoid superfluous information and cheap shots against the examinee.
- Keep all language professional, objective, and formal.
- Consider, if appropriate, documenting the following introductory information.
    - That the examinee was told that there would be no treating physician/patient relationship.
    - That the examinee was informed that the information shared by the examinee would be included in the examiner's report.
    - That the examinee was told he should not engage in any physical maneuvers that might cause injury and should immediately report any discomfort encountered during the examination. (If applicable, the fact that no discomfort was reported during the examination should also be documented.)
    - Whether anyone else, such as a member of the examiner's staff, a spouse, a significant other, an attorney, or a treating provider, was present during the evaluation.
    - The role and behavior of all present.
    - Whether the examinee was uncooperative; for example, by not providing a history or refusing to fill out pain inventories.
    - Whether the examinee drove himself to the examination.
    - Any requests to audiotape or videotape the examination should also be documented along with a note as to whether such taping occurred.
    - If the examinee's history was dictated in the presence of the examinee to ensure accuracy.
    - The beginning and ending times of the examination. (When times are documented, they should be precise and not rounded off.)
- Make sure cover letters are short, objective, and devoid of extraneous information. As a rule of thumb, any cover letter that is more than one sentence is too long.

Chapter 2 provides detailed information and examples of how to best present background and introductory information. It also discusses best practices in drafting transmittal letters for IME reports.

## 1.5 The Examiner's Qualifications

IME reports sometimes directly (e.g., curriculum vitae attached or qualifications summarized) or indirectly (e.g., credentials listed after the examiner's name or on the examiner's letterhead) contain statements or representations regarding the examiner's qualifications. The authors recommend the following regarding statements of the examiner's qualifications.

- An appropriate statement of qualifications must be included in the IME report if this is a requirement of the court or forum in question. Failure to do so may result in the disallowance of the examiner and her report.
- Any and all statements of the examiner's qualifications must be 100% accurate. This means actively proofing the qualifications to avoid unintentional mistakes.
- Examiners should be objective when stating qualifications. They should reword subjective, self-serving statements and characterizations (e.g., instead of calling oneself an "extremely prolific" writer, it would be better to objectively state that the examiner is an author or co-author of six texts and 47 articles).
- An examiner should not claim as a qualification a degree or designation that sounds like it was earned but was, in reality, bought from a "diploma mill."
- Wise examiners are careful when claiming knowledge of the current literature in their respective fields because there is *a lot* of literature out there.

Chapter 3 covers how to properly state the examiner's credentials.

## 1.6 The Examiner's True Area of Expertise

***IME reports should only express opinions that are within the examiner's true area of expertise.*** Examiners should be very careful to avoid expressing opinions in areas outside of their true area of expertise. Specifically, the authors recommend that examiners do the following.

- Avoid using legal terms (e.g., "informed consent," "grossly negligent," "proximate cause," etc.) and making legal conclusions (e.g., "this was a compensable injury").
- Only use terms for which they know the definitions.
- Not opine on cost estimates unless they are qualified to do so. Where cost estimates are made, these should be supported with objective evidence.
- Not opine on areas outside of their medical discipline, specialty, or sub-specialty.
- Not offer opinions in non-medical areas, such as machine design or accident reconstruction, where the examiner is not qualified to do so.

Chapter 4 details and demonstrates the importance of staying within the examiner's true area of expertise.

## 1.7 Formatting

The use of proper formatting is a low-cost, easy way to improve IME reports. Proper formatting makes IME reports easier to read and understand and more valuable to the reader. The authors recommend that examiners follow these guidelines when formatting their reports.

- Construct and use a cover page that provides basic information about the examinee, examiner, and examination.
- Use a 12-point font, which is easier to read than smaller fonts.
- Break up the IME report by using topic headings (and subheadings). These should be in bold.
- Use short, concise paragraphs and avoid long, run-on paragraphs. This may require a combination of improved dictation skills and a review of the report after transcription but prior to it being finalized and sent to the client.
- Consider using 1½ spaces between lines.
- Include page numbers in the following format: [page number] of [total number of pages in report]. For example, "page 5 of 19."

Chapter 5 explores proper and improper formatting.

## 1.8 Medical Records and Other Documents Reviewed

It is essential that the examiner organize, explicitly list, and precisely describe all of the medical records, reports, depositions, and other documents she has reviewed. This serves several purposes.

- It forces the examiner to account for all the material she has reviewed.
- It removes any ambiguity about what was and was not reviewed by the examiner.
- It permits the examiner to consult her report quickly when questioned as to what was and was not reviewed.

In terms of presentation of the list of medical records and other documents reviewed, the authors recommend the following.

- Each document should be precisely described, including, when appropriate, date, length, author, and other descriptive information.
- The list should be numbered.

- The documents should be listed chronologically or according to some natural, logical grouping (for example, all medical reports, all diagnostic studies, all depositions).[1]
- To make an IME report truly stand out and highly valuable to the referring client, the examiner should consider not merely listing the medical records reviewed, but summarizing each record reviewed as well.
- The following descriptives should be avoided: "including," "including, but not limited to," "relevant portions of," and "various."
- Examiners should not make opposing counsel's job easier by explicitly listing documents that were not available for review.
- Examiners should generally not produce reports in cases where there were few or no records available for review.
- Surveillance material should be described objectively and without any gratuitous language attacking the claimant.
- Illegibility should not be used as an excuse for the wholesale ignoring of records.
- Examiners should expect close questioning regarding the authenticity, accuracy, and completeness of medical records provided by the referral source.

Chapter 6 covers how to best document the medical and other records reviewed.

## 1.9 History

A precise, well-written, and accurate history is an essential part of a high-quality IME report. The authors recommend the following.

- Thorough IMEs address the following areas.
    - Pre-existing Status/Past Medical History
    - Description of Injury/Incident
    - Treatment History
    - Psychosocial/Socioeconomic/Social/Educational History
    - Family Medical History
    - Occupational/Employment/Work History
- The various parts of the history should each be addressed in their own section, each identified by a topic heading.
- To help ensure accuracy, the examiner should:
    - dictate the history in the presence of the examinee,
    - not rely on a staff member to take the history, and

[1] Thomas G. Gutheil, *The Psychiatrist As Expert Witness* (Washington, DC: American Psychiatric Press, 1998) 104-105.

  - use a translator, where needed.
- Objective, measured language should be used, especially when documenting inconsistencies.
- The examiner should not include superfluous verbiage or take subtle or overt cheap shots at the examinee.
- It is best that the examiner takes and documents a treatment history from the examinee and also creates a history from the available medical records. This will help ensure completeness and allow for the identification of potential inconsistencies.
- When opinions are expressed on work capacity in the occupational history section, the examiner will be in the best position to defend these opinions when he has as much accurate information concerning the job in question as possible.

Chapter 7 discusses documenting the examinee's history.

## 1.10 Physical Examination

A detailed, well-documented physical examination is an essential part of the IME report. All of the tests performed and all findings made should be clearly documented. Further advice regarding documenting the physical examination includes the following.

- Self-serving descriptions of the physical examination as "comprehensive" or "complete" should be avoided. If the numerous tests and measurements performed are documented in the report, the "completeness" of the examination will speak for itself.
- The physical examination section of the report should be broken up into subsections dealing with the various components of the examination, such as "Observation," "Structural Examination," "Range of Motion," "Neurological Examination," etc. This will make the report easier to read.
- The precise (not rounded off) starting and ending times of the physical examination should be documented.
- The behavioral assessment should be objectively documented.
- Examiners should be aware that IME reports are most believable when the "normal" results received are not universally "textbook perfect" figures.
- Test results and measurements should be formatted in an easy-to-read manner.
- The specific tests performed for nonphysiological findings should be carefully documented. Examiners should expect close questioning during cross-examination regarding any nonphysiological findings.

- Adding digital photos to an IME report is of great benefit to the client and will make the IME report stand out.
- Examiners should consider using the most common pain inventories. These include the following.
  - Medical Outcome Studies (MOS)
  - SF-36 Health Survey
  - Pain Drawing
  - Pain Disability Index
  - McGill Pain Questionnaire
  - West Haven-Yale Multidimensional Pain Inventory, Short Form - 36 Questions (SF-36)
  - Mensana Clinic Pain Validity Test
  - Center for Epidemiologic Studies - Depressed Mood Scale
  - Beck Depression Inventory
- The examiner should only use pain inventories he sufficiently understands and can defend during cross-examination.
- The *current status* (e.g., the examinee's current symptoms, pain status, and level of disability and impairment) should be elicited in detail and thoroughly documented.
- The location, intensity, frequency, pattern, and nature of the pain, as well as aggravating and relieving factors, need to be documented.
- Functional status should be thoroughly elicited and documented in detail.
- Examiners should not spy on examinees while they arrive at and leave the examination.

Chapter 8 contains detailed information on properly documenting the physical examination.

## 1.11 Citing Authority

Citations to a well-accepted authority that supports an examiner's opinions will bolster the credibility of the IME report. The authors recommend the following.

- The citations should be detailed and precise. They should include title, author, edition, publisher, and year published.
- A pinpoint cite should be used if specific pages are referenced.
- The examiner should be prepared to be cross-examined on any authority cited in the report.
- It is wise to avoid general statements that the examiner's conclusions are supported by the "weight of the literature" or "studies."

- Examiners should attempt to use authority that is as recent as possible and, where possible, avoid using outdated authority.
- Quoting authority may bolster the report's credibility, but the examiner should expect to be closely questioned not only about the quoted passage but other passages from the reference as well.
- Examiners should avoid describing any authority as "authoritative" or "reliable" because these terms may have special legal significance that can expand the scope of permissible cross-examination of the examiner.
- Examiners should be familiar with the ABIME guidelines for performing IMEs and be prepared to answer questions about these guidelines, especially if they are certified by ABIME or if the report cites the ABIME guidelines.

Chapter 9 discusses the optimum ways to cite authority in an IME report.

## 1.12 Opinions

One of the main reasons an examiner is involved in a case is to draft a report that states her opinion. The examiner's opinion should be communicated effectively and be expressed in a defensible manner. The authors recommend the following.

- State all opinions clearly, explicitly, and with confidence.
- Use the magic words "based upon a reasonable degree of medical certainty" or "based on a reasonable degree of medical probability" when expressing opinions in the report.
- Avoid hedge words, such as "it seems," "I think," and "I believe," when expressing opinions in the IME report.
- State the reasons that justify the opinion, preferably in concise bullet-point format.
- Avoid expressing net or summary opinions; that is, bare conclusions without supporting justification.
- State all of the opinions the examiner expects to express at hearing or trial.
- Document a detailed and reliable reasoning so that the report will not be challenged under *Daubert.*
- Prepare a list of the examinee's clinical diagnoses, including any need for further evaluation. For each diagnosis, indicate, where appropriate, which is acute, which is chronic or degenerative, and which is pre-existing.
- Carefully analyze the current diagnoses, the mechanism of injury, the diagnoses at the time of injury, the pre-existing status, and the clinical history to determine whether the injury was pre-

existing or caused by an event or occurrence that is not a subject of the claim. The examiner's analysis and conclusions regarding causation need to be clearly documented in the report.
- State objectively supported reasons for apportionment opinions.
- Properly use the terms "aggravation" and "exacerbation" and understand their legal significance in the jurisdiction in question.
- Provide objective justification for prognosis opinions and refrain from making extraneous comments about the examinee.
- Understand the meaning of "maximum medical improvement" in the jurisdiction in question. The term needs to be properly used and the examiner's written opinion needs to be accompanied by the reasons supporting it.
- Express permanent impairment ratings correctly by using the correct edition of the appropriate guidelines and by documenting precisely how the rating was calculated. If needed, the examiner should obtain training on conducting impairment ratings.
- Only opine on work capacity and disability when the examiner has sufficient information to do so. When opinions are made in this area, the examiner should have a thorough understanding of the examinee's job and correctly use terms from the *Dictionary of Occupational Titles.*
- Be careful when commenting on appropriateness of past care.
- Do not take "pot shots" at other providers or disciplines.
- Avoid, in most cases, using the terms "fraud" and "malingering."
- Document symptom magnification or lack of objective support for the examinee's subjective complaints with non-inflammatory language supported by specific, objective evidence.
- Be prepared for questions concerning the examinee's pain and questions accusing the examiner of trying to "trick" the examinee with distraction tests.

Chapter 10 explains best practices for expressing opinions in IME reports.

## 1.13 The Powerful, Persuasive, and Understandable Report

There are numerous techniques that can be used to make an IME report powerful, persuasive, and understandable. The authors recommend the following.

- State things clearly and directly.
- Do not speculate or guess.
- Document all reasons that support findings and conclusions.
- Take extra care when opining on future medical costs.
- Avoid, or at least minimize, the use of boilerplate language.

- If boilerplate language is used, carefully proof the report for internal inconsistencies before signing off on it.
- Avoid the use of absolute words, such as “always,” “completely” and “never.”
- Make sure the report is not vague, equivocal, or uncertain.
- Avoid emphatic language, exclamation points, boldface type, italics, and capital letters to emphasize findings, conclusions, and other information.
- Use the active and not the passive voice.
- Use precise language.
- Use the first person when referring to oneself in the report.
- Write with confident language and avoid hedge words, such as “it seems,” “could,” “apparently,” and “I believe.”
- Define all technical medical terms and jargon.
- Use objective language and avoid subjective characterizations to describe the examination, findings, and conclusions.
- Explain the meaning of any medical abbreviations used.
- Avoid argumentative language.
- Document all inconsistencies, but avoid opining on the credibility of the examinee.
- Make sure the report is internally consistent and consistent with any previous reports in the case or other cases.
- Avoid any appearance of bias in the report.
- Be very careful when using computer-generated standard language or report templates in IME reports.

Chapter 11 covers how to write a powerful, persuasive, and understandable IME report.

## 1.14 Extraneous Language

The only language that should appear in IME reports is language that objectively states or supports an examiner’s findings and conclusions or language that is otherwise relevant. All other information and language is extraneous and should not be included in the report.

Including superfluous language in an IME report is one of the most common mistakes independent medical examiners make. This mistake can cost the examiner’s (and the report’s) credibility dearly. Extraneous language often provides fertile grounds for cross-examination. The authors recommend the following.

- Avoid “friendly” language to counsel that thanks her for the assignment, invites comments or questions, offers further assistance, or includes personal salutations.
- Do not include speeches in IME reports.

- Make sure letterhead does not include references to being an "IME doctor."
- Cover letters accompanying reports should be short and formal. One sentence is ideal.
- Do not document in the IME report discussions with counsel, adjusters, or brokers unless they are relevant.
- Examiners should aggressively self-edit their reports to remove all other superfluous language (including offers to provide treatment, piling on against a party in the case, the examiner's personal feelings, the name of any third-party broker or expert witness service, solicitation of future assignments, and snide comments directed at the examinee, opposing counsel, the examinee's providers, or anyone else).

Chapter 12 demonstrates the importance of avoiding extraneous language in IME reports.

## 1.15 Words to Avoid

The use of certain words in IME reports will raise red flags with the attorney whose job it is to undermine the examiner, her credibility, and her opinions. Such red-flag words should be avoided. Chapter 13 discusses some of the most common red-flag words found in independent medical examination reports. Red-flag words include the following.

- "Authoritative" to describe a medical text or journal. This term has special legal significance that may allow a cross-examining attorney to question the examiner about everything in the text.
- "Legal" or "legally." What is and is not legal is usually outside of the area of expertise of most examiners.
- "Draft." This term alerts counsel to the existence of draft reports that are usually extremely fertile grounds for cross-examination.
- "Work product," "confidential," or "privileged." These terms make it appear as though the examiner is trying to hide something. These are also legal terms that the examiner may have difficulty defining properly.
- "Probable" and "possible." These ambiguous words should be avoided.
- "Substantially." This is another ambiguous word to avoid.
- "Obviously" and "clearly." These terms can be used to make the expert appear patronizing or presumptuous.
- "Appears," "presumably," "supposedly," "is said," and "evidently." These terms imply uncertainty.

- "He," "she," "it," "they," and other pronouns. Pronouns are uncertain. It is best to use a proper noun. For example, it is best to write "Mrs. Jane Smith."
- Royal "we." This can be used to make the expert look silly, pompous, or even dishonest.
- "It seems," "could," "apparently," "I believe," and other hedge words. It is always best to use confident language.
- "Complete," "thorough," "meticulous," "exhaustive," and other such words to describe the examiner's chart review, research, or examination. These self-serving words will hold the examiner and her report to an extremely high standard.
- "Patient." The person being examined is an "examinee" or a "claimant," not a patient. There is no doctor/patient relationship.
- "Malingering." In the majority of cases, it is usually better for the examiner to merely document exaggerated pain behaviors, inconsistencies, non-organic findings, and lack of objective findings rather than making a diagnosis of malingering.
- "Alleged," "credible," and other words that directly or indirectly opine on the credibility of the examinee. The examiner is a medical expert, not a credibility expert.
- "Dictated but not read" and "electronic signature." These practices make the examiner appear to be more interested in cranking out reports and collecting fees than in precision and accuracy.

Chapter 13 contains detailed advice on red-flag words to avoid.

## 1.16 The Influence of the Referring Client

An examiner's credibility can be severely damaged if opposing counsel can show that the examiner's client improperly influenced the examiner and his report. The authors recommend the following.

- Do not circulate draft reports to the referral source. If a draft report is circulated, opposing counsel will attempt to show that the final report's contents were improperly influenced by the referral source.
- Do not discard circulated draft reports or cover letters from the referral source. Destroying these may be illegal and will certainly have a negative influence on the examiner's credibility.
- Do not agree to change the substance of the report at the request of the referral source. If a mistake was made, issue a supplemental report and explicitly correct the previous mistake. If additional information is requested, write an addendum and label it as such.

- If the referral source is pressing for improper changes in a report, ask the referral source to make its request in writing.
- Review and sign all reports personally.
- Do not work for referral sources that "improve" and "finalize" the IME report and attach the examiner's on-file electronic signature.

Chapter 14 explains the importance of not allowing the referring client to improperly influence an IME report.

## 1.17 Proofreading

Examiners need to carefully proof their IME reports for mistakes. Each and every mistake made in an IME report will lessen the report's persuasive value and the credibility of the examiner who wrote it. Opposing counsel will argue that if the examiner could make one mistake in his report, he may have made other mistakes and his entire report may be suspect. Opposing counsel will also use the mistakes to show that the examiner was sloppy or even ill-informed. Common mistakes that need to be corrected in the proofreading process include:

- substantive mistakes,
- bad grammar,
- typographical or transcription errors, and
- misspelled words.

Mistakes can and should be avoided. They are best avoided by careful proofing before the report is finalized and sent to the client. When an examiner is confronted with an apparent mistake, he should either gracefully admit the mistake or explain to counsel why no mistake was made.

Chapter 15 demonstrates the importance of thorough proofreading.

## 1.18 Defending the IME Report

Examiners need to be prepared to defend their IME reports at hearings, trials, and depositions. Advice on how to truthfully and artfully defend IME reports is contained throughout Chapters 2–15. This is generally accomplished by telling the truth and actively disputing counsel's mischaracterizations and misleading questions. Chapter 16 provides detailed advice on how to defeat counsel's tactics used during cross-examination. Chapter 17 lists the most difficult questions examiners may face on cross-examination and analyzes how to deal with each question effectively.

## 1.19 Model Reports

One of the best ways to draft a quality IME report is to study and emulate other quality IME reports. Chapter 18 contains ten complete model IME reports. The model reports in Chapter 18 have been annotated in an attempt to make them more helpful to the reader. Examiners should study reports from their colleagues and adapt the best features of these reports into their own reports.

# Chapter 2 Background Information and Transmittal Letters

## 2.1 Executive Summary

Examiners should expect the reader to focus extra attention on the beginning of the IME report. This is only natural. To make the beginnings of reports effective and defensible, the authors recommend the following.

- Document identifying information, such as the name of the examinee, the date of the evaluation, the date of the injury, the file number, and the referral source, in an easy-to-read, professional-looking format.
- Include an "Executive Summary" or "Summary of Diagnoses" at the beginning of lengthy reports.
- Avoid superfluous information and cheap shots against the examinee.
- Keep all language professional, objective, and formal.
- If appropriate, document the following introductory information.
    - That the examinee was told that there will be no treating physician/patient relationship.
    - That the information shared by the examinee will be included in the examiner's report.
    - That the examinee should not engage in any physical maneuvers that may cause injury and should immediately report any discomfort encountered during the examination. (If applicable, the fact that no discomfort was reported during the examination should also be documented.)
    - Whether anyone else, such as a member of the examiner's staff, a spouse, a significant other, an attorney, or a treating provider, was present during the evaluation.
    - The role and behavior of all present.
    - Whether the examinee was uncooperative; for example, by not providing a history or refusing to fill out pain inventories.
    - Whether the examinee drove himself to the examination.
    - Any requests to audiotape or videotape the examination should also be documented along with a note as to whether such taping occurred.
    - If the examinee's history is dictated in the presence of the examinee to ensure accuracy.
    - The beginning and ending times of the examination are given in order. (When times are documented, they should be precise and not rounded off.)

- Make sure cover letters are short, objective, and devoid of superfluous information. As a rule of thumb, any cover letter that is more than one sentence is too long.

## 2.2 Preliminary Identifying Information

It is customary at the beginning of the report to include the name of the examinee, the date of the evaluation, the date of the injury, the file number, and the referral source. This is best done in an easy-to-read, professional-looking format. Well-written reports also contain an executive summary or summary of diagnoses and a table of contents if the report is lengthy. These features make the report easier to use and more valuable to the reader.

**Example 2.21: Introductory information includes list of diagnoses and table of contents**

*Report States:*

| | |
|---|---|
| Examinee: | Martha Jane Formaggio |
| Identification Number: | 123456789 |
| Date of Birth: | 01/24/40 |
| | |
| Date of Examination: | 04/25/01 |
| | |
| Examining Physician: | Thomas S. Eagan, M.D., P.C. |
| Examination Location: | 215 County Highway 128, Gloversville, NY 12078 |
| | |
| Date of Injury: | 11/26/99 |
| | |
| Client Organization: | Buntz Claims Services, Ltd. |
| Referral Source: | Judy Buntz |
| Date Exam Requested: | 04/06/01 |

**<u>Summary</u>**

**Diagnosis**

1. Dislocation Right Shoulder.
2. Lower Brachial Plexus Injury Right Shoulder.
3. Chip Fracture Nasal Bone.
4. Diabetes.
5. Hypertension.
6. Morbid Obesity.
7. Degenerative Arthritis Right Shoulder (pre-existing).
8. Rotator Cuff Tear Right Shoulder.
9. Fracture Left Clavicle.
10. Cervical Spondylosis.
11. Carpal Tunnel Syndrome Right.

**Table of Contents**



**Comment:** The introductory information in this report is presented in an easy-to-read format. The summary of diagnoses and table of contents add value to the report.

Some reports are written in the form of correspondence addressed to the client. Such reports simply reference the relevant information. In any case, the relevant identifying information should be provided in a straightforward, professional manner and superfluous information should be omitted from the report.

**Example 2.22: Level of examination: Comprehensive**
*Report States:*

| | |
|---|---|
| **Examinee:** | James Sample, IV |
| **Date of Birth:** | December 27, 1960 |
| **Date of Evaluation:** | August 28, 2003 |
| **Date of Injury:** | October 1, 2001 |
| **Referral Organization:** | Unified Mutual |
| **Referral Individual:** | Marge Smith |
| **Referral Reference No.:** | WC112-456-1 |
| **Examining Physician:** | James A. Smith, MD |
| **Location of Examination:** | Peabody, Maine |
| **Type of Examination:** | Workers' Compensation |
| **Level of Examination:** | Comprehensive |

*Resulting Cross-examination:*
**Q.** Doctor, you performed a comprehensive IME in this case, correct?
**A.** Yes. I stated that in the report, "level of examination: comprehensive."
**Q.** So sometimes you just do a down and dirty quickie IME and sometimes you do a comprehensive one?

**Comment:** It is not advisable to include superfluous comments and information in IME reports. Superfluous information by its very nature fails to support the opinions of the examiner. In addition, superfluous information often raises new issues and invites additional, damaging cross-examination. For more information on the importance of avoiding superfluous information in an IME report, please see Chapter 12.

**Defending the Report As Written:** Some jurisdictions and venues may require the physician to specify the level of examination. In this case, the physician is absolutely correct to do so.

**Q.** So sometimes you just do a down and dirty quickie IME and sometimes you do a comprehensive one?

**A.** Counsel, as you should know, in this jurisdiction when an IME physician is presented with over 100 pages of medical records to review, the IME is considered "comprehensive." All my IMEs are high quality. Some just require reviewing more medical records than others and evaluating more areas and functions of the body.

**Example 2.23: "Dear Johnny"**

*Report States:*

John E. Cochoran, Esq.
Cochoran, Bailey & Shapiro
60 State Street
Boston, MA 02110

RE:

| | |
|---|---|
| Examinee: | John Sample |
| D.O.I.: | 3/6/02 |
| Your File No.: | 1807 |
| Our File No.: | 03-123 |
| Claim No.: | 1234-95T |
| Insurer: | Lloyds' of Londonderry |

Dear Johnny:

*Resulting Cross-examination:*

**Q.** Doctor, your IME report was impartial and done without bias, correct?
**A.** That's correct.
**Q.** You are a personal friend of Attorney John E. Cochoran, are you not?
**A.** Not really.
**Q.** Have you worked with him before this case?
**A.** Yes.
**Q.** How often?
**A.** That would be hard to say.
**Q.** Do you have other cases pending with him?
**A.** I believe I do.
**Q.** How many?
**A.** That's hard to say.
**Q.** You golf with him?
**A.** Yes, but not too well.
**Q.** And you attended his daughter's recent wedding?
**A.** Yes, I did.
**Q.** You referred to him as "Dear Johnny" in the IME report, correct?
A. Yes.
**Q.** You are a personal friend of John E. Cochoran. Is that too hard for you to say?

**Comment:** Independent medical examiners should refer to their referral sources in a formal, business-like manner and not by a nickname that implies an ongoing relationship or friendship. The failure to do so will result in cross-examination concerning the nature and extent of the relationship, as in the above example.

The denial of the obvious relationship in this example serves to compound the error because it demonstrates the physician's dishonesty.

**Defending the Report As Written:** Many times, a personal greeting, salutation, or passing comment is merely the independent medical examiner's way of being friendly, informal, or courteous. While opposing counsel may try to imply a bias, the examiner may be able to easily neutralize this type of attack by pointing out objective reasons why the examiner is not biased.

**Q.** You are a personal friend of Attorney John E. Cochoran, are you not?
**A.** Even though I am usually on the other side of his cases, I am proud to say he is a personal friend. I call them as I see them. That has been my reputation for the past 27 years.

## 2.3 Preliminary and Introductory Information

Certain preliminary information should be documented in the report. This includes the fact that the examinee was told that there will be no treating physician/patient relationship, the fact that the information shared by the examinee will be included in the examiner's report, that the examinee should not engage in any physical maneuvers that may cause injury, and that she should immediately report any discomfort encountered during the examination. If applicable, the fact that no discomfort was reported during the examination should also be documented. If discomfort was reported, the examiner should document that that part of the physical examination was stopped and no apparent residual symptoms were observed or were communicated to the examiner by the examinee.

The examiner should also document whether anyone else, such as a member of the examiner's staff, a spouse, a significant other, an attorney, or a treating provider, was present during the evaluation. The role and behavior of all present should be noted. If the examinee is uncooperative (for example, by not providing a history or refusing to fill out pain inventories), this should also be documented in the report. The examiner should also note whether the examinee drove herself to the examination.

Any requests to audiotape or videotape the examination should be documented along with documentation as to whether such taping occurred. Furthermore, if the examinee's history is dictated in the presence of the examinee to ensure accuracy, this should also be documented in the beginning of the report.

Some examiners also document the beginning and ending times of the examination in order to insulate against "all he did was look at me for five minutes" attacks. When times are documented, they should be precise and not rounded off.

All of the above information needs to be documented in an objective, professional, non-judgmental way. Superfluous information and "cheap shots" against the examinee need to be avoided. Such cheap shots could include documenting the type of car driven by the examinee, flashy jewelry, the nature of tattoos, etc.

**Example 2.31: "A…fair historian"**
*Report States:*

> This 42-year-old right-handed man was referred for an independent medical evaluation at the request of the above client. The IME process was explained to the examinee, and he understands that no patient/treating physician relationship exists and that a report will be sent to the requesting client. History was provided by the examinee, who was a cooperative, fair historian. He arrived on time for the appointment, driven by his wife, who often answered for him and reinforced statements of disability. Approximately 1½ hours were spent directly with the examinee, with an additional 45 minutes in review of clinical information and preparation of the report. The examinee reported no difficulties associated with the examination.

*Resulting Cross-examination:*
**Q.** You classify examinees as poor historians, fair historians, or good historians?
**A.** Yes, I do.
**Q.** This is not a hard and fast scientific classification—just your subjective impression, correct?
**A.** Yes.
**Q.** Thank you.

**Comment:** When IME examiners comment on the examinee as a historian, vague subjective descriptions are of little value. If the examinee had difficulty relating a portion of the history, the examiner should state the problem with specificity.

> The history was provided by the examinee, who had difficulty relating the names of his treating physicians and the dates he underwent surgery and physical therapy.

**Defending the Report As Written:** When being cross-examined, physicians need not agree with the characterizations of opposing counsel. Just because the question seems reasonable does not mean one needs to agree with it.

**Q.** This is not a hard and fast scientific classification, just your subjective impression, correct?
**A.** No, it's the traditional method used by experienced IME examiners to describe the examinee as a historian. My 27 years of experience make it much more than a "subjective impression."

**Example 2.32: Cheap shot, superfluous information**
*Report States:*

> Mr. Sample was accompanied by his spouse, who is currently on Social Security disability.

*Resulting Cross-examination:*
**Q.** Your IME report is impartial and unbiased, correct?
**A.** Yes, it is.
**Q.** The issue you addressed is whether the examinee's ruptured cervical disc was the result of his car accident?
**A.** That's correct.
**Q.** You wrote in your IME report that the examinee's spouse is currently on Social Security disability, correct?
**A.** Yes, I did.
**Q.** Did that fact influence your opinion on the issue of causation?
**A.** No, not really.
**Q.** You recorded that fact in your unbiased IME report because you wanted to color the fact finder's impression of the examinee, correct?

**Comment:** The IME physician who shows bias and lack of impartiality in her report instantly loses credibility. Some IME physicians consciously or subconsciously make passing denigrating comments about the examinee and his lifestyle. Comments about driving a fancy car, jewelry, or a spouse's source of income may fall into this category. Opposing counsel may go through each and every one of these comments to show a pattern of bias. When done effectively, the IME physician is eventually unmasked as an advocate for a position and not an impartial examiner. Her IME report then becomes worthless. The keys to avoiding the appearance of bias and lack of impartiality are knowing the science that supports one's conclusions and knowing the information in the report.

**Defending the Report As Written:** IME physicians may have very legitimate reasons for their passing comments. If so, they should not be afraid to state them.

**Q.** You recorded that fact in your unbiased IME report because you wanted to color the fact finder's impression of the examinee, correct?
**A.** I stated that fact because that is how the examinee introduced his spouse. "This is Nancy, my wife. She is on Social Security disability." I did find it curious as Nancy is only 29 years old.

Or, alternatively:

**A.** No. I am aware of medical studies that demonstrate that disability can be influenced by learned behavior patterns and that the most common risk factor for this learned behavior pattern is family members who have experienced a disability in the past or who are currently classified as disabled.

**Example 2.33: Round numbers used on time documentation**
*Report States:*

> Ms. Formaggio arrived at 3:00 PM, the interview commenced at 4:00 PM, followed by the physical examination, which started at 4:30 PM and was completed by 5:00 PM.

*Resulting Cross-examination:*
**Q.** Doctor, your IME report is unbiased and accurate, correct?
**A.** Yes, it is.
**Q.** When you say the examinee arrived at 3:00 PM, that is an approximation?
**A.** Yes. It was around 3:00 PM.
**Q.** Your interview didn't commence at exactly 4:00 PM either, correct?
**A.** That's correct.
**Q.** The same for the time of the physical examination starting at 4:30 PM and ending at 5:00 PM?
**A.** Yes.
**Q.** So when you testified that your IME report was accurate, that's not true. All of the times are approximate. Are your medical findings and impairment ratings also just mere approximations?

**Comment:** Examiners are best served by using precise times (as opposed to approximate round numbers) when time is documented. This serves two purposes:

1. the more precise the time noted, the more believable the time documentation, and
2. precisely documented times permit the examiner to testify that the times were accurate and not "mere approximations."

**Defending the Report As Written:** When attorneys have little to attack, they try to split hairs on cross-examination. There is no reason examiners have to engage in these games with counsel.

**Q.** When you say the examinee arrived at 3:00 PM, that is an approximation, is it not?
**A.** Counsel, we don't have examinees punch a time clock. That is the time the receptionist noted on the file. Are you going to argue our clock is slow or fast, Counsel? I guess you prefer not to discuss the medical-legal issues in the case.

## 2.4 Transmittal/Cover Letters

If the report is not written in the form of a letter, it will usually be sent to the referral source along with a transmittal or cover letter. Transmittal/cover letters should be as short as possible, formal, and devoid of any superfluous information. ***As a general rule of thumb, any cover letter that is more than one sentence probably contains superfluous information.***

**Example 2.41: "Detective-like instincts"**
*Cover Letter States:*

Dear Ms. Smith:

Thank you for referring this fascinating and challenging case to me. It really forced me to put my substantial detective-like instincts to work. Please do not hesitate to contact me if I can be of any further assistance.

*Resulting Cross-examination:*

**Q.** In addition to your medical training, you have received training as a detective as well?

**A.** No, I have not.

**Q.** So the "substantial detective-like instincts" you have are self-taught?

**A.** I picked them up along the way.

**Q.** Do the "substantial detective-like instincts" you have, Doctor, tell you when an examinee is not telling you the truth?

**A.** Very often they do.

**Q.** You pride yourself on this ability to detect the truth, don't you?

**A.** Yes, I do.

**Q.** Sometimes you are wrong about the veracity of the examinee?

**A.** Not very often.

**Q.** How would you know that, Doctor?

**A.** Experience, Counselor.

**Q.** You watched this examinee exit his car on his way into your office?

**A.** I did.

**Q.** You wrote in your report he moved freely without difficulty?

**A.** Yes, it was very informative.

**Q.** Do you watch many of your examinees exit their cars on the way into your office?

**A.** As many as I can.

**Q.** How many IMEs have you done, Doctor?

**A.** Over 2,000.

**Q.** Can you show me one IME report in which you wrote, "I observed the examinee exit his vehicle on the way into my office. He did so with great difficulty?"

**Comment:** When opposing counsel can portray the IME physician as an advocate (as opposed to an impartial examiner), the physician and his report lose credibility and believability. The superfluous self-description "substantial detective-like instincts" opens this door and invites unnecessary cross-examination.

**Defending the Report As Written:** The ability to recover from a potentially damaging comment is the hallmark of an experienced IME examiner.

**Q.** Do the "substantial detective-like instincts" you have, Doctor, tell you when an examinee is not telling the truth?

**A.** As a forensic psychiatrist, I am trained to question the examinee and elicit information. I then compare the information given by the examinee to the medical, hospital, and other records available. This obtaining and comparing information is part of my job. You need detective instincts to do it well. Otherwise, the examinee would tell me information and I would just record it as being accurate. You then would be questioning me about why I took everything at face value.

**Example 2.42: "In compliance with F.R.C.P. 26(a)(2)(b) and with local standards of my profession regarding the preparation of expert reports"**
*Cover Letter States:*

> In compliance with F.R.C.P. 26(a)(2)(b) and with local standards of my profession regarding the preparation of expert reports, I have attached the following....

*Resulting Cross-examination:*

**Q.** Is your IME report in compliance with F.R.C.P. 26(a)(2)(b)?
**A.** Yes, it is.
**Q.** What is F.R.C.P. 26(a)(2)(b)?
**A.** The rule dealing with expert reports.
**Q.** What does F.R.C.P. stand for?
**A.** I don't know.
**Q.** Have the Federal Rules of Civil Procedure been adopted in your jurisdiction, Doctor?
**A.** Well, I thought...I don't know.
**Q.** Have you attached all of the cases you have testified in the past four years as required by the Rule?
**A.** All of the trials.
**Q.** What about the depositions?
**A.** No.
**Q.** Are you aware that the Rule states: "...and a listing of any other cases in which the witness has testified as an expert at trial or by deposition within the preceding four years"?
**A.** No, I didn't know that.
**Q.** So, when you stated in your cover letter, "In compliance with F.R.C.P. 26 (a)(2)(b) and with local standards of my profession regarding preparation of expert reports," that was not accurate? Let's now talk about the so-called "local standards."

**Comment:** The above is a good example of how superfluous language in a cover letter can get the examiner in trouble. There was no need to put this language in the cover letter.

**Defending the Report As Written:** When legal terminology is used, the examiner needs to understand it and be able to explain it easily.

**Q.** What does F.R.C.P. stand for?
**A.** Federal Rules of Civil Procedure.

# Chapter 3 Stating the Examiner's Qualifications Accurately and Objectively

## 3.1 Executive Summary

IME reports sometimes directly (e.g., a curriculum vitae is attached or qualifications are summarized) or indirectly (e.g., credentials are listed after the examiner's name or on the examiner's letterhead) contain statements or representations regarding the examiner's qualifications. The authors recommend the following regarding statements of the examiner's qualifications.

- An appropriate statement of qualifications must be included in the IME report if this is a requirement of the court or forum in question. Failure to do so may result in the disallowance of the examiner and her report.
- Any and all statements of the examiner's qualifications must be 100% accurate. This means actively proofing the qualifications to avoid unintentional mistakes.
- Examiners should be objective when stating qualifications. It is best to reword subjective, self-serving statements and characterizations (e.g., instead of calling oneself an "extremely prolific" writer, it would be better to objectively state the examiner is an author or co-author of six texts and 47 articles).
- An examiner should not claim as a qualification a degree or designation that sounds like it was earned but was, in reality, bought from a "diploma mill."
- Wise examiners are careful when claiming knowledge of the current literature in their respective fields because there is *a lot* of literature out there.

## 3.2 Legal Requirements

An examiner who fails to provide her curriculum vitae (CV) as required by applicable discovery rules[1] or court orders can jeopardize not only the admissibility of her testimony but, in some instances, the case itself. Consider the following examples.

**Example 3.21: Failure to provide CV prior to testifying**
*Seivewright v. State*, 7 P.3d 24 (Wyoming 2000)
In this criminal case, the expert, Dr. Huben, failed to provide his CV before he testified. The court pointed out the importance of the CV, which is relevant to

[1] For example, expert reports prepared pursuant to Federal Rule of Civil Procedure 26(a)(2)(B) must contain "...the qualifications of the witness, including a list of all publications authored by the witness within the preceding ten year..."

qualifications and credibility. "In the case of an expert witness, in which qualifications go to both admissibility and weight, a vitae is material information by which the opposing party's counsel can challenge the expert's qualifications and credibility."

The Wyoming Supreme Court found that the trial court committed reversible error by allowing the expert to testify without producing his CV and report. The court stated:

> In accordance with W.R.Cr.P. 26.2, if a party elects not to comply with an order to deliver a statement, the district court has three options for sanctioning that behavior. The rule requires that the trial court *"shall* order" (1) that the witness not be permitted to testify; or (2) that the testimony of the witness be stricken from the record; or (3) if the attorney for the State elects not to comply, the court *shall* declare a mistrial if required in the interest of justice. W.R.Cr.P. 26.2(e). The rule is mandatory in all respects; it does not allow the district court any discretion to refuse to act in the face of uncontradicted allegations of discovery violations in a criminal prosecution. Allowing Seivewright to object to "particular questions" at trial is not one of the sanctions mandated by the rule. Thus, it cannot be argued that the district court's ruling was within the parameters of the rule despite its failure to determine if the discovery order has been violated.
>
> When Seivewright alleged the State failed to comply with W.R.Cr.P. 26.2, the district court should have ordered the State to submit the document for *in camera* inspection or held a hearing to determine whether the report and the curriculum vitae fell within the purview of the rule or the pretrial discovery order. Failure to take any action at all violated the rule and was reversible error. At 27.

**Example 3.22: Report without qualifications insufficient, expert must supplement or be barred from testifying**

*Nguyen v. IBP, Inc.,* 162 F.R.D. 675 (D. Kansas 1995)

This case involved an insufficient Rule 26 report in federal court. The court stated:

> The disclosures served by plaintiff clearly and indisputably do not comply with Fed.R.Civ.P. 26(a)(2)(B). The only document signed by the expert witness was a letter addressing the expert's opinions and the basis therefor, the data considered by the expert, and exhibits to be used as a summary of or support for the opinions. While a curriculum vitae was provided, it was not signed by the witness and did not include publications authored by the witness within the past 10 years. Although plaintiff, by interrogatory answer, provided the compensation agreement, this agreement was not a part of the report signed by the witness. Plaintiff's counsel supplied a list of 137 patients about whom the witness had apparently testified during the 34 month period prior to October 28, 1994, and the dates of the deposition testimony. No identification of the "cases" in which these depositions were given is provided. The court or administrative agency in which the depositions were taken is not provided. Although an attorney's name is provided as to most of the patients, in many instances the first or last name of the attorney is missing. The telephone numbers are not supplied for the attorneys for 55 patients. The list is not signed by the witness. It includes entries for less than three years rather than for four years as required by the rule. At 679.
>
> Plaintiff's failure to provide a report including a statement of the expert's compensation agreement, the expert's qualifications, or an identity of the publications authored by the expert during the past 10 years, in light of the lack of any such publications, is harmless since the facts were otherwise supplied and the

> failure may be cured by simply having the witness sign a disclosure to these facts. As noted above, the failure to provide the listing of cases is not harmless. The court will allow the plaintiff to provide a supplemental disclosure which corrects the deficiencies identified herein within 40 days from the date of the filing of this order, otherwise, Dr. Shechter will not be permitted to testify at the trial of the action. At 682.

## 3.3 Accuracy

The statement of qualifications must be 100% accurate. Even honest mistakes in stating an examiner's qualifications can have a devastating effect on the examiner's credibility. Opposing counsel can make very good use of mistakes in an IME report dealing with the examiner's own qualifications. Opposing counsel will try to show that the examiner was either so incompetent or sloppy that he couldn't even get his own qualifications correct. Even worse, counsel may be able to show that the examiner exaggerated his qualifications and was dishonest in doing so. Mistakes regarding an examiner's qualifications are completely avoidable. Consider the following example.

**Example 3.31: Incorrect use of "Diplomate" instead of "Board Certified by"**

*Report States:*

Diplomate, American Board of Independent Medical Examiners

*Resulting Cross-examination:*

**Q.** Doctor, your report indicates on page 3, second paragraph, that you are a Diplomate of the American Board of Independent Medical Examiners or ABIME, correct?
**A.** Yes, that's right.
**Q.** For how long have you been a Diplomate of ABIME?
**A.** Two years.
**Q.** During that time, how many expert reports have you issued?
**A.** I am not sure.
**Q.** Approximately, Doctor.
**A.** 100 or more.
**Q.** Did you list your ABIME Diplomate status on these reports?
**A.** Yes.
**Q.** Doctor, you carefully check your report for mistakes or errors, do you not?
**A.** Yes, as best I can within my time constraints.
**Q.** What do you think of doctors who claim credentials they do not possess?
**A.** That's not right.
**Q.** What about their credibility?
**A.** They would have none as far as I am concerned.
**Q.** Doctor, I show you a letter from the American Board of Independent Medical Examiners and ask you if you would read the highlighted portion.
**A.** "I am the Executive Director of ABIME and state that the American Board of Independent Medical Examiners has no current, nor has ever had, any Diplomates." There must be some mistake.

**Q.** Apparently so, Doctor. Are you going to continue to use this Diplomate status of ABIME in the future?
**A.** Absolutely not.
**Q.** Do you intend to correct the 100+ reports in which you previously claimed these credentials?
**A.** Huh? I am not sure. I think I need to consult with counsel.

**Comment:** The doctor in question was, in fact, board certified by ABIME. He mistakenly—and innocently—claimed to be a Diplomate. This simple error destroyed the examiner's credibility. The examiner should have verified that the qualifications stated in his report were 100% accurate. He should have stated:

> Board Certified as an Independent Medical Examiner by the American Board of Independent Medical Examiners

**Defending the Report As Written:** IME physicians need to carefully prepare before testifying. During this in-depth preparation, the physician may be able to identify many of his mistakes and be able to correct them quickly, efficiently, and with as little damage as possible.

**Q.** Doctor, your report indicates on page 3, second paragraph, that you are a Diplomate of the American Board of Independent Medical Examiners or ABIME, correct?
**A.** No, that's a mistake on my part. It should state Board Certified by ABIME. I have corrected my current CV to reflect this change.

**Example 3.32: Examiner inaccurate regarding status as author**
*Report States:*

> I am the author of two texts in the field of impairment and disability.

*Resulting Cross-examination:*
**Q.** Doctor, on page 12 of your IME report you state your qualifications, correct?
**A.** Yes, that's correct.
**Q.** You state, "I am the author of two texts in the field of impairment and disability," correct?
**A.** Yes, that's correct.
**Q.** You stated that under the penalty of perjury?
**A.** Yes, I did.
**Q.** How many times have you stated this in your IME reports?
**A.** Hundreds, maybe more.
**Q.** Even though you know that the statement is not true?
**A.** Pardon me?
**Q.** Doctor, on your 1997 book, how many authors are listed on the title page and spine?
**A.** Well, three.
**Q.** So, you are not the author of the text, but one of three co-authors?
**A.** Yes, but I wrote most of it.
**Q.** On your 1999 book, how many authors are listed?

**A.** Four. But again, I wrote most of the material.
**Q.** Doctor, when you intentionally stated in your IME report, "I am the author of two of the texts in the field of impairment and disability," you did so knowing that this was not true but because you felt you deserved most of the credit?

**Comment:** Examiners often get into trouble when listing their writings and publications in the qualifications portion of their reports. The examiner should carefully distinguish if he was an "author," a "co-author," or a "contributor" to a text or article. Failure to do so will make it appear as if the examiner is exaggerating his qualifications to impress the fact finder or jury. Offering weak excuses for the action will just make the situation worse.

> I am a co-author of two texts in the field of impairment and disability.

**Defending the Report As Written:** As soon as the examiner detects an error in his report, he should endeavor to correct it.

**Q.** You state, "I am the author of two texts in the field of impairment and disability," correct?
**A.** That's what it says, but that is not accurate. I am a co-author of these texts. Sorry for the mistake.

## 3.4 Objectivity

Subjective, self-serving statements and characterizations should be left out of reports. Such subjective characterizations of an examiner's qualifications will almost invariably lead to trouble on the witness stand. Qualifications need to be stated objectively and accurately.

**Example 3.41: "Internationally recognized expert"**
*Report States:*
> I am an internationally recognized expert on impairment evaluations and am frequently interviewed and quoted in *Impairment Evaluation Monthly.*

*Resulting Cross-examination:*
**Q.** You state in your report that you are an internationally recognized expert on impairment evaluations.
**A.** That's correct.
**Q.** When you say "internationally recognized," what percentage of the world's four billion people do you think would recognize your name?
**A.** Counsel, obviously I meant by my peers.
**Q.** How many people read and would recognize your name from *Impairment Evaluation Monthly?*
**A.** At least 1,000.
**Q.** So you consider yourself internationally recognized because 1,000 members of the world's population have heard of your name?

**Comment:** Subjective statements to the effect that the examiner is "nationally recognized" or is a "leading authority" should be avoided. As can be seen in this example, counsel will use such statements to make the examiner appear to be exaggerating her own qualifications and importance. This will result in a loss of credibility. This particular examiner would have been better served by including the following *objective* evidence of her qualifications.

**Journal and Press Quotations**
"Challenging Examinees," *Impairment Evaluation Monthly,* July 2002
"Fibromyalgia," *Impairment Evaluation Monthly,* September 2001
...

**Awards**
2003 Lifetime Achievement Award

**Defending the Report As Written:** Opposing counsel may attempt to lead the IME physician down the primrose path. Alert examiners should develop a sense of when this is occurring and attempt to head it off when possible.

**Q.** When you say "internationally recognized," what percentage of the world's four billion people do you think would recognize your name?
**A.** Counsel, I have taught over 2,400 physicians about impairment. I taught physicians in the United States, Canada, Australia, and thirteen other countries. *Impairment Evaluation Monthly* is distributed worldwide as well. I am an internationally recognized expert in this area.

## 3.5 Unearned Designations or Degrees

It is unwise to claim as a qualification a degree or designation that sounds as though it was earned but was, in reality, bought. Examiners should not claim such status unless they have truly earned it. For example, such designations are earned by passing a serious examination and having appropriate and qualifying experience. Listing a bought-and-paid-for designation or degree from a "diploma mill" will lessen an examiner's credibility, not increase it.

**Example 3.51: Bought-and-paid-for designation**
*Report States:*
Board Certified, International Board of Forensic Medicine and Science
Diplomate, International Board of Forensic Medicine and Science

*Resulting Cross-examination:*
**Q.** You state in your report, do you not, that you are board certified by the International Board of Forensic Medicine and Science?
**A.** That's correct.
**Q.** You also state that you are a Diplomate of the International Board of Forensic Medicine and Science?
**A.** Yes.
**Q.** You never took a written examination to earn your board certification, did you?
**A.** It wasn't required.
**Q.** You never took an oral examination to earn your board certification, did you?

**A.** No, it wasn't required.
**Q.** You never took a written examination to earn your Diplomate status, did you?
**A.** No.
**Q.** You never took an oral examination to earn your Diplomate status, did you?
**A.** No.
**Q.** You did apply for the Diplomate status and the board certification, did you not?
**A.** Yes, I did.
**Q.** And when you sent in your application, there was an application fee?
**A.** Yes.
**Q.** Isn't it a fact that the "application" fee was $1,250 for the board certification and $1,500 for the Diplomate status?
**A.** Yes.
**Q.** You sent them the money and they gave you the designations. That about sums it up, doesn't it?
**A.** I met all their requirements, sir.
**Q.** What requirements were there beyond sending the money?

**Comment:** Unearned, "bought" certifications should not be included in a CV. They are not relevant to an examiner's qualifications and can be used to lessen an examiner's credibility.

**Defending the Report As Written:** When faced with questions about credentials, the IME physician can defend the credentialing process if he has the information available. This defense should only be attempted when the physician truly believes in the credentialing process.

**Q.** What requirements were there beyond sending the money?
**A.** The requirements include graduation from an accredited medical school, current valid license, minimum 10 years experience, copies of a deposition, a trial transcript, a sample report, a copy of your current curriculum vitae, and two letters of reference from judges. All of these are submitted to the committee.

## 3.6 Knowledge of Literature

Wise examiners are careful when claiming knowledge of the current literature in their field. There is a *lot* of literature out there. It is easy for counsel to use a statement that an examiner is current with the literature against the expert.

**Example 3.61: "Current with the literature"**
*Report States:*
I keep current with the literature in this field.

*Resulting Cross-examination:*
**Q.** You state in your report that you keep current with the literature in "this field," meaning shoulder dystocia, is that correct?
**A.** Yes.

**Q.** Did you read the article entitled "What is shoulder dystocia?" in the February 2001 issue of the *Journal of Reproductive Medicine?*
**A.** I can't recall.
**Q.** Did you read the article entitled "Shoulder dystocia: The event that wraps a midwife's heart in cold terror" in the Autumn 2000 issue of *Midwifery Today?*
**A.** No.
**Q.** Did you read the article entitled "Shoulder dystocia" in the December 2000 issue of the *Journal of Reproduction Medicine?*
**A.** Yes.
**Q.** Could you please summarize the conclusions of that article?

**Comment:** If an examiner claims in her report to keep current with the literature, she can expect a cross-examination similar to that provided above. It would be extremely difficult for even the most brilliant expert to do well in this type of a cross-examination. This report would have been much better had it not included the statement regarding keeping current with the literature in the examiner's field.

**Defending the Report As Written:** Counsel, when cross-examining the IME physician, will try to build momentum and then finish with a flourish. Knowing this fact, experienced IME physicians will often intentionally interrupt or slow counsel down. The more disjointed the questions and eventual answers, the less power the tactic will have.

**Q.** Did you read the article entitled, "What is Shoulder Dystocia?" in the February 2001 issue of the *Journal of Reproductive Medicine?*
**A.** I subscribe to the *Journal of Reproductive Medicine* and read the article some time ago. I do a Medline search on the topic each time I write an article. In the last year, I wrote three journal articles. Each time I collected all of the articles written in English over the past months. There are dozens of articles written each year, Counsel. Are you going to ask me about each one and expect me to recite from memory the article and its conclusions? That doesn't seem particularly fair, does it?

# Chapter 4 The Importance of Staying within the Examiner's True Area of Expertise

## 4.1 Executive Summary

***IME reports should only express opinions that are within the examiner's true area of expertise.*** Examiners should be very careful to avoid expressing opinions in areas outside of their true areas of expertise. Specifically, the authors recommend that examiners use the following guidelines.

- Avoid using legal terms (e.g., "informed consent," "grossly negligent," "proximate cause," etc.) and making legal conclusions (e.g., "this was a compensable injury").
- Only use terms for which they know the definitions.
- Not opine on cost estimates unless they are qualified to do so. Where cost estimates are made, these should be supported with objective evidence.
- Not opine in areas outside of their medical discipline, specialty, or sub-specialty.
- Not offer opinions in non-medical areas, such as machine design or accident reconstruction, where the examiner is not qualified to do so.

## 4.2 Legal Terms and Opinions

One of the many traps that examiners often walk into is the use of legal terms and conclusions in their reports. An examiner can expect to be closely questioned about any and all legal terms and conclusions in her report.

This is an easy trap to avoid. The best practice is to simply avoid using legal terms and drawing legal conclusions. Where the examiner insists on reporting on legal concepts, these should be stated without the use of legal terminology. For example, instead of using the term "malpractice," the examiner could discuss a violation of the standard of care that resulted in harm to the patient. If legal terms are used or legal conclusions are made, the examiner needs to be prepared to define and defend these terms and conclusions.

When an examiner uses legal terms or makes legal conclusions, the cross-examiner will attempt to show that the examiner didn't really know what she was talking about when she employed the legal terms. This can be used to lessen the examiner's credibility by demonstrating that because the examiner did not know what she was talking about in one area of her report, the rest of the report should also be called into question.

**Example 4.21: Informed consent**

*Report States:*

The signed statement qualifies as informed consent for dental therapy.

*Resulting Cross-examination:*

**Q.** You found the statement sufficient legally for informed consent, correct?
**A.** Yes.
**Q.** Can you explain the four elements of informed consent?
**A.** No, not off-hand.
**Q.** The dentist would have to explain the nature of the procedure and treatment, correct?
**A.** Yes.
**Q.** Did that take place here?
**A.** I don't know.
**Q.** The patient should be informed about the expectations of the treatments and the likelihood of success?
**A.** Yes.
**Q.** Is that contained in the form?
**A.** No.
**Q.** What about reasonable alternatives and probable outcome? Are those in the form?
**A.** No.
**Q.** What about the known inherent material risks? Is that in the form?
**A.** No.
**Q.** So, when you concluded that the signed, nonspecific statement qualified as informed consent for dental therapy, you were wrong, weren't you?

**Comment:** A statement less vulnerable to cross-examination would avoid the legal term "informed consent." This can be done without taking anything away from the report or opinion by simply substituting non-legal words for the legal term "informed consent." For example, consider this:

> In my opinion, Dr. Jones fully and effectively communicated to Ms. Bailey all the information necessary for Ms. Bailey to make an intelligent decision on her course of treatment.

**Defending the Report As Written:** The examiner should pay careful attention to the specific words chosen by opposing counsel conducting the cross-examination. Frequently, counsel will make slight but crucial changes in what was said in the report. The examiner can easily overlook these changes.

**Q.** You found the statement sufficient legally for informed consent, correct?
**A.** That's not what I said at all. What I said in my report is, "The signed statement qualifies as informed consent for dental therapy." In my opinion as a practicing dentist, it does qualify. I was not giving a legal opinion because I am not a lawyer. May I explain further?

**Example 4.22: "Draft Copy. Attorney Work Product."**
*Report Cover Page States:*

Draft Copy. Attorney Work Product.

*Resulting Cross-examination:*
**Q.** Your report is labeled "Draft Copy. Attorney Work Product," correct?
**A.** Yes.
**Q.** This was your attempt to keep it out of the hands of opposing counsel, the judge, and jury?

**Comment:** This superfluous statement should be avoided. It serves no use and can create a multitude of problems. The term "draft" is a red flag for attorneys and should be avoided (see Section 13.4). "Draft" implies that the report was changed after discussions with the referral source. This can be problematic. "Work product" is an extremely complex legal term dealing with the discovery process. Writing "work product" on the document does not, as a matter of law, magically make the document work product. It does, however, make it look like the examiner is trying to hide something from the other party in the case.

**Defending the Report As Written:** When dealing with legal issues, the examiner who understands the law in question is in the best position to defend them. When an examiner does not know or understand the issue, he should consult with his own counsel and obtain an explanation.

**Q.** This was your attempt to keep it out of the hands of opposing counsel, the judge, and jury?
**A.** No. When I wrote the report, I was a consulting expert and was not expected to testify. As you know, the opinions of and the facts known by an expert retained in anticipation of litigation but not expected to testify (a non-testifying expert) are exempt from discovery unless the other side makes a showing of exceptional circumstances under which it is impracticable for them to obtain facts or opinions on the same subject by other means.

**Example 4.23: Grossly negligent**
*Report States:*

Based on the above findings, it is my opinion that the nursing staff was grossly negligent in the care of Mrs. Wilson.

*Resulting Cross-examination:*
**Q.** What is the legal definition of negligence?
**A.** I am not sure.
**Q.** What is the legal definition of gross negligence?
**A.** I am not sure.
**Q.** So, you used the term "gross negligence" in your report even though you don't know what it means?

**Comment:** The expert can expect to be cross-examined on the meaning of gross negligence, which is a technical legal term. The expert would have been better served by rephrasing her statement as follows.

> It is my opinion that the nursing staff was far below the applicable standard of care in its care of Mrs. Wilson.

**Defending the Report As Written:** The examiner may not have the precise, legal answer to opposing counsel's questions. This does not mean she must act like a sheep being led to the slaughter.

**Q.** So, you used the term "gross negligence" in your report even though you don't know what it means?
**A.** I may not be able to recite verbatim the precise *Black's Law Dictionary* definition of gross negligence, Counsel, but I know a surgeon leaving a heart operation in the middle of the operation to cash his paycheck at a bank is gross negligence.

**Example 4.24: "The claim should be allowed"**
*Report States:*

> In my opinion, the claim should be allowed.

*Resulting Cross-examination:*
**Q.** Doctor, you were retained to perform an Independent Medical Examination?
**A.** Yes.
**Q.** Was part of your role rendering legal advice to the workers' compensation insurer?
**A.** No.
**Q.** What about rendering claims advice?
**A.** No. I was just performing an Independent Medical Examination and reporting my findings.
**Q.** When you wrote in your IME report, "In my opinion, the claim should be allowed," was that your legal advice, claims advice, or just reporting your findings?

**Comment:** The examiner who strays from strictly performing an examination and offering his legal opinion has overstepped the traditional bounds of the IME process. IME physicians may or may not be experts on the state workers' compensation statute regulations and case law. Examiners who offer opinions about whether a particular claim should be allowed are vulnerable to cross-examination about their workers' compensation expertise as well as questions regarding potential bias. Examiners are better served by offering their medical opinions and letting others decide whether to allow claims.

**Defending the Report As Written:** When faced with a statement such as the one in the above example, the IME physician should explain what he actually meant to say.

**Q.** When you wrote in your IME report, "In my opinion, the claim should be allowed," was that your legal advice, claims advice, or just reporting your findings?
**A.** It just was my shorthand way of saying that in my medical opinion the

examinee's condition is a direct result of her industrial injury of 8/1/2003.

**Example 4.25: "Conclusive evidence"**
*Report States:*

> I do not find any conclusive evidence to suggest that trigger point injections would help or are indicated.

*Resulting Cross-examination:*
**Q.** Doctor, you expressed several medical opinions in your IME report, correct?
**A.** Yes.
**Q.** Your opinion that conservative treatment was reasonable and necessary was expressed to what degree of certainty?
**A.** More probable than not.
**Q.** Your opinion that the examinee did not sustain any major structural damage to the cervical spine was expressed to what degree of certainty?
**A.** More probable than not.
**Q.** How would you express that as a percentage?
**A.** 51% or more.
**Q.** When you expressed an opinion on trigger point injections, you wrote in your IME report, "I do not find any conclusive evidence to suggest that trigger point injections would help" the examinee, correct?
**A.** Yes, that's what it says.
**Q.** What degree of certainty is conclusive evidence, Doctor?
**A.** That's hard to say.
**Q.** Is it more than "more probable than not"?
**A.** Yes.
**Q.** Would that be 100% certainty?
**A.** No.
**Q.** So somewhere between 51% and 99% certainty?

**Comment:** Examiners should avoid using terms they cannot readily explain. The term "conclusive evidence" used in the above example is such a term. Examiners should be particularly careful to avoid using a legal term when they do not have a complete understanding of the term's true meaning and usage.

**Defending the Report As Written:** Examiners, when faced with their own loosely drafted opinions, need not become defensive when questioned about them. For physicians, the medicine is paramount, not some opposing lawyer later parsing each and every word or phrase in a lengthy, detailed report. When the examiner keeps that perspective in mind, he will be much better positioned to reply to opposing counsel's cross-examination.

**Q.** When you expressed an opinion on trigger point injections, you wrote in your IME report, "I do not find any conclusive evidence to suggest that trigger point injections would help" the examinee, correct?
**A.** This examinee has undergone multiple injections in the neck including cervical epidural steroid injection, facet anthography, nerve root blocks, facet injections, and trigger point injections without success. As these have not

worked in my opinion, it is not medically reasonable or necessary to proceed with further trigger point injections.

**Example 4.26: Precise legal term dealing with causation**

*Report States:*

> There is no question that this claimant had a pre-existing left shoulder condition which was aggravated by the 9/13/2002 accident at work. There are no records indicating that the patient was symptomatic prior to the injury of 9/13/2002. The pre-existing condition is the predominant cause for the need for surgery.

*Resulting Cross-examination:*

**Q.** Your opinion stated in your IME report is that the claimant's pre-existing left shoulder condition was aggravated by the 9/13/2002 accident at work, correct?
**A.** Yes, that's correct.
**Q.** Prior to the 9/13/2002 accident the claimant was working, correct?
**A.** Yes, that is the history that I have.
**Q.** The accident at work made the shoulder worse, correct?
**A.** Yes.
**Q.** In fact, it increased his disability and prolonged his rehabilitation?
**A.** Yes, it did.
**Q.** When did the claimant recover from his 9/13/2002 injury?
**A.** He has not recovered.
**Q.** In fact, the aggravation was a permanent worsening of the shoulder injury, correct?
**A.** Yes.
**Q.** You have no records indicating that the claimant was symptomatic prior to the 9/13/2002 injury, isn't that true?
**A.** That's true.
**Q.** The reason for the need for surgery is the accident of 9/13/2002?
**A.** That and the pre-existing condition.
**Q.** Had the claimant not had the 9/13/2002 accident, would he need surgery?
**A.** That's hard to say.
**Q.** Can you say with a reasonable degree of medical certainty that if the claimant did not have the 9/13/2002 accident he would currently need surgery?
**A.** I can't honestly say.
**Q.** But you were able to say that the predominant cause of the need for surgery was the asymptomatic pre-existing condition?
**A.** Yes, that's my opinion.
**Q.** What does "predominant cause" mean, Doctor?
**A.** I am not really sure.

**Comment:** The IME physician who uses medical-legal terminology (e.g., "predominant cause," "proximate cause," "contributory cause," "major contributing cause," or "cause-in-fact") should understand the meaning and usage of the term, be able to define it, and defend its use.

**Defending the Report As Written:** When faced with questions concerning medical-legal determinations, the IME physician who can combine her medical findings with an understanding of the medical-legal terms is in the strongest position to defend her report.

**Q.** Had the claimant not had the 9/13/2002 accident, would he need surgery?
**A.** Yes. It was just a matter of time. Prior to the 9/13/2002 accident, the claimant had pre-existing degenerative disease of the acromioclavicular joint as well as type 2 acromion and impingement as well as supraspinatus tendinopathy. The accident made it symptomatic but the vast majority of the problem was pre-existing. Thus my opinion that the pre-existing condition was the predominant cause.

**Example 4.27: Informed consent/State Statute 490**

*Report States:*

> *Informed Consent:* At the first visit for the purpose of completing the various questionnaires, Mr. Plaintiff 2 was informed as to the limits of confidentiality, i.e., that this was not a therapeutic relationship, and that as his mental status was placed at issue as part of his claim he was not entitled to the protections of privilege as might otherwise be afforded by *S.S. 490.*

*Resulting Cross-examination:*
**Q.** Your IME report indicates that the examinee was not entitled to the privilege under *S.S. 490*, correct?
**A.** That's correct.
**Q.** Are you aware of the new regulations 206.24 which make *S.S. 490* applicable to IME examinees?

**Comment:** The examiner in the above example ensnared himself unnecessarily in legal issues in which he was not an expert and did not have the latest information.

**Defending the Report As Written:** When faced with this type of surprise, the examiner should not just roll over.

**Q.** Are you aware of the new regulations 206.24 which make *S.S. 490* applicable to IME examinees?
**A.** I have not seen the new regulations. I wonder why you waited until now to raise this issue, Counsel. You have had the report for months.

## 4.3 Costs, Value, and Money

Examiners should generally not offer opinions regarding costs. Most times, making an estimate regarding costs or value is outside of the examiner's true area of expertise. When cost estimates are made, they should be objectively supported. When an examiner makes an unsupported financial prediction, she will suffer a loss of credibility. Please consider the following examples.

**Example 4.31: Examiner's cost estimate of future medical care**

*Report States:*

> The permanent injuries described above will most likely require physician-directed supportive care conservatively estimated at an ongoing cost of $1,200.00 to $1,500.00 per year for a minimum of two years and on a possible lifetime basis.

*Resulting Cross-examination:*

**Q.** Your estimate is that the future medical expenses could be $2,400 or $3,000 or $95,000 for this 25-year old?

**A.** Yes.

**Q.** Can you tell us if he will need this medical care for 1 year or 2 years or 50 years?

**A.** No.

**Q.** Could you explain on what you based your $1,200–$1,500 per year estimate?

**A.** My years of training and experience.

**Q.** What training do you have in the accurate projection of future medical expenses?

**A.** None.

**Q.** Did you consult with an expert in the field before you came up with your estimate?

**A.** No.

**Q.** So, in fact, you have no objective guidelines or support for your figures, is that correct?

**Comment:** This examiner's cost estimate is on extremely shaky ground. This examiner did not appear to be qualified to comment in this area and he failed to provide *objective* justification for the cost estimates. This examiner should have either refrained from offering an opinion in this area or should have provided objective evidence for his cost estimates.

**Defending the Report As Written:** When dealing with estimates of future medical care, the examiner should defend his report as an "estimate" and not a projection of fact.

**Q.** Can you tell us if he will need this medical care for 1 year or 2 years or 50 years?

**A.** I am not a fortune-teller. I am a doctor. No one can predict precisely how long he will need the care for. My opinion, based upon a reasonable degree of medical certainty, is a minimum of two years. However, he may need this for the rest of his life expectancy. That is why I put the 50 years in my report.

## 4.4 Different Medical Discipline, Specialty, or Sub-Specialty

IME reports should only express opinions that are within the examiner's true area of medical expertise. This can frequently be a problem when opinions are offered in disciplines, specialties, and sub-specialties in which the examiner is not a true expert. Examiners should refrain from offering opinions in any areas in which they are not truly experts. When the examiner expresses opinions that are beyond her true area of expertise, opposing counsel can then argue to the fact finder that the examiner will say anything and opine on any topic to help the referral source that is paying her bill.

**Example 4.41: Refusal to opine beyond area of expertise**
*Report States:*

> This is a very complex case as related to the medical course pre-dating her acquired brain injury. I will defer the etiology of her cardiac tamponade to those appropriately qualified to make this determination. Clearly, the examinee's hypoxic ischemic brain injury resulted from her cardiac arrest which was secondary to her cardiac tamponade. Her current permanent vegetative state is 100% apportionable to the sequela of her hypoxic ischemic brain injury, based upon information available to this examiner at the time of this report.

*Resulting Cross-examination:*
**Q.** You admit that you are not qualified to offer opinions on the etiology of the cardiac tamponade?
**A.** Yes and I stated that in my report, Counselor.

**Comment:** This expert acted wisely in limiting her opinions to those areas where she is truly qualified. This prudent self-restraint will help insulate the expert's opinions against attack on cross-examination.

**Example 4.42: Orthopod opining on depression**
*Report States:*

> The examinee does not have a significant orthopedic problem but does suffer from a major depression.

*Resulting Cross-Examination:*
**Q.** Doctor, you are an orthopedic surgeon, correct?
**A.** Yes.
**Q.** You are not a psychiatrist?
**A.** Correct.
**Q.** You diagnosed the examinee as suffering from a major depression?
**A.** Yes, I did.
**Q.** Is this a single episode or a recurrent major depressive disorder?
**A.** I am not sure.
**Q.** Can you tell us the difference?
**A.** No, I cannot.
**Q.** You are familiar with DSM IV—*The Diagnostic and Statistical Manual of Mental Disorders?*
**A.** Somewhat.
**Q.** Can you tell us what section covers major depression?
**A.** Not without seeing the text.
**Q.** Can you tell us the diagnostic criteria for 296.3X major depressive disorder, recurrent?
**A.** No, I cannot.
**Q.** What about the diagnostic criteria for 296.2X major depressive disorder,

single episode?
**A.** No, I cannot.
**Q.** Doctor, if you had a family member with a major depressive disorder, would you diagnose and treat them yourself or refer them to a qualified psychiatrist?

**Comment:** When examiners offer opinions outside their area of specialty and expertise, they become vulnerable to challenges to their opinions and reports. The further they venture, the more vulnerable they become.

**Defending the Report As Written:** An examiner who has training and expertise in allied specialties may feel comfortable in diagnosing conditions outside of her specialty. Such an examiner needs to be familiar with the diagnostic criteria.

**Q.** Is this a single episode or a recurrent major depressive disorder?
**A.** It is a single episode, moderate (296.22). Would you like me to explain the meaning and the use of the digits and the recording procedure, Counsel?

## 4.5 Commenting on Non-medical Areas of Expertise

Examiners need to be particularly careful to avoid expressing *non-medical* opinions outside of their true area of expertise. As a general rule, most examiners should never express non-medical expert opinions in their IME reports. Opposing counsel can be expected to zero-in on any such non-medical opinions and attempt to show that the expert was not qualified to give that opinion. If counsel is successful at this, he will be able to easily damage the examiner's credibility and show that the examiner will say anything to help the referral source. When non-medical opinions are proffered, examiners should be prepared to justify their qualifications to give such non-medical opinions and be equally prepared to defend the opinions.

**Example 4.51: Hand surgeon opines regarding saw blade**
*Report States:*

> It is further my opinion that had the miter saw in question included a wraparound blade guard, or a more complete guard that would have prevented exposure to the rotating blade in a kickback incident, Mr. Garcia would have received no injuries. (Written by hand surgeon.)

*Resulting Cross-examination:*
**Q.** You are a medical doctor by training, correct?
**A.** Yes.
**Q.** You are not a mechanical engineer or a safety engineer, correct?
**A.** That's correct.
**Q.** Have you ever actually designed or helped to design guards on power tools?
**A.** No.
**Q.** Despite your lack of formal training and practical experience, you are willing to offer an "expert" opinion on what kind of safety guard was

appropriate and would have prevented this accident?

**Comment:** As the above cross-examination shows, an examiner is extremely vulnerable to cross-examination when he opines in areas beyond his true area of expertise. This expert would have been far better off had he not addressed the issue of the design of the saw at all and left that issue to qualified experts.

**Defending the Report As Written:** Examiners should generally stick to their own true areas of expertise. Through experience, however, some examiners become quite familiar with related areas of expertise. When an examiner opines on areas that appear to be beyond his true area of expertise, he needs to be prepared to explain why he is in fact knowledgeable in this area.

**Q.** Despite your lack of formal training and practical experience, you are willing to offer an "expert" opinion on what kind of safety guard was appropriate and would have prevented this accident?
**A.** Unfortunately, I have 27 years of repairing hand injuries like this one as a result of a lack of a proper guard. I have studied each of these injuries and my article on injuries, safety guards, and hands will be appearing in *Industrial Safety* next month. I am frequently asked to consult on safety guards to help prevent accidents such as this one.

**Example 4.52: Kinetic energy and dollar damage**
*Report States:*

Kinetic energy is proportional to dollar damage. Understandably, the occupant of a vehicle requiring $100 in repairs would be less likely injured than one in a vehicle sustaining $1,000 in damage, and the latter less likely injured than the occupant of a vehicle with $10,000 in damage.

*Resulting Cross-examination:*
**Q.** Doctor, would you agree if you backed up a Ferrari into a parking meter you could do damage running into the thousands of dollars?
**A.** Yes, you could.
**Q.** Various bumper systems could impact the dollar amount of damage to a vehicle in an accident?
**A.** Yes, that's true.
**Q.** Are you an expert on piston, foam, and honeycomb bumper systems?
**A.** No.
**Q.** Are you aware of the different stiffness and energy absorption properties of vehicles?
**A.** No.
**Q.** Are you familiar with the vehicle's 5 m.p.h. impact test damage testing done by the National Institute for Safety?
**A.** No.
**Q.** Do you know what a basher test is, Doctor?
**A.** No.
**Q.** Do you know what the ATB results were for this vehicle?
**A.** No.
**Q.** Do you know what the normalized impact acceleration was for this vehicle?

**A.** No.
**Q.** Would you agree that you are not an expert on automotive issues, Doctor?
**A.** I am not.
**Q.** So when you said in your IME report that, "Kinetic energy is proportional to dollar damage," you were not expressing an opinion as an expert, correct, Doctor?

**Comment:** Examiners should stay within their true areas of expertise when expressing their opinions and writing their reports. The further examiners stray "out of their sandbox," the more vulnerable they are to cross-examinations such as the one in the above example.

**Defending the Report As Written:** IME physicians who wish to expound in their reports on areas other than medicine need to be able to "walk the walk" when they "talk the talk."

**Q.** Would you agree that you are not an expert on automotive issues, Doctor?
**A.** I said in my IME report that I readily admit that I am not an automotive engineer or accident reconstructionist. That said, however, I have had 27 years experience as a trauma surgeon treating patients in motor vehicle accidents and, as such, I have a keen interest in automotive medicine. I have found the most important determinant of bodily injury is kinetic energy which is expressed by the equation KE=1/2 mass x velocity$^2$. The fact that velocity is squared indicates the primary determinant of kinetic energy is speed. Would you like me to explain what happened in this case, Counsel?

**Example 4.53: Examiner not an automotive expert**
*Report States:*
The claimant was seat-belted and driving a Dodge Intrepid, a large car.

*Resulting Cross-examination:*
**Q.** Doctor, how long is the Dodge Intrepid?
**A.** I don't know.
**Q.** How much does it weigh?
**A.** I couldn't say.
**Q.** Do you know how high it is or how wide it is or what its wheelbase is?
**A.** I am a physician, not an automotive expert.
**Q.** So when you said in your IME report, "The claimant was seat-belted and driving a Dodge Intrepid, a large car," you were offering an opinion outside your area of expertise?

**Comment:** Examiners should not make comments or render opinions outside of their true areas of expertise. The further the IME physician moves from his true area of expertise, the more vulnerable he becomes to cross-examination. Examiners should stick to the facts when taking and reporting a history.

The claimant was seat-belted and driving a Dodge Intrepid.

**Defending the Report As Written:** When an examiner inadvertently strays outside of his area of expertise, he can still defend his choice of language in his report. There is no need for an examiner to roll over and play dead during cross-examination just because he is missing a few facts or cannot answer a few pointless questions.

**Q.** Do you know how high it is or how wide it is or what its wheelbase is?
**A.** Counsel, I know it seats five to six comfortably, has a large trunk, and can tow a powerboat comfortably. I don't have the specs for the vehicle in front of me. That's what I meant by a large car, the terminology generally used is "full-sized." Smaller vehicles would be those that are "mid-sized," "compact," and "sub-compact."

# Chapter 5 Formatting

## 5.1 Executive Summary

The use of proper formatting is a low-cost, easy way to improve IME reports. Proper formatting makes IME reports easier to read and understand. They are, therefore, more valuable to the reader. The authors recommend that examiners format their reports in the following manner.

- Construct and use a cover page that provides basic information about the examinee, examiner, and examination.
- Use a 12-point font, which is easier to read than smaller fonts.
- Break up the IME report by using topic headings (and subheadings). These should be in bold.
- Use short, concise paragraphs and avoid long, run-on paragraphs. This may require a combination of improved dictation skills and a review of the report after transcription, prior to it being finalized and sent to the client.
- Consider using 1½ spaces between lines.
- Include page numbers in the following format: [page number] of [total number of pages in report].

## 5.2 Cover Page

Some examiners construct a simple cover to their IME reports. This is well worth the minimal time involved. A well-drafted cover page will readily provide basic identifying information about the examinee, the examiner, and the examination to the reader. It may also demonstrate to the reader that the examiner is a methodical person and that the examiner produces high-quality work. This will help to increase the value of the examiner's reports and bolster the examiner's credibility. Consider the following example.

**Example 5.21: Well-drafted cover page**
*Report States:*

**Steven Babitsky, 12/30/02**

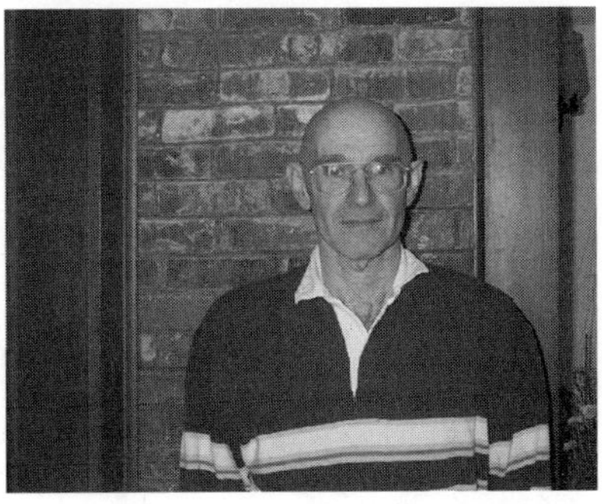

# INDEPENDENT MEDICAL EXAMINATION

| | |
|---|---|
| EXAMINEE: | Steven Babitsky |
| EXAMINEE'S DATE OF BIRTH: | 08/25/62 |
| DATE OF EXAMINATION: | 6/30/02 |
| DATE OF INJURY: | 11/01/99 |
| REFERRING INDIVIDUAL: | Mr. James J. Mangraviti, Jr. |
| REFERRING ORGANIZATION: | ACME Claims Services |
| REFERRING ORGANIZATION'S ADDRESS: | Post Office Box 729<br>Falmouth, MA 02541 |
| REFERENCE NO.: | 10100 |
| EXAMINING PHYSICIAN: | Preston B. Fitzgerald, Sr., D.C., CDE I, CICE, CIFCME |
| LOCATION OF EXAMINATION: | Manning, South Carolina 29102 |
| TYPE OF EXAMINATION: | Workers' Compensation |

**Comment:** A well-drafted cover page is helpful to the user and makes an IME report look as if it were carefully written. This report even contains a digital photo of the examinee, which is a nice touch. This will serve to bolster the examiner's credibility and increase the value of the report.

## 5.3 Font

The authors recommend that examiners use a 12-point font in their reports. This is a simple and virtually cost-free thing to do. Smaller fonts can be very difficult to read. This is especially true if the report is faxed one or more times. Some examiners may be tempted to use a smaller font to help get more information onto a page. Examiners should resist this temptation.

Attorneys and adjusters spend a large portion of their day reading. Much of what they need to read are medical records, which are often barely legible, if not illegible. Attorneys, adjusters, and other clients will appreciate when an examiner helps make her IME reports easy to read by using a 12-point font.

**Example 5.31: Font too small**
The following example shows a report with text in a 10-point font. It is less easy to read than it could be if a larger font were used and needlessly takes away from the effectiveness of the report.

*Report States:*

These complaints are symptoms or problems the patient states she did not experience prior to the accident or are obvious exacerbations of symptoms the patient reports she experienced prior to the accident. Ms. X XX states she currently experiences the following symptoms:

1. Occasional stiffness in the neck. This is worse in the morning. "I can't sleep well due to my neck pain. Sometimes this gets worse than at other times. It has gotten some better with treatment but it still bothers me every day. My neck hurts more when I have to read or study for my nursing exam." The patient rates this pain level as 2-4.

2. Frequent soreness and dull aching in the spinal column area of the low back and on the muscles on the right side and on the left side. A reduction of the normal ability to bend and twist at the waist is reported. She states that moving from a seated position to a standing position and back again is difficult now. The pain is reportedly increased by minimal physical activity that involves the use of this area. The patient rates this pain level as 4-5. "This is my worst pain. I can't stand for long without a lot of pain."

3. A sensation of numbness in the posterior…

**Comment:** The examiner would have been better served by using the following larger, easier-to-read font.

*Report States:*

These complaints are symptoms or problems the patient states she did not experience prior to the accident or are obvious exacerbations of symptoms the patient reports she experienced prior to the accident. Ms. X XX states she currently experiences the following symptoms:

1. Occasional stiffness in the neck. This is worse in the morning. "I can't sleep well due to my neck pain. Sometimes this gets worse than at other times. It has gotten some better with treatment but it still bothers me every day. My neck hurts more when I have to read or study for my nursing exam." The patient rates this pain level as 2-4.

2. Frequent soreness and dull aching in the spinal column area of the low back and on the muscles on right side and on the left side. A reduction of the normal ability to bend and twist at the waist is reported. She states that moving from a seated position to a standing position and back again is difficult now. The pain is reportedly increased by minimal physical activity that involves the use of this area. The patient rates this pain level as 4-5. "This is my worst pain. I can't stand for long without a lot of pain."

3. A sensation of numbness in the posterior…

## 5.4 Topic Headings

IME reports should have topic headings (and subheadings). Topic headings should be in bold. This will help them stand out.

Some lengthy IME reports go on and on with few or no topic headings. This is a mistake. Topic headings break up the report and allow the reader to put the entire report in context more easily. Topic headings also allow the reader to focus on the sections of the report that are of most interest.

Reports without topic headings can be incredibly boring to read. There are few things worse for an attorney or adjuster than to have to read through a 20-page, single-spaced IME report with no topic headings. The reader of such a report cannot easily jump to the sections she is most interested in and has no idea where the report is going and how it is getting there.

Topic headings may also directly help the examiner. If the examiner is called to testify in the case, the examiner may use the report to refresh his recollection. The use of topic headings will make it easy for the examiner to quickly locate the needed information.

**Example 5.41: Failure to use topic headings**
The following report has not been broken down into topic headings.

*Report States:*

> At the request of Ms. Mary Miller, senior claims representative of ABC Insurance Company, I did review the extensive medical file that had been sent to me. This file consisted of the office notes (not complete) of Dr. Stevens, Healthy Orthopedic Group, cardiology notes of Dr. Riley of Browning University, as well as extensive physical therapy notes and in-hospital records and numerous test results.
>
> Mr. Hall sustained injuries to his neck, upper back, and lower back when in the course of his employment on 4/25/99, he attempted to break up a fight between the students at the school where he is a vocational teacher.

## FORMATTING

Mr. Hall was initially seen at the Best Medical Center by Dr. Stanton, who after evaluation, prescribed medication and a course of physical therapy. The patient did begin a course of physical therapy but was unable to complete this due to increase in pain.

Sometime in June or July of 1999, Mr. Hall sustained a massive anterior myocardial infarction involving the anterior wall of the heart. He was treated for this by Dr. Andersen of the Browning Cardiology Department. Dr. Stevens did see Mr. Hall again on 9/11/99 following his myocardial infarction and did continue to recommend physical therapy.

One note throughout the multiple evaluations by Dr. Stevens that there was not any focal neurologic signs—either objective sensory losses or reflex abnormalities. Evidently the x-rays of the entire spine were eventually taken and these are reported as being negative.

Mr. Hall continued with neck, upper and lower back pain and was unable to return to work throughout the Fall of 1999. One notices a marked lack of any objective findings with respect to his neck, upper and lower back. An MRI of the lumbar spine was obtained (? location) on 12/21/99 and was consistent with "mild changes" of degenerative disease at L1-2, L4-5, and L5-S1. There is no evidence of disc herniation. An MRI of the thoracic spine was obtained on 3/11/2000 (? location) and was interpreted as "within normal limits." An MRI of the cervical spine was performed on 12/29/99 (? location) and interpreted as:

1. Multilevel changes of bulging degenerative intervertebral discs;
2. Mild central disc protrusion at C3-C4;
3. Acquired canal and foraminal stenosis at C5-6 "greater on the left."

It is further noted throughout that the patient never presented with any localizing signs or specific neurologic signs.

On January 10, 2000, Dr. Stevens allowed Mr. Hall to attempt to return to work on "about 2 hours per day" basis which was all that Mr. Hall could tolerate due to the pain.

On 2/26/00, Mr. Hall was reported by Dr. Stevens as "having undergone open heart surgery a couple of weeks ago." "His complaint is a persistent pain in his back which has always been his major complaint." Once again there was a lack of any objective findings.

It is inconceivable to me that without any more objective findings than the minimal ones that are present (cervical spine-MRI which may be a normal variant) that the event of 4/25/99 may be a factor in Mr. Hall's inability to work and continued complaints of back pain.

It is obvious that this patient's severe cardiac status coupled with his myocardial infarction and open heart surgery are the major factors in prohibiting his return to work and his ongoing problems.

It appears that Mr. Hall's problems particularly with his upper and lower back are related to a chronic weakness of the musculature coupled with what appears to be some sort of fibromylasia syndrome. The patient has had more than an extensive course of physical therapy and he must accept his present condition and be assured that symptoms should improve, if honestly reported, with time.

Once again I stress the lack of orthopedic findings within this entire case.

It is impossible to state at the present time what Mr. Hall's work capacity is as I have not had the advantage of examining myself.

Once again, it is to be noted that the patient's problems are due in only the most minimal manner to the events of 4/25/99 and are due to his cardiac problems with the deconditioning of the muscles following all of his cardiac problems as well as the minimal degenerative changes present throughout his entire spine present prior to the event of 4/25/99.

**Comment:** The same IME report can be made *much* more valuable with a little rewriting, some careful proofreading, and the addition of topic headings.

**Documents Reviewed**
At the request of Ms. Mary Miller, senior claims representative of ABC Insurance Company, I reviewed the extensive medical file that had been sent to me. This file consisted of the office notes (not complete) of Dr. Stevens, Healthy Orthopedic Group, cardiology notes of Dr. Riley of Browning University, as well as extensive physical therapy notes and in-hospital records and numerous test results.

**History of Injury**
Mr. Hall sustained injuries to his neck, upper back, and lower back when in the course of his employment on 4/25/99, he attempted to break up a fight between the students at the ACES school where he is a vocational teacher.

**Initial Treatment**
Mr. Hall was initially seen at the Best Medical Center by Dr. Stanton, who, after evaluation, prescribed medication and a course of physical therapy. The patient began a course of physical therapy but was unable to complete this due to increase in pain.

**Physical Therapy**
Mr. Hall was then referred for evaluation and treatment to Dr. Stevens, an orthopedic surgeon in Cary, CT. Dr. Stevens's initial evaluation has not been available to me but Dr. Stevens's appears to have an extensive course

of physical therapy. Dr. Stevens refers repeatedly to "muscular ligamentitis sprain strain syndrome."

**Subsequent Myocardial Infarction**
Some time in June or July of 1999, Mr. Hall sustained a massive anterior myocardial infarction involving the anterior wall of the heart. He was treated for this by Dr. Andersen of the Browning Cardiology Department. Dr. Stevens saw Mr. Hall again on 9/11/99 following his myocardial infarction and continued to recommend physical therapy.

**Lack of Objective Findings**
One note throughout the multiple evaluations by Dr. Stevens was that there was not any focal neurologic signs of either objective sensory losses or reflex abnormalities. Evidently the x-rays of the entire spine were eventually taken and these are reported as being negative.

Mr. Hall continued with neck, upper and lower back pain and was unable to return to work throughout the fall of 1999. There was a marked lack of any objective findings with respect to his neck, upper and lower back. An MRI of the lumbar spine was obtained (? location) on 12/21/99 and was consistent with "mild changes" of degenerative disease at L1-2, L4-5, and L5-S1. There is no evidence of disc herniation. An MRI of the thoracic spine was obtained on 3/11/00 (? location) and was interpreted as "within normal limits." An MRI of the cervical spine was performed on 12/29/99 (? location) and interpreted as:

1. Multilevel changes of bulging degenerative intervertebral discs;
2. Mild central disc protrusion at C3-C4; and
3. Acquired canal and foraminal stenosis at C5-6 "greater on the left."

It is further noted throughout that the patient never presented with any localizing signs or specific neurologic signs.

**Return to Work**
On January 10, 2000, Dr. Stevens allowed Mr. Hall to attempt to return to work on "about 2 hours per day" basis which was all that Mr. Hall could tolerate due to the pain.

**Continued Lack of Objective Findings**
On 2/26/2000, Mr. Hall was reported by Dr. Stevens as "having undergone open heart surgery a couple of weeks ago." "His complaint is a persistent pain in his back which has always been his major complaint." Once again there was a lack of any objective findings.

**Conclusions**
In my opinion, based on a reasonable degree of medical certainty, the event of 4/25/2000 is not a factor in Mr. Hall's inability to work and continued complaints of back pain. This is based on the lack of objective findings

other than the minimal ones that are present (cervical spine-MRI, which may be a normal variant).

In my opinion, based on a reasonable degree of medical certainty, this patient's severe cardiac status coupled with his myocardial infarction and open heart surgery are the major factors in prohibiting his return to work and his ongoing problems.

In my opinion, based on a reasonable degree of medical certainty, Mr. Hall's problems, particularly with his upper and lower back, are related to a chronic weakness of the musculature coupled with a fibromyalgia syndrome.

It is impossible to state at the present time what Mr. Hall's work capacity is as I have not had the advantage of examining him myself. The patient's problems are due in only the most minimal manner to the events of 4/25/99 and are due to his cardiac problems with the deconditioning of the muscles following all of his cardiac problems as well as the minimal degenerative changes present throughout his entire spine present prior to the event of 4/25/99.

## 5.5 Short, Concise Paragraphs

Long paragraphs should be avoided. Short, concise paragraphs are most effective in IME reports because they are easier to read and understand.

Long, run-on paragraphs are often a product of poor dictation technique. The examiner is advised to either include "new paragraph" directions in his dictation or to edit the report post-transcription to eliminate any lengthy, run-on paragraphs. Replacing long paragraphs with shorter ones will improve the quality and value of an IME report.

**Example 5.51: Run-on "History" paragraph**
The following report contains a run-on "History" paragraph. This was most likely caused by a combination of poor dictation technique and a failure to review and edit the report after it was transcribed but before it was sent to the client.

*Report States:*

History

The examinee is a right-hand dominant 51-year-old male who is here for evaluation of a neck injury sustained in a motor vehicle accident on 01/14/2003. Prior to that time he never had any significant neck problems. On the date of injury, the examinee was on the way to a doctor's appointment for follow-up of a gastrointestinal condition (see Past Medical History). The examinee was driving a 1997 full-size pickup truck. As he was going through an intersection, he was hit broadside on the driver's side of his vehicle. He says he never saw the other vehicle coming. There were stop signs at the intersection for the cross traffic, but not for the examinee. He was wearing his seat belt with shoulder harness. The vehicle that hit him was a compact car and its front end went under the back end of the examinee's pickup truck, lifting up the back end of the truck such that the back wheels of the pickup truck went over the front of the compact car. The impact caused the examinee's pickup truck to spin around about 270 degrees, landing against the opposite curve. The bolts of the pickup truck's left rear tire were sheared off from the impact. The examinee recalls being thrown forcefully forward and to the right against his shoulder strap. This resulted in a large bruise across his left chest wall. The examinee was stunned after the impact. He dialed 911 on his cell phone, and remained in the pickup truck for about five or six minutes. Then he got out of the pickup truck around the same time emergency assistance arrived. The examinee recalls being "numb and stunned by the whole thing." He was interviewed by emergency personnel and was determined to be medically stable. He called his wife and she came to pick him up. She took him to the medical clinic where he was heading towards originally for his doctor's appointment. At the medical clinic they took some x-rays of his right shoulder, as he was complaining of immediate pain in the right shoulder and right upper extremity. A suspicious finding of a fracture in the shoulder blade was noted, and he was placed in a right arm sling for the next couple of weeks. Since that time, he continued to suffer from the effects of this motor vehicle accident. Within a day or two after the accident, he started to experience numbness and tingling in his right hand. He also began to experience neck pain. Because of these symptoms, he decided to go to a chiropractor. He had never been to one before, and decided to try one. The chiropractor took x-rays and told him he had a whiplash injury of the neck. He proceeded to adjust the examinee about six or seven times, but the examinee notes that he really wasn't making much improvement. He notes that because of his lack of response to chiropractic treatment he stopped going to the chiropractor and just hoped it would get better on its own. However, it did not and he continued to have symptoms of persistent neck pain, and in particular numbness and difficulty using his right hand, especially in performing fine manipulation. He subsequently again sought medical treatment with his physician because of his persistent symptoms, particularly in the neck and right hand, and his doctor referred him to an orthopedic specialist at the University of Maine. Carpal Tunnel Syndrome was suspected. He was treated conservatively with wrist braces and anti-inflammatory medication, but his condition never improved. In fact, he says it got worse. By this time, he was not only having the numbness in the right hand, but also a dull aching pain extending down the inside of his right upper extremity. EMGs revealed a problem with a pinched nerve in the neck. He was referred to a spinal specialist at the UM Spine Clinic. An MRI scan of the cervical spine was performed showing problems with 2 disks in the neck. He was diagnosed with a cervical radiculopathy of the right upper extremity caused by abnormalities with the discs in the neck. He was treated conservatively with physical therapy and traction devices, and has continued a daily home exercise program. This has helped his condition somewhat in that he has increased range of motion in his neck. However, he remains with persistent numbness, tingling, and difficulty using the right hand. He has been told that should his condition deteriorate or become intolerable, the next step would be surgery. Currently, he is functionally limited in use of his right hand. He does work with power tools such as table saws, and he has to take special amounts of caution because of the lack of sensation and inability to finely manipulate the right hand. He has trouble sleeping at night because he frequently wakes up with numbness in his entire right upper extremity. He says last night's sleep was a good example of what he suffers with: he woke up every hour or so with his right upper extremity feeling numb. He experiences daily chronic pain in the right upper extremity which is treated with Vioxx, making it more tolerable. He used to be an avid fisherman, but has not fished since this condition developed because he has difficulty feeling the line or the hook. He used to enjoy golf, but no longer is able to play because he has no control of his swing. Performing any work activity at shoulder or above height is particularly difficult for him. He avoids this type of work activity whenever he can. Driving the car for prolonged periods of time causes an exacerbation of symptoms. Simple things like buttoning his shirt buttons with his right hand are difficult to perform because he has trouble feeling and manipulating the buttons with his right hand. Any physical activities such as pushing a lawnmower or shoveling snow exacerbate the pain in his neck and the numbness, tingling, and pain in the right upper extremity. Prior to the accident he lived in a house that required a lot of these activities. After the accident, he decided to sell the house and move to a condo in order to avoid these types of activities. One of the hobbies he used to enjoy was woodworking. He continues to do woodworking to the best extent that he is able. However, simple activities he formerly was able to perform are now much more difficult, and this is a source of frustration for him. For example, several weeks ago he was building a crib for the anticipated arrival of his new grandchild. It was extremely frustrating for him to perform such simple activities as inserting slats into a small groove to make the crib railing. Even brushing his teeth is done with some difficulty since the accident. Every morning he awakens with his neck extremely stiff and he requires a long, hot shower to loosen it up. He also does daily physical therapy exercises and uses a home traction unit.

**Comment:** Breaking up this run-on paragraph makes the IME report easier to read and much more interesting and valuable to the reader. Adding a few subheadings improves the report even more.

**History**

The examinee is a right-hand-dominant 51-year-old male who is here for evaluation of a neck injury sustained in a motor vehicle accident on 01/14/2003. Prior to that time he never had any significant neck problems.

*Motor Vehicle Accident of 01/14/2003*

On the date of injury, the examinee was on the way to a doctor's appointment for follow-up of a gastrointestinal condition (see Past Medical History). The examinee was driving a 1997 full-size pickup truck. As he was going through an intersection, he was hit broadside on the driver's side of his vehicle. He says he never saw the other vehicle coming. There were stop signs at the intersection for the cross traffic, but not for the examinee. He was wearing his seat belt with shoulder harness. The vehicle that hit him was a compact car and its front end went under the back end of the examinee's pickup truck, lifting up the back end of the truck such that the back wheels of the pickup truck went over the front of the compact car.

The impact caused the examinee's pickup truck to spin around about 270 degrees, landing against the opposite curve. The bolts of the pickup truck's left rear tire were sheared off from the impact. The examinee recalls being thrown forcefully forward and to the right against his shoulder strap. This resulted in a large bruise across his left chest wall.

The examinee was stunned after the impact. He dialed 911 on his cell phone, and remained in the pickup truck for about five or six minutes. Then he got out of the pickup truck around the same time emergency assistance arrived. The examinee recalls being "numb and stunned by the whole thing." He was interviewed by emergency personnel and was determined to be medically stable. He called his wife and she came to pick him up.

His wife took him to the medical clinic where he was heading towards originally for his doctor's appointment. At the medical clinic they took some x-rays of his right shoulder, as he was complaining of immediate pain in the right shoulder and right upper extremity. A suspicious finding of a fracture in the shoulder blade was noted, and he was placed in a right arm sling for the next couple of weeks.

*Post-Accident Treatment*

He continued to suffer from the effects of this motor vehicle accident. Within a day or two after the accident, he started to experience numbness and tingling in his right hand. He also began to experience neck pain.

Because of these symptoms, he decided to go to a chiropractor. He had never been to one before, and decided to try one. The chiropractor took x-rays and told him he had a whiplash injury of the neck. He proceeded to adjust the examinee about six or seven times, but the examinee notes that he really wasn't making much improvement. He notes that because of his lack of response to chiropractic treatment he stopped going to the chiropractor and just hoped it would get better on its own. However, it did not and he continued to have symptoms of persistent neck pain, and in particular numbness and difficulty using his right hand, especially in performing fine manipulation.

He subsequently again sought medical treatment with his physician because of his persistent symptoms, particularly in the neck and right hand, and his doctor referred him to an orthopedic specialist at the University of Maine. Carpal Tunnel Syndrome was suspected. He was treated conservatively with wrist braces and anti-inflammatory medication, but his condition never improved. In fact, he says it got worse.

By this time, he was not only having the numbness in the right hand, but also a dull aching pain extending down the inside of his right upper extremity. EMGs revealed a problem with a pinched nerve in the neck. He was referred to a spinal specialist at the UM Spine Clinic. An MRI scan of the cervical spine was performed showing problems with 2 disks in the neck. He was diagnosed with a cervical radiculopathy of the right upper extremity caused by abnormalities with the discs in the neck.

He was treated conservatively with physical therapy and traction devices, and has continued a daily home exercise program. This has helped his condition somewhat in that he has increased range of motion in his neck. However, he remains with persistent numbness, tingling, and difficulty using the right hand.

He has been told that should his condition deteriorate or become intolerable, the next step would be surgery. Currently, he is functionally limited in use of his right hand. He does work with power tools such as table saws, and he has to take special amounts of caution because of the lack of sensation and inability to finely manipulate the right hand. He has trouble sleeping at night because he frequently wakes up with numbness in his entire right upper extremity. He says last night's sleep was a good example of what he suffers with: he woke up every hour or so with his right upper extremity feeling numb. He experiences daily chronic pain in the right upper extremity which is treated with Vioxx, making it more tolerable.

*Effects of Conditions on Daily Activities*
He used to be an avid fisherman, but has not fished since this condition developed because he has difficulty feeling the line or the hook. He used to enjoy golf, but no longer is able to play because he has no control of his swing. Performing any work activity at shoulder or above height is particularly difficult for him. He avoids this type of work activity whenever he can. Driving the car for prolonged periods of time causes an exacerbation of symptoms. Simple things like buttoning his shirt buttons with his right hand are difficult to perform because he has trouble feeling and manipulating the buttons with his right hand. Any physical activities such as pushing a lawnmower or shoveling snow exacerbate the pain in his neck and the numbness, tingling, and pain in the right upper extremity.

Prior to the accident he lived in a house that required a lot of these activities. After the accident, he decided to sell the house and move to a condo in order to avoid these types of activities. One of the hobbies he used to enjoy was woodworking. He continues to do woodworking to the best extent that he is able. However, simple activities he formerly was able to perform are now much more difficult, and this is a source of frustration for him. For example, several weeks ago he was building a crib for the anticipated arrival of his new grandchild. It was extremely frustrating for him to perform such simple activities as inserting slats into a small groove to make the crib railing. Even brushing his teeth is done with some difficulty since the accident. Every morning he awakens with his neck extremely stiff and he requires a long, hot shower to loosen it up. He also does daily physical therapy exercises and uses a home traction unit.

## 5.6 Spacing

Examiners may want to consider using 1½ lines of space between lines. This makes the IME report easier to read and easier for the reader to make notes on. Using 1½ lines of space can also help in making concise reports seem longer and more impressive.

**Example 5.61: 1½ lines of space**
The following report is presented in single-space format.

*Report States:*
*Behavioral Observations & Interview:*

*Informed Consent:* At the first visit for the purpose of completing the various questionnaires, Mr. Plaintiff 2 was informed as to the limits of confidentiality, i.e., that this was not a therapeutic relationship and that as his mental status was placed at issue as part of his claim, he was not entitled to the protections of privilege as might otherwise be afforded by *F.S. 490.* Mr. Plaintiff 2 was given a written statement concerning these limitations and was advised to review them with his attorney.

*Appearance:* Mr. Plaintiff 2 is a well groomed, muscular, and handsome but grim-looking African-American male, who is forty-two years of age.

He arrived early for his testing and interview sessions and at each appeared initially put out or impatient that he was here at all. Throughout, he spoke in a *soto voce* [soft voice] that was at times difficult to hear at first listening. His responses to questions were given with just sufficient information to be acceptable but nothing of his personal history or feelings were forthcoming without continued or repeated inquiry.

He was easily engaged despite his continued emotional distance and guardedness. He apparently felt comfortable enough to take and make a business call initiated during a brief break and continued even though signals were given that it was time to resume.

*History:* Mr. Plaintiff 2 is currently employed by XYZ Corp. in Halley, a company not dissimilar to Defendant where he had worked previously. Prior to his work in the XYZ manufacturing industry he did *"nothing steady"* having worked for ACME, Inc. and for his father's night club business *"collecting tickets at the door."*

Mr. Plaintiff 2 was born in the Caribbean and raised in France, coming to live in Florida as a late teen.

He reports that his parents are not divorced, but separated since 1985, his father living in Caribbean where he owns a retail business, having formerly been a policeman; and, his mother lives with him [Mr. Plaintiff 2]. She is not working because she is disabled having suffered a stroke in 1983.

He has three older sisters. The oldest ran away from home at age sixteen and hasn't been seen in years; the middle sister, age 47, lives in France; and the youngest [but older than Mr. Plaintiff 2] is a nurse, living in Florida.

Mr. Plaintiff 2 reports having completed his A.A. degree at the College of Education, in Taylor, Florida.

Early in the interview I asked Mr. Plaintiff 2 where or how he had developed such a soft voice. He replied, initially, that he had learned to talk softly so as not to be perceived as *"talking back to my father."* His father was *"strict,"* prone to *"yelling and hitting."*

Mr. Plaintiff 2 reports not having very many close friends because *"I don't trust a lot of people," "I see what people do."* Mr. Plaintiff 2 is not married, *"Everybody has problems."* During the inquiry about significant relationships, family, and marriage, Mr. Plaintiff 2 did not initially disclose that he had two children [out of wedlock from a previous relationship], aged eleven and eight, who he only spoke about later in the interview when he was being asked about perceived changes in his affective life.

Much like his delayed disclosure of having children, he delayed reporting any history of sexual victimization. When asked about any psychiatric history in his family, he briefly reported that he *"had a cousin in France that liked to mess with kids."* Only on further inquiry did Mr. Plaintiff 2 reveal that he had been sexually victimized by his cousin.

**Comment:** The report is easier to read in the following 1½-line spacing format. It is also easier for the user to make notes on the report.

*Behavioral Observations & Interview:*

*Informed Consent:* At the first visit for the purpose of completing the various questionnaires, Mr. Plaintiff 2 was informed as to the limits of confidentiality, i.e., that this was not a therapeutic relationship and that as his mental status was placed at issue as part of his claim, he was not entitled to the protections of privilege as might otherwise be afforded by *F.S. 490.* Mr. Plaintiff 2 was given a written statement concerning these limitations and was advised to review them with his attorney.

*Appearance:* Mr. Plaintiff 2 is a well groomed, muscular, and handsome but grim-looking African-American male, who is forty-two years of age.

He arrived early for his testing and interview sessions and at each appeared initially put out or impatient that he was here at all. Throughout, he spoke in a *soto voce* [soft voice] that was at times difficult to hear at first listening. His responses to questions were given with just sufficient information to be acceptable but nothing of his personal history or feelings were forthcoming without continued or repeated inquiry.

He was easily engaged despite his continued emotional distance and guardedness. He apparently felt comfortable enough to take and make a business call initiated during a brief break and continued even though signals were given that it was time to resume.

*History:* Mr. Plaintiff 2 is currently employed by XYZ Corp. in Halley, a company not dissimilar to Defendant where he had worked previously. Prior to his work in the XYZ manufacturing industry he did *"nothing steady"* having worked for Acme, Inc. and for his father's night club business *"collecting tickets at the door."*

Mr. Plaintiff 2 was born in the Caribbean and raised in France, coming to live in Florida as a late teen.

He reports that his parents are not divorced, but separated since 1985, his father living in Caribbean where he owns a retail business, having formerly been a policeman; and, his mother lives with him [Mr. Plaintiff 2]. She is not working as she is disabled having suffered a stroke in 1983.

He has three older sisters. The oldest ran away from home at age sixteen and hasn't been seen in years; the middle sister, age 47, lives in France; and the youngest [but older than Mr. Plaintiff 2] is a nurse, living in Florida.

Mr. Plaintiff 2 reports having completed his A.A. degree at the College of Education, in Taylor, Florida.

> Early in the interview I asked Mr. Plaintiff 2 where or how he had developed such a soft voice. He replied, initially, that he had learned to talk softly so as not to be perceived as *"talking back to my father."* His father was *"strict,"* prone to *"yelling and hitting."*
>
> Mr. Plaintiff 2 reports not having very many close friends because *"I don't trust a lot of people," "I see what people do."* Mr. Plaintiff 2 is not married, *"Everybody has problems."* During the inquiry about significant relationships, family, and marriage, Mr. Plaintiff 2 did not initially disclose that he had two children [out of wedlock from a previous relationship], aged eleven and eight, who he only spoke about later in the interview when he was being asked about perceived changes in his affective life.
>
> Much like his delayed disclosure of having children, he delayed reporting any history of sexual victimization. When asked about any psychiatric history in his family, he briefly reported that he *"had a cousin in France that liked to mess with kids."* Only on further inquiry did Mr. Plaintiff 2 reveal that he had been sexually victimized by his cousin.

## 5.7 Page Numbering

IME reports need to have numbered pages. Ideally, the page numbers will list the page number and the total number of pages (e.g., "page 7 of 15"). Failure to number the pages makes the report appear unprofessional and sloppy.

**Example 5.71: Failure to number pages**

The following cross-examination regarding page numbers is an example of the way an expert can needlessly lose credibility by preparing a sloppy report without page numbers.

*Cross-examination:*

**Q.** I am looking at what appears to be page six of your report. You didn't number the pages, sir?
**A.** Let me see, I guess not.
**Q.** Was that done intentionally?
**A.** No. My secretary probably forgot.
**Q.** Did you write this report or did your secretary?
**A.** I did.
**Q.** Did you read the report carefully before you signed it?
**A.** Of course.

**Q.** You didn't notice that there were no page numbers?
**A.** Is there a point to this?
**Q.** Did you carefully prepare and read over this report?
**A.** Page numbers were not and are not important. It's a little detail. My report is my report and I stand by it.
**Q.** What other little details that you didn't think were important did you omit from your report?

**Comment:** The examiner would have avoided this needless distraction by proofing the report carefully and making sure page numbers were included.

**Defending the Report As Written:** When an examiner is confronted by his mistake or oversight, he should admit the error, not try to blame someone else, and attempt to correct it as simply and as quickly as possible.

**Q.** I am looking at what appears to be page 6 of your report. You didn't number the pages, sir?
**A.** No. That is my mistake. Can we take a moment now and number them?

# Chapter 6 Properly Disclosing Precise Medical Records and Other Documents Reviewed

## 6.1 Executive Summary

It is essential that the examiner organize, explicitly list, and precisely describe all of the medical records, reports, depositions, and other documents he has reviewed. This serves several purposes.

- It forces the examiner to account for all the material he has reviewed,
- it removes any ambiguity about what was and was not reviewed by the examiner, and
- it permits the examiner to consult his report quickly when questioned regarding what was and was not reviewed.

In terms of presentation of the list of medical records and other documents reviewed, the authors recommend the following.

- Each document should be described precisely, including, where appropriate, date, length, author, and other descriptive information.
- The list should be numbered.
- The documents should be listed chronologically or according to some natural, logical grouping (for example, all medical reports, all diagnostic studies, all depositions).[1]
- To make an IME report truly stand out, the examiner should consider not merely listing the medical records reviewed, but summarizing each record reviewed as well.
- The following descriptives should be avoided: "including," "including but not limited to," "relevant portions of," and "various."
- Examiners should not make opposing counsel's job easier by explicitly listing documents that were not available for review.
- Generally, examiners should not produce reports in cases where there were few or no records available for review.
- Surveillance material should be described objectively and without any superfluous language attacking the claimant.
- Illegibility should not be used as an excuse for the wholesale ignoring of records.

[1] Thomas G. Gutheil, *The Psychiatrist as Expert Witness* (Washington, DC: American Psychiatric Press, 1998) 104-105.

- Examiners should expect close questioning regarding the authenticity, accuracy, and completeness of medical records provided by the referral source.

## 6.2 Precisely Listing Medical Records and Other Documents Reviewed

The thoroughness of the examiner's evaluation is directly related to which medical records and other documents the examiner reviewed and the thoroughness of that review. Failure to review key medical records and other documents can reduce the weight the examiner's report is given. The examiner will also be vulnerable on cross-examination.

The records reviewed should be described precisely. For example, instead of stating "Examinee's MRI was reviewed," it would be far better to state, "Examinee's MRI from East Coast Imaging, Inc., 4/15/2003, was reviewed." Failure to use precise language when describing the medical and other documents reviewed will cause the examiner to lose credibility.

Ideally, the records in question should be read thoroughly and not merely skimmed. The medical records in question may contain important information that is impossible to glean absent a careful review. Any words which may indicate that the records were only casually reviewed should be avoided.

A good way to present the medical records and other records reviewed is through a numbered list. A numbered list is visually pleasing and will make the report appear to be drafted carefully and precisely. The records should also be organized chronologically, by the type of record (e.g., medical records, imaging reports, depositions, etc.), or in some other logical manner.

Perhaps the best way to present the medical records reviewed in the IME report is to not merely list the records reviewed, but to summarize the key points in each record. Doing this clearly demonstrates that the records were carefully reviewed by the examiner and this will bolster the examiner's credibility. Summarizing the medical records also provides a significant value-added benefit to the examiner's attorney or claims manager client. A summary of the medical records should be presented in the report chronologically. Please consider the following examples.

**Example 6.21: Deposition "perused"**

*Report States:*

The deposition of John Sly was perused.

*Resulting Cross-examination:*

**Q.** Doctor, in your IME report you indicate that you reviewed the claimant's medical records, correct?

**A.** Yes, that's correct.

**Q.** You comment extensively on the deposition of John Sly as well in your report.

**A.** Yes, I do.

**Q.** But you didn't review the deposition.
**A.** I certainly did.
**Q.** Your report said, "the deposition of John Sly was perused," isn't that what you wrote, Doctor?
**A.** That's what it says.
**Q.** So you reviewed all of the records, but you only "perused" the deposition you comment on so extensively in your IME report?

**Comment:** Examiners are best served by carefully reviewing the records and other documents that serve as part of the basis for their written opinion. Any language in IME reports relating to a review of the documents in the case should reflect a careful review of those records.

> I also reviewed the deposition of John Sly.

**Defending the Report As Written:** When opposing counsel plays word games during cross-examination, the examiner can, when appropriate, respond in kind.

**Q.** So, you reviewed all of the records, but you only "perused" the deposition you comment on so extensively in your IME report?
**A.** Counsel, perhaps you are unaware of the fact that the *American Heritage Dictionary* defines "peruse" as "to read or examine especially with great care." Would you care to review, read, or peruse the dictionary, sir?

**Example 6.22: Imprecise description of medical record**
*Report States:*

> Documents reviewed:
> MRI report

*Resulting Cross-examination:*
**Q.** Which MRI report did you review?
**A.** The one in my file.
**Q.** Who sent the MRI report?
**A.** I don't know.
**Q.** When was the MRI report dated?
**A.** I can't remember.
**Q.** How long was the MRI report?
**A.** I'd have to check my file on that.

**Comment:** *Precise* descriptions of the medical records reviewed will help examiners prepare for deposition or trial and avoid having to answer a seemingly endless series of questions about what was reviewed with "I don't know" or "I can't recall." Precise descriptions will also make the report appear to have been carefully drafted.

**Example 6.23: Vague description of medical records**
*Report States:*

> I reviewed the examinee's medical records, including diagnostic studies, physical therapy, primary care, and chiropractic.

*Resulting Cross-examination:*
**Q.** Your report indicates that, "I reviewed the examinee's medical records, including diagnostic studies, physical therapy, primary care, and chiropractic," correct?
**A.** Yes.
**Q.** Did you review the MRI of 2/17/2001?
**A.** If I was sent it.
**Q.** As you sit here today, you have no recollection of reviewing it?
**A.** Correct.
**Q.** So you don't know the results, either?
**A.** Correct.
**Q.** Here is a list of 13 other diagnostic studies. Which ones did you review and what were the results?

**Comment:** This IME report would have been far better had it listed precisely what medical records had been reviewed.

**RECORDS REVIEWED**
1. John Smith, MD 3/6/02-4/2/03 (34 pages)
2. Joe Jones, DC 9/18/02-6/15/03 (62 pages)
3. MRI, ACME Imaging, Inc. 2/17/01
4. Physical Therapy Associates, Inc. 3/10/02-6/28/02 (61 pages)

**Defending the Report As Written:** When the examiner does not specify the records he reviewed in his IME report, he will have to "work around" this problem on cross-examination.

**Q.** Did you review the MRI of 2/17/2001?
**A.** Give me a moment. Yes, here it is in my file. I reviewed it. It was negative.

**Example 6.24: Imprecise description of documents**
*Report States:*
I have reviewed the following documents:
1. OSHA Citation to Acme Construction Company
2. Accident Report, Acme Construction
3. Admission Form, Falmouth General Hospital

**Comment:** A more precise description makes the report and the examiner appear more careful, more thorough, and thus, more credible.

I have reviewed the following documents:
1. OSHA Citation #01-1234 to Acme Construction Company, dated 3/6/2001
2. Accident form dated 8/7/2000, Acme Construction
3. Admission Form, Falmouth General Hospital, Falmouth, Massachusetts, 1 page, dated 8/7/2000

**Example 6.25: "I did review"**

*Report States:*

I did review the MRI study from 1999 with her and she had plain films that I have seen from the chiropractor which are unremarkable.

*Resulting Cross-examination:*

**Q.** In your report you note and I quote, "I did review the MRI study from 1999." Am I reading that correctly?
**A.** Yes.
**Q.** You found it noteworthy to document in your report that you did in fact review the MRI?
**A.** Yes.
**Q.** What records didn't you review?
**A.** I can't recall. I believe I reviewed them all.
**Q.** Apparently not, Doctor. You said you "did" review the MRI. That implies that there are other records that you "did not" review, does it not?
**A.** I guess it does.

**Comment:** This needless loss of credibility occurred because of the examiner's use of the seemingly innocuous "I did review" preface. The expert would have been better served with a straightforward list of what was reviewed.

MRI report, 1 page, dated 7/6/01, signed by M. Jones, MD

**Example 6.26: Precise, numbered list of documents reviewed**

*Report States:*

The following documents were reviewed:

1. Amended Complaint [Home County]
2. Amended Complaint [Federal]
3. Defendant's Answer to Plaintiffs' Amended Complaint
4. Plaintiff 2's Response to Defendant's First Set of Interrogatories
5. Plaintiffs' Second Amended Complaint
6. Second Amended Complaint [Federal]
7. Defendant's Answer to Plaintiffs' Second Amended Complaint
8. Memorandum of Law in Support of Motion for Summary Judgment & Appendix of Evidence
9. Defendant's Answer to Plaintiff's Second Amended Complaint
10. Defendant's Motion for Summary Judgment
11. Expert's [Dr. Skinner, Ph.D.] report, c.v. & deposition [June 20, 2003]
12. Collateral empirical research review, including:
    a. Articles referenced by Plaintiffs' expert
    b. APA Psych Info Search
13. Materials related to *"APT Test,"* including:
    a. Document: *"Validation of the APT Management Trainee-Executive Profile,"* and
    b. Sub Test components
14. Deposition transcripts of:

a. Lyle Lovett
b. Barry Gibbs
c. Nicholas Claus
d. Walt Disney
e. Larry the "Plaintiff" #1
f. Eddie the "Plaintiff" #3

15. Personnel Records of three [3] plaintiffs: Plaintiff 1, Plaintiff 2, & Plaintiff 3
16. Defendant's Motion to Compel Rule 35 Mental Examination of Plaintiff 1, Plaintiff 2 and Plaintiff 3 and Brief in Support of Plaintiff's Memorandum of Law in Opposition to Motion to Compel Rule 35 Mental Examination of Plaintiffs
17. Defendant's Reply to Plaintiff's Memorandum of Law in Opposition to Motion to Compel Rule 35 Mental Examination of Plaintiffs
18. Plaintiff's Appeal of and Objection to Magistrate Judge O'Connor's Order of October 24, 2003
19. Defendant's Memorandum in Response to Plaintiff's Appeal of and Objections to Magistrate Judge O'Connor's Order of October 24, 2003

**Comment:** This is an effective listing. The documents reviewed are numbered and described precisely. This suggests that the documents were carefully reviewed and that the report was drafted by a meticulous individual. The IME report appears to have been carefully drafted, which will bolster the report's credibility and value.

**Example 6.27: Review of unspecified medical records**
*Report States:*

I reviewed the medical records, which were enclosed.

*Resulting Cross-examination:*
**Q.** Doctor, which medical records did you review before writing your IME report?
**A.** The records that were enclosed.
**Q.** Do you have the records in your file?
**A.** No, I returned them to the insurance company.
**Q.** Can you tell me if you reviewed the 9/14/2001 UMass Medical Center record?
**A.** If it was enclosed.
**Q.** You don't have an independent memory of reviewing the record?
**A.** No, I don't.
**Q.** What about Dr. Jensen's records?
**A.** I don't know.
**Q.** Here is a list of 27 medical and hospital records that I will mark as an exhibit. Could you tell us which ones you reviewed, Doctor?

**Comment:** A well-written IME report should include a section that lists precisely the medical records reviewed. In this section the IME physician will list the records reviewed including the date of the record and the name of the physician or other provider. The best IME reports will also include a brief summary of what occurred during the visit, lab work, or testing performed. (Please see Example 6.28.)

**REVIEW AND SUMMARY OF MEDICAL RECORDS**

1. Records from Corrine Daley, D.C., of Daley Rehab Clinic, 4009 N. Doyle Ave., Dixon, Iowa, dated 11/02/99 through 12/15/99.

2. Records from Karl Petersen, Sr., M.D., of Midwestern Health, 1515 W. Shawnee Rd., Morristown, Iowa, dated 11/05/99 through 04/11/01.

3. MRI reports from Maria Lorenz, M.D., Ph.D., and Holly Folgam, M.D., of MRI Specialists, 4028 Doyle Ave., Dixon, Iowa, dated 11/08/99 and 01/04/00.

4. History and Physical from St. Elizabeth's Hospital, 1001 W. Lincoln Ave., Dixon, Iowa, dated 01/06/00.

5. Report of Operation from St. Elizabeth's Hospital, 1001 W. Lincoln Ave., Dixon, Iowa, dated 11/23/99 through 01/09/00.

6. Discharge Summary from St. Elizabeth's Hospital, 1001 W. Lincoln Ave., Dixon, Iowa, dated 01/09/00.

**Defending the Report As Written:** When faced with no list of medical records reviewed in a report, the examiner will have to rely on the records in the file (if they are still there) or the records commented on in his IME report.

**Q.** Doctor, which medical records did you review before writing your IME report?
**A.** The ones I commented on in my IME report. The Midwestern Health record of 2/14/2001, and the two office notes of Dr. Lorenz dated 1/13/2001 and 1/17/2001.

**Example 6.28: Report provides chronological summary of medical records**
*Report States:*

**Medical Record Review**

Type of Encounter: C=Consult, H=Hospital, I=IME/Impairment Assessment, M=Medical Visit, O=Operation, R=Report/Letter, P=PT/OT Visit, S=Diagnostic Study, X=X-ray (Imaging) Study, *=Other

| Date | Provider | Type | Summary |
|---|---|---|---|
| 11/26/ 1999 | Prehospital Care Report | * | Pt states she tripped and fell landing on R shoulder....she can't feel her hand. |
| 11/26/ 1999 | Everett Hospital | H | ...R shoulder pain... |

| | | | |
|---|---|---|---|
| 11/26/ 1999 | Everett Hospital | H | …diagnosis…R shoulder dislocation axillary nerve injury. |
| 11/26/ 1999 | Arsenault, MD | X | Right Shoulder–Routine, Right Clavicle and Right Humerus.…anterior dislocation…no…fracture… |
| 11/26/ 1999 | Flogger, MD | X | Right Shoulder Routine. Normal position post reduction right humerus. Nasal Bones Routine. Chip fracture anterior aspect nasal bones. |
| 11/26/ 1999 | Arsenault, MD | X | Right Ankle Routine.… no…fracture…no significant soft tissue swelling… |
| 11/26/ 1999 | Arsenault, MD | X | Right Tibia/Fib Uni. Right Lower Leg…no…fracture… |
| 11/27/ 1999 | Everett Hospital | H | …R arm feeling “dead.” |
| 11/27/ 1999 | Everett Hospital | H | …no movement in RUE. Brachial plexus injury. |
| 11/29/ 1999 | Lancaster, MD | M | She had immediate numbness in the arm and it felt dead… brachial plexus palsy secondary to a dislocation... probably contused. |
| 11/29/ 1999 | Lancaster, MD | M | …R breast tumor (benign). |
| 11/30/ 1999 | Lancaster, MD | M | She has US Healthcare which we don’t participate…She had gone to Acton Med Emergency …they are going to schedule her for an MRI…she had almost complete brachial plexus neuropraxia. |
| 11/30/ 1999 | Sanders, MD | X | Shoulder, Right-Routine. Degenerative changes of the AC joint…irregularity about the greater tuberosity most likely from a previous trauma. |
| 11/30/ | Sanders, MD | X | Spine Cervical 4-5 Views… |

| | | | |
|---|---|---|---|
| 1999 | | | chronic disc disease at C5-C6…fracture of the mid-shaft of the left clavicle. |
| 12/02/1999 | Laramy, MD | S | MRI Shoulder-Right…tear…supraspinatus tendon…inferior labral…injury/tear…tear…long head biceps… |
| 12/02/1999 | Davies, MD | S | MRI Spine-Cervical. Spondylosis…biforaminal encroachment at C5-6… |
| 12/06/1999 | Smith, MD | M | She…fell…had immediate pain as well as noticing that strength in the arm and sensation were just not there ....lot of discomfort in the shoulder…can't move her hand…can't lift her arm…no evidence of vascular injury …She does not volitionally move at all at the elbow or shoulder…no volitional movement of the hand…no sensation in the C6, C7, C8 or T1 distributions. I cannot elicit any deep tendon reflexes …MRI of the cervical spine…spondylotic changes…brachial plexus injury….active Tinel's …suggests that there is at least some continuity of fibers in the brachial plexus…wait and see how much of this returns…plan…EMG's…five or six for this to be a valid test…I am hopeful that this is an injury that will improve on its own without any need for surgery. |
| 12/06/1999 | Casazza, MD | M | …injury to the brachial plexus. |
| 12/08/1999 | Casazza, MD | M | …MRI…tears of the rotator cuff… |
| 12/21/1999 | Zigler, MD | M | …immediate severe pain in the right shoulder…severe electric shock-like pain down the right upper extremity…pain and |

| | | | |
|---|---|---|---|
| | | | hyperesthesia in the forearm and hand…MRI…full thickness tear of the supraspinatus tendon and…infraspinatus tendon. MRI…cervical spondylosis …borderline canal stenosis …arthroscopic knee…bilateral carpal tunnel release…history of an irregular heartbeat… chronic heartburn, hiatal hernia…good range of motion of the cervical spine…patchy sensory loss in the right upper extremity, most dense in the ulnar distribution of the hand …infraclavicular stretch/ contusion injury of the brachial plexus…effects multiple cords and nerves…arrange for evaluation in our anesthesia pain clinic for treatment of her severe neuropathic pain…she will improve significantly in the proximal upper extremity, but the lower cord function may be most seriously impaired on a long term basis. |
| 12/21/ 1999 | Browning, MD | * | Severe diffuse right brachial plexus injury, especially… lower trunk…NCS and EMG findings indicate that the radial, musculocutaneous, median and ulnar nerves are in partial continuity. This has favorable prognosis implications. |
| 01/04/ 2000 | Berchowitzc, MD | M | Brachial plexus injury especially of the lower cords including the ulnar nerve distribution, some involvement of the median nerve distribution. The radial nerve appears to be spared at least partially. Rotator cuff tear…Gerald Williamson …recommended rotator cuff |

| | | | |
|---|---|---|---|
| | | | repair surgery…recommend …rotator cuff repaired… |
| 01/04/ 2000 | Winer, MD | X | Shoulder…Right…mild degenerative changes of the glenohumeral joint and of the acromioclavicular joint. Clavicle left. No clavicular fracture is seen. |
| 01/04/ 2000 | Williamson, MD | M | …most of her ability to not raise her arm has to do with her rotator cuff and not her brachial plexus…her weakness in her shoulder is primarily the responsibility of her rotator cuff. |
| 01/12/ 2000 | Benson, MD | S | MRI Right Shoulder. Rotator cuff tear which involves the supraspinatus tendon and a part of the infraspinatus tendon. |
| 01/21/ 2000 | Berchowitzc, MD | M | …improved…biceps is 4/5…wrist extension is also about 3+-4/5…EDS and EDP function at the fingers which is improved…3/5 pronator strength, 3/5 supinator strength as well…hand is still somewhat numb to light touch throughout the median and ulnar nerve distributions… MRI…Some of the brachial plexus nerves…appear to be normal in size…infraspinatus …torn…put her in touch with our hand therapists… |
| 02/02/ 2000 | Williamson, MD | O | The biceps tendon was completely absent. We then identified the rotator cuff tear…two traction sutures… and mobilized…by bluntly lysing adhesions on the superficial surface. We then incised the rotator interval all the way to the base of the |

| | | | |
|---|---|---|---|
| | | | coracoid…also released the undersurface of the tendon and muscle belly by releasing the capsule just distal to the labrum…placed a longitudinal incision between supra and infraspinatus at the area of retraction… |
| 02/24/ 2000 | Daniels, MSN/ Vickers, MD | M | …MRI performed on January 12, 2000, of the brachioplexus, revealed no gross abnormality of the right brachioplexus…bilateral carpal release in the 1990's, irregular heartbeat… hypertension, chronic heartburn, hiatal hernia, diabetes… appendectomy…chronic pain as the result of…right brachial plexus injury and status post rotator cuff tear. |
| 03/02/ 2000 | Zigler, MD | M | …underwent operative repair of her right rotator cuff… progressive improvement in function of the right upper extremity…recovered quite strong biceps and triceps strength, good supination and pronation, reasonably good wrist extension and wrist flexion…moderate improvement in median nerve function in the hand…FCU now has 3+ function…chronic pain in the ulnar aspect of the forearm and hand…making excellent progress in terms of spontaneous recovery of her brachial plexus injury. |
| 03/06/ 2000 | Williamson, MD | M | …passive range of motion is excellent. |
| 03/24/ 2000 | Chisolm, MD | M | Right rotator cuff tear status post-repair. Right brachial plexopathy with main involvement of the lower trunk by exam and early EMG. |

| | | | |
|---|---|---|---|
| 03/31/ 2000 | Sanders, MD | O | Colonoscopy; Upper Endoscopy…Duodenitis. |
| 04/07/ 2000 | Browning, MD | * | EMG. Strength in the right was deltoid 3, extensor digitorum communis 5, ulnar hand muscles 3- and median hand muscles 2…diminished pinprick perception over the inner 2/3 of the right hand and forearm. Right median motor studies were normal… prolonged median distal motor latency…mild chronic denervation…axillary…muscu locutaneous…radial …median …very severe denervation in ulnar muscles. Generalized brachial plexopathy…lower trunk most affected…modest but defined improvement in ulnar nerve function… |
| 04/12/ 2000 | Berchowitzc, MD | M | …weakness in extension and finger flexion is improved. …pain in her right hand…3/5 strength in finger adduction. …positive Froment's sign. Two point discrimination is intact to approximately 5-6 mm spacing in a median and ulnar nerve distribution in the hand…improvement with regard to her electrodiagnostic findings. This is quite reassuring…in terms of the regaining of strength, as well as for prognostic reasons. |
| 04/17/ 2000 | Williamson, MD | M | …no lag sign with her arm at 90…fairly reasonable external rotation strength… |
| 06/19/ 2000 | Williamson, MD | M | …active flexion to 90 degrees …strength is actually a good 4/5. |
| 08/25/ 2000 | Beachum, MD | M | …complains of edema… probably at this point due to |

| | | | her obesity… |
|---|---|---|---|
| 10/06/ 2000 | Bird, MD | * | EMG. Right median motor…prolonged distal motor latency. Right brachial plexopathy…only minimal abnormalities at the upper and middle trunk level…chronic denervation in muscles innervated by lower trunk… collateral sprouting from remaining motor axons. Moderate right median neuropathy at the wrist (carpal tunnel syndrome). |
| 10/11/ 2000 | Berchowitzc, MD | M | …numbness and tingling in the ulnar aspect of her hand… medial aspect of her forearm …she appears to be quite symptomatic, even though her function is not significantly impaired. |
| 12/18/ 2000 | Williamson, MD | M | …really don't know what the cause of her pain is…she has virtually complete overhead function… |
| 01/09/ 2001 | Zigler, MD | M | …fairly dense sensory loss in the ulnar aspect of the right hand…weakness of selected ulnar innervated intrinsic hand muscles. Her thumb functions quite well…Dr. David Kline…New Orleans…he recommended…possible proximal ulnar nerve neurolysis and transposition of the ulnar nerve at the elbow. |
| 03/09/ 2001 | Sanders, MD | O | Mild gastritis. |

**Comment:** This is a superb listing of the medical records reviewed. The summary is provided chronologically, which makes it easiest to understand for the reader. The type of each record is readily identified. No self-serving, limiting, or superfluous language was added describing the review (e.g., "comprehensive," "including, but not limited to," "relevant portions of," etc.).

Finally, this listing also provides a summary of the records reviewed. This provides an extremely valuable extra benefit to the examiner's client.

**Example 6.29: Identifying records reviewed**

*Lorca-Merono v. Yokes Washington Foods, Inc.,* 50 P.3d 461 (2002)

An examiner who is unable to identify the medical records he has reviewed before issuing his report can expect to be closely questioned about the issue. In the case *Lorca-Merono v. Yokes Washington Foods, Inc.,* the Idaho Supreme Court was asked to exclude the testimony of an IME examiner who could not identify the records he reviewed before his examination. The Court sustained the overruling of the objection to the testimony and stated:

> Claimant next argues that Dr. Linder's deposition testimony should have been excluded because Dr. Linder could not insure that his testimony a based upon records he had reviewed before the hearing. Dr. Linder examined Claimant on March 14, 1996, on November 14, 1996, on June 13, 1997, and on September 28, 1998. When cross-examined at his deposition taken on December 7, 1999, Dr. Linder testified that he did not have copies of the medical records he had reviewed prior to these examinations because they were retained by the business that had retained him to perform the examinations. The day before his deposition, he reviewed some medical records that had been provided by Employer/Surety's counsel. When reviewing those records, he testified that he focused on his own work and skimmed the other records, particularly the orthopedic and Neurologic reports. Claimant's counsel asked him to identify the particular records he had before each of his examinations of Claimant, and Dr. Linder stated that he was unable to do so. Claimant's counsel then objected to Dr. Linder's testimony because there was no showing that his opinion was based solely upon information provided him before the hearing. Employer/Surety's counsel responded by stating that the medical records provided to Dr. Linder were simply a complete set of Claimant's medical records that were prepared and disclosed prior to the hearing, and he offered claimant's counsel an opportunity to examine them and match them with records admitted during the hearing. Claimant's counsel declined to do so.
>
> Claimant bases her objection upon Rule X(E) which provides, "[T]he evidence presented by post-hearing deposition shall be evidence known by or available to the party at the time of the hearing and shall not include evidence developed, discovered, or manufactured following the hearing." She argues that if Dr. Linder formed an opinion based upon documents that he had not seen prior to the hearing, then his opinion would have been developed after the hearing in violation of the rule. The Commission overruled Claimant's objection to Dr. Linder's deposition testimony on the grounds that Claimant had failed to identify any document provided to Dr. Linder after the hearing that was not known at the time of the hearing, that on direct examination Dr. Linder essentially repeated the diagnoses and conclusions contained in his medical reports that had been admitted into evidence at the hearing, and that the majority of his deposition testimony was developed during cross-examination by Claimant's counsel. On appeal, Claimant has not identified any diagnosis or opinion rendered by Dr. Linder during his deposition testimony that differed from the diagnoses and opinions contained in his earlier reports. The Commission did not err in overruling Claimant's objection to the deposition testimony of Dr. Linder. At 408.

## 6.3 "Including" and "Including, but not limited to"

The word "including" is a red flag for attorneys. It should be avoided when describing medical and other records reviewed. The word "including" implies that other records were reviewed but (intentionally or unintentionally) not listed. Alternatively, it implies that not all of the medical records were received. In either case, the examiner will unnecessarily open herself up to cross-examination.

**Example 6.31: "These include"**

*Report States:*

> I have reviewed the medical records of Jane Doe. These include the following:….

*Resulting Cross-examination:*

**Q.** On page 1 of your report you state that the documents you reviewed prior to forming your opinion include a history and then you list several documents. Is that correct?

**A.** Yes, that's what I stated.

**Q.** What documents did you review prior to forming your opinion that you did not include in the listing on page 1 of your report?

**A.** I don't know if there were any.

**Q.** Are you sure?

**A.** No, I am not. I'd have to check my file.

**Comment:** Use of the word "include" has given counsel an opportunity to make the expert appear unsure of herself.

**Defending the Report As Written:** The examiner should have a list of the medical records she reviewed prior to forming her opinion and writing the IME report. Ideally, the list should be specified in the report itself (see Section 6.2, above). If the report does not include such a list, the examiner can still defend herself.

**Q.** What documents did you review prior to forming your opinion that you did not include in the listing on page 1 of your report?

**A.** None, only the ones listed on page 1.

**Example 6.32: "Including, but not limited to"**

*Report States:*

> In preparing this independent medical evaluation report, I have reviewed medical records of Mr. Smith including, but not limited to, the following:…

**Comment:** The use of "including, but not limited to" should be avoided. The examiner should list all of the medical records reviewed.

Prior to preparing this initial report, I have reviewed the following documents:...

## 6.4 "Relevant portions of"

Another red flag for attorneys is using the descriptive "relevant portions of" prior to the list of medical records and other documents reviewed. Including the descriptive term "relevant portions of" prior to a list of medical records is a serious error. How is the examiner to know what is and is not relevant unless he reviews the document in its entirety? Was the examiner rushing and not reviewing everything? Worst of all, did retaining counsel, an adjuster, or another referral source screen out the "irrelevant" portions of the documents for the examiner?

**Example 6.41: "Relevant portions of"**
*Report States:*
Depositions reviewed:
Relevant portions of deposition transcripts of John Jones and Peter Peters.

*Resulting Cross-examination:*
**Q.** Your report states that prior to forming your opinion you reviewed the relevant portions of the Jones and Peters depositions, is that correct?
**A.** Yes.
**Q.** You would agree, wouldn't you, that it is important that you do in fact review all relevant information?
**A.** Yes, that was done in this case.
**Q.** I see. But the irrelevant portions of those depositions you didn't review?
**A.** Correct.
**Q.** I was wondering if you could help me with something. In regards to the Jones and Peters depositions, how can you possibly have determined which portions of the depositions were relevant if you didn't review the entire depositions?
**A.** I can't. Retaining counsel sent me the relevant portions.
**Q.** You reviewed what counsel wanted you to review, correct?
**A.** Yes.
**Q.** And you didn't see the portions of the depositions counsel didn't want you to see?
**A.** Correct.
**Q.** Did you ever ask counsel to provide you with the entire depositions?
**A.** No, they weren't relevant.
**Q.** Do you know what was contained in the portions of the depositions that counsel didn't send you?
**A.** No.
**Q.** That's because you never reviewed them, correct?
**A.** Correct.

**Comment:** Examiners should review all of the available documents and explicitly list the documents that were reviewed. Examiners are wise to avoid "relevant portions of" language in IME reports.

**Defending the Report As Written:** It is preferable for the examiner to personally review the complete medical records, depositions, etc. Occasionally, due to the volume of material, the referring client may send only portions of the record to the examiner. The referral source does this at his own risk. The examiner can still defend himself even if he has not personally reviewed all of the documents.

**Q.** You reviewed what counsel wanted you to review, correct?
**A.** As you know, there were over 3,500 pages of deposition transcripts in this claim. I was sent the portions dealing with multiple chemical sensitivity. I have listed what I reviewed. If you feel that I have missed something, please share that with me so I can review it now.

## 6.5 "Various"

It is wise to avoid the word "various" in an examiner's list of medical records and documents reviewed. "Various" communicates the idea that the examiner is not thorough and precise. Documents reviewed should be listed precisely. (Please see Examples 6.27 and 6.28.)

**Example 6.51: "Various"**
*Report States:*

I have reviewed the following documents:
1. Various photos of the accident scene…

**Comment:** A better way to list the photos would be to say:

I have reviewed the following documents:
1. 27 4" x 6" photos of the accident scene, taken June 4, 2001 by Insurance Co.'s investigator.
These photos are copied and attached to this report as exhibits #1 through #27…

**Example 6.52: "Various"**
*Report States:*

I have reviewed the following documents:
1. Various medical records from John Smith, DC, Joe Jones, MD, and Acme Rehab. Associates, Inc.

**Comment:** It is much better practice to explicitly list and describe each document reviewed.

**Records Reviewed**

1. John Smith, DC. 9/28/2001-3/6/2002. 95 pages.
2. Joe Jones, MD. 10/6/2002-3/1/2003. 28 pages.
3. Acme Rehab. Associates, Inc. 4/1/2003-7/5/2003. 72 pages.

## 6.6 Missing Medical Records and Documents Not Reviewed

Failure to receive and review all relevant medical records makes an examiner vulnerable during cross-examination. An examiner's opinion can easily be called into question if the examiner did not have access to or did not review all of the medical records in the case.

Some examiners explicitly state in their reports which records they did not have access to. This makes opposing counsel's job a lot easier. It may be better practice to simply list all medical records that were reviewed and let opposing counsel figure out for herself what the examiner did not review. The best practice of all is to demand and then review all relevant medical records prior to issuing the IME report. If all available relevant documents are not made available to the expert, the examiner should strongly consider refusing to offer an opinion in the case.

**Example 6.61: No records have been made available to me**

*Report States:*

> Dr. Z. performed some sort of surgical procedure on the back of her neck in late 1998. No records have been made available to me by Dr. Z. nor are there any operative notes. This procedure appears to have been some sort of a surgical procedure on the occipital nerve.

*Resulting Cross-examination:*

**Q.** You don't know what surgery Dr. Z. performed on the patient, do you?
**A.** That's correct.
**Q.** That's because the records were not provided to you before you reached your conclusions and formed your opinions?
**A.** True.
**Q.** Would you have liked to have had the operative notes and medical records?
**A.** Yes.
**Q.** Would they have changed your opinion in this case?
**A.** I don't know.
**Q.** So, your opinion may be incorrect?
**A.** I did the best I could with what I had.
**Q.** Could you have refused to reach a conclusion and form an opinion until the records were provided to you?

**Comment:** An examiner who bases her opinion on incomplete medical records places that opinion in question. This examiner made opposing counsel's job much easier by explicitly noting that she did not review the records from Dr. Z. A better practice would have been to list all of the medical records reviewed and let opposing counsel figure out for herself what is missing from the list.

**Defending the Report As Written:** It is not unusual for examiners to be provided with a file that has some missing medical records. Sometimes the reason is innocent; for example, the records are unavailable, were lost, or have been misplaced. Other times, the reason is not so innocent; for example, the record does not help the retaining party.

The examiner should not be flustered when counsel raises "missing records." Usually it is a ploy to imply a conspiracy. The examiner should stay calm and make counsel "put up or shut up."

**Q.** Would they have changed your opinion in this case?
**A.** I doubt it since I am commenting on impairment and work capacity. If you do have records you would like me to see, please show them to me and I will be happy to tell you if they change my opinion.

**Example 6.62: Many key records missing**
*Report States:*

> I did not have school records or records from the psychologist who treated Ms. X after the alleged sexual harassment. Dr. Jones's monthly handwritten notes were illegible. I did not have any previous medical or employment records.

*Resulting Cross-examination*:
**Q.** When you start treating patients you like to see their past medical and other records, don't you?
**A.** Yes.
**Q.** That is because they are part of the puzzle you are looking into?
**A.** Yes.
**Q.** Here there were crucial parts to the puzzle missing, correct?
**A.** Records were missing.
**Q.** Are the school records important?
**A.** They could be.
**Q.** No way of knowing without looking at them?
**A.** That's right.
**Q.** The same for the psychologist records?
**A.** Yes.
**Q.** The same for Dr. Jones's records?
**A.** No, I have them.
**Q.** But you say you can't read them, correct?
**A.** True.
**Q.** So they are of no help?
**A.** Correct.
**Q.** The prior medical records are important to establish a baseline, correct?
**A.** Yes.
**Q.** But you didn't have them so you could not establish a baseline?
**A.** True.
**Q.** The same for the employment records?
**A.** Correct.
**Q.** So you have five crucial parts to this puzzle that are missing?
**A.** Yes.
**Q.** Did you ever consider holding off forming an opinion until counsel provided you with these crucial missing records?

**Comment:** This examiner's opinion can be easily questioned because she did not have access to key documentation. In a situation like this, the examiner may have been better off to list all the records she reviewed and not red-flag the missing records for opposing counsel.

**Defending the Report As Written:** Examiners will often be faced with missing records in their IME reports.

> Review of medical records is a prime component of the independent medical evaluation, and the objective document confirming history and treatment. A modern medical record may include office notes, hospital records, nursing assessment, therapy notes, radiological studies, depositions, and accident reports. The consistency of the record is valuable in assessing validity of complaints and ultimately causal relationship.[2]

Many examiners develop an office policy regarding missing records.

> A report and bill is sent at the time of the IME irrespective of missing or illegible records. It is stated the opinion rendered is based on the history, if factual, the physical examination, and the records available. The missing records are requested noting that a supplemental report, opinion, and bill will be rendered upon receipt.[3]

Examiners should develop their own techniques for dealing with counsel's missing records gambit.

**Q.** Here there were crucial parts to the puzzle missing, correct?
**A.** There are almost always parts to the puzzle missing, Counsel. In my 28 years of experience, I have rarely seen a case in which all of the records are provided. As to whether records are crucial, we should probably let the judge decide that issue.

**Example 6.63: Lack of medical records**
*Report States:*
There are no medical records to review.

*Resulting Cross-examination:*
**Q.** You performed an IME on the examinee, whose chief complaint was back and neck pain, correct?
**A.** Yes.
**Q.** What did the x-rays reveal, Doctor?
**A.** As I stated in my IME report, there were no medical records to review.
**Q.** How long was it between the time of the accident and the time of your examination and report?
**A.** Approximately seven months between the alleged accident and my examination.
**Q.** Do you know why you were not provided with the hospital records, the x-rays, the treatment records from the orthopedic surgeon, the CT scan results, or the physical therapy records, Doctor?
**A.** No.

---

[2] SEAK, Inc., *IME Summit Handbook*, Stephen F. Freifeld, MD, p. 151 (2000).
[3] Ibid. at 151.

**Q.** Did you request the records?
**A.** Yes.
**Q.** Would you have liked to have them when you performed your IME?
**A.** Yes.
**Q.** Would the records have assisted you in forming your opinions as to your diagnosis, as to causation, and work capacity?
**A.** They may have. As I haven't seen them, I can't say.
**Q.** Are you at all suspicious as to why, even after you requested them, *no* medical records of any kind were provided to you?
**A.** It's curious.
**Q.** Could the records have changed or modified the opinions you expressed in your IME report?
**A.** I don't know as I haven't seen them.
**Q.** But you did swear under the penalty of perjury that the statements were true and correct without having seen any medical records, Doctor?

**Comment:** Examiners are often faced with some missing medical records when performing IMEs and writing their reports. As a practical matter, it is not always possible to wait until all the records are provided before proceeding. When, however, as in the above example, *no* medical records are provided, the examiner who proceeds with his examination and an IME report does so at his peril. Does he rely on the examinee for the results of x-rays, CT scans, or treatment? What if the examinee is a poor historian?

For example, the AMA *Guides to the Evaluation of Permanent Impairment,* fifth edition (2001), suggests that a physician preparing a report should:

> List diagnostic study results and outstanding pertinent diagnostic studies. These may include laboratory tests, electrocardiograms, exercise stress studies, radiographic and other imaging studies, rehabilitation evaluations, mental status examinations, and other tests or diagnostic procedures. (2.6a.4)

The examiner may be better served by refusing to write an IME report until he is provided with the available medical records.

**Defending the Report As Written:** The examiner who proceeds with an examination and report without the benefit of any medical records can still defend himself and his actions.

**Q.** But you did swear under the penalty of perjury the statements were true and correct without having seen any medical records, Doctor?
**A.** First, I said that the statements contained herein are true and correct to the best of my knowledge and belief. Secondly, I specifically recommended on page 5 of my report that the medical records be obtained for background, documentation, and a supplemental report.

## 6.7 Surveillance Material

Examiners may be called upon to review surveillance material of the examinee. The surveillance material reviewed should be documented objectively without any superfluous language attacking the examinee or the examinee's credibility. Depending on the forum and jurisdiction, the examiner may be strictly limited as to what surveillance she can and cannot review and comment on in the IME report. The following example is illustrative.

**Example 6.71: Subjective characterization of surveillance material**
*Report States:*

> It also must be noted that I had occasion to review a most remarkable and damning surveillance video. This video shows the plaintiff carrying heavy groceries in and out of his car, twisting and bending. All of these activities the examinee stated to me he was incapable of doing without pain.

*Resulting Cross-examination*:
**Q.** You viewed the plaintiff carrying heavy groceries, Doctor?
**A.** Well, I saw a video of him lifting them.
**Q.** How much did they weigh?
**A.** I couldn't say exactly, but they looked heavy.
**Q.** Could you see what was in the bags?
**A.** No.
**Q.** They looked heavy because the plaintiff was struggling lifting them?
**A.** Yes, exactly.
**Q.** Do you know how many days the investigator followed the plaintiff before he filmed the video?
**A.** No, I don't.
**Q.** Do you know how the plaintiff felt the day after he lifted the bags?
**A.** No, I don't.
**Q.** Do you know if the plaintiff was in pain when he lifted the groceries?
**A.** He looked OK.
**Q.** As a trained examiner, you know that someone could be dying from cancer and look OK, correct?
**A.** Yes, that's true.
**Q.** Do you know why the plaintiff had to go to the grocery store that day, Doctor?
**A.** No.
**Q.** How long did you observe the plaintiff lift the bags for?
**A.** About a minute or so.
**Q.** Do you know how many days he was in bed for after getting the groceries for his sick child, Doctor?
**A.** No, I don't.
**Q.** Would you want to know these things before you decide how damning the tape is?

**Comment:** This report would have been more effective had the reference to the reviewed surveillance material been more objective and precise. One way to do this is to document a representative sample of the specific activities performed on the tape along with the time each activity was performed.

Medical Records and Other Documents and Materials Reviewed
1. VHS Surveillance Video. 3-minute running time. Shot 9/28/2003 by Acme Investigations, Inc., lifting bags of groceries

**Defending the Report As Written:** Examiners can expect opposing counsel to attack surveillance material. The harder they attack, the more they are concerned about the impact the video may have on the judge or other fact finder. Examiners need not back down from commenting on what they have seen.

**Q.** They looked heavy because the plaintiff was struggling lifting them?
**A.** No. They looked heavy because they were large paper bags bulging and overflowing and large bags of dog food. They looked heavy, Counsel, because they were heavy. The judge will see what I am talking about when she views the video.

## 6.8 Illegible Records

IME reports are based to a large degree on a review of the examinee's medical records. A common problem with medical records is that they often contain much illegible information. Examiners should be prepared to answer questions about illegible medical records and what effect, if any, this has on the accuracy of the examiner's opinion. The examiner faced with records that are illegible due to poor copying should request clean copies he can read. Where portions of records are illegible, the examiner should specifically document this in his IME report.

**Example 6.81: Whole series of illegible records**
*Report States:*
The records of Dr. Walter Carlson, 1/14/2002-3/17/2003, are handwritten and illegible.

*Resulting Cross-examination:*
**Q.** The records you can't read cover some 4 pages and over one year, correct?
**A.** Yes, that's correct.
**Q.** They are handwritten and more difficult to make out than neatly typed records?
**A.** Absolutely.
**Q.** Medical records are important and should be typed?
**A.** Correct.
**Q.** You shouldn't have to spend your valuable time deciphering handwritten notes?
**A.** I should not.
**Q.** You could read some of the records, correct?
**A.** Some of it, yes.
**Q.** But it was quicker and easier to just say they were all illegible so you didn't have to bother with them?
**A.** I did the best I could.
**Q.** If the health of a family member was at stake, would you have taken the time to read them then, Doctor?

**Comment:** Examiners who state that large numbers of records are illegible should expect to be questioned closely on this issue. Examiners should be careful not to use illegibility as an excuse for avoiding reviewing handwritten records.

**Defending the Report As Written:** When faced with cross-examination, the IME examiner needs to be able to stand his ground.

**Q.** They are handwritten and more difficult to make out than neatly typed records?
**A.** No, not more difficult…illegible. I couldn't read them, so I was unable to comment on them. I am not going to sit and try to guess what they mean.

**Example 6.82: Portion of specific record illegible**
*Report States:*

> On June 13, 1997, Dr. Albertson noted "…episodes over the last three [illegible] of a sharp, shooting pain in the right [illegible]…if she gets into certain positions, either sitting or twisting. Between episodes, she has [illegible] pain…Her neck is overall better. She is still having problems with…bilateral knees [and]…cannot kneel on either one…and the right is much worse than…left." Abnormal exam findings included mild tenderness over right thoracolumbar junction and patellar tendons and "positive patellar apprehension…bilaterally but mostly in the distal poles of the patellae." Assessments were neck pain doing well, mild soft tissue pain in thoracolumbar junction, and bilateral patellar tendonitis. Plan was "physical therapy to work on her knees," the orthopedist adding "…this could be a long-term problem. The key will be her program afterwards. I will see her back prn [as needed]."

*Resulting Cross-examination:*
**Q.** Your IME report contains the notes of Dr. Albertson, correct?
**A.** Yes.
**Q.** You included these because they were instructive and important?
**A.** Yes. They were helpful.
**Q.** There were a few words that you noted were illegible?
**A.** Yes.
**Q.** For example, "episodes over the last three [word illegible]"?
**A.** Yes.
**Q.** You don't know if that said years, months, weeks, or days?
**A.** No, I don't.
**Q.** Could that be of significance?
**A.** It could.
**Q.** The next one, "between episodes she has [word illegible] pain"?
**A.** That's correct.
**Q.** That word could be a description of the pain…mild, moderate, or severe?
**A.** Yes.
**Q.** It could be the body part also?
**A.** Yes, it could be.
**Q.** It could be something else?

**A.** Yes.
**Q.** Could that be of significance?
**A.** Yes, it could be.
**Q.** Did you make any attempt to find out what these potentially crucial words were, Doctor?

**Comment:** Examiners can expect to be cross-examined about words they noted as illegible. Counsel will try to show that the words could be of significance and that the examiner made little or no attempt to find out what they were.

**Defending the Report As Written:** While counsel can try to make "something" out of a few illegible words, the examiner need not play this game.

**Q.** Did you make any attempt to find out what these potentially crucial words were, Doctor?
**A.** Counsel, there are approximately 375 pages of medical and hospital records in this case. I did not call each doctor, physical therapist, and nurse and try to get them to interpret their handwriting. That is not a reasonable request.

## 6.9 Records Supplied by the Referral Source

The medical records and other documents reviewed by the examiner are often sent to the examiner by the attorney, adjuster, broker, or other referral source. Where this is the case, examiners can expect close questioning during cross-examination. Opposing counsel will try to show that the referral source could have withheld or even altered the medical records the examiner relied upon. If a cover letter was sent with the records, this cover letter could become a source for close questioning as well.

**Example 6.91: Records supplied by referral source untrustworthy?**
*Report States:*

I reviewed the medical records submitted to me, including the following:

1. Admission note and discharge note, Stanley Williams, MD, Neurosurgeon, dated 3/3/89 and 3/10/89.
2. Operative note, Stanley Williams, MD, 3/4/89.
3. Admission note and discharge note, Stanley Williams, MD, 5/12/89 and 5/17/89.
4. Operative note, Stanley Williams, MD, 5/12/89.
5. Admission note and discharge note, Stanley Williams, MD, 4/23/91 and 5/5/91.
6. Admission note, Laurence P. Foley, MD, FACS, Neurosurgeon, 1/19/01.
7. Operative report, Thomas R. Lewis, MD, Neurosurgeon, 1/24/01.
8. Discharge note, Thomas R. Lewis, MD, 1/26/01.
9. Office notes, Thomas R. Lewis, MD, from 2/21/01 through 11/22/02.
10. Physical therapy progress notes, Fitness Plus, Inc., 5/14/01 through 4/5/02.
11. Office notes and procedure notes, St. John's Clinic, 5/29/02,

6/6/02, 6/28/02, 7/19/02 and 10/24/02.
12. Correspondence from Thomas R. Lewis, MD, to Steven Kaye dated 7/8/02.
13. Independent Medical Examination report of Brandon J. Coens, MD, Neurologist, dated 10/4/02.

*Resulting Cross-examination:*
**Q.** You reviewed the 13 records submitted to you before you issued your IME report, correct?
**A.** Yes.
**Q.** You relied in part on these records in forming your opinion?
**A.** Yes, I did.
**Q.** Are these all of the records in this case?
**A.** All I have.
**Q.** Who put together the package of these records that were sent to you?
**A.** The workers' compensation insurance company adjuster.
**Q.** The adjuster's job is to resolve the case as cheaply as possible?
**A.** Yes.
**Q.** That is the same insurance company that will have to pay the benefits if the claim is lost?
**A.** Yes.
**Q.** You would agree that the workers' compensation insurance company has a vested interest in this case?
**A.** Yes.
**Q.** Do insurance company adjusters sometimes hide or "deep six" some unhelpful records?
**A.** It happens.
**Q.** They do this to try to win the case?
**A.** Yes, sometimes they do.
**Q.** Do insurance companies sometimes decide to remove pages from hospital records or nurse's notes so the examiner doesn't have them?
**A.** Rarely, but it does happen.
**Q.** Did you make any attempt to make sure that you had a complete, accurate, and unaltered set of records?
**A.** No, I did not.
**Q.** Could you tell us why the workers' compensation insurance company did not send you the emergency room record of 2/14/89 when the examinee was taken directly from the job site to the hospital?

**Comment:** Counsel here is trying to show that the examiner should not have relied exclusively on the workers' compensation insurance adjuster to put together the "complete" package of medical records. Getting the examiner to justify the actions of the insurer is an effective technique.

**Defending the Report As Written:** When counsel plays the missing record game, the examiner can refuse to play.

**Q.** Are these all the records in the case?
**A.** I listed the records I reviewed in my report. If you have any additional

records, I would be happy to review them.

**Example 6.92: Cover letter/opinions sought**
*Report States:*
> According to your introductory letter, he is claiming an injury to his neck and temporo mandibular joint as a result of this accident.

*Resulting Cross-examination:*
**Q.** You start off your IME report of 3/21/2001 by stating, "According to your introductory letter, he is claiming an injury to his neck and temporo mandibular joint as a result of this accident," correct?
**A.** Yes.
**Q.** You accepted his characterization of the issues?
**A.** Yes.
**Q.** Attorney Butler sent you an introductory letter, the medical records, and the opinions he was seeking from you, correct?
**A.** I did receive the cover letter and the medical records. He did not tell me the opinions he was seeking.
**Q.** He asked you to express your opinion as to whether the claimant's neck and TMJ injuries were the result of the accident, correct?
**A.** Yes.
**Q.** You knew, of course, that he was representing the workers' compensation carrier?
**A.** Yes.
**Q.** You expressed an opinion that the neck and TMJ were not the result of the accident, correct?
**A.** Yes.
**Q.** He asked you for an opinion as to whether the claimant may be expected to suffer any future complications from the accident, correct?
**A.** Yes.
**Q.** You expressed an opinion that he is not expected to suffer any future complications from the accident, is that correct?
**A.** Yes.
**Q.** He asked you whether the claimant has any permanent injury from the accident?
**A.** Yes.
**Q.** You expressed the opinion that he has not?
**A.** Yes.
**Q.** Attorney Butler sent you the three opinions he was seeking from you in his cover letter and you provided the three opinions he needed to defend the workers' compensation insurer, correct?
**A.** I answered his questions, yes.
**Q.** So what you are saying, Doctor, is that there was nothing improper because Attorney Butler didn't say, "Please give me your opinion that the claimant's neck and TMJ injuries were not the result of the accident?" Instead he said, "Please give me your opinion whether the claimant's neck and TMJ injuries were the result of the accident."
**A.** I just answer the questions, Counsel.

**Q.** Did Attorney Butler tell you the opinions he was seeking?
**A.** He asked me for my opinions and I provided them.

**Comment:** When the IME physician is sent a cover letter by retaining counsel outlining the case and the issues, the physician should anticipate questions about the letter and its intent. Counsel will try to imply or prove that the attorney gave the doctor his "marching orders" and the examiner was all too happy to comply.

**Defending the Report As Written:** When faced with the implication or allegation that retaining counsel improperly influenced the IME physician with his cover letter, the physician is not without recourse.

**Q.** Attorney Butler sent you an introductory letter, the medical records, and the opinions he was seeking from you, correct?
**A.** I did receive the medical records and the cover letter. As to your insinuation that there was something wrong with the cover letter, I ask that you attach the cover letter to the deposition and let the judge decide if there is anything wrong with it. If you refuse to do so, please explain to the judge what you are trying to hide, Counsel.

# Chapter 7 The Examinee's History

## 7.1 Executive Summary

A precise, well-written, and accurate history is an essential part of a high-quality IME report. The authors recommend the following.

- The following areas should be addressed in thorough IMEs.
  - Pre-existing Status/Past Medical History
  - Description of Injury/Incident
  - Treatment History
  - Psychosocial/Socioeconomic/Social/Educational History
  - Family Medical History
  - Occupational/Employment/Work History
- The various parts of the history should each be addressed in their own section, identified by a topic heading.
- To help ensure accuracy, the examiner should:
  - dictate the history in the presence of the examinee,
  - not rely on a staff member to take the history, and
  - use a translator, where needed.
- Objective, measured language should be used, especially when documenting inconsistencies.
- The examiner should not include superfluous verbiage or take subtle or overt cheap shots at the examinee.
- It is best for the examiner to take and document a treatment history from the examinee and to also create a history from the available medical records. This will help ensure completeness and allow for the identification of potential inconsistencies.
- When opinions are expressed on work capacity in the occupational history section, the examiner will be in the best position to defend these opinions when he has as much accurate information concerning the job in question as possible.

## 7.2 Overview

*Areas addressed*

A detailed and complete history will increase an IME report's value and make the report more readily defensible. The history should, depending upon the particular case, include the following.

1. Pre-existing Status/Past Medical History
2. Description of Injury/Incident
3. Treatment History
4. Psychosocial/Socioeconomic/Social/Educational History

5. Family Medical History
6. Occupational/Employment/Work History

Sections 7.3 to 7.8 discuss each of these six areas in detail.

*Organization*
The history can be organized in many different ways. Depending upon the complexity of the case, all of the above six items could be included in a narrative that does not explicitly break out the various parts of the history (see Example 7.21). The authors prefer a format in which each of the portions of the history is broken out into its own subsection and identified by its own topic heading (see Example 7.22). For further examples of some of the many appropriate ways to organize the "History" section or sections of an IME report, please see Chapter 18.

**Example 7.21: Injury and treatment history combined into one section**
*Report States:*

**HISTORY OF PRESENT INJURY**

The patient indicates that her history of low back problems dates back to June of 1998, when she injured her low back in the course of her work as a preloader at ACME Shipping. She recalls twisting while trying to catch a computer that was falling to the floor. She apparently had abrupt onset of pain in her low back.

She reports that following this injury she remained off work until about December of 1998. She went through a work hardening program as she attempted to return to her job.

She indicates that between December of 1998 and August of 2001, she was able to keep up with her work responsibilities at ACME, although she had ongoing problems with her low back.

She indicates that her situation deteriorated substantially in August of 2001. She recalls that she was loading a 40-pound box onto a truck. She advanced her right leg and felt a jolt of pain in the lumbosacral region with radiation over the right buttock. She says that she lost control of her bowels.

She says that she reported the event to her supervisor and was referred to "a company doctor." This physician apparently ordered an MRI scan. He then indicated that she could return to her ACME job, although she should have light duty restrictions. She says that her supervisor told her that she needed to continue working on the conveyor belt where she had worked before, although she was given the opportunity of sitting down and resting if she needed to do this. She indicates that she continued working (apparently for a couple of weeks), but then went off work sometime in September. She has been consistently out of the workforce since then except for one day in about December of 2001, when she tried to return to work. She says that when she made this attempt, she was told that she needed to be able to function 100% before she could go back to ACME. She went off work again and says that she is currently receiving time loss benefits through a workers' compensation claim.

She indicates that she has been seeing Dr. A since September of 2001. He referred her to physical therapy, but the patient says that this made her symptoms worse so that therapy was discontinued in about January. She does have a self-directed exercise program that she learned as she went through her 1998 injury. She recalls undergoing several injection procedures. An epidural injection done shortly after onset of her symptoms in August provided no benefit. She recalls undergoing three nerve root blocks (right S1 selective nerve root blocks) performed by Dr. A. She says that these helped for about three or four hours. She reports that she has recently undergone a three level discography. She indicates that she experienced severe pain during injections of two of the three discs and at least moderate pain during injection of the third disc. She says that she had a marked flare-up of pain that lasted for days after the discography. She indicates that a physician (presumably Dr. A) has now recommended either an IDET procedure or a spinal fusion.

**MEDICAL HISTORY:**

CURRENT MEDICAL PROBLEMS: As far as her general health is concerned, she indicates that she has undergone a hysterectomy and ovariectomy. She is taking Estratest for this. She reports that she has had pneumonia on several occasions.

CURRENT MEDICATIONS: Currently, her medications consist of Vicodin, 4-6 tablets per day, and Estratest.

ALLERGIES: She describes herself as allergic to Penicillin, Codeine, Morphine, and aspirin.

PREVIOUS INJURIES: The patient denies any significant problems with her low back prior to 1998.

PRIOR HOSPITALIZATIONS/SURGERIES: She has also undergone a Mumford procedure on her right shoulder and some procedure on her right knee. She can't give any details.

HABITS: She smokes about a pack and a half of cigarettes per day. She describes herself as an occasional drinker and denies a history of drug or alcohol abuse.

**SOCIOECONOMIC:**

The patient indicates that she has worked as a preloader for ACME Shipping for more than four years. She indicates that she is divorced and has two dependent children. She has a tenth-grade education. (She indicates that she subsequently got a GED.)

**Comment:** This report combines the history of the injury with the treatment history provided by the examinee. The socioeconomic and previous medical history are provided in separately marked sections. This is an acceptable format given the relative brevity of the history.

**Example 7.22: Different portions of the "History" section broken out into their own labeled sections**
*Report States:*

**History (per Examinee)**

**Pre-Existing Status**
She denies any previous problems or injuries, including any other work- or liability-related injuries. Ms. Formaggio also denies having any difficulties similar to those she is now experiencing until the injury.

**Injury**
She reports that on 11/26/99 she came in contact with a cart at WalMart located at the Lancaster Farms Shopping Center. She was inside the store. It was very crowded. All she can remember is making contact with something hitting her right shin and she flew through the air. She came down landing flat on her nose with her right arm stretched over her head.

She could not move. There was no loss of consciousness. She had excruciating pain in her right shoulder and the right shin and ankle. Her left shoulder was also painful. Her nose was bleeding. Her arm was paralyzed. She couldn't move her right arm.

Following the injury, she was taken by ambulance to Everett Hospital.

**Clinical Chronology**
She was in a great deal of pain at Everett ER. She was x-rayed and told her right shoulder was dislocated. It was reduced. Dr. Lancaster, Schenectady orthopedic surgeon came in. Pain medication was given. A sling was given. She was sent home. She was told she had a fracture of the nose.

She continued to experience pain and electroshocks radiating up her entire arm. Because of this she returned to Everett Hospital Emergency Room. She was met by Dr. Lancaster. He gave her stronger medication and told her to follow up in his office.

## THE EXAMINEE'S HISTORY

The pain was still so bad that she went to Acton Medical Center Hospital. Her arm "wouldn't do anything." She went to AMCH within the next couple of days.

She was seen by Dr. Smith, neurosurgeon at AMCH. She was sent for an MRI and x-rays. She followed up with Dr. Smith in his office. She was set up for EMG's. She was also referred to Dr. Casazza, Acton orthopedic surgeon. Dr. Casazza told her that she would never be able to move the arm again and might need an arthrodesis procedure of the right arm.

She previously lived in the Acton area, several of her children continued to live in the Acton area. She was visiting them from her new home in Nottingham, PA.

She had a lump on the right anterior leg, which got larger. There was throbbing. She returned to Pennsylvania. This was evaluated and she was told that it was not a blood clot. Her home in Pennsylvania is 260 miles from Acton.

She went to the University of Pennsylvania in Philadelphia and saw Dr. Zigler, neurosurgeon. He had EMG's performed. He said that she also needed orthopedic care because a rotator cuff tear was noted on the MRI. She saw a hand surgeon and also Dr. Williamson a shoulder surgeon.

Dr. Williamson said that there was a very bad rotator cuff injury. He said that he couldn't promise what kind of result she would have but that she should have surgery.

On February 2, 2000, she had surgery performed on her right shoulder.

She was in physical therapy prior to and after this surgery. Her leg continued to bother her. She had a test for a blood clot but this was okay.

She was depressed because of the loss of use of her hand. She was seen by a psychiatrist. She was treated with pills. Her stomach became irritated from this medicine. She subsequently had gastroscopy. She had to cut back on these medications.

Her psychiatrist is now deceased. She sees a psychotherapist every two weeks. "I am a very depressed person. It's like living with a tourniquet around my arm, like someone is pulling on it. It's like sleeping on your arm and not being able to wake it up."

She has tried acupuncture on two occasions, physiatry, and pain management. She had a second opinion with a neurosurgeon in New Orleans. He offered to "cut the nerves in her neck."

She saw Dr. David Kline, a specialist in New Orleans. He performed testing and evaluation. He told her that success from a surgical procedure would be low. He discouraged surgery.

She returned to Dr. Zigler, neurosurgeon in Philadelphia. He placed her back in therapy. Eventually physical therapy told her that it made no sense for her to come anymore, because she was not improving.

She asked Dr. Zigler to amputate her hand. He told her that this would not work because she would still get phantom pain in her hand.

She now sees Dr. Fried in Nottingham. Dr. Williamson said to come back if her arm is hurting.

The physical therapy ended a week ago.

She is also seeing a Dr. Niescien for a dietary program.

**Occupational History**
At the time of the injury she was not employed. She had previously worked eight years ago as a bank teller. She worked there for less than one year. Prior to that she worked in her father's store for fifteen to twenty years. She previously sold real estate. She and her husband also have real estate properties, which she states she takes care of. She then corrected herself and stated that she used to take care of these. She has a high-school-graduate education. In terms of current work status, she is not working. She reports no work restrictions placed upon her.

**Social History**
The examinee lives in Nottingham, Pennsylvania with her husband. The activities of a typical day include getting up, watching television, going to doctor visits and going for rides in the car once in a while. She denies performing any other work activities or vigorous recreational pursuits. The examinee does not smoke. She denies any problems with alcohol or illicit drug usage.

**Past Medical History**

Medical: Hypertension. (Controlled)
Diabetes.
Hiatal hernia.
Chronic heart burn.
History of irregular heart beat.

Surgery: Cholecystectomy.
Complete hysterectomy age 48.
Appendectomy.
Bilateral carpal tunnel releases.
Bilateral arthroscopic knee surgery.

| Medications (other): | Catapress.<br>Prevacid.<br>Lipitor.<br>Aceybutolol. |
|---|---|
| Allergies: | None known. |

**Family History**
Mother alive at age 82 with Diabetes Mellitus. Father deceased age 64 with cancer of the urethra.

**Comment:** This "History" section provided by the examinee is very well organized and written precisely. Each portion of the history is broken out into its own section. This makes the report very easy for the client to read and thus more valuable to the client. It also makes the report easier to use as a tool for the examiner to refresh his recollection prior to (or while) testifying. The dates of the medical treatment are provided by the examiner in his review of the medical records.

*Potential problem areas*
It is important that a reliable and complete history is taken and documented. Many examiners dictate the history in the presence of the examinee (and document this in the report) to help ensure the accuracy of the history. Three common problem areas regarding histories follow.

1. *The history is taken by an assistant, such as a nurse, not by the examiner.* It is preferable that the examiner, and not an assistant, take the history. When an assistant takes the history, the report should document this. It is best that procedures are followed that help guarantee the accuracy of the history. For example, the assistant might dictate the history in the presence of the examinee and the examiner could confirm the history with the examinee before proceeding with the examination.

2. *The examiner makes superfluous or inappropriate negative comments concerning the examinee's truthfulness or editorializes on the history by using emphasis or making snide comments.* Superfluous or inappropriate negative comments and characterizations dealing with the examinee's credibility should be avoided. Inconsistencies should be objectively documented using professional, measured language. Accusatory or judgmental language or editorializing in the history can potentially be used against the examiner to show bias.

3. *The history is unreliable due to a language barrier between the examinee and the examiner.* Reliable and qualified interpreters are a must if there is a language barrier. It should be the referring client's responsibility to provide an

interpreter where needed. Examiners should not perform exams where they are unable to communicate with the examinee.

Please consider the following examples.

**Example 7.23: History taken by staff member**
*Report States:*
Information as given by Paula DeSoto.

*Resulting Cross-examination:*
**Q.** The first three pages of your IME report are listed under the heading "Information as given by Paula DeSoto," correct?
**A.** Yes.
**Q.** Is this the history that was elicited?
**A.** Yes.
**Q.** Did you take the history yourself or did a staff member do that for you?
**A.** It was done by a staff member.
**Q.** Was your failure to state that an attempt to conceal the fact that you did not take the history yourself?
**A.** No.
**Q.** You didn't think it was important enough to put in the report?
**A.** That's correct.
**Q.** Do you know if the staff member took the history verbatim or paraphrased it?
**A.** It was, as I understand it, pretty much verbatim.
**Q.** Of course you were not present, correct?
**A.** That's correct.
**Q.** Do you have the contemporaneous notes that were taken by your staff member?
**A.** No.
**Q.** Have you seen the notes?
**A.** No.
**Q.** Do you know for a fact that they exist?
**A.** Well….she would have had to take notes.
**Q.** We subpoenaed your complete file and there were no such notes, so, Doctor, where are the missing notes?
**A.** I don't know.
**Q.** When the history says, "She recalls them checking her eyes with a light," what does that mean to you?
**A.** They checked her eyes with a light.
**Q.** The next sentence says, "She clearly recalls that she hit her head on the steering wheel"?
**A.** Correct.
**Q.** Does her "clear recollection" differ from "her recollection" in accuracy, in your mind, Doctor?
**A.** No, it's just a choice of words.
**Q.** Do you know if your staff member helped or added any words to the history on pages one to three of your IME report?
**A.** No, she did not, to the best of my knowledge.

**Q.** Of course, you weren't there, so you can't say for sure.
**A.** That's correct.
**Q.** Now, the history is in her own words?
**A.** Yes. I already said that.
**Q.** Could you explain then why some of it is in quotes? For example, page 2, line 8, "She tried to work for two weeks but 'she couldn't do the work.'"
**A.** Some key phrases are emphasized by the quotes.
**Q.** Your staff member determined the portions of the detailed history which were "key phrases"?
**A.** Yes. She is a trained case manager.
**Q.** Just so I understand, the history is taken "pretty much verbatim" but some of the phrases are in quotes because they are key phrases?
**A.** Yes.
**Q.** Well, if it's verbatim, isn't the entire three-page history made up of quotes?
**A.** Yes, to the best of my knowledge.
**Q.** Did the case manager also correct the history when she felt it was mistaken?
**A.** Absolutely not.
**Q.** I refer you to page 2, line 13, "she then met with a psychologist that she refers to as Dr. Williamson. His name in fact is Jon K. Williams, PhD." Is that what your report says, Doctor?
**A.** Yes.
**Q.** Is that a correction of the history by your case manager?
**A.** It's a clarification or correction, as you choose.
**Q.** How many other corrections of the history did your case manager make?
**A.** I don't know if she made any.
**Q.** So as you sit here today, you don't know how many "corrections" the case manager made correcting the history taken.

**Comment:** The taking of the history is a crucial aspect of all IME reports. The examiner who takes the history directly from the examinee, preserves his notes, and clearly differentiates the history from his impressions, is in the best position to defend the history portion of his IME report. If the history is taken by a nurse, assistant, or third party, it should be accurately recorded, and, if possible, the IME physician should verify it with the examinee.

**Defending the Report As Written:** IME physicians who have case managers, nurses, or others taking histories need to be able to explain and defend the history in the report.

**Q.** Do you know if the staff member took the history verbatim or paraphrased it?
**A.** My case manager records what the examinee tells her and then dictates the history portion in the presence of the examinee. The examinee is instructed to stop the dictation if any mistakes are made. This is done to ensure accuracy.

**Example 7.24: Causal relationship dependent on accuracy of history**
*Report States:*

> The above diagnoses are all causally related to the injury <u>if the history is accurate.</u>

*Resulting Cross-examination:*
**Q.** Doctor, who took the history contained in your IME report?
**A.** I did.
**Q.** You took it accurately, did you not?
**A.** Yes.
**Q.** The history of the auto accident, immediate medical care for a cervical sprain, injury to the right shoulder, physical therapy, and surgery to the shoulder was well documented, was it not?
**A.** It is documented.
**Q.** Did you find any inconsistencies in the history in any of the medical, physical therapy, or hospital records?
**A.** I did not.
**Q.** As you sit here today, Doctor, do you have any reason to question the accuracy of the history?
**A.** No.
**Q.** Were you suspicious of the history when you wrote "The above diagnoses are all causally related to the injury <u>if the history is accurate</u>"?
**A.** No.
**Q.** Despite the fact that the history was taken by you, was well documented in all the records, that you were not suspicious of the history, and you had no reason to question it, you wrote an opinion conditional on the history being accurate?

**Comment:** Examiners who question the accuracy of the history given to them by examinees should put their objective reasons for their suspicions in their reports. This should be done with nonjudgmental, objective language.

> The examinee gave a history of sustaining an injury to his right shoulder in an auto accident of 9/10/2002. He did not seek medical treatment for this injury for 11 days. He denies prior injury. This is inconsistent with the medical records in the case. An 11/17/2002 physical therapy note and x-ray of 7/9/1993 indicate that he fractured this shoulder in July 1993.

**Defending the Report As Written:** When questioned about the accuracy of the history, the examiner should point out that he relied on the information provided by the examinee and then compared it to the records.

**Q.** Doctor, who took the history contained in your IME report?
**A.** I did.
**Q.** You took it accurately, did you not?
**A.** I recorded what the examinee told me, but found marked inconsistencies between what he said and what the records showed. Would you like me to go through all the discrepancies, Counsel?

**Example 7.25: Lack of interpreter**
*Report States:*

> There is a language barrier in this case.

*Resulting Cross-examination:*
**Q.** What was the language barrier you mention in your IME report, Doctor?
**A.** The examinee spoke Spanish only.
**Q.** How much Spanish do you speak?
**A.** None.
**Q.** You have been performing IMEs in the Bronx for 10 years but have not learned any Spanish?
**A.** That's right. Let them learn to speak English.
**Q.** You did have a translator, correct?
**A.** Not correct—no translator.
**Q.** If the examinee spoke only Spanish, you speak only English, and there was no translator, how did you obtain the history in your report which starts with "The claimant informs me…"?
**A.** Sign language.
**Q.** You used sign language to determine that he was "an unrestrained passenger involved in a motor vehicle accident on 6/6/2001"?
**A.** Yes.
**Q.** You used sign language to determine he is being treated by physical therapy two times a week and under chiropractic care once a week?
**A.** Yes.
**Q.** You used sign language to determine he "can comfortably lift 30 pounds"?
**A.** Yes.
**Q.** How did you do that, Doctor?
**A.** It wasn't easy.
**Q.** I understand you find this amusing. What is not so funny is that you affirmed under the penalties of perjury that the statements contained in your IME report are true and, even worse, are accurate. Is that what you did, Doctor?

**Comment:** Examiners who are faced with a serious language problem at an IME are best served by insisting that an interpreter be present before they proceed.

**Defending the Report As Written:** The authors are reluctant to even attempt to defend the report as written.

**Q.** What was the language barrier you mention in your IME report?
**A.** The examinee spoke only Spanish and did not come with an interpreter. To avoid having him make another long trip back, I took the history from the medical records that I was provided and did the best I could with the examination and report.

## 7.3 Pre-existing Status/Past Medical History

The cause of the injury in question is often an area that the examiner is asked to address in the report. It is, therefore, imperative that the examiner document what, if any, problems were pre-existing. The examiner should ask the examinee if she had any previous problems or dysfunction at the time of the injury and document the response. If the history provided by the examinee is inconsistent with the medical documentation, this should be objectively documented in the report. The examinee's pre-existing status should be documented with objective language that does not imply subtle or overt bias on the part of the examiner. As always, extraneous comments, such as those concerning the outcome of prior lawsuits, should be avoided.

A detailed IME report will also include the past medical history of the examinee. This is helpful to determine the overall well-being of the individual and is potentially relevant to the issue of causation of the injury in question. In appropriate cases, some examiners choose to simply list the past medical history as "none" or "noncontributory." Please consider the following examples.

**Example 7.31: Past medical history**

*Report States:*

> The examinee notes traumatic fever during childhood with consequent mitral valve prolapse. She notes no prior work-related injury and no prior involvement in motor vehicle accidents. She denies any prior chiropractic care and specifically denies any prior body aching, visual or hearing disturbances, or difficulty with memory.
>
> The examinee notes multiple allergies/sensitivities including Elavil, Penicillins, anti-inflammatories, lotions, detergents, molds, Prednisone, aspirins, Cortisones, perfumes, dust, heat, plants, and sun. She has had no prior surgery.

*Resulting Cross-examination:*

**Q.** You would agree that this examinee's past medical history is noncontributory to her current back condition?
**A.** Yes, I would.

**Comment:** The judge or fact finder and the attorneys will look to the past medical history to see if a pre-existing condition, susceptibility, or past injury will affect causation, disability, impairment, recovery, and/or return to work. If the past medical history is contributory, the examiner may have to deal with the issues of aggravation, exacerbation, and/or impairment.

**Defending the Report As Written:** Even when the past medical history appears to be noncontributory, it may play an important part in the IME process.

**Q.** You would agree that this examinee's past medical history is noncontributory to her current back condition?
**A.** While it did not cause the back condition, her multiple allergies, especially to anti-inflammatories, have made it more difficult to treat the back pain.

**Example 7.32: "He denies....There was no settlement"**
*Report States:*

> Mr. Sample denies any prior similar injury or problems. He had a previous work-related injury to his left shoulder while employed by Smith Trucker. He was out of work for two months and was treated with a sling. He had complete resolution. There was no settlement. He denies any symptoms or dysfunction immediately prior to this injury.

*Resulting Cross-examination:*
**Q.** Your IME report indicates that the examinee had a prior workers' compensation injury and that "there was no settlement"?
**A.** That's correct.
**Q.** The issue of settlement or no settlement of the workers' compensation injury is not really germane to the examinee's pre-existing status, is it?
**A.** Well, not directly.
**Q.** Can you explain how it is even remotely germane, Doctor?

**Comment:** This report would have been more persuasive if it were written in a nonjudgmental way that does not give the impression of bias.

> Mr. Sample states that he has not had any prior similar injury or problems. He states that he had a previous injury to his left shoulder while employed by Smith Trucker. He was out of work for two months and was treated with a sling. He had complete resolution. He stated that he did not have any symptoms or dysfunction immediately prior to this injury.

**Defending the Report As Written:** Examiners may comment on issues they feel can be part of the "big picture." When doing so, they need to be able to explain or defend their explanation.

**Q.** The issue of settlement or no settlement of the prior workers' compensation injury is not really germane to the examinee's pre-existing status, is it?
**A.** I find that it is. The examinees who do not settle their cases are likely to return to work for the same employer as soon as they are able. The examinees who wait for settlements certainly don't return to work for the same employer and are usually out for longer periods of time.

**Example 7.33: Objective pre-existing status description**
*Report States:*

> HISTORY OF PAST HEALTH
>
> Ms. Borgatti has been diagnosed with diabetes mellitus since age 26. Adverse effects of diabetes have mainly affected her eyes.
>
> In the early 1990s, Ms. Borgatti underwent bowel and bladder surgery.

> Ms. Borgatti stated that she has not had any other serious medical illnesses, operations, accidents or injuries.
>
> Current medications include Glucovance 2.5/500 mg one bid, Glucophage XR 500 mg one qhs, Actos 30 mg one qam, Protonix 40 mg one qam, and captopril 25 mg two qam and one qhs.
>
> She has no known allergies.

**Comment:** This report is well written. It is nonjudgmental and does not give the impression of bias.

## 7.4 Injury/Incident

The report should document the injury or incident as reported by the examinee. This documentation should include the referenced mechanism of injury and reported problems at that time and be as specific as possible. The examiner should review any and all other information available (such as first report of injury, the accident report, and reports to other health care providers). Any inconsistencies between the examinee's recollection of the injury and that contained in other documents should be documented objectively in the report without any superfluous or judgmental comments by the examiner. Please consider the following examples.

**Example 7.41: "This so-called work-related injury"**

*Report States:*

> His description of this so-called work-related injury is that, while emptying the office's three-pound wastepaper basket, "I twisted and got pain in my back. Later that day it went down my right leg." Frankly, this examiner finds the reported mechanism of injury very thin.

*Resulting Cross-examination:*

**Q.** You are an impartial examiner, correct?
**A.** Yes, absolutely.
**Q.** Were you present at the examinee's office on 2/17/2002?
**A.** No, I was not.
**Q.** Can you sit here under oath and say the examinee is lying when he says he injured his back at work on 2/17/02 emptying the office's wastepaper basket?
**A.** No, I cannot.
**Q.** But, as an impartial examiner, you refer to the 2/17/2002 injury as "this so-called work-related injury"?

**Comment:** This report would have been more persuasive if it were written in a nonjudgmental way that does not give the impression of bias. Examiners who review the mechanism of injury with the examinee may have reason to be skeptical about the injury. The most effective way to make this point is by objective facts, not snide comments. Snide passing comments make the examiner look like an advocate. The objective facts are much more powerful.

> In terms of how the injury in question occurred, the examinee stated to me that, while emptying the office's three-pound wastepaper basket, "I twisted and got pain in my back. Later that day it went down my right leg." He lifted the box from floor level and twisted to the left. The pain was in his right low back. In my opinion, to a reasonable degree of medical certainty, the lifting of a three-pound basket is not medically consistent with the injury he describes.

**Defending the Report As Written:** Examiners expressing an opinion on the mechanism of injury should be prepared to defend their opinion.

**Q.** But, as an impartial examiner, you refer to the 2/17/2002 injury as "this so-called work-related injury"?
**A.** Yes. He told me the little basket weighed three pounds. The lifting of a three-pound basket is not consistent with the injury he describes.

**Example 7.42: Detailed and objective history of injury**
*Report States:*

> She reports that on September 26, 2003, at 1:30 P.M., she bent down to crank up a bed, which she describes as "scooching." She states that her right knee "felt weird," and that the patella seemed to move to the outside of her knee. This was associated with mild pain. She was able to stand up, and the kneecap returned to its normal position. While kneeling she heard a "pop." Initially the pain seemed to be relatively mild. She was scheduled to work until 2 P.M. and left work at her scheduled time. Over the next couple of hours the knee became more painful and swollen, "about three times normal size," after several hours. She had the following day off and took it easy, but had ongoing knee pain.
>
> Two days after the injury, because of ongoing symptoms, she went to the emergency room. The first report of injury indicates that she bent down to crank up a bed, felt a pop followed by pain, and the knee popped again the next day at home. She states that this is inaccurate and the knee simply stayed painful and swollen.
>
> The examinee states that there didn't seem to be anything unusual about the way she was kneeling at the time of the event. She doesn't feel her knee twisted in any manner and she believes she was using good posture.

**Comment:** This is a well-written section. It is detailed and objective and does not contain any statements that may suggest bias on the part of the examiner.

**Example 7.43: Vague history of injury**
*Report States:*

> He was struck from the back while driving his car on 9/19/2003.

*Resulting Cross-examination:*
**Q.** The history of the accident contained in your IME report is that, "He was struck from the back while driving his car on 9/19/2003." Is that correct?
**A.** Yes.
**Q.** Would you agree that in formulating your opinion on the causal relationship between the 9/19/2003 motor vehicle accident and the examinee's shoulder injury, the amount of force would be significant?
**A.** It could be.
**Q.** What kind of car was the examinee driving at the time of the accident?
**A.** I was not given that information.
**Q.** Did you ask for it?
**A.** No.
**Q.** Why not?
**A.** It doesn't seem that significant.
**Q.** Was his vehicle struck by an 18-wheeler, dump truck, or a Yugo?
**A.** I don't know.
**Q.** You again didn't ask because it didn't seem "significant"?
**A.** That's correct.
**Q.** How fast was the 18-wheeler, dump truck, or Yugo going when it struck the examinee's vehicle?
**A.** I don't know.
**Q.** Didn't ask, didn't tell?
**A.** That's correct.
**Q.** Your opinion is that a collision between the examinee's vehicle, make and weight unknown, and the defendant's vehicle, size and weight unknown, traveling at an unknown speed, did not cause the examinee's shoulder injury?

**Comment:** The physician in the above IME report lacked critical information when he formulated and attempted to defend his opinion and report. He would have been better served with a more precise history and report.

> The examinee was driving a 2002 Ford Explorer on 9/19/2003 when he was stopped and his vehicle was struck from behind by a 1998 Toyota Corolla traveling at 5 m.p.h.

**Defending the Report As Written:** IME physicians need not act like sheep being led to the slaughter when replying to questions concerning their IME reports.

**Q.** Would you agree that in formulating your opinion on the causal relationship between the 9/19/2003 motor vehicle accident and the examinee's shoulder injury, the amount of force would be significant?
**A.** No, not in this case. The examinee is suffering from pre-existing degenerative disease of the AC joint and impingement. If this was traumatic in nature, one would look for AC separation. This was not present. Would you like me to explain further, Counsel?

## 7.5 Treatment History

It is usually helpful to present the chronology of the examinee's treatment from the date of injury to the present. This is usually best done by summarizing the examinee's treatment to date in chronological order.

Some examiners prefer to separate information from the initial clinical encounter into its own section. This is done because the initial clinical encounter is often of particular significance.

The specificity and length of the treatment history provided depends in part on the issues for evaluation and the complexity of the case. For example, if the issue in an evaluation is primarily permanent impairment assessment, the review of the treatment history may be relatively brief. If, however, the issues are causation and the significance of various injuries over time, the history may need to be quite lengthy and should document the various encounters with health care providers.

Some examiners present the treatment history by summarizing the medical records provided. Although this can provide detailed and helpful information, it is best to do this in combination with the taking of a treatment history from the examinee. This will help ensure that the examiner has complete information. For example, without eliciting a treatment history from the examinee, the examiner may easily miss treatment from providers whose records where not made available to the examiner.

As always, the examiner should avoid superfluous comments and taking cheap shots at the examinee. The treatment history should be documented with objective language. Please consider the following examples.

**Example 7.51: "I was not convinced by this performance"**

*Report States:*

> Mr. Sample described at length the numerous clinicians he has sought treatment from since this injury. He stated emphatically that none of this extensive treatment has had "any effect whatsoever" on his alleged pain and that there's no way "anyone should have to go back to work" being in as much pain as him. I do have to say that I was not convinced by this performance.

*Resulting Cross-examination:*

**Q.** You characterized the examinee's description of his pain and how the treatment has not helped him as a "performance," Doctor?

**A.** Well, yes. I didn't believe him.

**Q.** Who is the only person who knows how much pain the examinee is really in?

**A.** The examinee.

**Q.** Were you aware that the examinee worked for 17 straight years for this employer without missing one sick day before his accident?

**A.** No, I was not aware of that.
**Q.** Do you think the 17 years were also a performance?

**Comment:** This report would have been more persuasive if it were written in a nonjudgmental way that does not give the impression of bias.

> Mr. Sample stated that he has sought treatment from numerous providers since his injury. He stated that none of this treatment has helped him.

**Defending the Report As Written:** Examiners who make caustic comments in their reports should be prepared to defend them.

**Q.** You characterized the examinee's description of his pain and how the treatment has not helped him as a "performance," Doctor?
**A.** His description was just one small part of the performance. He limped dramatically, grimaced, and had the presence of 5 of 5 Waddell's non-organic signs, which is consistent with symptom exaggeration and inappropriate illness behavior. Would you like me to explain further, Counsel?

**Example 7.52: Brief, imprecise history**
*Report States:*

> Mr. Sample sought chiropractic care with Debbie Manca, DC, within a week of the injury and was manipulated for approximately six weeks without improvement. Dr. Manca obtained an orthopedic consultation with Dr. Smart two months postinjury. He ordered an MRI which revealed a herniated disc at L4-5 with compression to the right. On December 10, 2001 the examinee was seen by neurosurgeon Fred Calipari, MD, who felt it was appropriate to proceed with surgery. On December 24, 2001 he underwent a lumbar diskectomy at L4-5, with findings of a herniated nucleus pulposus compressing the right L5 nerve root. The surgery was uncomplicated.
>
> Since surgery, his primary treatment has been passive physical therapy and analgesics. He did perform exercises for two weeks in August 2002, but these were discontinued because of pain. As discussed under Occupational History, he has been out of work since his injury.

*Resulting Cross-examination:*
**Q.** When did the examinee start chiropractic care with Dr. Manca?
**A.** About a week after the injury.
**Q.** Do you know the date of the first treatment?
**A.** No, I don't.
**Q.** What was the date of his last manipulation?
**A.** I don't have that date. He was treated for about six weeks.
**Q.** Are you missing these dates because you didn't bother to look them up in

the records or because you didn't feel it important to be that precise in your IME report?

**Comment:** This report would have been more persuasive if it were written more precisely.

> Mr. Sample first sought chiropractic care with Debbie Manca, DC, four days after injury on March 6, 2000. He was manipulated for approximately six weeks without improvement. The last manipulation occurred on April 15, 2000. Dr. Manca obtained an orthopedic consultation with Dr. Smart two months post-injury. Dr. Smart ordered an MRI which revealed a herniated disc at L4-5 with compression to the right. On December 10, 2001 the examinee was seen by neurosurgeon Fred Calipari, MD, who felt it was appropriate to proceed with surgery. On December 24, 2001 he underwent a lumbar diskectomy at L4-5, with findings of a herniated nucleus pulposus compressing the right L5 nerve root. The surgery was uncomplicated.
>
> Since surgery, his primary treatment has been passive physical therapy and analgesics. He did perform exercises for two weeks in August 2002, but these were discontinued because of pain. As discussed under Occupational History, he has been out of work since his injury.

**Defending the Report As Written:** When "missing" some dates, examiners can let themselves be beaten up on cross-examination or they can choose to fight back.

**Q.** What was the date of his last manipulation?
**A.** It was on April 15, 2000. The original record was illegible so I called Dr. Manca for the date.

**Example 7.53: History summarizes the medical records provided**
*Report States:*

> I reviewed the medical records you sent to me regarding C.B. Among these records is an initial WC-2 report dated 7/22/94 concerning treatment rendered to Mr. B. by Dr. W. beginning on 7/2/94 for an injury occurring on 7/1/94. The report indicates "pain in left lower back radiating down left leg while lifting one end of engine." Mr. B. was noted to have pain at the L2-3 level with radiation of pain in the L3 nerve distribution. He had difficulty standing and bending at the waist. A CT scan of the low back was recommended. Vicodin was prescribed. The assessment was herniated nucleus pulposus with radiculopathy. Mr. B. was placed on temporary total disability beginning on 7/22/94.
>
> On 9/8/94 an initial physical therapy evaluation report was submitted by S.T. of the Rehab Center regarding evaluation and treatment of Mr. B. at the request of Dr. X. Symptoms at that time included an intermittent mild

> central low back pain with constant numbness, paresthesias, and sensitivity referred down the posterior left lower extremity to the toes and intermittently to the right buttock. The treatment program was initiated.
>
> * * *
>
> On 10/27/94 a report was submitted by Dr. Y., a neurosurgeon, regarding independent medical evaluation on Mr. B. Dr. Y. summarized Mr. B.'s history concerning the 7/1/94 injury and his subsequent clinical course. Mr. B. continued to have some functional limitations associated with complaints of back pain. Dr. Y. documented his examination of Mr. B. and reviewed imaging studies and medical records. Dr. Y.'s impression was that Mr. B. had a midline herniated left L5-6 extruded disc. The prognosis was said to be fairly good except for slight numbness in the left leg, now in a stocking distribution distally. Dr. Y. felt this would still improve in the future but that the subsequent numbness should be tolerable. Mr. B.'s clinical course was felt to be consistent with that expected following surgical treatment for a large herniated disc.

*Resulting Cross-examination:*

**Q.** You reviewed the medical records you were sent?

**A.** Yes.

**Q.** Did you receive all of C.B.'s medical records?

**A.** I don't know.

**Q.** Did you analyze the records you did receive, or did a member of your staff assist you?

**A.** I did the analysis myself.

**Q.** When you "analyzed" these records, did you give your opinion about the meaning of the records or did you merely summarize what the doctors said?

**A.** For the most part, I summarized the pertinent parts of the medical records.

**Q.** Of course, you are not in a position to vouch for the accuracy of what is in the records?

**A.** That's correct.

**Q.** You did attempt to characterize the records you reviewed, correct?

**A.** No, I don't agree with that.

**Q.** In the 09/08/1994 initial physical therapy evaluation report your summary says, "intermittent <u>mild</u> central low back pain," does it not?

**A.** Yes.

**Q.** Here is the actual 09/08/1994 physical therapy evaluation. Where does the word "mild" appear?

**A.** Well, it's not stated in that way.

**Q.** You summarize the prognosis in Dr. Y.'s IME report as "fairly good except for slight numbness in the left leg." Is that what you said?

**A.** Yes.

**Q.** Where in the actual IME report does the word "slight" appear?

**A.** Well, it doesn't.

**Q.** You repeatedly added or deleted key words in the reports you summarized in an attempt to minimize the extent of injury, pain, and disability, did you not, Doctor?

**Comment:** The summary of the medical records provided should be accurate and precise and not used to "make the case" for a desired outcome. Failure to do so will call into question the integrity of the process and the credibility of the examiner. It is also a good idea to take the medical history from the examinee as well as from the records. This will help ensure that information is not missed.

**Defending the Report As Written:** IME physicians should be prepared to defend their summaries of medical records. The examiner needs to be cognizant of the "tricks" counsel may play to confuse or rattle the examiner during cross-examination.

**Q.** Here is the actual 09/08/1994 physical therapy evaluation. Where does the word "mild" appear?
**A.** Counsel, the sentence before in the physical therapy evaluation says that "the examinee states his pain is a 2 on a scale of 1-10." I think it is very fair to characterize that as mild, don't you?

**Example 7.54: Treatment history taken from examinee and objectively documented**
*Report States:*

> **HX:** Mr. Charles is a 53-year-old right-handed Caucasian male who confirmed his identity with the picture on his driver's license. He states that on 12/1/00 he noted symptoms of pain and numbness in his left arm extending up into his left shoulder and neck that occurred after a fall. He was working on a step-up platform that was 12 inches above the floor. He stepped back and fell onto the floor using his left hand to catch himself. He does not remember if there was any swelling or bruising of the left upper extremity. Over the next two weeks, the pain moved down his arm into his fingers. He is uncertain which fingers were affected. He states that he believes that his pain became worse because he does repetitive work. He shared his concerns with his supervisor the next day who suggested that he see the company physician. The company physician examined Mr. Charles and obtained X-rays. His treatment included Motrin and heat. Mr. Charles states that he had no improvement over the next 4 weeks and was referred to Dr. Jones for an NCT/EMG, which was completed on 03/30/01. The NCT/EMG was reported electrophysiologic evidence for cervical polyradiculoneuropathy (roots C6 through T1), sensory and motor, predominantly axonal with some demyelinating features, chronic with evidence of active denervation. Over the next 4 weeks, little improvement was experienced. He says he was frustrated by Workers' Comp and elected to get an attorney. He says his attorney referred him to Dr. Smith for a disability rating and work restrictions so he could be off work.
>
> The employer wanted a second opinion and he was sent to Dr. Adams. Dr. Adams told him that he had a pinched nerve in his elbow but suggested a cervical MRI. The cervical MRI was completed on 05/03/01 with a report of degenerative change greatest at C5-6 with central and lateral stenosis,

marrow changes along the end-plates of C5-6 are probably related to degenerative change, and left posterolateral disc bulge at C6-7. On return to Dr. Jones, he was started on a 6-week physical therapy program for his neck.

At the suggestion of his attorney, he saw Dr. Smith again. Dr. Smith's diagnosis was neck pain secondary to polyradiculopathy and left carpal tunnel syndrome. Mr. Charles was provided an impairment rating of 25% based on cervical DRE category IV page 104 and was given light-work-only guides.

He was then referred to a neurosurgeon for possible surgery. Treatment included 3 epidural injections for the cervical spine without improvement. Surgery with diskectomy and fusion was discussed.

The company physician suggested medium-level work and limit hand over shoulder activities on the left. He has continued in this work pattern with persistent but not progressive symptoms. His current work activities are outlined below.

**Comment:** This is a fairly detailed treatment history. It is objectively written. It was obtained from the examinee and is combined with the injury history. When combined with a well-documented summary of the available medical records, it will show the thoroughness of the examiner's investigation and bolster the credibility of the IME report.

## 7.6 Occupational History

Depending upon the issues at hand, some examiners include an occupational, employment, or work history. An occupational history should be provided if the disorder is work-related or if disability is an issue in the case.

The occupational history can begin with a detailed description of the job at the time of injury and include the physical demands of the job. For toxicology cases, a detailed review of exposures at the current and previous jobs is required to help determine causation.

The events relative to disability, from the injury to the present, are explored. If the examinee is not working, the reasons for this, the involvement of vocational rehabilitation, possibilities for work in the future, and the patient's plans for the future are identified. If the examinee is working, the details of this position are explored. Any work restrictions that have been imposed are identified along with the rationale for them. If a functional capacity assessment has been performed, the results from the assessment should be documented.

The examinee's previous work experiences, educational background, and future work plans can be documented as well. Work histories should be precise and accurate or else the examiner can expect close questioning in this area. If opinions are expressed regarding the ability of the examinee to work at a particular job, the examiner should expect close questioning on exactly what the examinee's job requires.

**Example 7.61: Occupational history of truck driver**
*Report States:*

> The examinee was employed by Jones Trucking beginning August 1, 1999. At the time of the injury he was working full time as a truck driver. According to the description provided by the examinee, this involved long-haul driving of a tractor trailer and helping with loading and unloading. The physical demands included sitting for three hours at a time, standing for two hours at a time, walking for one hour at a time, and frequent lifting. The heaviest object he usually had to lift was a box weighing 200 lbs. The examinee reports enjoying the job but having only a fair relationship with his direct supervisor, who was not friendly to him. He also rates his employers as only fair, stating that they were not sympathetic.
>
> He previously worked at Smith Trucking from 1992 to 1999, leaving for more money. He belongs to a labor union and is a high school graduate. He has a driver's license. He is currently receiving workers' compensation and disability loan payments. He has no specific long-term occupational plans.
>
> The examinee has been out of work for almost two years, and is currently not working. He is not currently receiving vocational rehabilitation counseling, but previously worked with Jane Simpcoe in evaluation and job search. Records of this are not available. There is no projected return to work date, and the examinee does not expect to return to work in the near future. He hopes to be retrained. He does not know what work is available.
>
> He reports that Dr. Cutter imposed work restrictions of four hours per day, five days per week, with no frequent bending and no lifting over 10 lbs. A functional capacity evaluation has not been performed. A functional job description is not available; however, I am familiar with its demands from having viewed similar jobs.

*Resulting Cross-examination:*
**Q.** You obtained all the information you have regarding the examinee's job duties directly from the examinee, correct?
**A.** Yes.
**Q.** Did you compare the duties he told you about to his actual written job description?
**A.** No.
**Q.** Why is that?
**A.** I didn't have a written job description.
**Q.** Did you ask for one?
**A.** No, I did not.

**Q.** In your experience, do examinees sometimes exaggerate about how difficult their job is and how much they had to lift, for example?
**A.** Yes, sometimes they do.
**Q.** Are you familiar with the physical demands listed in the *Dictionary of Occupational Titles* for truck drivers at 904.383-010?
**A.** No, I am not, Counsel.
**Q.** Do you know what the labor contract says about how many pounds a truck driver has to lift unassisted?
**A.** No, I don't.
**Q.** The contract provides a maximum of 120 lbs. lifting unassisted, does it not?

**Comment:** The issue of job duties is a difficult one for the IME examiner. There are often differing descriptions of what the job actually entails. For example, there may be:

- a written job description,
- an oral description from the employer,
- an oral description from the examinee,
- labor agreements, and
- a description from the *Dictionary of Occupational Titles.*

The examiner should obtain as much information as possible on this issue and identify the source of the information in his report.

**Defending the Report As Written:** When faced with questions concerning "job requirements," the examiner should not forget the big picture when defending his opinion and report.

**Q.** Are you familiar with the physical demands listed in the *Dictionary of Occupational Titles* for truck drivers at 904.383-101?
**A.** Counsel, whether it's 100 pounds, 150 pounds, or 200 pounds makes little difference in this case because his treating doctor has restricted his lifting to 10 pounds.

**Example 7.62: Occupational history of mechanic**
*Report States:*

> At the time of the injury the examinee had been employed by Gordon Outboard, Inc. since 1997. He was working full time as a mechanic. According to the description provided by the examinee, this involved picking up outboard motors, snow machines, trailers, and operating a forklift. The physical demands included standing for up to 8 hours at a time, walking for up to 6 hours, repetitive use of the hands, climbing stairs and ladders, overhead work, frequent lifting and neck movement, and awkward positioning. The heaviest object he usually had to lift was a 150-lb. motor.
>
> He previously worked at AuCoin's Sales & Services, at Unitrode Corp., as a supervisor, and at other places. He is a high school graduate and has a current driver's license.

> The examinee was most recently employed by Naples Marina as a mechanic, but was laid off for a seasonal shutdown. In April 2002 Dr. Fiore imposed work restrictions of no lifting over 25 lbs. A functional capacity evaluation has not been performed. Functional descriptions of his job at the time of injury and his current job are not available; however, I am familiar with the physical demands from having viewed similar jobs.

*Resulting Cross-examination:*
**Q.** You stated in your IME report that you are "familiar with the physical demands from having viewed similar jobs," correct?
**A.** Yes, that is what I said.
**Q.** What is the examinee's job title?
**A.** Marine mechanic?
**Q.** Is that an answer or a question?
**A.** My answer.
**Q.** What kind of boats does the examinee work on?
**A.** All kinds, I assume.
**Q.** Do you know the tonnage of the boats he works on?
**A.** No, I don't.
**Q.** Did you view the examinee or his replacement doing his job?
**A.** No, I did not.
**Q.** You viewed a similar job?
**A.** Yes.
**Q.** How could you tell it was similar if you never viewed the original job being done, Doctor?

**Comment:** IME physicians who claim to be familiar with the physical demands of the examinee's job should have a substantive basis for the claim. In some significant cases the client will pay the examiner personally to go to the jobsite to view the job being done. In many instances, however, the economics of the cases do not permit this. IME physicians who are familiar with the job being performed are in the best position to defend their reports.

**Defending the Report As Written:** When opposing counsel makes the mistake of asking a "why" question, examiners should seize the opportunity this creates.

**Q.** How could you tell it was similar if you never viewed the original job being done, Doctor?
**A.** Counsel, I own a 36-foot boat that has spent the better part of the last two summers at the marine mechanic being repaired. During these two summers I have spent countless hours watching marine mechanics working on my boat as well as many others. I am, unfortunately, intimately knowledgeable about the duties of a marine mechanic.

**Example 7.63: Vague work history**
*Report States:*

As previously stated, she has been off work now for about one year.

*Resulting Cross-examination:*
**Q.** Doctor, on page 4 of your IME report, paragraph 2, you stated "as previously stated, she has been off work now for about one year." Is that correct?
**A.** Yes, that is what I stated.
**Q.** Could you point to where in your April 1999 IME report you previously stated that?
**A.** Well, I didn't say it in so many words, but I did report she moved to Arizona in January 1998 and tried to work for two weeks but couldn't do it.
**Q.** What you actually said on page 3 was, "she moved to Arizona in January 1998." You then stated, "she had a job in advertising but couldn't do the work." Is that correct?
**A.** Yes.
**Q.** Can you tell us, Doctor, when she worked in Arizona?
**A.** Well, not specifically. It would presumably be after January 1998 when she moved there.
**Q.** Can you tell us where she worked?
**A.** No.
**Q.** Can you tell us what she did? Was she an administrative assistant or an account executive?
**A.** I don't know.
**Q.** Can you tell us when she started there?
**A.** No.
**Q.** Can you tell us when she last worked there?
**A.** No, I can't.
**Q.** Would it be fair to say, Doctor, that your statement on page 4 of your IME report under the heading Work History, "as previously stated, she has been out of work now for about one year," is sloppy, misleading, and inaccurate?

**Comment:** The work history contained in an IME report is usually significant when a physician is evaluating disability, impairment, or work capacity. The above description of the examinee's work history lacked the precision found in excellent IME reports. The physician would have been better served with the following.

> The examinee last worked in Phoenix, Arizona, at the ACT Advertising Agency from January 4, 1998, to January 21, 1998. She left due to her inability to take the stress of working as an account executive in a high-pressure environment.

**Defending the Report As Written:** IME physicians need to be able to "recover" from their omissions to properly defend their reports.

**Q.** Can you tell us, Doctor, when she worked in Arizona?
**A.** Yes. She started to work in Arizona in January 1998 and lasted

approximately six months according to her history. She did not give me the exact dates. She said she didn't remember them.

## 7.7 Psychosocial History

Depending on the issues in the report and the level of detail desired, the examiner may document the examinee's psychosocial history. Psychosocial information includes an understanding of the home and family structures of the examinee and how the examinee spends his day. Activities of daily living and recreational activities before and after the injury should also be documented. It may also be worthwhile (and useful to the report's end-user) to document health habits, such as the use of tobacco, alcohol, other drugs, and the level of physical exercise. Specific, precise, and objective information is most helpful.

**Example 7.71: Psychosocial history**

*Report States:*

The examinee has been married for four years and lives in a two-story house in Old Town with his wife and 17-year-old child. His wife works outside the home. During the day he rests, watches TV, reads, does light chores, and visits friends or family. He denies being able to do heavy chores, clean house, or work. He describes his average day as: "Get up at 7, have breakfast, walk my dog, visit friends, get coffee, get lunch, watch soaps, eat dinner, watch TV, go to bed at 11." Prior to the injury his recreation consisted of fishing, hunting, and bowling, but he reports only fishing a little now. He is not involved in any community or religious activities. He states that "I can't do anything—my wife and daughter have to do all the chores."

He has smoked one pack of cigarettes a day for 20 years, and has three or four alcoholic drinks a week. He reports that on rare occasions he uses alcohol to help with the pain, and that there is a family history of alcoholism. He consumes six caffeinated beverages per day, but denies the use of recreational drugs.

*Resulting Cross-examination:*

**Q.** Your IME report indicates that the examinee denied "being able to do heavy chores, clean house, or work," correct?
**A.** Yes, that's correct.
**Q.** What exactly are heavy chores?
**A.** Chores requiring physical exertion and/or lifting.
**Q.** Is that your definition or one that the examinee used?
**A.** That's mine.
**Q.** Do you know what the examinee meant when he used that phrase?
**A.** Not exactly.
**Q.** So, you don't exactly know what he denied being able to do, correct?

**Comment:** Examiners who take a psychosocial history should be careful to define and be able to explain the terms they use in the history. Vague, undefined terms, such as "heavy chores," are more difficult to defend.

**Defending the Report As Written:** While it is best to define terms in an IME report, the failure to do so need not damage the examiner's credibility.

**Q.** What exactly are heavy chores?
**A.** The examinee told me he is unable to put out the trash barrels, vacuum, and carry grocery bags. These are the heavy chores I am referring to.

**Example 7.72: Examinee's spouse collecting workers' compensation**
*Report States:*

> The examinee smokes one pack of cigarettes per day and has done so for 21 years. She denies alcohol intake. She does have daily caffeine intake.
>
> The examinee has been married for five years. This is her fourth marriage. She indicates that she has one adopted daughter and two stepsons who are on their own. The examinee notes that her husband continues to do poorly following his problems related to his work-related motor vehicle accident and continues to collect workers' compensation benefits. The patient also notes that her mother-in-law died the night of their motor vehicle accident and there was another death in the family two weeks prior to their accident.
>
> The examinee completed high school and has a college degree. She enjoys fishing, truck driving, car driving, hiking, cooking, reading, sewing, and painting. Primarily due to her visual problems, "blackouts," and dizziness, she is no longer able to enjoy these activities.

*Resulting Cross-examination:*
**Q.** You mentioned in your IME report that the examinee's husband is on workers' compensation benefits?
**A.** Yes, I did.
**Q.** You felt that fact was significant?
**A.** Well, yes. It's indicative of the family dynamics.
**Q.** The examinee may be staying home to help her husband?
**A.** It's possible.
**Q.** Can you point to any facts supporting that allegation?
**A.** I cannot.
**Q.** You made the comment about the spouse being on workers' compensation to influence the judge and cast aspersions on the family unit, didn't you?

**Comment:** Examiners may feel that the dynamics of the family situation may play an important role in disability, impairment, motivation, and return to work. Examiners should be careful not to appear to be making snide passing comments about the examinee's family in an attempt to discredit the examinee and his claim. If counsel can paint the examiner with this brush, the examiner will be successfully portrayed as an advocate and not a truly impartial examiner.

**Defending the Report As Written:** Examiners should be prepared to defend the significance of the psychosocial history they take. Examiners who are well prepared can be extremely effective.

**Q.** The examinee may be staying home to help her husband?
**A.** It's not that simple, Counsel, but it goes to motivation and social network support for illness. The AMA *Guides,* fifth edition, deals with this issue and I quote,

> "Motivation is a difficult issue for assessment since it is multifactorial in nature, involving the following potential factors: (1) lack of motivation as a sign of illness such as depression or schizophrenia; (2) fear of losing entitlement or other benefits of being ill; (3) a side effect of some neuroleptic medications; (4) conscious malingering; (5) a consequence of demoralization of persons with any chronic illness; (6) social network support for illness; and others. Thus, the determination of motivation is often non-empirical, and conclusions are all too often drawn on the basis of prejudice. Many times, an individual's motivation is not well understood even after careful assessment.
>
> Nevertheless, motivation is a link between impairment and disability. For some people, poor motivation is a major cause of poor functioning. An individual's underlying character may be important in determining whether he or she is motivated to benefit from rehabilitation. Personality characteristics usually remain unchanged throughout life. However, internal events and psychological reactions can influence the course of illness. An individual who tends to be dependent, for example, may become even more dependent as his or her illness proceeds." (Section 14.2B, page 360.)

So, yes, I think that a spouse being on workers' compensation benefits is of significance.

**Example 7.73: Social history: drinking every other week**

*Report States:*

The examinee reports perhaps drinking every other week.

*Resulting Cross-examination:*

**Q.** Doctor, you felt it was important to take a social history and report the history in your IME report?
**A.** Yes.
**Q.** This is because the use of alcohol and tobacco can impact the examinee's health and recovery?
**A.** Yes, the examinee reports perhaps drinking every other week.
**Q.** Do you know if she drank a beer, a 12-pack, or a quart of vodka?
**A.** I do not know that information.
**Q.** Could it be significant?
**A.** It could be.
**Q.** So the social history you took was incomplete?

**Comment:** When the examiner decides to take a social history, it should be done in a meaningful fashion. Failing to do so may be worse than not taking one at all.

> The examinee has two to three alcoholic drinks every week.

**Defending the Report As Written:** Often, failure to record a detailed social history is not the fault of the examiner.

**Q.** So the social history you took was incomplete?
**A.** No. I recorded what the examinee told me. She refused to be more specific about her alcohol consumption.

## 7.8 Family Medical History

Including a brief but precise family medical history will make the IME report appear to be thorough. In addition, the family history may have a bearing on relevant issues in the report, such as causation. It may also be relevant to the psychosocial history.

**Example 7.81: "Remarkable" family medical history**
*Report States:*

> Remarkable for mother and grandparents with hypertension and also heart disease.

*Resulting Cross-examination:*
**Q.** Family history of heart disease is a known risk factor for heart attack, correct?
**A.** Correct.
**Q.** What about hypertension in the family?
**A.** That is also a risk factor.
**Q.** This examinee had both of these risk factors in addition to obesity before his heart attack at work, correct?

**Comment:** The family history can be crucial in cases where the issue is causation. In these cases, the IME examiner should take care to develop these issues fully and document them with as much specificity as possible.

> Remarkable for mother and grandparents with hypertension and also heart disease. Maternal grandparent died at 52 and paternal grandparent died at 53 of heart attacks. Mother died at age of 47 of heart attack.

**Defending the Report As Written:** Examiners need to be able to defend their opinions and reports with detailed information.

**Q.** Family history of heart disease is a known risk factor for heart attacks, correct?
**A.** Heart disease is just one of many risk factors. These include

smoking, obesity, age, male gender, hypertension, high blood cholesterol, physical inactivity, and diabetes mellitus.

# Chapter 8 Physical Examination

## 8.1 Executive Summary

A detailed, well-documented physical examination is an essential part of the IME report. All of the tests performed and all findings should be clearly documented. Further advice regarding documenting the physical examination follows.

- Although commonly used to support EM (Evaluation and Management) coding, self-serving descriptions of the physical examination as "comprehensive" or "complete" should be avoided. If the tests and measurements performed are documented in the report, the "completeness" of the examination will speak for itself.
- The physical examination section of the report should be broken up into subsections dealing with the various components of the examination (such as "Observation," "Structural Examination," "Range of Motion," "Neurological Examination," etc.). This will make the report easier to read.
- The precise (not rounded off) starting and ending times of the physical examination should be documented.
- The behavioral assessment should be objectively documented.
- IME reports are most believable when the "normal" results received are not universally "textbook perfect" figures.
- Test results and measurements should be formatted in an easy-to-read manner.
- The specific tests performed for nonphysiological findings should be carefully documented. Examiners should expect close questioning during cross-examination regarding any nonphysiological findings.
- Adding digital photos to an IME report is of great benefit to the client and will make the IME report stand out.
- The most commonly used pain inventories are:
    - Medical Outcome Studies (MOS)
    - SF-36 Health Survey
    - Pain Drawing
    - Pain Disability Index
    - McGill Pain Questionnaire
    - West Haven-Yale Multidimensional Pain Inventory, Short Form - 36 Questions (SF-36)
    - Mensana Clinic Pain Validity Test
    - Center for Epidemiologic Studies - Depressed Mood Scale
    - Beck Depression Inventory

- The examiner should only use pain inventories that she sufficiently understands and can defend during cross-examination.
- The *current status* should be elicited in detail and thoroughly documented.
- The location, intensity, frequency, pattern, and nature of the pain, as well as aggravating and relieving factors, need to be documented.
- Functional status should be thoroughly elicited and documented in detail.
- Examiners should not spy on examinees while they arrive at and leave the examination.

## 8.2 Physical Examination

A detailed physical examination is essential. All of the tests performed and findings should be clearly documented. Appropriate normal examination findings should also be recorded and, when possible, a comparison to the opposite extremity should be made. If the tests performed are not documented, counsel may try to imply on cross-examination that the tests were not done. Self-serving descriptions of the physical examination as "comprehensive" or "complete" should be avoided. Such descriptions will needlessly open up the examiner to cross-examination. If the numerous tests and measurements are documented in the report, the "completeness" of the examination will speak for itself.

The physical examination section of the report should be broken up into subsections dealing with the various components of the examination (such as "Observation," "Structural Examination," "Range of Motion," and "Neurological Examination"). This will make the report easier to read.

It is good practice to note the starting and ending times of the physical examination and to make sure that the examination is not rushed or hurried. A common line of questioning used against independent medical examiners is to try to show that the examination was too brief. Times should be noted precisely to the minute and not rounded off. (See Example 11.104.)

### *Behavior assessment*

Some examiners also perform a behavioral assessment as a supplement to the physical examination. This commences when the examinee is greeted. Pain behavior and inconsistencies are documented as part of this behavioral assessment. All findings should be documented in an objective, professional, and nonjudgmental manner. The examiner's behavioral assessment is likely to be an area of close questioning because this assessment is subjective and may be outside of the examiner's true area of expertise.

## PHYSICAL EXAMINATION

*Musculoskeletal conditions*
If the problem is musculoskeletal in nature, posture and structural examinations are made. The general observations include factors such as level of cooperation, appearance, presence or absence of multiple tattoos, use of assistive appliances (noting whether they appear used), affect, vital signs, height, and weight. The examiner should also document observed tolerances (e.g., for sitting) and any pain behaviors, such as guarding, rubbing, sighing, grimacing, or rigidity. Any inconsistencies should be objectively documented.

*Regional examinations*
Regional examinations will help ensure reliability in the evaluation process. The examiner should document all positive, negative, and nonphysiologic findings. For example, in an examinee with low back pain, the examination should include a detailed assessment of gait, observation of the back (lordotic curves, pelvic symmetry, surgical scars), palpatory findings (localized tenderness, spasm, trigger points), and range of motion.

*Neurologic examinations*
A neurologic examination includes, among other evaluations, sensory assessment, motor evaluation (strength and atrophy), and straight-leg raising in both sitting and supine positions. Specific maneuvers also should be performed to determine the presence of suspected problems, such as sacroiliac problems, piriformis syndrome, somatic dysfunction syndrome, and problems that may masquerade as low back pain.

*Range of motion*
Range of motion of the spine should be determined using an inclinometer, measuring true cervical, thoracic, and lumbosacral angles. All measurements obtained, such as range of motion measurements, grip strength measurements, and girth measurements, should be documented. IME reports are most believable when the "normal" results received are not universally "textbook perfect" figures. (Please see Example 11.105.) Test results and measurements should be formatted in an easy-to-read manner. (Please see Example 8.24.)

*Pain*
Complaints of pain during the examination should be noted. The absence of pain complaints should also be documented. Use of a pain drawing and pain scales are helpful.

*Nonphysiologic findings*
The examination should also include tests for nonphysiologic findings or symptom magnification. The specific tests performed should be carefully

documented. Examiners should expect close questioning during cross-examination regarding any nonphysiologic findings.

*Photos*

Some examiners supplement the physical examination section of their report with digital photos of the affected area or tracings of the hand. For example, if the injury in question is to a finger, a digital photograph of this finger is taken and inserted into the report. (Please see Example 5.21 and the hand tracing at end of the book.) Adding digital photos to an IME report is of great benefit to the client and will make the IME report stand out.

**Example 8.21: "The examinee appeared healthy"**

*Report States:*

The examinee appeared healthy and had no callus on the hands. He was overweight, with a protuberant abdomen. He reported his weight as 204 lbs. and his height at 5 ft., 9 in. His resting pulse rate was 72, and it remained at 72 when reporting pain.

Behavioral Examination

The examinee was cooperative and attentive, although somewhat irritable. Affect was normal and he maintained eye contact. He appeared comfortable during the interview, sitting continuously for 45 minutes, but uncomfortable during the exam, displaying guarding, bracing, and grimacing. There was more pain behavior during the exam than at other times. Nonphysiologic findings were present and are detailed in the exam.

Structural Examination

In the standing neutral position, cervical and thoracic curves were well-maintained. There was no loss of lower cervical lordosis or exaggeration of upper thoracic kyphosis, but lumbar hypolordosis was present. There was no scoliosis or protraction of the shoulders. The upper and lower extremities appeared grossly normal. The pelvis appeared symmetric.

Gait was normal, with no antalgia. There was normal gluteal participation in weight-bearing and leg-clearing phases. There was no tendency to asymmetric external rotation at the hips. Heel and toe walking were intact.

Low Back Examination

There were surgical scars. There was generalized tenderness over the low back, but no paraspinal muscle tenderness or spasm. There were no vertebral, sciatic, sacroiliac, or coccygeal tenderness. Active trigger points were identified in the right gluteus medius.

| Lumbar Motion | True Lumbar Angle (degrees) | Sacral Angle (degrees) |
|---|---|---|
| Flexion forward | 6-17 | 0-5 |
| Extension backward | 7-18 | 0-5 |
| Left lateral flexion | 13-25 | 5 |
| Right lateral flexion | 5-29 | 5 |

Range of motion measurements were made with an inclinometer and were not reproducible. The sacral components were inconsistent with straight-leg raising as noted. Specific individual results are shown on Fig. 79, Lumbar Range of Motion, attached. Sacroiliac tests were negative for pain bilaterally.

Lower Extremity Neurologic Examination

Patellar reflexes were +1/4 L, +1/4 R; Achilles were +1/4 L, +1/4 R.

There was normal strength symmetrically of hip flexion, knee flexion and extension, ankle dorsi- and plantar flexion, and great toe plantar flexion. There was mild weakness of great toe extension on the right. There was no muscle atrophy. Mid-thigh circumferences 15 cm above the patella were 51 cm L and 51 cm R. Mid-calf circumferences in extension were 32 cm L and 32 cm R.

Sensation was diminished to light touch and pinprick on the right, in a distribution consistent with the L5 dermatome. Straight-leg raising sitting was negative bilaterally, limited to 80° L and 80° R by hamstring tautness. Straight-leg raising supine, however, was positive for back pain at 40° L and 30° R.

Nonphysiologic Findings

Numerous nonphysiologic findings were present: light pressure on the skull caused complaints of increased back pain, rotation of the trunk as a unit resulted in complaints of increased pain, superficial touch resulted in severe pain, superficial pressure resulted in radicular pain complaints, range of motion measurements were

> inconsistent, range of motion was inconsistent with straight-leg raising, and SLR supine measurements were inconsistent with SLR sitting.

*Resulting Cross-examination:*
**Q.** Doctor, the examinee was cooperative, correct?
**A.** Yes, he was.
**Q.** When you say he "appeared healthy," you don't mean to say you can tell what is wrong with an examinee just by looking at him, do you?
**A.** That's not what I meant.
**Q.** Did you weigh him, Doctor?
**A.** No.
**Q.** So you don't know what he actually weighed?
**A.** Only what he told me.
**Q.** He was cooperative but exhibited pain behavior?
**A.** Yes, he did.
**Q.** Could the pain behavior he exhibited be due to his pain?
**A.** It's possible.
**Q.** His nonphysiologic findings made you suspect pain behavior or symptom magnification?
**A.** Yes, they did.
**Q.** Did you test for nonphysiologic findings using Waddell tests?
**A.** No.
**Q.** Did you have the examinee fill out a pain drawing?
**A.** No.
**Q.** Did you perform the Patric test?
**A.** No.
**Q.** The Gaensler test?
**A.** No.
**Q.** The Milgram test?
**A.** No.
**Q.** Did you have the examinee complete one or more of the pain status inventories?
**A.** No.
**Q.** So, just like he "appeared healthy," he appeared to you to have nonphysiologic findings?

**Comment:** Examiners who are faced with nonphysiologic findings and suspect symptom magnification or malingering should carefully document their findings. The more specific and detailed the findings, the better position the examiner will be in to defend his report.

> Mr. Johnson's examination today is significant for the absence of objective signs of neurologic impairment and is significant for the absence of objective signs of musculoskeletal impairment. Mr. Johnson's examination specifically revealed no muscle spasm, no muscle atrophy, no loss of relevant reflexes, no atrophy of one arm or leg in comparison with the opposite arm or leg, no non-verifiable radicular complaints, no radicular complaints and no nonuniform loss of range of motion.

> Mr. Johnson's examination today, including marked pain behavior and the presence of 5 of 5 Waddell's nonorganic signs, is consistent with symptom exaggeration and inappropriate illness behavior.

**Defending the Report As Written:** Examiners should expect opposing counsel to directly attack findings of pain behavior, symptom magnification, or malingering. The successful examiner can defend himself during these attacks.

**Q.** His nonphysiologic findings made you suspect pain behavior or symptom magnification?
**A.** It was not just the nonphysiologic findings, but also the exaggerated grimacing, limping, and grabbing his back. It was also not just one nonphysiologic finding. As I said in my report:

> "Numerous nonphysiologic findings were present: light pressure on the skull caused complaints of increased back pain, rotation of the trunk as a unit resulted in complaints of increased pain, superficial touch resulted in severe pain, superficial pressure resulted in radicular pain complaints, range of motion measurements were inconsistent, range of motion was inconsistent with straight-leg raising (SLR), and SLR supine measurements were inconsistent with SLR sitting."

Taking all this into consideration, I concluded that both pain behavior and symptom magnification were present.

**Example 8.22: The "complete, detailed, and lengthy physical examination"**
*Report States:*

> A complete, detailed, and lengthy physical examination was performed.

*Resulting Cross-examination:*
**Q.** Your IME report indicates that you performed a complete, detailed, and lengthy physical examination, correct?
**A.** Yes, it does.
**Q.** Are you familiar with the saying in medicine that "If it's not documented, it's not done," Doctor?
**A.** I have heard it.
**Q.** What does that mean?
**A.** If the physician doesn't properly document the medical record, it will be presumed that the procedure was not done.
**Q.** Doctor, where in your ½-page IME report do you document the complete, detailed, and lengthy physical examination that you allegedly performed?

**Comment:** Examiners who do not adequately document their reports are particularly vulnerable to cross-examination. It will be difficult to defend an undocumented report.

**Defending the Report As Written:** Even a poorly documented IME report can be defended. The examiner will have to focus on what he did do as opposed to what he failed to do.

**Q.** Doctor, where in your ½-page IME report do you document the complete, detailed, and lengthy physical examination that you allegedly performed?
**A.** I was asked to answer one simple question in my report, which I have done. I am sure the judge would prefer that we concentrate on my findings and opinions than engage in personal attacks. Would you like me to discuss my medical findings and opinion, Counselor?

**Example 8.23: "Personally" examined**
*Report States:*
I personally examined the claimant.

*Resulting Cross-examination:*
**Q.** Doctor, you personally examined the claimant in this case?
**A.** Yes, I did.
**Q.** Is there any difference between examining and personally examining a claimant?
**A.** Not really.
**Q.** Why did you state in your IME report, then, that you personally examined the claimant?

**Comment:** Examiners are best served by not characterizing their examinations or review of records as "personal," "thorough," "careful," etc. This leads to avoidable cross-examinations about why sometimes the examiner is thorough and sometimes she is not.

**Defending the Report As Written:** When confronted with her own characterization, the examiner needs to be able to explain what she meant.

**Q.** Why did you state in your IME report, then, that you personally examined the claimant?
**A.** I did the exam myself, as opposed to one of the other four physicians in my group. That's what I meant by "personally examined."

**Example 8.24: Well-formatted and documented physical examination—second example**
*Report States:*

**Physical Examination**

**Vital Signs**

Temperature - 97.4
Pulse - 70
Blood Pressure - 130/74

**Observations**

Mr. Babitsky is a well-developed male who was in obvious pain and distress.

## PHYSICAL EXAMINATION

### Behavioral Observations

Mr. Babitsky was pleasant and cooperative during the examination. He demonstrated a normal affect. During the visit he appeared comfortable and demonstrated pain behaviors that were appropriate and confirm clinical findings of the lower back and right leg. The pain behavior that was observed was mild limping right leg.

He scored a +1 in pain behavior assessment. This indicates that the pain behaviors are appropriate and tend to confirm the clinical findings of the lumbar spine and lower extremities (legs).

### Structural Examination:

His observed gait was mild limp right leg. There was no antalgic posture noted. There was significant loss of lumbar lordosis and deconditioning of the lumbosacral muscles. There was a surgical scar of 10 cm.

### Range of Motion

Range of motion was tested using dual inclinometers and the results of the maximal ROM in each plane follows. The ROMs indicated below in Table 1 meet the validity criteria as delineated in the AMA's *Guides to the Evaluation of Permanent Impairment,* 5th edition, in all ranges.

| Lumbar ROM | | |
|---|---|---|
| Flexion | 20 | 33% of Normal (60°) |
| Extension | 12 | 50% of Normal (25°) |
| Left Lateral Bend | 8 | 33% of Normal (25°) |
| Right Lateral Bend | 8 | 33% of Normal (25°) |

## ORTHOPEDIC EXAMINATION:

### <u>Lumbar Spine</u>:

### Lumbar palpation examination:

Muscle spasms and tenderness detected to palpation in the lumbar paraspinal musculature on range of motion with pain.

Muscle spasms and tenderness detected in the gluteus musculature on range of motion with pain.

Tenderness to palpation detected in the lumbar spinous processes of L2, L3, L4, and L5.

Tenderness detected in the lumbar facets of L2, L3, L4, and L5 bilaterally.

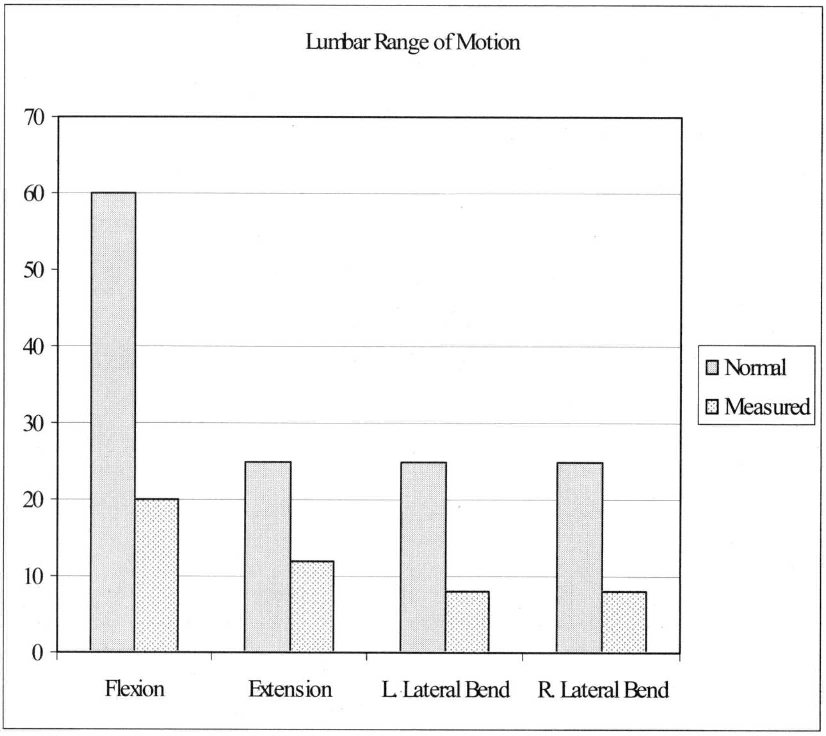


| | Flexion | Extension | L Lateral Bend | R Lateral Bend |
|---|---|---|---|---|
| Normal | 60 | 25 | 25 | 25 |
| Measured | 20 | 12 | 8 | 8 |

## PHYSICAL EXAMINATION

Lumbar joint pain and tenderness, joint asymmetry, range of motion joint abnormality, connective tissue tone, texture, and temperature abnormality was detected.

Deconditioning to the lumbar spine, loss of lumbar lordosis and loss of muscle tone.

SI joint pain and tenderness, joint asymmetry, range of motion joint abnormality, connective tissue tone, texture, and temperature abnormality was detected bilaterally.

Limited mobility of the SI joint with pain noted bilaterally.

**Lower Extremity Right Lower Thigh and Calf**

The patient exhibited a mild limp on toe off and heel off.

Circumferential mensuration was as follows:

| | | Left | Right |
|---|---|---|---|
| **leg:** | **10 cm above superior pole of patella:** | **51 cm** | **47 cm** |
| | **10 cm below inferior pole of patella:** | **44½ cm** | **42 cm** |

There are 4 cm of atrophy noted in the right thigh.

There are 2½ cm of atrophy noted in the right lower calf.

There is a 60% 3/5 right muscle strength deficit and sensory loss.

| | |
|---|---|
| Supraspinatus tendonitis test | NEGATIVE |
| Codman arm drop | NEGATIVE |
| Apprehension test | NEGATIVE |
| Yergason's test | NEGATIVE |
| Apley's test | NEGATIVE |
| Drawer test | NEGATIVE |
| McMurray's test | NEGATIVE |

**RELIABILITY TESTS:**

| | |
|---|---|
| Libman's | NEGATIVE |
| Mannkopf's | NEGATIVE |
| Burn's Bench | NEGATIVE |
| Waddel's | NEGATIVE |

## NEUROLOGICAL TESTING:

Neurological testing consisted of 1) muscle testing, 2) reflex testing and 3) sensation testing.

### SENSORY DERMATOME LEVELS:

A hypoesthesia was noted along the L5 right nerve distribution.

Upper extremities along the sensory dermatome distribution, sensory dermatome level testing was within normal diagnostic perimeters for upper appendages.

### DEEP TENDON REFLEXES:

The Deep Tendon Reflexes tested as follows:

| | |
|---|---|
| Patellar Reflexes 1+/3 right | 2+/3 left |
| Achilles Reflexes 0+/3 right | 2+/3 left |

### MUSCLE TESTING:

C5, C6, C7, C8 and T1 upper extremity strengths of the muscles involved were tested and found to be symmetrical and equal.

L4, L5, S1 lower extremities strengths of the muscles involved were tested and found to be weaker on the right leg and unequal compared to the left leg.

### ORTHOPEDIC TESTING

Valsalva's test was positive L2, L3, L4, and L5.
Kemp's was positive L2, L3, L4, and L5.
Straight leg raise was painful at greater than 60 degrees, positive on the right.
Confirmatory straight leg raise test was positive on the right.
Soto-Hall's test was positive in the lumbar spine.

### VASCULAR TESTING:

The following tests were done to determine any abnormalities of the lower extremities:

There were no abnormal clinical signs of the arteries of the lower extremities.

**Jamar Dynamometer**

Mr. Babitsky was tested for grip strength using the Jamar Dynamometer. Mr. Babitsky is right-hand dominant. His best performance was obtained at position 4 and the data are presented in Table 1.

**Table 1**
**Grip Strengths of Right and Left Upper Extremities**

| | Left Hand | Mean Value Left Hand | Right Hand (Dominant) | Mean Value Right Hand |
|---|---|---|---|---|
| **1** | 54 lbs | | 60 lbs | |
| **2** | 56 lbs | 58 lbs | 60 lbs | 60 lbs |
| **3** | 58 lbs | | 60 lbs | |
| **4** | 60 lbs | | 60 lbs | |
| **5** | 60 lbs | | 60 lbs | |

Mr. Babitsky made a concentrated and maximal effort to comply with this test protocol. This is evidenced by the minimal variance between trials for each hand. His grip strength fell well within the average ranges for males in his age group.

Mr. Babitsky's performance on the five-position Jamar Dynamometry tests produced curves that demonstrate symmetry between the efforts of the right and left hands, Figure 1. These curves represent the expected research trends and indicate a maximal attempt at the task and the ability to use repeated grip mechanics. I concluded that Mr. Babitsky gave maximum effort to provide grip strength data.

**Figure 1**

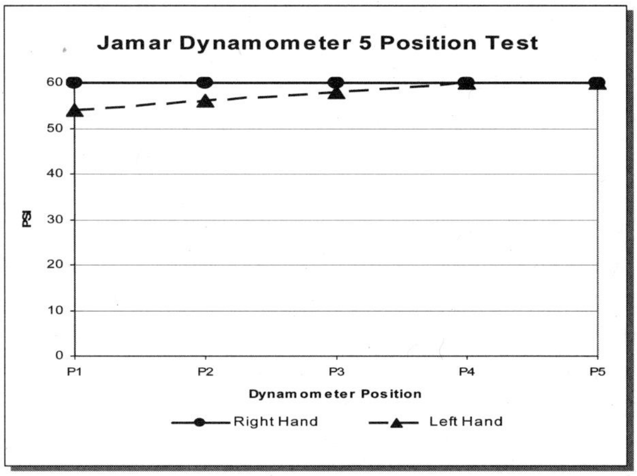

**Pain Status Inventories**

Mr. Babitsky completed the following self-report questionnaires:

. **Pain Drawing**

Mr. Babitsky completed a Pain Drawing. Using the scoring mechanisms for this diagram, he scored a 2 which suggests good psychometrics. Scores of less than "2" are considered indicative of normal psychometrics.

. **CES-D**

The CES-D is a psychometric instrument designed to screen for depression and an affective overlay that may result in symptom magnification. Scores of greater than "16" suggests depression and may suggest a need for additional investigation. The examinee scored a 22.

**Comment:** This is another example of a well-documented, clearly written, and easy-to-read section.

## 8.3 Pain Status Inventories

Pain and functional status inventories may supplement the evaluation. This is especially true of someone with pain complaints. Pain status inventories include instruments to assess behavioral and psychological factors. The most commonly used inventories are as follows.

- Medical Outcome Studies (MOS)
- SF-36 Health Survey
- Pain Drawing
- Pain Disability Index
- McGill Pain Questionnaire
- West Haven-Yale Multidimensional Pain Inventory, Short Form - 36 Questions (SF-36)
- Mensana Clinic Pain Validity Test
- Center for Epidemiologic Studies - Depressed Mood Scale
- Beck Depression Inventory

The examiner should choose a battery of pain inventories consistent with the needs of the assessment. These inventories provide information on the perceived level of function and disability and offer information concerning behavioral overlay and psychological problems. When selecting an inventory, the examiner should consider its intended use, appropriateness to the examinee, validity, and reliability. The examiner should only use pain inventories that he sufficiently understands and can defend during cross-examination.

The report should briefly explain the findings and significance of the inventories in an objective, supportable manner. If the examinee refuses to complete the inventories, this should be documented in the report.

**Example 8.31: Pain inventories confirm non-organic cause of pain**

*Report States:*

The patient was provided a battery of pain inventories. These confirm my suspicion of the non-organic cause of the so-called pain.

*Resulting Cross-examination:*

**Q.** Your report indicates that the "patient was provided a battery of pain inventories. These confirm my suspicion of the non-organic cause of the so-called pain," correct?
**A.** Yes, that's what it says.
**Q.** You interpreted the MMPI-2 yourself?
**A.** Yes, I did.
**Q.** What did the L-Scale show, Doctor?
**A.** I am not sure.
**Q.** Do you know what the L-Scale tests for?
**A.** Not specifically.
**Q.** What about the F-Scale?
**A.** I don't know.
**Q.** Can you explain how the F Minus K-Scale measures "faking bad" and "faking good"?
**A.** I cannot.
**Q.** What did the meta-analysis of the research reports show that an F-K score less than or equal to -8 is a strong indicator of?
**A.** I don't know.
**Q.** The only thing that you really do know is that the pain inventories which you do not understand confirm your suspicion of a non-organic cause of the examinee's so-called pain?

**Comment:** Examiners who use pain inventories in their IME reports should understand the inventories, how and what they test, how the numbers are arrived at, and what they mean. Examiners who do this will be in the best position to defend their IME reports. For example:

The most commonly used pain inventories are: Pain Disability Index, Oswestry Low Back Pain Disability Questionnaire, Short Form McGill Pain Questionnaire, and the West Haven-Yale Multidimensional Pain Inventory.

*Pain Disability Index*

The Pain Disability Index was developed by Tait et al and focuses on pain-related disability. The index uses 0 (no disability) to 10 (total disability) ratings of disability in seven areas of activity. These areas are family/home responsibilities, recreation, social activity, occupation, sexual activity, self-care, and life-support activities. They are scored by identifying the percentage of perceived disability for each category and the overall level of perceived disability. An individual who reported being totally disabled in all areas would have a score of 70 (10 x 7). Levels of reported disability disproportionate to impairment and clinical assessment suggest behavioral overlay. According to Tait, high scores relate to "time spent in bed, psychosomatic symptoms, stopping activities because of pain, work status, pain duration, usual pain intensity, quality of life, pain extent, and education." The Pain Disability Index appears to possess both test-retest reliability and validity for pain-based disability.[1]

*Oswestry Low Back Pain Disability Questionnaire*

The Oswestry Low Back Pain Disability Questionnaire includes ten six-point scales. The first section rates the intensity of pain and the remaining nine cover the disabling effect of pain on typical daily activities. The examinee marks the statement in each section that most accurately describes the effect of his or her pain. The sum of the total scores is expressed as a percentage of the maximal score. If the examinee fails to complete a section, the percentage is adjusted. Scores from 0 to 20% represent minimal disability, 20 to 40% represent moderate disability, 40 to 60% represent severe disability, while scores of 60% or more indicate that the examinee reports being severely disabled in several areas of life.[2]

*Short-Form McGill Pain Questionnaire*

The McGill Pain Questionnaire (MPQ) was designed to provide a quantitative profile of pain. It is the leading instrument for describing the diverse dimensions of pain. This instrument is available in long and short forms. The short-form MPQ includes 15 descriptive words, 11 of which are sensory and four of which are affective. Sensory descriptors describe the sensory qualities of the experience in terms of temporal, spatial, pressure, thermal, and other properties. In the short-form MPQ each word or phrase is rated on a four-point intensity scale. The MPQ is scored by determining if sensory descriptors are predominately used, suggesting less emotional overlay, or whether affective descriptors are used, suggesting behavioral overlay. The process of scoring the MPQ is detailed in the *Handbook of Pain Assessment* by Turk and Melzack.[3]

*West Haven-Yale Multidimensional Pain Inventory*

The (West Haven-Yale) Multidimensional Pain Inventory focuses on the pain's impact on the individual's life, the responses of others to the individual's communication of pain, and the extent to which the individual participates in common daily activities. It groups individuals into categories of adaptive cooperative, dysfunctional, or interpersonally distressed. This instrument and the software to score the inventory are available at minimal cost through the University of Pittsburgh.[4]

---

[1] *The Comprehensive IME System,* SEAK, Inc. p. 52 (1997).
[2] Ibid. at 52.
[3] Ibid. at 53.
[4] Ibid.

**Defending the Report As Written:** Examiners who are not intimately familiar with pain inventories but who insist on using them can still defend their reports.

**Q.** So you interpreted the MMPI-2 yourself?
**A.** No. I have a forensic psychologist who I use to interpret and score psychological tests. I reviewed her scoring.

**Example 8.32: Pain inventories clearly documented**
*Report States:*

Pain Drawing
The examinee completed a pain drawing (enclosed), using symbols to describe sensations. This drawing received a score of 8, suggesting poor psychometrics.

Pain Disability Index
The Pain Disability Index uses rating scales to measure the extent of perceived disability in seven areas of life. The results are as follows:

| Area | Perceived Disability |
|---|---|
| Family/home responsibilities | 90% |
| Recreation | 90% |
| Social activity | 90% |
| Occupation | 100% |
| Sexual activity | 80% |
| Self-care | 60% |
| Life-support activities | 70% |

The overall score is 58 out of 70, for a high level of perceived disability (83%), with the highest level of reported disability being for occupation.

McGill Pain Questionnaire
The patient completed the McGill Pain Questionnaire (Short Form), rating 15 pain descriptors on a scale from 0 (none) to 3 (severe). The sum of 11 sensory descriptors was 25, averaging 2.3. The sum of 4 affective descriptors was 11, averaging 2.75. The total of all descriptors was 36 (an elevated score). The descriptors were primarily affective, suggesting exaggerated pain. The descriptors rated as severe were stabbing, hot-burning, aching, tender, splitting, tiring-exhausting, sickening, and punishing-cruel. The overall pain intensity was rated at 4 (horrible) on a scale of 0-5.

Multidimensional Pain Inventory
The results of the University of Pittsburgh School of Medicine Multidimensional Pain Inventory are attached. The examinee rated the impact of the pain in several areas on a 0-6 scale. The first page reports the scores and statistical analysis, and the second page

gives a graphic representation of the results compared with a control group.

This profile is that of a dysfunctional individual. Compared with the control group, these individuals report a higher severity of pain, greater interference with their lives, a higher degree of psychological distress, a lower perceived ability to control their lives, and lower activity levels. They are labeled dysfunctional because the pain has affected a broad range of their functioning.

<u>CES-D</u>
The Center for Epidemiologic Studies Depressed Mood Scale was administered. The examinee scored 34, suggestive of a depressed mood.

<u>Oswestry Function Test</u>
His score on the Oswestry Function Test was 27 out of a possible 50 (54th percentile), indicating a perception of severe disability.

*Resulting Cross-examination:*
**Q.** Doctor, you scored the examinee's pain drawing as an 8 in your IME report?
**A.** Yes, I did.
**Q.** That's because he made too many Xs and went outside the line?
**A.** It's not that simple, Counsel.
**Q.** Had the examinee not "colored outside the lines," would you have scored him as an 8?
**A.** Well, no.
**Q.** Did anyone explain to this examinee, with his third-grade education, that he should stay within the lines?
**A.** No. That's part of the test.
**Q.** The pain indexes utilized do have their shortcomings, don't they, Doctor?
**A.** Well, no test is perfect.
**Q.** Are you familiar with the critique of the Pain Disability Index done by Hebben?
**A.** What are you referring to, Counsel?
**Q.** Hebben, N., *Toward the Assessment of Clinical Pain in Adults*, in Aronoff G.M., (ED) *Evaluation of Chronic Pain*, William and Wilkins, 1992, p. 384-393?
**A.** No, I am not.
**Q.** Would you like to see this before you continue to use this index?
**A.** Yes.
**Q.** Are you familiar with the problems using the McGill Pain Questionnaire?
**A.** No.
**Q.** There is significant disagreement over the accuracy of the test and its ability to discriminate diagnostic groups of patients, correct?
**A.** I have not heard of that criticism and I doubt it exists.
**Q.** Doctor, I am showing you the chapter by Hinnant, D.W., "Psychological Evaluation and Testing," from *Tollison Handbook of Pain Management*, 2nd

edition, 1994, pp. 18-35. Would you like some time to review it before we proceed?

**Comment:** Examiners who make extensive use of pain inventories should study the inventories and understand their strengths and weaknesses. Only then will they be in the best position to defend their opinions and reports.

**Defending the Report As Written:** Physicians who are ready to respond excel at defending their opinions and reports.

**Q.** Are you familiar with the critique of the pain disability index done by Hebben?
**A.** Hebben found that the Pain Disability Index possessed both test-retest reliability and validity with regard to pain-based disability.

## 8.4 Current Status

The current status should be elicited in detail and thoroughly documented. This process usually commences with identification of the examinee's primary concern. Most often the complaint is pain. The location, intensity, frequency, pattern, and nature of the pain, as well as aggravating and relieving factors, need to be documented. Associated symptoms, such as numbness, tingling, weakness, morning stiffness, and other physiologic difficulties, should be assessed and documented. It is important to identify not only positive attributes but negative attributes as well. Anxiety, discouragement, depression, and sleep disturbance should be referenced. Any inconsistencies should be documented.

**Example 8.41: Current complaints documented**
*Report States:*

The examinee's major concern is that his "back hurts and I can't lift." He reports that since the injury he has remained the same. The pain is located primarily in the right low back, and is described as nagging. It radiates down the right leg posterior to the knee.

Aggravating Factors: Significantly worsened by forceful use, movement, lifting, cold or damp weather, and sitting; somewhat by exercise, coughing, or sneezing, standing, walking, and "driving my car."

Relieving Factors: The pain is improved somewhat with rest. On a scale from 0 (no pain) to 10 (excruciating pain), initially it was a 10. During the past month it averaged a 7, with a low of 4 and a high of 10. Today the pain is a 7.

He has numbness on the outside of the right leg to the knee, and rare tingling. He reports weakness of his back and right leg, and morning stiffness lasting an hour or so. He admits feeling

> discouraged at times and depressed, although he denies suicidal thoughts. His sleep is disturbed, with primary and secondary insomnia due to pain. He mentions as another problem that "my neck is occasionally stiff."

*Resulting Cross-examination:*
**Q.** Doctor, do you believe the examinee when he reports that his back hurts and he can't lift?
**A.** I have no reason not to believe him.
**Q.** Depending on the intensity and frequency, pain can be disabling?
**A.** In some cases.
**Q.** Did you ask him about the frequency of his pain?
**A.** No, I did not.
**Q.** Do you know if his pain is intermittent, occasional, frequent, or constant?
**A.** I do not.
**Q.** You would agree that the frequency of his pain is of significance, would you not?

**Comment:** Examiners who comment on pain should do so in a detailed manner. Both the intensity and frequency of the pain should be documented.

**Defending the Report As Written:** Examiners can expect to be questioned about the nature, extent, and impact of the pain reported by the examinee. The examiner needs to be able to defend his comments on pain and its impact on the examinee. When given an "opening," some examiners capitalize on it.

**Q.** Depending on the intensity and frequency, pain can be disabling?
**A.** In my experience, the motivation and not the pain is what is crucial. I have seen workers who lost a finger return to work in two hours and others who complain of pain from a simple laceration be out of work for months. This is not a pain issue. It is a question of motivation.

## 8.5 Functional Status

Functional status should be thoroughly elicited and documented in detail. This is particularly true for those functions that are most problematic. The physician should have the examinee express her capacity to perform various activities of daily living, such as exercising, sitting, standing, household chores, driving, etc. This is helpful in understanding the difficulties perceived or reported by the examinee and may be useful in assessing work ability. If the examinee is quoted in the report, the physician should be careful not to misquote her.

The functional status may also be considered in terms of whether it fits with the diagnoses in question and is consistent with other observations. The person's reported tolerances for sitting, standing, walking, lifting, and carrying are noted. Also noted is the ability to carry out a variety of tasks associated with activities of daily living. In a credible examinee, these representations may be accurate. In an examinee with symptom magnification behavior, the representations may be inconsistent with observations during the visit, surveillance material, and the medical condition.

Some examiners include observations of the claimant arriving at and leaving the examiner's office. This is not recommended because it will likely result in close questioning on cross-examination in an attempt to show that the examiner was spying or looking for anything to help the insurance company.

All findings should be objectively and carefully documented in the report. Ideally, functional status is addressed in a separate section of the report that is identified with a topic heading. Please consider the following examples.

**Example 8.51: Functional status**
*Report States:*
**FUNCTIONAL STATUS**

He feels he can sit for half an hour, stand for one hour, walk for half an hour, and lift up to 10 lbs. occasionally. He reports being unable to lift heavy weights, and has major difficulty lifting a heavy bag of groceries, bending, lifting from floor to waist or waist to shoulder, lifting above shoulder level, climbing stairs, or driving. He indicates minor problems lifting a light bag of groceries, reaching above shoulder level, pulling, pushing, sweeping or vacuuming, and moving his neck. He is unsure of his ability to climb ladders. His most difficult task is "driving my car over bumpy roads."

*Resulting Cross-examination:*
**Q.** Doctor, the functional status portion of your IME report is just what the examinee told you, correct?
**A.** Well, yes.
**Q.** You didn't perform a functional capacity evaluation to determine if the examinee has the ability to return to work?
**A.** No, I did not.
**Q.** Thank you.

**Comment:** The examiner can obtain significant information from the examinee by asking him about his limitations. These self-reported limitations are another part of the IME puzzle.

**Defending the Report As Written:** Examiners need not apologize for the fact that the functional status is the examinee's perception of his ability and limitations.

**Q.** Doctor, the functional status portion of your IME report is just what the examinee told you, correct?
**A.** The examinee's perceived functional status expressed in his own words is very important in clarifying work capacity and potential behavioral issues.

**Example 8.52: "He cannot articulate"**
*Report States:*

> **Functional Status**
>
> He states he cannot be as active as he would like when performing activities such as hunting, riding horses, riding in the mountains, jogging, swimming, or fishing secondary to the pain. He denies any problems with household or yard work or preparing meals, but states he has problems pulling on his shoes and socks and picking things up once he has dropped them. Most of his yard work and household work is done by his relatives. He is able to sit for only 20 minutes. He cannot articulate how long he could stand, drive, or walk.

*Resulting Cross-examination:*
**Q.** Doctor, you said in your IME report that the examinee could not articulate how long he could stand, drive, or walk, correct?
**A.** Yes.
**Q.** When you asked him how long he could stand, he didn't say, "I cannot articulate," did he?
**A.** No.
**Q.** He said he wasn't sure, didn't he?
**A.** Something like that or words to that effect.
**Q.** You didn't put in his answer but your characterization of what he said, correct?

**Comment:** Examiners are better served by using the examinee's verbatim response or non-response to questions regarding his functional status.

> When asked how far he could drive, the examinee replied, "I don't know. I haven't driven in two years."

**Defending the Report As Written:** Examiners need not take criticism for the failure of the examinee to reply to simple, direct questions.

**Q.** When you asked him how long he could stand, he didn't say, "I cannot articulate," did he?
**A.** No, Counsel. He said, "I couldn't say."

**Example 8.53: Observation in parking lot**
*Report States:*

> Mrs. Buckner was observed entering a blue Toyota Camry, which includes bending and turning, including her neck, without difficulty or limitations. She operates it without any identifiable problems.

*Resulting Cross-examination:*
**Q.** Doctor, you observed the claimant in your parking lot?
**A.** Yes.

**Q.** Do you normally observe claimants get into their cars as part of your IME exam?
**A.** Sometimes I do.
**Q.** Is this intentional or by accident?
**A.** Mostly by accident.
**Q.** How far away were you from the claimant when you observed her?
**A.** About 75-100 feet.
**Q.** Which part of the car was closest to you?
**A.** The rear.
**Q.** When she got into the car, you were looking at the back of her head, correct?
**A.** Yes.
**Q.** If she grimaced in pain you could not see that, correct?
**A.** She seemed to be OK.
**Q.** Could you see if her back went into spasms after she sat down?
**A.** I didn't see anything like that.
**Q.** You couldn't see it because her back was against the seat, correct?
**A.** Her back was against the seat.
**Q.** You observed her operate her vehicle "without any identifiable" problems. Is that what you wrote in your independent medical report?
**A.** Yes.
**Q.** You observed her as she pulled out of the parking lot?
**A.** Yes.
**Q.** How long did that take, Doctor?
**A.** 20-30 seconds.
**Q.** You didn't follow her…or did you?
**A.** No, I did not and I do not appreciate your sarcasm, Counselor.
**Q.** Based on those 20-30 seconds, you formed an opinion about her ability to operate a motor vehicle without problems?
**A.** I reported what I saw.
**Q.** You did not observe her for the rest of her 45-minute drive?
**A.** That's correct.
**Q.** Do you normally observe patients you treat getting in and out of their cars?
**A.** Once in a while.
**Q.** Do you report your observations in their medical records, Doctor?
**A.** No.
**Q.** That's because in those cases you are not working for an insurance company and trying to build a case that there is nothing wrong with the patient, correct?
**A.** I call them as I see them, Counselor.
**Q.** It's just the IME examinees that you "accidentally" see getting in and out of their cars and driving out of the parking lot so you can report your observations in your independent medical report?

**Comment:** When examiners stretch to find items that will help them show that the examinee is "normal," they run the risk of being perceived as an advocate. The reporting of objective medical test results is much more effective and does not smack of partiality. When, as in the above example, the examiner tries to argue that in a brief observation he can determine the examinee's true health status, he undermines his credibility and even the appearance of his impartiality. The examiner would have been better served by either omitting the sentence completely or at least reporting the observations without drawing opinions directly from his observation.

> The examinee entered her Toyota Camry, twisted her neck, and backed out of the driveway without apparent difficulty.

**Defending the Report As Written:** The IME physician, when faced with questions on his observations, should give the simple facts that he observed without embellishment or characterization.

**Q.** Doctor, you observed the claimant in your parking lot?
**A.** I saw her enter her Toyota Camry, turn her neck around to back up, and drive out of the lot without apparent difficulty.

# Chapter 9 How to Use Citations to Texts, Journals, Guidelines, and Other Authority to Bolster a Report's Credibility

## 9.1 Executive Summary

Citations to well-accepted authorities that support an examiner's opinions will bolster the credibility of the IME report. The authors recommend the following.

- The citations should be detailed and precise. They should include title, author, edition, publisher, and year published.
- A pinpoint cite should be used if specific pages are referenced.
- The examiner should be prepared to be cross-examined on any authority cited in the report.
- Avoid general statements that the examiner's conclusions are supported by the "weight of the literature" or "studies."
- Examiners should attempt to use authority that is as recent as possible and avoid the use of outdated authority.
- Quoting authority may bolster the report's credibility, but the examiner should expect to be closely questioned not only about the quoted passage, but on other passages from the reference as well.
- Examiners should avoid describing any authority as being "authoritative" or "reliable" because these terms may have special legal significance that can expand the scope of permissible cross-examination of the examiner.
- Examiners should be familiar with the ABIME guidelines for performing IMEs and be prepared to answer questions about these guidelines, especially if they are cited in the examiner's report.

## 9.2 Citing Authority Properly

Citations to authority that supports an examiner's opinions will bolster the authoritativeness of the IME report. Citations to authority should be made with as much specificity as possible. The citations should include title, author, edition, publisher, and year published. A pinpoint cite should be used if specific pages are referenced.

The list of authorities should be detailed and precise. Such a detailed list makes the report much more credible than it would have been had the examiner instead made a general statement that the literature in the field was reviewed. Of course, if the examiner does list the authority specifically, she can expect to be cross-examined on the authority. The examiner must be prepared for such cross-examinations by doing her homework. Please consider the following examples.

**Example 9.21: Failure to explicitly list articles reviewed**
*Report States:*

Various scientific/medical articles and references were consulted and reviewed.

**Comment:** This report would have been more credible if it had explicitly and precisely listed the articles and references that were consulted. Consider the following. Note the detailed citations used. Such detailed citations add credibility to the report.

The following scientific/medical articles and references were consulted and reviewed:

1. Pierce, DA, et al., Joint Effects of Radiation and Smoking on Lung Cancer Risk among Atomic Bomb Survivors. Radiat Res. 2003 Apr; 159(4):511-520.
2. Kouides, P.A., and Bennett, J. M., The Myelodysplastic Syndromes, *in* Abeloff, M.D., et al Clinical Oncology Churchill Livingstone, New York. 2000.
3. Stone, R.M., and Mayer, R.J., Acute Myeloid Leukemia in Adults, *in* Abeloff, M.D., et al Clinical Oncology Churchill Livingstone, New York. 2000.
4. Upton, Arthur C. The Linear-Nonthreshold Dose-Response Model: A Critical Reappraisal. Proceedings of the Thirty-Fifth Annual Meeting of the National Council on Radiation Protection and Measurements. Bethesda, MD, National Council on Radiation Protection and Measurements, 1999, pp 9-31.
5. Gundestrup, M., and Storm, H.H. Radiation-induced acute myeloid leukemia and other cancers in commercial jet cockpit crew: a population-based cohort study. Lancet: 354: 2029-2031, 1999.
6. Upton, A.C. The linear-nonthreshold dose-response model: a critical reappraisal. Proc. of the thirty-fifth annual meeting of the National Council on Radiation Protection and Measurements. Bethesda, MD. National Council on Radiation Protection and Measurements, 1999, pp 9-31.
7. Gundestrup, M., Storm, H.H. Radiation-induced acute myeloid leukemia and other cancers in commercial jet cockpit crew: a population-based cohort study. Lancet: 354: 2029-2031, 1999.
8. Dollinger, M.R., Rosenbaum, E.H., and Cable, G. Everyone's Guide to Cancer Therapy. Somerville House/Toronto and Andrews-McMeel/Kansas City, 1998.
9. Fairlie, I., and Resnikoff, M. No Dose Too Low. Bulletin Atomic Scientists. Nov.-Dec.1997, pages 52-56.
10. Ellenhorn, M.J. Medical Toxicology: Diagnosis and Treatment of Human Poisoning. Chapter 70: Radiation poisoning. 2nd Ed. Williams & Wilkins, Baltimore, 1997.
11. Little, J. B. Ionizing Radiation *in* Holland, et al, Cancer Medicine,

Fourth Edition, Williams and Wilkins, Baltimore, 1997.
12. Schottenfeld, D., and Fraumeni, Jr., J.F. Cancer Epidemiology and Prevention, 2nd ed, Oxford University Press, New York, 1996.
13. Band, P.R., et al. Cohort study of Air Canada pilots: mortality, cancer incidence, and leukemia risk. Am. J. Epid. 143: 137-143, 1996.
14. Fairlie, I. Risk of radiation-induced cancer at low doses and low dose rates for radiation protection purposes. National Radiological Protection Board. Vol. 6: No. 1, 1995.
15. Straume, T. High-energy gamma rays in Hiroshima and Nagasaki: Implications for risk and $W_R$. Health Phys. 69: 954-956, 1995.
16. Bonin, S.R., et al. Treatment-related myelodysplastic syndrome following abdominopelvic radiotherapy for endometrial cancer. Gynec. Oncology. 57: 430-432, 1995.
17. Pederson-Bjergaard J. Radiotherapy- and chemotherapy-induced myeloysplasia and acute myeloid leukemia. A review. Leuk Res. 16:61, 1992.
18. Warren, G.S., and Dreyer, N.A. Leukemia among nuclear workers with protracted exposure to low-dose ionizing radiation. Epidemiology 2: 305-309, 1991.
19. Wing, S., et al. Mortality among workers at Oak Ridge National Laboratory: Evidence of radiation effects in follow-up through 1984. J.Am. Med.Assn. 265: 1397-1402, 1991.
20. Hall, E.J. Risk of Cancer Causation by Diagnostic X-rays. Cancer Prevention [DeVita, Hellman, and Rosenberg, eds], p 1-9, March 1990.
21. Stewart, A.M. Low-level radiation: the cancer controversy. Bull. Atomic Scientists. Sept. 1990, pp. 15-19.
22. Hall, E.J. Risk of Cancer Causation by Diagnostic X-rays. Supplement to Cancer Prevention, eds. DeVita, V.T. Hellman, S., and Rosenberg, S.A. March 1990.
23. Flodin, U., et al. Acute myeloid leukemia and background radiation in an expanded case-referent study. Arch. Env. Health. 45: 364-366, 1990.
24. Dreyer, N.A., and Friedlander, E. Identifying the health risks from very low-dose sparsely ionizing radiation. Am. J. Pub. Health. 72: 585-588, 1982.
25. Wallace, R.W., and Sondhaus, C.A. Cosmic radiation exposure in subsonic air transport. Aviat. Space Environ. Med. 49: 610-623, 1978.
26. Martland, H.S, et al. Some Unrecognized Dangers in the Use and Handling of Radioactive Substances: J. Am. Med. Assn. 85: 1769-1776, 1925.
27. Portions of CFR: Department of Veterans Affairs, Ch.1 (7-1-97 Edition), pages 221-226 [alternatively sections 3.309 to 3.312], dealing with radiation exposure – related cancers in veterans exposed to radiation.

**Example 9.22: Explicit list of authority reviewed**

*Report States:*

- Chin, DH and Jones, NF, Repetitive Motion Hand Disorders. J. Calif. Den Assoc. 2002 Feb;30(2):149-60.
- Pascarelli, EF and Hsu, YP, Understanding Work-related Upper Extremity Disorders: Clinical Findings in 485 Computer Users,

Musicians, and Others. J. Occup. Rehabil. 2001 Mar;11(1):1-21.
- Abbas, MA et al., Meta-Analysis of Published Studies of Work-Related Carpal Tunnel Syndrome. Int. J. Occup. Environ. Health. 1998 Jul-Sep;4(3):160-7.
- Melhorn, J.M., Understanding the types of carpal tunnel syndrome. J Workers Comp. 1988 7(3): 52-73.
- Szabo, RM, Carpal Tunnel Syndrome as a Repetitive Motion Disorder. Clin Orthop. 1998 Jun;(351):78-89.
- Rempel, D, et al., The Effect of Wearing a Flexible Wrist Splint on Carpal Tunnel Pressure During Repetitive Hand Activity. J Hand Surg [AM]. 1994 Jan;19(1):106-110.
- Eisma, TL, Ergonomic Design Protects Hands from Repetitive Motion Stress, Vibration. Occup Health Saf. 1990 Apr;59(4):75-77,80-82.

**Comment:** This detailed list shows that the report was the product of significant research. The author of this report would also need to prepare herself for cross-examination based on each of these references.

## 9.3 Consequences of Failure to Cite Authority Specifically

The failure to research and cite specific supporting literature is a potential area of close questioning on cross-examination. Examiners sometimes state that their conclusions are supported by the "weight of the literature" or "studies." Examiners may be called upon during cross-examination to give specific examples of the supporting studies or literature. This may be difficult to do under the pressure of giving testimony. It is, therefore, better practice to list at least a representative sampling of the specific literature relied upon. The examiner can then consult his IME report when questioned about the authorities upon which he relied. Please consider the following examples.

**Example 9.31: Failure to cite specifically**

*Report States:*

Impairment was calculated according to the AMA criteria.

*Resulting Cross-examination:*

**Q.** In forming your opinion and writing your report, you relied upon certain publications by the American Medical Association, did you not?

**A.** Yes.

**Q.** Did you note in your report what year the edition that you relied upon was published?

**A.** No.

**Q.** You didn't think that was important either?

**A.** Not particularly.

**Q.** Are you aware of the fact that there have been seven different editions of that book?

**A.** No, I wasn't.

**Q.** Do you know why a book like that is updated periodically with a new edition?

**A.** To keep it current.
**Q.** Is that because things change?
**A.** Yes.
**Q.** Were you aware that the latest edition of the AMA *Guides* (5th edition) specifically states:

> "The fifth edition includes most of the common conditions, excluding unusual cases that require individual consideration. Since this edition encompasses the most current criteria and procedures for impairment assessment, it is strongly recommended that physicians use this latest edition, the fifth edition, when rating impairment?"[1]

**A.** No, I was not.
**Q.** So, if you didn't use the 5th edition, you utilized outdated information and the wrong text?
**A.** It appears so.

**Comment:** Use of a fuller citation makes the examiner and his report more credible. Consider the following.

> Permanent impairment was rated according to the American Medical Association's *Guides to the Evaluation of Permanent Impairment* (4th edition, 1993).

**Defending the Report As Written:** Just because counsel says something during cross-examination doesn't make him correct. IME examiners need to be prepared to counter counsel's tactics by bringing forward the key information that counsel conveniently failed to disclose.

**Q.** So, if you didn't use the 5th edition, you utilized outdated information and the wrong text?
**A.** That's not correct. My state workers' compensation statute requires that we use the 4th edition of the *Guides*. We have not yet adopted the 5th edition.

**Example 9.32: The "literature is in agreement"**
*Report States:*

> The literature is in agreement with this principle.

*Resulting Cross-examination:*
**Q.** Your IME report indicates that the literature is in agreement with your opinion, correct?
**A.** Yes, it does.
**Q.** How many texts have been written about low back pain?
**A.** I don't know exactly, but quite a few.
**Q.** How many medical journal articles have been written about low back pain?
**A.** I am not sure, but I would imagine thousands of articles.
**Q.** How many of the books and thousands of articles on low back pain have you read?
**A.** I am not sure, but quite a few.

---

[1] AMA *Guides*, Sec. 1.1.

**Q.** Here is a Medline list of 493 medical journal articles on low back pain. How many of them have you read, Doctor?
**A.** Well, it's hard to remember. All the titles are so similar.
**Q.** So, despite the fact that there are numerous texts and hundreds of journal articles you either haven't read or can't remember reading, you are willing to testify under oath that the literature is in agreement with your opinion?

**Comment:** If an examiner broadly claims that the literature or "many studies" agree with his opinion, he can expect to be asked, as above, to cite specific examples. Such a difficult question will be much easier to answer when the specific citations of supporting literature are listed explicitly.

**Defending the Report As Written:** Examiners who non-specifically cite "the literature" in their IME reports should be prepared to cite specific articles during cross-examination.

**Q.** Your IME report indicates that the literature is in support of your opinion, correct?
**A.** Yes, it does. Here is a list of four texts and 37 journal articles that support my opinion. The list is current and I would be pleased to make it part of the record and discuss it with you.

**Example 9.33: "Studies consistently demonstrate"**
*Report States:*

> Studies consistently demonstrate that reported mold on surfaces, water damage, and excessive moisture are strongly associated with excess reporting of upper and lower respiratory symptoms—wheeze, asthma, and other conditions.

*Resulting Cross-examination:*
**Q.** In your report you state on page 3 that, and I quote, "Studies consistently demonstrate that reported mold on surfaces, water damage, and excessive moisture are strongly associated with excess reporting of upper and lower respiratory symptoms—wheeze, asthma, and other conditions." Am I reading that correctly?
**A.** Yes.
**Q.** Specifically, which studies are you referring to?
**A.** I'd have to look them up.
**Q.** Sitting here today in front of this jury, you can't specifically cite ANY study to support your conclusion, can you?
**A.** No, but if I could have some time to research this, I'd get you what you are looking for.

**Comment:** If an examiner generally cites "studies" or "the literature," she can expect to be asked to cite the specific studies or the specific literature.

> Studies consistently demonstrate that reported mold on surfaces, water damage, and excessive moisture are strongly associated with excess

> reporting of upper and lower respiratory symptoms—wheeze, asthma, and other conditions. Examples of such studies follow.
>
> 1. Excessive building moisture and prevalence of lower respiratory distress, *New England Journal of Medicine*...

**Defending the Report As Written:** Examiners should review their reports in detail before testifying. When an examiner notes an omission in her report, she should be prepared to "fill in" the missing information when given an opportunity during cross-examination.

**Q.** Specifically, which studies are you referring to?
**A.** The most recent study was done at Johns Hopkins and was reported in the *New England Journal of Medicine* on 3/15/03. The other study was done at the Massachusetts General Hospital and reported in *JAMA* on 2/12/03.

**Example 9.34: Opinion based on general scientific seminars/studies**
*Report States:*

> This opinion is based upon educational seminars given by engineers who have analyzed rear-end collisions.

*Resulting Cross-examination:*
**Q.** You expressed the opinion in your IME report that in a rear-end collision there is no forceful opening or closing of the jaw, correct?
**A.** Yes.
**Q.** You stated that, "This opinion is based upon educational seminars given by engineers who have analyzed rear-end collisions" in your report?
**A.** That's correct.
**Q.** Can you give me the names, dates, and locations of the seminars you based your opinion on?
**A.** The industry is replete with them, Counsel. I don't know where to start.
**Q.** Just give me the names of six of them?
**A.** As I sit here today I can't do that.
**Q.** Can you name two or three of them?
**A.** No.
**Q.** Can you name one of them, Doctor?
**A.** Not at this time.
**Q.** Can you name the engineers who you relied on to form your opinion?
**A.** No.
**Q.** So your opinion is based upon educational seminars for which you cannot provide names, dates, or locations and upon engineers whom you cannot identify?

**Comment:** When an IME physician bases his opinion in part or in whole on scientific seminars or studies, he should anticipate being closely questioned about them. Making general references to the science is certainly the quickest and easiest way to draft an IME report. If the examiner cannot back up such general references, however, use of general, non-specific references is a recipe for disaster.

**Defending the Report As Written:** An omission in a report can be turned into an opportunity to excel during cross-examination.

**Q.** Can you give me the names, dates, and locations of the seminars you based your opinion on?
**A.** There are 12 seminars and studies I reference. The first one was held on 7/2/2002 in New York City by the American Society of Biomechanical Engineers. I attended the conference. The second seminar…

## 9.4 Outdated Authority

An examiner should attempt to use authority that is as current as possible. Use of authority that is outdated can and will be seized upon by opposing counsel.

**Example 9.41: 1972 edition**

*Report States:*

> For some time, the American Medical Association has published a *Guide to Evaluating Permanent Impairment.* They point out in their 1972 edition of this *Guide* the following:…

*Resulting Cross-examination:*

**Q.** In your report you rely on the 1972 edition of the AMA *Guides,* is that correct?
**A.** Yes, I do.
**Q.** That was published in 1972 when Richard Nixon was president?
**A.** Yes.
**Q.** The United States was still at war in Vietnam?
**A.** Yes.
**Q.** Cars ran on leaded gas?
**A.** Yes.
**Q.** How old are you, sir?
**A.** Thirty-six.
**Q.** How old were you when this was published?
**A.** Four.
**Q.** Did you cite in your report any more recent publications?
**A.** No.
**Q.** Were you practicing medicine in 1972?
**A.** No, of course not.
**Q.** There have been significant changes in medicine since 1972, have there not?
**A.** Certainly, yes.

**Comment:** Relying on outdated authority will undermine an expert's credibility. The expert should rely on recent authority.

> For some time, the American Medical Association has published a *Guide to Evaluating Permanent Impairment.* They point out in their 5th edition (2000) of this *Guide* the following:…

**Defending the Report As Written:** Prior to testifying, the examiner should thoroughly review his report and file with a critical eye. The examiner should anticipate being questioned about "weak areas" of the report and be prepared to reply to questions during cross-examination.

**Q.** Did you cite in your report any more recent publications?
**A.** I failed to mention the 5th edition of the AMA *Guides*, which, on this issue, remains essentially unchanged from the 1972 edition. This is obviously a well-proven principle that has stood the test of time.

## 9.5 Quoting Authority

IME reports may quote from one or more authorities. Such quotations, if taken in context, will help to bolster the report. The examiner needs to be prepared, however, to be closely questioned on other portions of the authority that may not support her opinion.

**Example 9.51: Statements from text quoted**
*Report States:*

The following statements from the current edition of Campbell's *Urology* would support Dr. Doe's management of Mr. Clark:

~ It is uncertain whether residual urine volume indicates impending bladder or renal damage.
~ Large residual urine volumes may predict a slightly higher failure rate with a strategy of watchful waiting. However, the threshold volume defining a poorer outcome is uncertain.
~ There are no data documenting that the incidence of urinary tract infection is related to postvoid residual volume.

*Resulting Cross-examination:*
**Q.** In your report you quote three statements from Campbell's *Urology* that support your opinion, is that correct?
**A.** Yes.
**Q.** Do you consider that work authoritative?
**A.** Yes.
**Q.** How big is that book?
**A.** I'm not sure, but it's quite thick.
**Q.** Maybe 200,000 words?
**A.** Maybe, yes.
**Q.** Would you agree that there likely are statements in Campbell's that do not support your opinion?
**A.** Probably.
**Q.** For example, page 237 of Campbell's *Urology* indicates that for some individuals, the presence of urinary tract infection can be related to post-void residual volume, correct?
**A.** That's what it says.
**Q.** You didn't quote that or any of the other statements that didn't support your opinion, did you?
**A.** No.

**Q.** And out of the 200,000-word treatise, you carefully chose only the 60 words that most support your opinion?
**A.** That's right.

**Comment:** Citing authority will bolster an expert's credibility and help defend against *Daubert*[2] attacks. There are two important caveats, however. One, the authority should in fact stand for the proposition that the examiner asserts that it does. Second, the examiner should be prepared to be cross-examined on the entire authority, not just the sections specifically used by the expert. Examiners need to assume that opposing counsel (with the help of her own expert) will thoroughly review the authority that the expert is relying on to verify that it does in fact stand for what the expert claims it does. Counsel will then review the authority and look for contradictory statements to use as ammunition for cross-examination. This particular citation would have been better had it listed the year and edition of Campbell's instead of saying the "current edition."

**Defending the Report As Written:** Examiners should be ready, willing, and able to support their opinions, especially when they are being cross-examined. Skillful counsel, by carefully choosing her questions, can try to make the examiner seem to leave a false impression with the fact finder or jury. Experienced examiners see through this strategy and do not let this happen.

**Q.** You didn't quote that or any of the other statements that didn't support your opinion, did you?
**A.** Counsel, you choose 17 words out of the 200,000-word text to attack my testimony. The portion I quoted is the gold standard on this issue. The 17 words you chose describe an extremely rare exception. As to alleged other statements in the text that are contrary to my opinions, I don't believe there are any. If there are, I would like to see them.

## 9.6 Authoritative

An examiner should not use the words "authoritative," "reliable authority," and the like to describe any resources the examiner relied upon in forming her opinion. These terms may have a special legal significance under the Federal Rules of Evidence. Under the Federal Rules (and many state rules), examiners may be cross-examined on any work that has been established as a reliable authority by expert testimony.[3]

---

[2] See *Daubert v. Merrell Dow Pharmaceuticals, Inc.,* 509 U.S. 579, 113 S.Ct.2786 125 L.E.2d 469 (1993); *General Electric Co. v. Joiner,* 522 U.S. 136, 118 S.Ct. 512, 517, 139 L.E.2d 508 (1977); and *Kumho Tire Co. Limited v. Carmichael,* 526 U.S. 137, 119 S.Ct. 1167, 143 L.E. 2d 238 (1999).

[3] "The following are not excluded by the hearsay rule, even though the declarant is available as a witness. **Learned Treatises.** To the extent called to the attention of an expert witness upon cross-examination or relied upon by the expert witness in direct examination, statements contained in published treatises, periodicals, or pamphlets on a subject of history, medicine, or other science or art, established as a reliable authority by the testimony or admission of the witness or by other expert testimony

**Example 9.61: "Recognized to be authoritative"**

*Report States:*

> Attached as Exhibit L are excerpts from Demeter's *Disability Evaluation.* This text is recognized to be authoritative in the field of disability evaluation and is used by many disability evaluating physicians in the United States.

*Resulting Cross-examination:*

**Q.** In your report you relied upon the Demeter *Disability* text, did you not?
**A.** Yes.
**Q.** You state in your report that this text is "recognized to be authoritative in the field of disability evaluation," is that correct?
**A.** Yes.
**Q.** Is this the book?
**A.** Yes.
**Q.** I direct your attention to page 274, third paragraph.

**Comment:** Calling the text that was relied upon "authoritative" was an engraved invitation by the examiner to be cross-examined on the text. The examiner may have been better served by omitting the "authoritative" language:

> In forming my opinion, I used, in part, *Disability Evaluation* written by Demeter. Particularly relevant portions of this text are attached to this report as Exhibit L.

**Defending the Report As Written:** Examiners need to be fully versed in any text they cite in their report as being authoritative. Examiners who know more about the text than the lawyer cross-examining them are in the best position to defend their reports and opinions.

**Q.** I direct your attention to page 274, third paragraph.
**A.** Counsel, you are referring to the old edition of Demeter. My report references the 2003 edition, which is the most current and up-to-date edition.

## 9.7 American Board of Independent Medical Examiners Guidelines

The American Board of Independent Medical Examiners has promulgated Guidelines for the Conduct of IMEs and the preparation of IME reports. Some examiners state that they followed the ABIME Guidelines. This can be helpful. Once the examiner cites the ABIME Guidelines, however, he needs to be prepared for questioning about those Guidelines.

**Example 9.71: Exam conducted according to Guidelines**

*Report States:*

> The exam was conducted according to the American Board of Independent Medical Examiners Guidelines of Conduct.

---

or by judicial notice. If admitted, the statements may be read into evidence, but may not be received as exhibits." Federal Rule of Evidence 803(18).

*Resulting Cross-examination:*
**Q.** Doctor, you say on page 2 of your IME report that, "The exam was conducted according to the American Board of Independent Examiners Guidelines of Conduct," correct?
**A.** Yes, exactly.
**Q.** Can you tell me how many ABIME Guidelines of Conduct there are, Doctor?
**A.** I don't have them memorized. I know there is one about introducing yourself to the examinee.
**Q.** Did you follow the six actions the Guidelines call for the IME doctor to do at the medical examination?
**A.** Well, again, it's hard for me to remember exactly what's listed in the Guidelines.
**Q.** Doctor, how can you swear under oath that you followed the Guidelines of Conduct if you don't know what they are?

**Comment:** The examiner in the above example let himself be bullied unnecessarily by opposing counsel. There was nothing wrong with his report referencing the ABIME Guidelines of Conduct. The doctor could have and should have consulted his ABIME directory as a reference to reply to the question. IME physicians are not expected to memorize documents such as the ABIME Guidelines.

**Defending the Report As Written:**
**Q.** Can you name the Guidelines that you say you followed?
**A.** (Doctor takes out ABIME directory) I am referencing the latest edition of the ABIME directory. I have incorporated the following Guidelines of Conduct into my IME practice and follow them in each IME. The Guidelines of Conduct are:

> Each physician certified by the American Board of Independent Medical Examiners (ABIME) must agree to comply with these guidelines of conduct:
>
> Physicians shall:
>
> 1. Be honest in all communications.
> 2. Respect the rights of the examinees and other participants, and treat these individuals with dignity and respect.
> 3. At the medical examination:
>     a. Introduce himself/herself to the examinee as the examining physician
>     b. Advise the examinee they are seeing him/her for an independent medical examination, and the information provided will be used in the assessment and presented in a report
>     c. Provide the examinee with the name of the party requesting the examination
>     d. Advise the examinee that no treating physician-patient relationship will be established

e. Explain the examination procedure
f. Provide adequate draping and privacy if the examinee needs to remove clothing for the examination
g. Refrain from derogatory comments, and
h. Close the examination by telling the examinee that the examination is over and ask if there is further information the examinee would like to add

4. Reach conclusions that are based on facts and sound medical knowledge and for which the independent medical examiner has adequate qualifications to address
5. Be prepared to address conflict in a professional and constructive manner
6. Never accept a fee for services which are dependent upon writing a report favorable to the referral service and maintain confidentiality consistent with the applicable legal jurisdiction.

# Chapter 10 Stating Opinions and Conclusions in a Defensible Manner

## 10.1 Executive Summary

One of the main reasons an examiner is involved in a case is to draft a report stating her opinion. The examiner's opinion should be communicated effectively and should be expressed in a defensible manner. The authors recommend the following.

- State all opinions clearly, explicitly, and with confidence.
- Use the magic words "based upon a reasonable degree of medical certainty" or "based on a reasonable degree of medical probability" when expressing the opinion in the report.
- Avoid hedge words, such as "it seems," "I think," and "I believe" when expressing opinions in the IME report.
- State the reasons that justify the opinion, preferably in concise, bullet-point format.
- Avoid expressing net opinions; that is, bare conclusions without supporting justification.
- State all of the opinions the examiner expects to express at hearing or trial.
- Document a detailed and reliable reasoning so that the report will not be challenged under *Daubert.*
- Prepare a list of the examinee's clinical diagnoses, including any need for further evaluation. For each diagnosis, indicate, where appropriate, which are acute, which are chronic or degenerative, and which are pre-existing.
- Carefully analyze the current diagnoses, the mechanism of injury, the diagnoses at the time of injury, the pre-existing status, and the clinical history to determine whether the injury was pre-existing or caused by an event or occurrence that is not a subject of the claim. The examiner's analysis and conclusions regarding causation need to be clearly documented in the report.
- State objective, supportive reasons for apportionment opinions.
- Properly use the terms "aggravation" and "exacerbation" and understand their legal significance in the jurisdiction in question.
- Provide objective justification for prognosis opinions and refrain from making extraneous comments about the examinee.
- Understand the meaning of maximum medical improvement in the jurisdiction in question. The term needs to be properly used and the examiner's written opinion needs to be accompanied by the reasons supporting it.

- Express permanent impairment ratings correctly using the correct edition of the appropriate guidelines and by documenting precisely how the rating was calculated. If needed, the examiner should obtain training on conducting impairment ratings.
- Only opine on work capacity and disability when the examiner has sufficient information to do so. Where opinions are made in this area, the examiner should have a thorough understanding of the examinee's job and correctly use terms from the *Dictionary of Occupational Titles*.
- Be careful when commenting on appropriateness of past care.
- Do not take "pot shots" at other providers or disciplines.
- Avoid, in most cases, using the terms "fraud" and "malingering."
- Document symptom magnification or lack of objective support for the examinee's subjective complaints with non-inflammatory language and specific evidence.
- Be prepared for questions concerning the examinee's pain and questions accusing the examiner of trying to "trick" the examinee with distraction tests.

## 10.2 State Opinions Clearly and with Confidence

One of the main reasons an IME report is prepared is so that the medical expert can express her medical opinions. These opinions should be stated clearly, explicitly, and confidently. It is best to avoid the passive tense.

For expert opinions to be admissible in most civil cases, the expert generally must believe that it is more likely than not that her opinion is correct (51% or more certainty). There are "magic words" that are commonly accepted as expressing the idea that the expert is 51% or more certain of her opinion. These include the expressions "based upon a reasonable degree of medical certainty" and "based on a reasonable degree of medical probability." It is good practice to use one of these phrases when stating an expert opinion in an IME report.

Hedge words, such as "it seems," "I think," and "I believe," should be avoided. Such words suggest that the examiner does not have confidence in her opinion. Failure to state opinions clearly and with confidence will make the report and opinion vulnerable to attack on cross-examination and could possibly result in the report being stricken by the judge or hearing officer. Where opinions are not stated clearly in the IME report, the examiner should be prepared to express them clearly during testimony. Please consider the following examples.

**Example 10.21: Overly vague opinion insufficient**
*Piascyk v. City of New Haven,* 64 F. Supp2d.19 (D.Conn. 1999)
This case dealt with an ADA case filed by a police officer. The expert report was written by a physician, Shine. In support of the plaintiff's claim that he was substantially limited with regard to carrying, the plaintiff offered only Dr.

Shine's statement in his report to the New Haven Workers' Compensation Division that the plaintiff would have difficulty "carrying heavy loads...." The court rejected the indefinite language "carrying heavy loads" and stated:

> This statement is too vague to support a finding that plaintiff is significantly restricted in his ability to carry compared to the average person. *See Colwell,* 158 F.3d at 644 (testimony that plaintiff could not lift "very heavy objects" did not support a finding of substantial limitation). At 29.

**Example 10.22: Failure to state opinion confidently: "Cannot be ruled out"**
*Report States:*

> Therefore, based upon the foregoing and to a reasonable degree of medical certainty, it is my opinion that the 2/8/2003 workplace accident cannot be ruled out as a possible aggravation of the examinee's multiple sclerosis.

*Resulting Cross-examination:*

**Q.** So, your opinion is that the workplace accident aggravated Ms. Jones's multiple sclerosis?
**A.** No, that's not what I said.
**Q.** You qualified your opinion, correct?
**A.** Yes.
**Q.** In fact, you used three qualifiers in your opinion?
**A.** Three?
**Q.** A reasonable degree of medical certainty would be what expressed in a percentage form?
**A.** 51 percent.
**Q.** Your use of the term "possible" indicates less than 51% certainty, correct?
**A.** Yes.
**Q.** And the phrase "cannot be ruled out" indicates even less certainty.
**A.** That's true.
**Q.** Would it be fair to say that there were several potential causes of the MS?
**A.** Yes.
**Q.** In fact, how many potential causes of the MS could you "not rule out"?
**A.** Approximately seven.
**Q.** You're not even certain about this, sir?
**A.** Well, there are various degrees of certainty.
**Q.** Would it be fair to say that you cannot truthfully testify with a reasonable degree of medical certainty as to what in fact aggravated the MS?
**A.** Yes, that's true.

**Comment:** Not only is this opinion highly vulnerable to cross-examination, the opinion may also be vulnerable to legal challenges.

> Therefore, based upon the foregoing and to a reasonable degree of medical certainty, it is my opinion that the 2/8/2003 workplace accident aggravated the examinee's multiple sclerosis.

**Defending the Report As Written:** When opposing counsel gets on a "roll" during cross-examination, the experienced examiner waits for an opportunity to break the momentum and reinforce his report and opinion.

**Q.** Would it be fair to say that there were several potential causes of the MS?
**A.** The underlying etiology of multiple sclerosis generally is unknown. In this case, where the examinee had no symptoms whatsoever prior to the work accident, the workplace accident either aggravated or precipitated the MS in the examinee. That is the opinion I hold to a reasonable degree of medical certainty.

**Example 10.23: "It would seem to me" language takes away from opinion**
*Report States:*

> It would seem to me, therefore, that the treatment rendered from August 31, 1998, to present was not reasonable or necessary.

*Resulting Cross-examination:*
**Q.** Are you certain that the treatment rendered from August 31, 1998, to present was not reasonable or necessary?
**A.** Yes.
**Q.** Sir, how old are you?
**A.** 53, but I don't see how that is relevant, Counselor.
**Q.** Why didn't you say *"it would seem to me* I am 53 years old"?
**A.** Because I know precisely how old I am.
**Q.** As opposed to your opinion on the reasonableness of the treatment when you said, "it seems to me it was not reasonable or necessary"?

**Comment:** The weight the examiner's opinion will be given is greatly lessened by his inclusion of the "it would seem to me" language. This language suggests uncertainty. This IME report would most likely be given more weight had the examiner used confident language to express his opinion:

> It is my opinion, based upon a reasonable degree of medical certainty, that the treatment rendered from August 31, 1998, to present was neither reasonable nor necessary. I base this opinion on the following:
> 1. (state the fact)
> 2. (state the fact)

**Defending the Report As Written:** When opposing counsel is afraid to question a medical report or opinion, he may resort to "word games" to aggravate or fluster the examiner. Counsel's goal is to pressure the examiner into making a mistake. Experienced examiners stay cool, calm, and collected.

**Q.** Why didn't you say *"it would seem to me* I am 53 years old"?
**A.** I see, Counsel, we're playing lawyers' word games. Anytime you want to discuss the medical portion of the case, please let me know.

**Example 10.24: "I do not think" language lessens weight report will be given**
*Report States:*

> I do not think that the revision of the total knee arthroplasties that took place following his accident of 2/7/02 was necessitated by the accident itself.

**Comment:** This report would have been far better had it used more confident language:

> It is my opinion, based upon a reasonable degree of medical certainty, that the revision of the total knee arthroplasties that took place following his accident of 2/7/02 was necessitated by the accident itself. I base this opinion on the following reasons.
> 1. …

**Example 10.25: "I do not believe" language lessens weight report will be given**

*Report States:*

> I do not believe that the laminectomies at T5–T6 caused any significant increase in Mr. Collins's complaints.

**Comment:** The "I do not believe" language takes away from the examiner's opinion.

> It is my opinion, based upon a reasonable degree of medical certainty, that the laminectomies at T5-T6 did not cause any significant increase in Mr. Collins's complaints. I base this opinion on the following reasons:
> 1. …

**Example 10.26: "The following conclusions can be made"**

*Report States:*

> Based on the foregoing, and to a reasonable degree of medical certainty, the following conclusions can be made.

**Comment:** This examiner's conclusions would be more persuasive if the "can be made" language was replaced with more confident language.

> Based on the foregoing, and to a reasonable degree of medical certainty, I reach the following conclusions:
> 1. …

**Example 10.27: "It can be argued": Expert now an advocate?**

*Report States:*

> Thus, it can be argued that the vast majority of the treatment received to date was not necessary.

*Resulting Cross-examination:*

**Q.** You testified that "it can be argued that the vast majority of the treatment received to date was not necessary"?

**A.** Correct.

**Q.** It could also be argued that the treatment was necessary, correct?

**A.** Yes.

**Q.** Thank you, no further questions.

**Comment:** The "it can be argued" language should not have been used. This language may make the examiner either appear to be an advocate or unsure of herself. Better language follows.

> It is my opinion, based upon a reasonable degree of medical certainty, that most of the treatment received to date has not been medically appropriate.

**Defending the Report As Written:** Examiners may need to push back against counsel to help clarify opinions stated with less than complete confidence in their IME reports.

**Q.** It could also be argued that the treatment was necessary, correct?
**A.** In the same way that it can be argued that the moon is made of cheese, yes. This treatment was not necessary.

**Example 10.28: Indefinite opinion**
*Report States:*

> It would be my opinion that the examinee did incur a back injury as a result of his 9/19/2002 accident.

*Resulting Cross-examination:*
**Q.** As I understand it, you have a conditional opinion in this case, Doctor?
**A.** I don't follow you, Counselor.
**Q.** You said in your report, "It would be my opinion that the examinee did incur a back injury as a result of his 9/19/2002 accident," correct?
**A.** Yes.
**Q.** It would be your opinion if what, Doctor?
**A.** That's just an expression. I meant it is my opinion.
**Q.** That's not what your report actually says, correct?
**A.** That's what I clearly meant.
**Q.** Clear to whom, Doctor?
**A.** Any reasonable person.
**Q.** Would you agree that it would have been more precise and accurate to say, "It is my opinion" if that's what you meant?
**A.** Yes.
**Q.** In the future, Doctor, will you make this mistake again?

**Comment:** Examiners are best served by stating their opinions in a simple and direct fashion.

> It is my opinion based upon a reasonable degree of medical certainty that the examinee did incur a back injury as a result of his 9/19/2002 accident.

Examiners who state their opinions in a conditional or oblique manner may be forced to explain their formulation.

**Defending the Report As Written:** Examiners will frequently be faced with opposing counsel picking apart words or phrases in their lengthy and detailed IME reports. Counsel here is trying to get the examiner mad, to admit to a mistake, or to create confusion or ambiguities where there really aren't any. Keeping in mind that the fact finder in most of the cases will be an experienced administrative law judge, physicians can, when appropriate, put counsel in his place.

**Q.** That's not what your report actually says, correct?
**A.** My opinion is that the examinee did incur a back injury as a result of his 9/19/2002 accident. I don't think Her Honor is interested in your word games. I am interested in a search for truth, not whether you can look at a 7-page single-spaced medical report and waste everyone's time trying to create ambiguities where there are none.

**Example 10.29: Opinion that states nothing**
*Report States:*

> Based on my examination today, I would feel he is cleared for return to any type of work that he is fit for.

*Resulting Cross-examination:*
**Q.** Doctor, you stated in your IME report the opinion that, "based on my examination today, I would feel he is cleared for return to any type of work that he is fit for," correct?
**A.** Yes.
**Q.** Do you offer any other opinions on his ability to return to work in your report?
**A.** No.
**Q.** Thank you, Doctor. No further questions.

**Comment:** The examiner in the above example has offered an opinion that does not address the issues of disability or return to work. If he was attempting to opine that the claimant was able to return to work, he was unsuccessful. The opinion as written and offered is legally insufficient to sustain the burden of proof or going forward. The physician would have been better served with an opinion expressed more clearly and directly.

> Based upon my review of the medical records, the history, and the job description (appended), it is my opinion that the claimant has no restrictions on bending, lifting, and twisting, and can return to his job as a billiard mechanic.

**Defending the Report As Written:** IME physicians may be forced to use findings not expressed in the formal opinion paragraph of their reports to explain their findings.

**Q.** Do you offer any other opinions on his ability to return to work in your report?
**A.** Yes. On page 1, I stated his diagnosis was a healed fracture compression type, minimal T8, and that I found no evidence of neurological difficulties. On page 2, I stated he had a full range of motion cervical and thoracic spine with no

pain. That's why I released him to return to his normal work as a billiard mechanic.

**Example 10.210: Unintelligible opinion**
*Report States:*

> It is my medical opinion based upon reasonable medical degree of certainty, that no further orthopedic care is not indicated and will provide no benefit to this patient.

*Resulting Cross-examination:*
**Q.** Doctor, is your opinion that the examinee needs or doesn't need further orthopedic care?
**A.** I said quite clearly that it is not indicated, Counsel.
**Q.** What you actually said, Doctor, is that, "It is my medical opinion based upon reasonable medical degree of certainty, that no further orthopedic care is not indicated and will provide no benefit to this patient." Is that what your IME report says?
**A.** Yes, exactly.
**Q.** This claimant is not your patient, correct?
**A.** Yes.
**Q.** So, when you said "patient," you meant "claimant"?
**A.** Yes.
**Q.** That was a mistake?
**A.** Well, I said "patient," not "my patient," so technically you could say it was not a mistake.
**Q.** When you said, "no further orthopedic care is not indicated," you meant no further care is indicated?
**A.** Yes.
**Q.** Was that a double negative mistake?
**A.** Well, it was poorly worded.
**Q.** When you then made it a triple negative by then saying, "and will provide no benefit to this patient," was that a mistake or done intentionally to confuse the fact finder?

**Comment:** The examiner in the above example worded his opinion so poorly that it was unintelligible. He then compounded this error by refusing to admit he made any mistakes. His failure to admit the obvious errors further eroded his credibility. The examiner would have been better served with a simple declarative sentence.

> It is my opinion based upon a reasonable degree of medical certainty that further orthopedic care is not indicated because the care will provide no benefit for this claimant.

**Defending the Report As Written:** When faced with an obvious mistake, the examiner should graciously admit the mistake. This technique makes the physician appear humble, human, honest, and, in most cases, it forces opposing counsel to move on.

**Q.** Doctor, is your opinion that the examinee needs or doesn't need further orthopedic care?
**A.** I am sorry for the mistake and lack of clarity. Further orthopedic care is not indicated as the care will provide no benefit for this claimant.

**Example 10.211: Legally insufficient opinion**
*Report States:*

> Causation: The aforementioned diagnoses and their causes are stated on a more probable than not basis, where possible, but must be qualified by adding that most of the former are based primarily, if not exclusively, upon subjective complaints and/or physical findings which can neither be confirmed nor denied.

*Resulting Cross-examination:*
**Q.** Doctor, you arrived at 10 different diagnoses in your IME report, correct?
**A.** Yes.
**Q.** Your opinion on these diagnoses is stated as more probable than not for some of the 10, correct?
**A.** That's not exactly what I said in my report, Counsel.
**Q.** What you said exactly in your report is that, "Causation: The aforementioned diagnoses and their causes are stated on a more probable than not basis, where possible, but must be qualified by adding that most of the former are based primarily, if not exclusively, upon subjective complaints and/or physical findings which can neither be confirmed nor denied," correct?
**A.** That's what I said, yes.
**Q.** In your 17-page, single-spaced report, did you anywhere indicate which one(s) of the 10 are stated on a more probable than not basis?
**A.** Not in those words.
**Q.** That is a no, Doctor?
**A.** Correct.
**Q.** Let's go through each of the 10, Doctor, and have you tell us, if you can, which are stated on a more probable than not basis, which are merely possible, and which ones you can't say with any reasonable degree of certainty.

**Comment:** The opinion in the above example is legally insufficient because it does not indicate which diagnoses and causes are stated on a more probable than not basis. The examiner would have been better served by restricting his opinions to ones that can be given on a more probable than not basis.

**Defending the Report As Written:** Just because an IME report or a portion thereof is not perfectly written does not mean it cannot be properly defended. The examiner who keeps his cool and responds truthfully but artfully can often salvage a poorly worded report.

**Q.** Let's go through each of the 10, Doctor, and have you tell us, if you can, which are stated on a more probable than not basis, which are merely possible, and which ones you can't say with any reasonable degree of certainty.
**A.** OK. On a <u>more probable than not basis</u> are numbers 2 and 3.
#2 Lumbar sprain/strain caused by the motor vehicle accident.

> #3 Symptom magnification and abnormal pain behavior related to psychosocial factors including depression and anxiety.

The remaining diagnoses and causes cannot be stated with a reasonable degree of medical certainty due to the examinee's poor memory and historical inconsistencies.

**Example 10.212: "A reasonable cause"**

*Report States:*

> It is not clear precisely what caused the patient's injury, but his description today of the juggling/balancing of multiple pieces of tile that occurred as a result of the event he attributes to this injury is a reasonable cause for a cervical disc to be herniated.

*Resulting Cross-examination:*

**Q.** Doctor, you were asked to render an opinion as to whether the examinee's cervical disc herniation was work related, correct?

**A.** I was and I did.

**Q.** What you said in your IME report about the cervical disc herniation was, "It is not clear precisely what caused the patient's injury, but his description today of the juggling/balancing of multiple pieces of tile that occurred as a result of the event he attributes to this injury is a reasonable cause for a cervical disc to be herniated"?

**A.** Yes, that's what I wrote.

**Q.** So, the cause of the disc herniation is not clear?

**A.** That's correct, but the balancing of the tile could have caused the disc to become herniated.

**Q.** It is just one of a series of reasonable causes for the cervical disc to have herniated?

**A.** Yes, it is.

**Q.** As you sit here today, under oath, can you say with a reasonable degree of certainty that the incident recounted by the examinee actually caused his cervical disc to become herniated?

**A.** That would be difficult to say.

**Q.** Thank you, Doctor.

**Comment:** An examiner who intends to express an opinion on causation should do so in a legally sufficient manner. In addition, prefacing an opinion on causation with the phrase, "It is not clear precisely what caused the patient's injury," makes the opinion even less defensible. The opinion, whatever the physician decides it is, should be stated simply and directly.

> Based upon the available information to a reasonable degree of medical certainty, there is (is not) probable causal relationship between the balancing incident at work described above and the examinee's herniation of his cervical disc.

**Defending the Report As Written:** Examiners can expound on their written reports to explain any ambiguities. Even when the report is not clear or is legally insufficient, the physician should be prepared to clarify what he meant.

**Q.** So, the cause of the disc herniation is not clear?
**A.** It is not clear from the file. However, given the history of the examinee, which is consistent with two eyewitness statements, and the history in the ER record, it is my medical opinion expressed to a reasonable degree of certainty that the herniated cervical disc is causally related to the tile incident at work.

**Example 10.213: "Certain degree of medical certainty"**
*Report States:*

> With a certain degree of medical certainty, it appears that this examinee had pre-existing osteoarthritis of his lumbosacral spine in 1999.

*Resulting Cross-examination:*
**Q.** Doctor, you expressed your opinion in the IME report that the examinee had pre-existing osteoarthritis in 1999?
**A.** That's correct.
**Q.** Your opinion is based upon a certain degree of medical certainty?
**A.** Yes, it is.
**Q.** Thank you, Doctor.

**Comment:** An examiner performing IMEs and writing IME reports should be familiar with the "magic words" that have been held to be legally sufficient in her jurisdiction. A medical opinion is usually best expressed as:

- Based on a reasonable degree of medical certainty…
- Based on a reasonable degree of medical probability…
- On a more probable than not basis…
- On a more likely than not basis…

When an examiner fails to use one of the traditional sets of "magic words," her opinion and report are likely to come under attack. The test of whether a physician's report and testimony are admissible will be determined by the judge after he looks at the entire substance of the testimony. Examiners are best served by expressing their opinions in a way that clearly communicates that they are based upon a reasonable degree of probability and not just mere possibility.

> With a reasonable degree of medical certainty, this examinee had pre-existing osteoarthritis of his lumbosacral spine in 1999.

**Defending the Report As Written:** When the examiner notices a mistake or a poor choice of words in her report, she should endeavor to clarify and explain at the first opportunity.

**Q.** Your opinion is based upon a certain degree of medical certainty?
**A.** Based on a reasonable degree of medical certainty. That is a mistake in my report. My apologies.

**Example 10.214: Vague report cannot support finding for plaintiff**
*Piascyk v. City of New Haven*, 64 F.Supp.2d 19 (D.Conn. 1999)
The court dealt with an ADA case filed by a police officer. The expert report was written by a physician, Shine.

> In support of his claim that he is substantially limited with regard to carrying, plaintiff has offered only Dr. Shine's statement in his report to the New Haven Workers' Compensation Division that plaintiff would have difficulty "carrying heavy loads...." (Shine Report, Plaintiff's Exhibit 11.) At 29.

The court rejected the indefinite language "carrying heavy loads" and stated:

> This statement is too vague to support a finding that plaintiff is significantly restricted in his ability to carry compared to the average person. *See Colwell,* 158 F.3d at 644 (testimony that plaintiff could not lift "very heavy objects" did not support a finding of substantial limitation). At 29.

**Comment:** The courts continue to reject reports where the expert's opinion is expressed vaguely, equivocally, or with insufficient certainty or clarity.

## 10.3 State Reasons for Opinions

The opinions expressed in the IME report should be supported with the reasons that justify them. This will significantly increase the weight that will likely be given to the examiner's report and opinions. If possible, the supporting reasons should be listed as a concise bullet-point or numbered list.

**Example 10.31: Reasons to support opinions provided in numbered list**
*Report States:*

> It is my opinion, based upon a reasonable degree of medical certainty, that the motor vehicle accident of 3-6-03 is not causally related to the examinee's current complaints of neck pain. I base this on the following:
>
> 1. Evidence of pre-existing injury. The medical records from Dr. Thanning clearly document unresolved neck pain prior to 3-6-03.
> 2. Mechanism of injury. The examinee stated that he was sitting in his Lincoln Town Car in a parking lot when it was bumped by a shopping cart being pushed by an employee of the supermarket. The incident as described is not likely to have caused the alleged injury.
> 3. Imaging studies. All are negative.
> 4. Physical examination. Positive for symptom magnification.
> 5. History of pain provided by the examinee. This was consistently nonspecific and consisted of non-physiological pain distribution.

**Comment:** The examiner's conclusions in this report are made more persuasive by the expert's inclusion of the reasons for his opinion. The numbered list also makes the report easy to read and even more persuasive.

**Example 10.32: Reasons to support opinion stated**
*Report States:*

> The claimant sustained severe closed head injury with persistent cognitive defects and post-traumatic seizure disorder. The symptoms are all causally related to the claimant's last accident on June 14, 2003. The reason they are causally related are that the claimant sustained a head injury in the past. However, he never had any seizures as a result of any prior injury. Of note, one week following this last injury he suffered on the aircraft he did sustain seizures and they were poorly controlled.

**Comment:** The examiner's conclusions in this report are made more persuasive by the examiner's inclusion of the reasons for her opinion.

## 10.4 Conclusory or "Net" Opinions

Examiners need to state the reasons that support their opinions. Failure to state reasons for the examiner's expert opinion makes the IME report less credible and may make it particularly vulnerable to legal challenges. "An expert's report which offers only a bare conclusion—nothing more than a bottom line—is insufficient to prove the expert's point."[1] This is what is known as a *net opinion*. Net opinions are usually inadmissible. Even if they are held to be admissible, a net opinion can be easily challenged on cross-examination.

**Example 10.41: Overly vague opinion insufficient**
*Ohime v. Foresman,* 186 F.R.D. 507 (N.D.Ind. 1999)
In this case, the proffered report of a psychiatric social worker, Nott, was found to be deficient. The court stated:

> Mr. Nott's second report still is deficient under Rule 26(a)(2)(B). The report states a summary of Ms. Ohime's two meetings with Mr. Nott (arguably the data or other information on which Mr. Nott relied in making his report), but it contains only a three-sentence paragraph of vague conclusions as to his expert opinion of Ms. Ohime's condition. These conclusory determinations are insufficient under Rule 26(1).

**Example 10.42: Overly vague opinion insufficient**
*Hemmen v. Atlantic City Medical Center,* 758 A.2d 1145 (N.J.Super.L. 1999)
This was a medical malpractice case. The court found the expert's report an inadmissible net opinion and stated:

> I recognize that the expert may have been reporting that the medical community understands that of the cases of drug induced sciatic nerve damage, negligence is the most frequent cause. Such a report, however, must rest upon the expert's experience or upon textual support. *Connors v. University Associates*, 769 F.*Supp.* 578, 587 (D.Vt.1991) *aff'd* 4 *F.*3d 123 (2d Cir.1993). In the absence of such a basis, the

---

[1] *SMS Systems Maintenance Services v. Digital Equipment Corporation*, 188 F.3rd11 24 (1999).

> opinion of the relative frequency of negligent and non-negligently caused damage would be an inadmissible net opinion, bereft of any factual underpinning.

### Example 10.43: One-page conclusory report insufficient under Rule 26(a)(2)B

*Bank Brussels Lambert v. Credit Lyonnais,* 2000 WL 1762533 (S.D.N.Y. 2000)
The court stated:

> The Perkins Report is a one page report that states a conclusion and offers no support for it. While it states that the conclusion is based on the "review of the brokers' reports and borrowing base reports" it does not explain the rationale that led to the conclusion nor does it set forth the testimony that will be provided at trial. As a result, the amount of information provided in the Perkins Report is not sufficient under Rule 26(a)(2)(B). Further, the Perkins Report fails to state that it is responding to the Boothman Sherwin Report.

### Example 10.44: Conclusory report inadmissible in Texas medical malpractice case

*Hart v. Wright,* 16 S.W.3rd 872 (Tex.App.-Fort Worth 2000)
This was a Texas medical malpractice case. The Medical Liability and Insurance Improvement Act contains expert report writing standards and was enacted to curtail frivolous claims against physicians and related healthcare providers.[2] The court dealt with and rejected a written report in affidavit form.

> An expert report is defined as any report written by an expert that provides a fair summary of the expert's opinions as of the date of the report regarding: (1) the applicable standard of care; (2) the manner in which the care rendered by defendant failed to meet the standard of care; and (3) the causal relationship between that failure and the injury, harm, or damages claimed.
>
> Appellants offered this written report of Dr. Maewal in affidavit form to comply with their obligation under the Act:
>
>> My name is Hrishi K. Maewal. I am over the age of majority. I have never been convicted of a felony or a crime of moral turpitude, and I am in all things qualified to make this affidavit.
>>
>> I am a physician licensed to practice medicine in the State of Texas.
>>
>> I am currently practicing medicine and was practicing medicine on January 22, 1996.
>>
>> I am board certified in Internal Medicine, Pulmonary Disease, Cardiology, and Critical Care Medicine.
>>
>> I examined Bobby Hart at Harris Methodist Fort Worth Hospital on January 23, 1996.
>>
>> Based on the history obtained from the patient and his family members along with the supporting evidence of laboratory evaluation which showed an elevated creatine kinase of 1854 U/L, CK-MB 219.7 ng/ml and % relative index 11.9 at 10:41 a.m. along with an EKG which shows an inferior infarction with Q-waves, in my expert opinion, Mr. Hart was experiencing an acute myocardial infarction at approximately 5:00 p.m. on January 22, 1996 while a patient in the emergency room at Huguley Memorial Hospital.

[2] Tex. Rev. Civ. Stat. Ann. Art. 49501 Sec. 13.01(d)1.

> Based on the above analysis, Dr. Wright, the treating physician at Huguley Memorial Hospital, and Huguley Memorial Hospital departed from the acceptable standard of care for the diagnosis, medical care, and treatment of a patient with an acute myocardial infarction.

Appellants argue that even though Dr. Maewal's report does not include all of the information required by section 13.01(r)(6), it nonetheless satisfies the definition of an expert report. We disagree because Dr. Maewal's report does not address a standard of care, deviation from that standard, or that a deviation from the standard caused injury or damages. *See id.* The report merely concludes that Mr. Hart demonstrated signs and symptoms of a heart attack at a time and place with which Dr. Maewal had no connection. For Dr. Maewal to qualify as an expert, the report had to show that he had knowledge of the accepted standards of care for the diagnosis, care and treatment of the injury involved, how the applicable standard was breached, and how the alleged breach contributed to Appellants' injuries or damages. *See id.* §§ 13.01(r)(5), (6). While a party need not marshal all its proof, a good faith effort in preparing an expert report must, at a minimum, attempt to incorporate the three requirements found in section 13.01(r)(6). Here, the conclusory report is not the good faith effort required by the statute. We overrule issue one. At 876, 877.

**Example 10.45: No reasons stated for this conclusion**
*Report States:*

Care by paramedics and intermediate EMS staff was appropriate.

*Resulting Cross-examination*:
**Q.** Your conclusion in your report is that care by the paramedics and EMS staff was appropriate?
**A.** Yes.
**Q.** Where in your report do you explain your reasoning and provide facts and the scientific rationale for this conclusion?
**A.** It's not in there.
**Q.** So, you are asking this jury to just accept this naked conclusion without any basis in fact or science?

**Comment:** Conclusions without supporting reasoning are not persuasive. Conclusions should always be supported with reasoning.

> Care by paramedics and intermediate EMS staff was appropriate. I base this conclusion on the following...

**Defending the Report As Written:** Just because reasons were not explicitly stated in the report does not mean that the examiner did not have valid reasons for his opinion.

**Q.** Where in your report do you explain your reasoning and provide facts and the scientific rationale for this conclusion?
**A.** It's implied. The care was appropriate because nothing they did or failed to do was inappropriate. Would you like me to explain further?

## 10.5 State All Opinions to Which the Expert Will Testify

The IME report should contain all of the opinions the examiner expects to express at deposition, hearing, or trial. Failure to include all opinions may result in the preclusion of the examiner from offering at hearing or trial the opinions that were not included in the examiner's report. Failure to include all opinions may also be a subject of pointed cross-examination. Counsel may try to show that the examiner's report is incomplete or that the examiner intentionally withheld information.

**Example 10.51: Some opinions omitted from report**
*Report States:*
This letter contains some of my opinions in the above-referenced matter.

*Resulting Cross-examination:*
**Q.** You do have other opinions on this case that were not contained in your letter, correct?
**A.** Yes.
**Q.** Why did you omit these opinions?
**A.** I was asked to.
**Q.** By counsel who retained you?
**A.** Yes.
**Q.** This was after you shared these opinions with her?
**A.** Well...yes.
**Q.** So, these opinions are ones you and counsel decided should not be shared with Her Honor and the members of the jury?
**A.** I was just....
**Q.** Following orders?
**A.** Completing my assignment.
**Q.** Let's go through these opinions and see why it was decided that they should not be shared with the hearing officer.

**Comment:** This language should be avoided because it can be made to appear as though the examiner is intentionally withholding some of his opinions.

**Defending the Report As Written:** There may be many reasons that examiners do not express all of their opinions in their IME reports. These include:

- being asked to comment on only one or more issues,
- some issues in the case have already been decided, and
- instructions from the judge.

There is no need to be apologetic for only expressing the opinions requested.

**Q.** You do have other opinions on this case that were not contained in your letter, correct?
**A.** I was only asked to express an opinion on one issue and that is what I did. Before expressing any other opinions, I would have to review all of the records again and may need to perform another physical examination.

## 10.6 Documenting a Reliable Methodology

Examiners should be aware that their reports may be closely scrutinized under the *Daubert* doctrine to see if the reasoning stated by the examiner is reliable. (See *Daubert v. Merrell Dow Pharmaceuticals, Inc.,* 509 U.S. 579, 113 S.Ct.2786 125 L.E.2d 469 (1993); *General Electric Co. v. Joiner,* 522 U.S. 136, 118 S.Ct. 512, 517, 139 L.E.2d 508 (1977); and *Kumho Tire Co. Limited v. Carmichael,* 526 U.S. 137, 119 S.Ct. 1167, 143 L.E. 2d 238 (1999).) Under the *Daubert* line of cases, the judge in federal court and many other jurisdictions will act as a gatekeeper to screen out and exclude unreliable expert testimony and reports. The judge will consider several factors, including the following.

1. Whether the theory or technique used by the expert can be, and has been, tested.
2. Whether the theory or technique has been subjected to peer review and publication.
3. The known or potential rate of error of the method used.
4. The degree of the method's or conclusion's acceptance within the relevant scientific community.

An expert report will survive *Daubert* challenges if the report is based upon reliable methodology and if this methodology is spelled-out clearly in the report. Even if the examiner's report is not legally challenged, the examiner's methodology is a likely area of inquiry on cross-examination.

**Example 10.61: Minimal examination, report stricken**
*Minisan v. Danek Medical, Inc.,* 79 F.Supp. 2d 970 (N.D.Ind. 1999)
This was a pedicle screw medical device case. The plaintiff offered the report of Dr. Lance Yarus, an osteopath, as her only evidence. The court rejected the report and proposed testimony. The court stated:

> Dr. Yarus states that he arrived at his conclusions based solely on an examination of Minisan's numerous medical records. He apparently never examined her, met with her, or even spoke to her. Neither did he examine or test the TSRH device. Dr. Yarus concludes that "both surgical interventions were the proximate cause of the non-unions and subsequent development of pain." (Def's Mem. In Supp., Ex. 0 at 4.) He also concludes that Minisan's continued disability is directly related to the metallic devices. (*Id.*) Under *Daubert*, the expert "must explain precisely how [he] went about reaching [his] conclusions and point to some objective source…to show that [he] has followed the scientific method…" *Daubert v. Merrell Dow Pharm.,* 43 F.3d 1311, 1317 (9th Cir.1995) *(Daubert II)*. Similar to his reports provided in other bone screw cases, Dr. Yarus has failed to provide any explanation as to how he reached his conclusions. *See McCollin,* 50 F.Supp.2d 1119, 1126-27; *Hartwell*, 47 F.Supp.2d 703, 712-13; *Pulice,* 199 WL 613370 at * 5-9; *Moses v. Danek Medical, Inc.* No.CV 95-512, 1998 WL 1041279 at *7 (D.Nev. Dec. 11, 1998). Dr. Yarus has not met the standard set forth in *Daubert.* The court therefore concludes that Dr. Yarus' opinion is simply insufficient to create a material fact issue for trial with respect to the issue of causation. At 976, 977.

**Example 10.62: Causation opinion based on anecdotal case reports rather than epidemiological studies unreliable**
*Brumbaugh v. Dandot Pharmaceutical Corporation,* 77 F.Supp.2d. 1153 (D.Mont. 1999)
The court stated:

> The challenged expert, Dr. Iffy, opines that he believes Parlodel has caused a chronic seizure condition in plaintiff. To support his opinions, he relies not on epidemiological studies but on anecdotal case reports and his theory that Parlodel can act as a vasospastic agent instead of a vasodilator. At 1155.
>
> ...
>
> Dr. Iffy recognizes the insufficiency of reliance on case reports or ADE's to establish causation when he states that controlled studies are necessary to show that a particular drug causes an event or a particular reaction. Yet, he has developed a hypothesis that plaintiff's seizure and other seizures reported in ADE's and case reports were caused by Parlodel-induced vasospasms. He admits that it is "simply a hypothesis" which has not been tested and may be impossible to test. At 1156, or 1157.
>
> ...
>
> Dr. Iffy is, in essence, opining that plaintiff's seizures are due to Parlodel because he believes that. He admits that this causation opinion is "simply a hypothesis." Since they lack the rigor imposed by scientific methodology, Dr. Iffy's opinions do not have the evidentiary reliability to be admissible and are therefore excluded pursuant to Fed.R.Evid. 702 and 703. At 1157.

**Example 10.63: Methodology challenged on cross-examination**
*Report States:*

> It is my opinion that the examinee is not in pain. I base this on the fact that his blood pressure did not markedly increase when he reported he was in severe pain during the IME.

*Resulting Cross-examination:*

**Q.** Doctor, as I understand it, you took the examinee's blood pressure during your exam?
**A.** Yes, in the beginning of the exam and about 45 minutes into the exam when the examinee complained of severe pain.
**Q.** What were the readings you obtained?
**A.** 125/80 and then 130/85.
**Q.** From this you concluded that the examinee was in fact not in severe pain?
**A.** Yes. If he was in severe pain, his blood pressure would have been markedly increased.
**Q.** What do you base your opinion and conclusion on, Doctor?
**A.** On my medical training and expertise.
**Q.** Has your theory about the relationship between increased blood pressure and pain been tested, Doctor?
**A.** No, not in any formal way.
**Q.** Can you point to any peer review that has been done on this theory?
**A.** No.
**Q.** Can you point to any publications citing this theory?
**A.** No, I can't.
**Q.** What are the false/positives using your blood pressure/pain test?

**A.** I don't understand.
**Q.** What is your error rate?
**A.** None that I know of.
**Q.** How many other physicians are using this blood pressure/pain test?
**A.** I don't know.
**Q.** When you say, "markedly increased," do you have a chart or table you use?
**A.** No, just a case-by-case basis.
**Q.** So, you are asking this hearing officer to accept a blood pressure/pain test that has not been tested, has not been subject to peer review, has an unknown error rate, and is not accepted in the medical and scientific community?

**Comment:** When the examiner is offering new or unique theories to support his opinion, he should expect to have his methodology challenged under a *Daubert* analysis. It is likely that the examiner's opinion in the above example would be excluded after a finding that it is junk science or not scientifically valid.

**Defending the Report As Written:** When faced with this type of *Daubert* attack, the expert needs to either have all of his ducks in a row or meet the challenge head-on.

**Q.** What do you base your opinion and conclusion on?
**A.** For the past two years I have conducted 200 examinations of my private patients who have pain problems but are not in litigation. Approximately 87% demonstrate clearly an increase in blood pressure when their pain is increased. I am submitting my paper to the *New England Journal of Medicine.* Would you like to see the results and make it part of the record, Counsel?

## 10.7 Diagnoses

The IME report should usually list the specific diagnoses. This may best be done as a numbered problem list in decreasing order of severity. The significance of the clinical diagnoses and information supporting the diagnoses can also be discussed in this section of the report. It is also good practice to identify, where appropriate, which problems are acute, which are chronic or degenerative in nature, and which problems pre-date the injury in question.

**Example 10.71: Numbered list of diagnoses**
*Report States:*
Diagnoses:

1. Dislocation Right Shoulder.
2. Lower Brachial Plexus Injury Right Shoulder.
3. Chip Fracture Nasal Bone.
4. Diabetes.
5. Hypertension.
6. Morbid Obesity.
7. Degenerative Arthritis Right Shoulder (pre-existing).
8. Rotator Cuff Tear Right Shoulder.

9. Fracture Left Clavicle.
10. Cervical Spondylosis (degenerative).
11. Carpal Tunnel Syndrome Right.

**Comment:** This list of diagnoses is presented in an easy-to-read format. The pre-existing arthritis is clearly identified as such. It is an effective presentation.

**Example 10.72: Numbered list of diagnoses, each with further explanation and specificity**
*Report States:*

Diagnostic Impressions:

1. The examinee had a non-occupational acquired disc herniation at L4-5 in 1995 that required surgical intervention and stabilization.

2. The examinee sustained on 11/01/99, an occupationally acquired broad based disc re-herniation at L4-L5 that has migrated a free fragment of disc material located above the disc space on the right side requiring a microscopic hemilaminotomy with discectomy and removal of large free fragment L4-5, right on 11/23/99.

3. The examinee experienced a change of condition to his lower back and right leg for the worse (deterioration) in January 2000 resulting in a L4-L5 disc re-herniation requiring a third surgery with a redo laminectomy discectomy at L4-5 with interbody fusion on 01/06/00.

4. Occupationally acquired persistent recurrent low back and right leg pain with some clinical response to surgical repair (post laminectomy syndrome) which occurred on 11/01/99 and deteriorated (worsened) in January 2000.

5. Occupationally acquired on lumbar and right leg deconditioning which occurred on 11/01/99 and deteriorated (worsened) in January 2000.

6. Occupationally acquired sensory and motor deficits (weakness of the right leg) of the right L5 nerve of the right leg with atrophy (loss of size of upper thigh by 4 cm and 2 ½ cm in the calf) and gait impairment (mild limp of the right leg) which occurred on 11/01/99 and deteriorated (worsened) in January 2000.

**Comment:** This list of diagnoses is precise and well supported. It will buttress the examiner's opinions.

**Example 10.73: "Possible" diagnoses**
*Report States:*

**DIAGNOSES:**

1. Chronic intermittent headaches, possibly tension and/or cervicogenic in type, onset in or before January 1995.
2. Right posterolateral cervical disc herniation in January 1995, if present

possibly due to degenerative disc disease.

3. Recurrent neck pain with associated headaches in October 1996, possibly due to recurrence or worsening of the aforementioned disc herniation.
4. Multiple injuries due to the February 1997 motor vehicle collision (left frontal impact), including:
    a. cervical sprain/strain,
    b. contusion anterior right and probably left knees, and
    c. laceration medial right knee.
5. Bilateral carpal tunnel syndrome, possibly due to a combination of avocational or occupational activities or excess weight.

*Resulting Cross-examination:*

**Q.** Doctor, as I understand it, you reached five diagnoses in your IME report?
**A.** Yes, that's correct.
**Q.** In diagnosis #1, you found headaches that were possibly tension or cervicogenic?
**A.** Correct.
**Q.** So you are not sure if the headaches came from tension or are cervicogenic?
**A.** That's correct. It's not clear.
**Q.** In diagnosis #2, you found a disc herniation but you are not sure if it is from degenerative disc disease?
**A.** Correct.
**Q.** It's not clear to you?
**A.** Correct.
**Q.** In diagnosis #3, the neck pain with headaches is due to a recurrence or possibly worsening of the disc herniation?
**A.** Yes, that's correct.
**Q.** Not clear to you?
**A.** I am just trying to be honest.
**Q.** I appreciate your candor, Doctor. In diagnosis #4, the injuries are possibly due to the 1997 motor vehicle accident?
**A.** Yes.
**Q.** And finally, in diagnosis #5, the carpal tunnel syndrome possibly resulted from one of three causes?
**A.** Yes, that's correct.
**Q.** As you sit here today, under oath, can you testify with a reasonable degree of medical certainty as to the causes of your five diagnoses?

**Comment:** The repeated use of the term "possibly" in the IME report makes the report speculative, difficult to defend, and, most likely, legally insufficient. The examiner needs to express his opinions with a reasonable degree of medical certainty.

**Defending the Report As Written:** A report of this nature is difficult, if not impossible, to defend.

**Q.** As you sit here today, under oath, can you testify with a reasonable degree of medical certainty as to the causes of your five diagnoses?

**A.** Yes, I can. In my opinion, based upon a reasonable degree of medical certainty, the headaches were due to tension. May I explain?

## 10.8 Causation

Causation is frequently a critical issue in the workers' compensation and personal injury cases that generate IMEs. The attorney, adjuster, or other referral source needs to know whether the examinee's condition was caused by the accident or occurrence that is the subject of the claim.

In workers' compensation cases, the injury must have arisen from an accident "out of and during the course of employment." The question usually arises as to whether the condition was pre-existing or whether it was caused by an accident or occurrence that is not a subject of the claim in question. With an acute injury, such as a fracture, this determination may be simple. In other cases, such as those with pre-existing conditions and environmental exposures, the process is far more complex.

To properly render an opinion on causal relationship, the examiner needs to scrutinize the specifics of the case and compare this information to the known pathogenesis of a condition. This analytical process requires careful assessment and includes:

- determining the current diagnoses,
- the mechanism of injury,
- the diagnoses at the time of the injury,
- the pre-existing status, and
- the clinical history.

As always, the examiner's reasons for finding or not finding causation must be sound and clearly documented or else the examiner will have difficulty defending these conclusions.

**Example 10.81: Causation based on history**

*Report States:*

Based upon history, there would be causal relationship of his complaints and the May 14, 2002 incident at work.

*Resulting Cross-examination:*

**Q.** Doctor, you based your opinion on causation solely on the history the examinee gave you?

**A.** No, I did not.

**Q.** Don't you say in your IME report under the Conclusion heading, "Based upon history, there would be causal relationship of his complaints and the May 14, 2002 incident at work"?

**A.** That's what I said, yes.

**Q.** So, Doctor, if the history was incorrect or changed, you would change your opinion on causation, correct?

**Comment:** Examiners who are requested to express an opinion on causation should understand that this is frequently the key issue in the case. Without causation, there is no liability or legal responsibility. Examiners who understand the significance of their opinions on causation are best positioned to succeed. The American Medical Association's *Guides to the Evaluation of Permanent Impairment,* 5th edition (2001), states:

> Determining causation is important from a legal perspective, as it is a factor in determining liability....Medical or scientifically based causation requires a detailed analysis of whether the factor could have caused the condition, based upon scientific evidence and, specifically, experienced judgment as to whether the alleged factor in the existing environment did cause the permanent impairment. Determining medical causation requires a synthesis of medical judgment with scientific analysis. Sec. 1.6a p.11.

Thus, the examiner would have been in a better position to defend his opinion on causation had he worded it more carefully.

> Based upon the available information, to a reasonable degree of medical certainty, there is causal relationship between the examinee's right foot injury and complaints and the May 14, 2002 incident at work.

**Defending the Report As Written:** Even when an IME report is not artfully written, it can be defended.

**Q.** Doctor, you based your opinion on causation solely on the history the examinee gave you?
**A.** No. I based it on all the available information including the history, my examination, review of the medical records, and the accident report. I should have made that clearer in my report.

**Example 10.82: "Some" symptoms causally related**
*Report States:*

> Based on the information available to me, to a reasonable degree of medical certainty, there is a probable causal relationship between some of Mr. B's reported symptoms and his accident of July 1, 2002.

*Resulting Cross-examination:*
**Q.** How many symptoms of Mr. B did you identify?
**A.** Well, seventeen.
**Q.** There is probable causal relationship only between some of these seventeen and the accident of July 1, 2002?
**A.** That's correct.
**Q.** Thank you, Doctor.

**Comment:** Because neither the report nor the testimony specifies which of the symptoms are causally related to the accident, the examiner's testimony may be legally insufficient to establish causation.

**Defending the Report As Written:** Experienced and knowledgeable examiners can "repair" defective reports by supplementing them during their testimony.

**Q.** There is probably causal relationship only between some of these seventeen and the accident of July 1, 2002?
**A.** Numbers 1-9 are in my opinion causally related to the accident of July 1, 2002.

**Example 10.83: Plausible reasons provided for causation opinion**
*Report States:*

> Based upon the available information, to a reasonable degree of medical certainty, the current complaint and the occupational injury reported are not related. While kneeling and squatting can certainly contribute to wear and tear on the medial meniscus and can even cause a tear of this structure, to have both a tear of this structure and an anterior cruciate ligament tear from a simple kneeling incident is, in my opinion, unusual and unlikely.
>
> Additionally, the MRI report suggests that the anterior cruciate ligament tear might have been a pre-existing problem. It might be helpful to ask the radiologist to explain his impression in further detail.
>
> In summary, although there has been no information provided to me that would question this patient's credibility, it seems unlikely that the event she described would have caused such significant pathology in her right knee.
>
> Certainly the patient's obesity is a significant risk factor for knee problems.

*Resulting Cross-examination:*
**Q.** Doctor, it is possible according to your IME report that a kneeling incident could have caused both the tear on the medial meniscus and the anterior cruciate ligament tear, correct?
**A.** It's possible but unlikely.
**Q.** But you're not really sure, are you?
**A.** I have expressed my opinion to a reasonable degree of medical certainty.
**Q.** But you did say it would be helpful to ask the radiologist to explain his impression in further detail?
**A.** Yes, I did.
**Q.** That was to clear up the lingering doubts you have on the causation issue?
**A.** Just to clarify it.
**Q.** If you were sure, you wouldn't be seeking clarification, isn't that fair, Doctor?

**Comment:** The examiner in the above example offers an opinion and report with strong plausible reasons. He undermines the effectiveness of the report by inadvertently introducing elements of doubt—"unusual and unlikely" and "ask the radiologist."

> Based upon the available information, to a reasonable degree of medical certainty, the current complaint and the occupational injury reported are not related. While kneeling and squatting can contribute to wear and tear on the medial meniscus and can even cause a tear of this structure, to have both a tear of this structure and an anterior cruciate ligament tear from a simple kneeling incident is, in my opinion, extremely unusual and not what occurred in this case. The MRI report suggests that the anterior cruciate ligament tear might have been a pre-existing problem and the patient's obesity is a significant risk factor for knee problems.

**Defending the Report As Written:** Examiners who desire to maintain their opinions and reports should be prepared to fight for them. An examiner who is unable or unwilling to defend his report and opinion is of little value to the client.

**Q.** That was to clear up the lingering doubts you have on the causation issue?
**A.** No, I have no doubts whatsoever. The kneeling down to pick up a chocolate bar did not cause the rupture of the medial meniscus and the anterior cruciate ligament. In my 32 years of practicing orthopedic surgery, every single case like this one was caused by a major traumatic event, such as a serious football or skiing accident.

**Example 10.84: Causation stated with sloppy language**

*Report States:*

> It is my opinion that Mr. Brody's disability in his left leg is causally related to this file.

*Resulting Cross-examination:*

**Q.** Doctor, you find causal relationship between the left leg injury and a file?
**A.** Yes. The file I was sent by the insurer.
**Q.** Are you trying to say now there was causal relationship between Mr. Brody's left leg injury and the forklift accident of March 6, 2002 at work?
**A.** Yes. That's what I meant.
**Q.** Did you say that anywhere in your 7-page IME report?
**A.** Not in so many words.
**Q.** Actually, Doctor, you didn't say it at all. Isn't that correct?

**Comment:** One of the crucial aspects of an IME report is the doctor's opinion on causation or causal relationship. The client seeking the IME report needs to know if the medical condition(s) found at exam are related to the incident in question. The IME physician who does not express his opinion on causation in a clear, direct, and legally sufficient manner can expect to be closely cross-examined on this issue. The examiner in the above example would have been much better served with a clearer opinion.

> Based upon the history, the records reviewed, and my examination, it is my opinion to a reasonable degree of medical certainty that there is probable causal relationship between the March 6, 2002 accident at work when Mr.

> Brody was run over by a forklift and the resulting left leg complaints and disability.

**Defending the Report As Written:** When the examiner finds that he has been guilty of poor draftsmanship, he should correct his IME report at the earliest opportunity.

**Q.** Doctor, you find causal relationship between the left leg injury and a file?
**A.** Causal relationship between the left leg injury and his accident at work on March 6, 2002. When I said the file, I meant the industrial accident of March 6, 2002.

**Example 10.85: Clear, confident, well-substantiated causation opinion**
*Report States:*

> To a reasonable degree of medical certainty, the examinee's current cervical spine complaints are causally related to the August 6, 2003 M.V.A. There was no evidence of pre-existing injury and the August 10, 2003 MRI shows clear objective evidence of traumatic pathology. In addition, the examinee's injuries are consistent with a person who was rear-ended by a vehicle going 30-35 MPH.

**Comment:** This is a clearly written and well-substantiated causation opinion.

## 10.9 Apportionment

An issue in some examinations is *apportionment.* Apportionment refers to the extent to which a problem is caused by various factors. For example, a worker may have sustained an injury with one employer, then returned to work, then sustained a similar injury with a second employer. It may be necessary to apportion current dysfunction between two parties (e.g., between two different insurers of the employer). It also may be necessary to apportion responsibility between work- and nonwork-related conditions. The apportionment process is an art and depends largely upon the judgment, expertise, and experience of the evaluating physician. The most defensible reports are made with adequate information and explain the apportionment decision as objectively as possible.

**Example 10.91: "It is difficult to apportion"**
*Report States:*

> It is difficult to apportion back to his previous problems, particularly given the discrepancies between his review of the history and the medical records. These discrepancies are of concern, particularly related to issues of credibility and integrity. Some of his difficulties between January 26, 1999 and the present could be considered as shared responsibility with his prior work-related injuries; however, it does not appear that he has recently sought medical treatment for his low back. With his apparent return to baseline at this time, it may be more appropriate to approach his recent back difficulties as a temporary exacerbation associated with his activities on January 26, 1999.

> If further clarification concerning causation is needed, I would recommend obtaining all previous medical records, including those of Nichols Chiropractic and Dr. Stone.

*Resulting Cross-examination:*
**Q.** Doctor, you found it difficult to apportion the examinee's back injury here, correct?
**A.** Well, it is complex.
**Q.** There are the discrepancies between the history you obtained and the medical records?
**A.** Yes, there are.
**Q.** You're not really sure whether the examinee has undergone recent medical treatment for his back condition?
**A.** Correct.
**Q.** That treatment or lack thereof could be of significance in opining on apportionment?
**A.** That's true enough.
**Q.** You didn't make a medical timeline with dates and treatment to clarify the baseline issue?
**A.** I was unable to do so.
**Q.** Because of the difficulties we just discussed, you can't really say whether the activities of January 26, 1999 are an exacerbation or aggravation, correct?
**A.** Not with a reasonable degree of medical certainty.
**Q.** To give an honest opinion on apportionment you would need to see all of the previous medical records including those of Nichols Chiropractic and Dr. Stone?
**A.** That's correct.
**Q.** Thank you, Doctor, for your candor.

**Comment:** The examiner in the above example had neither adequate records nor sufficient information to reach an opinion on apportionment. He said as much and, in the process, kept his integrity, reputation, and credibility intact. For examiners who do this when necessary, there will be many cases in the future.

**Example 10.92: "Perhaps less than 10%"**
*Report States:*

> The pre-existing back injury is the major contributing cause of his residual impairment. A small portion, perhaps less than 10%, is due to the motor vehicle accident of 9/17/2001.

*Resulting Cross-examination:*
**Q.** Doctor, can you go to the blackboard and explain where you got the 10% figure in your IME report?
**A.** Well, there's no need to go to the board. It is my professional opinion, sir.
**Q.** So you didn't use a formula or scientific basis to arrive at this "perhaps less than 10%"?
**A.** Only my experience.

**Q.** When you say "perhaps less than 10%," that means it could also be a little more?
**A.** Exactly.
**Q.** "Exactly" how much more, Doctor?
**A.** Not much.
**Q.** 11% or 12%?
**A.** Yes.
**Q.** 13% or 14%?
**A.** I don't want to get into a numbers game.
**Q.** I think it's a little too late for that. Can you say with a reasonable degree of medical certainty the amount of the impairment due to the motor vehicle accident?
**A.** Not exactly, I can't.
**Q.** Did you perform an apportionment analysis in accordance with the AMA *Guides to the Evaluation of Permanent Impairment?*
**A.** No, I did not.
**Q.** Would you agree that to provide an accurate percentage of impairment for the motor vehicle accident, you would need to have examined the claimant before his motor vehicle accident?
**A.** No, not necessarily. When there is a prior impairment rating, we can use that figure as a guideline for the impairment from the pre-existing condition.
**Q.** Where is the impairment rating that you used in this case, Doctor?
**A.** I did not have one.
**Q.** Doctor, did you calculate the current spine impairment?
**A.** No.
**Q.** Did you calculate the pre-existing impairment?
**A.** No, but the pre-existing back injury is the major contributing cause of his residual impairment.
**Q.** If you didn't calculate it, Doctor, would you like to estimate it now?
**A.** No.
**Q.** As you don't know what the pre-existing impairment is and you don't know what the total current spine impairment is, you are in no position to state that "a small portion, less than 10% is due to the motor vehicle accident of 9/17/2002"?

**Comment:** The examiner in the above example would have been better served had he followed the admonition "less is more." His opinion would have been stronger and easier to defend had he simply stated, "The pre-existing back injury is the major contributing cause of his residual impairment." When the physician goes off into speculation, "a small portion, perhaps less than 10%," he brings into question his entire opinion.

**Defending the Report As Written:** When faced with a direct frontal attack, the examiner needs to stay calm and collected if he is to successfully defend his report.

**Q.** Doctor, can you go to the blackboard and explain where you got the 10% figure in your IME report?
**A.** My opinion is based on my examination, the history I took, my review of

the records, my training, 27 years of experience, and my clinical skills and judgment.

**Example 10.93: Complex apportionment analysis**

*Report States:*

**Apportionment:** The plaintiff's current condition is obviously multifactorial, being due in part to whatever was causing her head, neck, and radicular pains prior to the February 1997 collision, presumably a cervical disc herniation, or perhaps more than one. It is also due in part to the February 1997 collision, which likely caused temporary worsening of her pre-existing neck pain with new onset of bilateral anterior knee pain. Additionally, her present condition is due in part to the May 1998 and April 2002 bus accidents. While the first of these appears to be the least severe of all her traumas, Ms. Mant reported today she did not recover completely therefrom. "I still continue to have problems with my knees." Lastly, her physical symptoms are likely due in part to psychosocial factors, probably including anxiety manifested in increased muscular tension and tension myalgia.

It is difficult to provide a precise percentage apportionment. However, in anticipation of such a question, the examiner asked Ms. Mant to quantify her pain levels on a scale of 0 (no discomfort) to 10 (the worst pain imaginable) before the February 1997, May 1998, and April 2002 accidents, and at present, to enable at least a subjective numerical basis for apportionment. Her current head and neck pain are probably due to two factors, whatever was causing them before the February 1997 MVA, and the April 2002 bus accident. Supporting the collision as a primary cause are the "abnormal amount of headaches," and neck pain for which she began another course of physical therapy on December 10, 1996, which continued up to and including the day prior to the MVA. On February 20, 1997, Ms. Mant reported on page 4 of the Personal Health History at Dr. Albertson's office she "had just finished" therapy prior to the collision six days earlier. However, this is not corroborated by Ms. Rogers's February 13$^{th}$ Progress Summary. The therapist thought it "appropriate to continue [treatment] once a week or…every other week."

While there was increased neck pain after February 1997 MVA, the table reveals it was an exacerbation (temporary worsening) rather than aggravation (permanent worsening). In other words, Ms. Mant's neck pain had returned to its baseline by the time of the May 1998 bus accident. It remained at that level (reportedly 2 but actually 0-2 since it was intermittent) until the April 2002 bus accident, with another spike upwards in head and neck pain thereafter. At least historically Ms. Mant has not recovered to her pre-fall baseline, the previously intermittent cervicalgia now being constant, and increased in severity from 0-2 to 6-7, with new onset of left shoulder pain. Whether she will completely recover from the 2$^{nd}$ bus accident remains to be seen. Hence the fall on the bus would be considered the most proximate and another primary contributor to her current cervicalgia. At present her neck pain is probably due 50% to each, the pre-existing pathology and the April 2002 accident.

By contrast, statements from the plaintiff suggest her bilateral knee pain is due to the February 1997 and May 1998 accidents. She reportedly did not have knee pain before the subject MVA, and stated that discomfort was permanently worsened by striking her knees on the bus seat. However, the table indicates her current knee pain is less than it was both before and after the 1st bus accident, suggesting it was an exacerbation. Given the latter, and the greater magnitude of collision, the examiner would apportion her knee conditions 75% to the February 1997 MVA and 25% to the May 1998 bus accident.

*Resulting Cross-examination:*

**Q.** Doctor, the apportionment in this case was difficult and complex, was it not?

**A.** Yes, it was.

**Q.** That was because you were dealing with a pre-existing condition and three separate accidents, correct?

**A.** Yes, that's correct.

**Q.** You were not able to examine this claimant after all of these accidents and come up with an accurate percentage apportionment?

**A.** Yes, I did just that.

**Q.** Didn't you say in your report, "It is difficult to provide a precise percentage apportionment"?

**A.** Yes, I did.

**Q.** So, you then went to the examinee and asked her to remember how she felt prior to 2/97, pre-5/98, pre-4/02, and now and express that in a numerical basis 1-10?

**A.** Yes, that's the only way it could be done.

**Q.** Can you say with a reasonable degree of medical certainty that the examinee's numerical ratings up to five years after the fact were accurate?

**A.** I believe what she said.

**Q.** You did this apportionment analysis under the AMA *Guides,* 5th edition, correct?

**A.** Yes, I did.

**Q.** Did you follow the techniques set forth in Section 1.6, which states:

> "The apportionment analysis must consider the nature of the impairment and its possible relationship to each alleged factor, and it must provide an explanation of the medical basis for all conclusions and opinions.
>
> * * *
>
> For example, in apportioning a spine impairment rating in an individual with a history of a spine condition, one should calculate the current spine impairment. Then calculate the impairment from any preexisting spine problem. The preexisting impairment rating is then subtracted from the present impairment rating to account for the effects of the former. This approach requires accurate and comparable data for both impairments."[3]

**Comment:** The examiner in the above example did the best he could in a very difficult situation. When multiple accidents are involved and the conditions

---

[3] AMA *Guides to the Evaluation of Permanent Impairment,* 5th edition, p. 13.

overlap, it may be difficult or impossible to do an accurate apportionment. Examiners should consider refusing to do an apportionment when their conclusions cannot be supported medically and defined legally.

The following formula is helpful when a previous impairment is available for the same diagnosis and to the same anatomic level of involvement.[4]

**Apportionment Percentage of New =**

**(New Impairment - Previous Impairment) / New Impairment x 100%**

**Defending the Report As Written:** When faced with a frontal assault, the examiner should consider fighting back.

**Q.** Can you say with a reasonable degree of medical certainty that the examinee's numerical ratings up to five years after the fact were accurate?
**A.** Yes. The examinee was in the best position to know exactly how much pain she was in at the time.

## 10.10 Aggravation and Exacerbation

Evaluators must be familiar with the definitions of the terms "aggravation" and "exacerbation" as they relate to pre-existing injuries or conditions in workers' compensation. An *aggravation* is a long-standing effect due to an event, resulting in a worsening, hastening, or deterioration of a condition. *Exacerbation* is a temporary increase in the symptomatology of a pre-existing condition. The distinction between the terms is that an aggravation has an ongoing substantial impact on the physical condition, whereas an exacerbation results only in a flare-up of symptoms. These terms need to be used correctly. If they are not, the examiner may face problems during cross-examination. In most workers' compensation jurisdictions, aggravations are compensable as a new injury. To be compensable, it is enough if the employment was one of the contributing factors in causing the injury. These aggravations are usually the responsibility of the insurer "on the risk" at the time of the aggravation. An exacerbation is *merely a temporary flare-up of symptoms and will be treated as such.*

**Example 10.101: "Temporary aggravation"**
*Report States:*

Based upon the available information, to a reasonable degree of medical probability, the episode of January 26, 1999 resulted in his underlying back difficulties becoming symptomatic. Subsequent to his treatment program, and at this time, he has returned to his baseline. In retrospect, therefore, it would

[4] Melhorn, JM, Talmage, JB, Fries, BE, and Zeppieri, JP. "Impairment Evaluations for the Upper Extremities Using the AMA *Guides*." In: *Occupational Orthopaedics and Workers' Compensation: A Multidisciplinary Perspective*, edited by Melhorn, JM and Strain Jr., RE. (Rosemont, IL: American Academy of Orthopaedic Surgeons, 2002) p. 351-442.

appear that the injury of January 26, 1999 was causative in that it resulted in a temporary aggravation of his underlying back problems. Therefore, the most recent treatments would be causally related to the event of January 26, 1999.

*Resulting Cross-examination:*
**Q.** You found a temporary aggravation in this case?
**A.** Yes, I did.
**Q.** Is that the same as an exacerbation, Doctor?
**A.** I am not sure.
**Q.** You don't really know the difference, correct?
**A.** That's correct. I don't usually do workers' compensation claims.
**Q.** So this could have been an exacerbation?

**Comment:** Examiners who are not familiar with the medical-legal terminology frequently used in the workers' compensation arena are at a severe disadvantage in writing and defending their IME reports. To succeed, they must master the terminology.

**Defending the Report As Written:** When placed in the uncomfortable position of not knowing the definition of a term being used by counsel, the IME examiner can ask counsel to define it.

**Q.** Is that the same as an exacerbation, Doctor?
**A.** Counsel, I am new to these kinds of cases. Would you be good enough to define what you mean by exacerbation?

**Example 10:102: "Aggravated"**
*Report States:*
Turning and twisting aggravated his back condition.

*Resulting Cross-examination:*
**Q.** When you use the term "aggravated" his back condition, are you referring to a permanent worsening of the underlying pathology that was present prior to the alleged aggravating incident?
**A.** No, I am referring to the fact that his turning and twisting activity in the back of the truck brought on an increase in symptoms at that time.
**Q.** So that the aggravation that you speak of is limited in time to the period that these symptoms were increased. Once the increased symptoms quieted down to the pre-incident level where they had been, the aggravation ceased?
**A.** No. I think that, you know, I would have to examine him at the time to decide what the aggravation consisted of. All I can say is that it aggravated his back condition.
**Q.** Assuming for the moment that the claimant, with his underlying back condition, was at pain level A when he had the incident; that his pain increased to pain level B, and after two days reverted back to pain level A. Would you agree that there was no permanent worsening of his underlying back pathology except for the two- or one-day period that his pain level was increased?
**A.** Well, that would be hard to say because I haven't examined him. All I know is that he apparently continued to see his doctor after that and he had a

period of aggravation.
**Q.** And would it not be equally as difficult to say that there would be an aggravation on a permanent nature as well as it being difficult to say that there wasn't?
**A.** I don't think it limited the aggravation.
**Q.** When you said in your report that "turning and twisting aggravated his back condition," for how long of a period of time did it make it worse?
**A.** I know there was an aggravation and I couldn't put an actual limit on it. That's all I'm saying.
**Q.** So, what occurred here was a temporary increase in the symptomatology of the pre-existing condition?
**A.** Exactly.
**Q.** Are you aware, Doctor, that a temporary increase in the symptomatology of a pre-existing condition is, in fact, an exacerbation and not an aggravation?

**Comment:** Examiners should be familiar with the medical-legal terms that arise frequently in workers' compensation, liability, and personal injury litigation. For example, the distinction between aggravation and exacerbation in workers' compensation cases can determine the outcome. The terms normally deal with pre-existing conditions. An *aggravation* is a long-standing effect due to an event, resulting in a worsening, hastening, or deterioration of a condition. *Exacerbation* is a temporary increase in the symptomatology of a pre-existing condition. The distinction between the terms is that an aggravation has an ongoing substantial impact on the physical condition, whereas an exacerbation results only in a flare-up of symptoms.

**Defending the Report As Written:** The examiner who understands the medical-legal terminology is in a better position to see where counsel is going with his cross-examination.

**Q.** When you use the term "aggravated" his back condition, are you referring to a permanent worsening of the underlying pathology that was present prior to the alleged aggravating incident?
**A.** Because I did not examine him at the time, it is impossible for me to say if the increase in symptoms was permanent or transitory in nature. I used the term "aggravated" to merely indicate a worsening of symptoms, but I am unable to say how long this lasted for.

### Example 10.103: Aggravation

*Southwest Cupid v. Jackson,* 7 P.3d 515 (2000)
Examiners who are not familiar with medical-legal terms that arise frequently during IMEs are at a substantial disadvantage.

In the case *Southwest Cupid v. Jackson,* the Oklahoma Court struggled to find that the IME physician meant aggravation during his testimony.

> The trial court appointed an independent medical examiner (IME) on April 21, 1999. It directed the IME to determine whether Claimant's complaints were caused by a new injury, aggravation of a pre-existing injury, or a change of condition for the worse directly related to her prior injury and condition. The IME's written report stated the causation of Claimant's complaints was both aggravation of pre-existing

condition and change of condition for the worse directly related to her prior problems. However, at his deposition, the IME indicated he was not using these terms as legal terms of art. He testified as follows:

> (Cross-examination)
> **Q:** Is it possible that [Claimant's] current symptomatology could have just been a gradual progression of the underlying injury?
> **A:** I think it's a speculation. I cannot give you with medical certainty that that is the case.
>
> ***
>
> (Redirect examination)
> **Q:** Given her work activities that were repetitious and continue to be repetitious, can you say whether it might be more likely true than not true that the cause of her present condition is her work activities since June of 1998?
> **A:** Well, I would say that at least aggravated her condition.....
>
> ***
>
> **Q:** Could you tell the court that it's more likely true than not true that the cause of the claimant's present problems are due to the aggravation of her pre-existing condition from her activities at work relative to simply the prior surgery that she had had in 1997?
> **A:** That would be—I would be inclined to think it that way, sir.
> **Q:** That it's more likely true than not true that her aggravation is more the cause of her current problems than her pre-existing surgery?
> **A:** Yes, sir. And I think I give my opinion based on the amount of repetitious activity that she was doing and what she told me she was doing with so many garments every day. At 516.

## 10.11 Prognosis

The referral source may request that the examiner identify the examinee's prognosis (i.e., the probability and predicted time of recovery). Any and all objective bases for the examiner's prognosis should be provided. Subjective superfluous comments should be avoided. Please consider the following examples.

**Example 10.111: "Has actively resisted all opportunities to return to work"**
*Report States:*

> Mr. B. is one year, four months post-injury and post-surgery. He continues to report persistent symptoms which have not changed significantly for a period of months. Mr. B. has been off work since the time of the injury and has actively resisted all opportunities to return to work. Without his wanting to return to work, the examinee's prognosis is extremely poor.

*Resulting Cross-examination:*
**Q.** Doctor, the examinee may be reporting symptoms because he actually has them, correct?
**A.** It's possible, but not likely.
**Q.** Some people have symptoms that do not improve?
**A.** Mostly workers' compensation claimants.
**Q.** Would you be willing to sign a return-to-work slip for the examinee to return to his construction job, Doctor?
**A.** Well, that's not my function. I am just here to do an IME.

**Q.** I take that as a no, Doctor?

**Comment:** The examiner in the above report and testimony comes off with just a little too much edge. The more counsel can goad him into making caustic comments, the more the examiner looks like an advocate. Objective, supportable facts used by the examiner are much more effective.

> Mr. B. is one year and four months post-injury and post-surgery. He continues to report persistent symptoms which have not changed significantly for a period of months. He has been off work continuously since the time of the injury. The examinee has refused rehabilitation, training, additional education, and light work, which were offered by his employer. His prognosis is poor.

**Defending the Report As Written:** Examiners need to be able to counter any misimpressions opposing counsel is trying to leave with the fact finder.

**Q.** Would you be willing to sign a return-to-work slip for the examinee to return to his construction job, Doctor?
**A.** I am willing to sign a slip for the light work offered and for the examinee to begin rehabilitation and retraining.

**Example 10.112: Citation to texts, guidelines, and other sources**
*Report States:*

> Mr. Jones's prognosis is that a full recovery is more probable than not. According to Dr. Presley Reed, these types of injuries result in a full recovery and return to work in 67% of cases.

*Resulting Cross-examination:*
**Q.** Doctor, can you guarantee that Mr. Jones will fully recover from his injuries and be able to return to work?
**A.** Physicians don't give guarantees.
**Q.** So he might fully recover and he might not.
**A.** Yes, but the chances are that he will.
**Q.** You cited Dr. Presley Reed as the basis of your prognosis?
**A.** Part of the prognosis.
**Q.** That would be Reed's *Medical Disability Adviser?*
**A.** Yes.
**Q.** Dr. Reed says in the preface, "These guidelines should always be used in conjunction with the combined information available regarding the individual case and the nature of the job itself," does he not?
**A.** Yes, he does.
**Q.** Do you have information on the job itself?
**A.** No, not specifically.
**Q.** Do you agree with Dr. Reed when he says in the introduction, "There are numerous other factors associated with the workplace that may significantly impact an individual's ability to return to work after an injury or illness. Factors such as the work environment (e.g., noise levels, exposure to weather, heat, cold, or vibration); sensory requirements

> associated with a job (e.g., hearing, visual acuity, color vision, verbal abilities); and special physical activities (e.g., kneeling, balancing, fingering, and climbing), may influence when and if an individual can return to the job performed prior to illness or injury?"

**A.** Yes, I do.
**Q.** Let's go over the restrictions in this case and see if there actually is a 67% chance of full recovery and return to work.

**Comment:** Examiners who offer specific recovery rates in their prognoses will have difficulty defending their reports and opinions. When citing sources, examiners open themselves up to additional cross-examination regarding the texts.

**Defending the Report As Written:** Examiners who cite sources should be very familiar with the source material.

**Q.** Dr. Reed says in the preface, "These guidelines should always be used in conjunction with the combined information available regarding the individual case and the nature of the job itself," does he not?
**A.** That's in the old 1991 text, not the latest edition, Counsel.

**Example 10.113: "No doubt" that examinee would respond favorably to appropriate chiropractic treatment**

*Report States:*

> There is no doubt that the examinee has mechanical spinal dysfunction that would respond favorably to appropriate chiropractic treatment.

*Resulting Cross-examination:*
**Q.** You guarantee that the examinee would get better if she had chiropractic care, Doctor?
**A.** There are no guarantees in medicine, Counselor.
**Q.** So, when you said in your IME report, "There is no doubt that the examinee has mechanical spinal dysfunction that would respond favorably to appropriate chiropractic treatment," you didn't really mean it?
**A.** No. That's my opinion.
**Q.** Could the chiropractic treatment make the examinee worse?
**A.** It's possible, but not likely.
**Q.** Could you tell us how many chiropractic treatments would be required?
**A.** That's hard to say.
**Q.** The examinee already had 27 chiropractic treatments by Dr. Spring, correct?
**A.** Yes.
**Q.** These 27 chiropractic treatments consisted of spinal manipulation, applications of heat, and galvanic stimulation?
**A.** Yes, that's correct.
**Q.** These treatments didn't cure her, correct?
**A.** No, but there was temporary relief.
**Q.** Until the next treatment?
**A.** Apparently.

**Q.** So, when you say "respond favorably," do you mean a cure or temporary relief?
**A.** We hope for cure, but more likely, temporary relief.
**Q.** How long would the temporary relief last for?
**A.** That varies from one day to two weeks.
**Q.** As you sit here today, under oath, Doctor, can you predict this examinee's medical future with or without chiropractic manipulation and galvanic stimulation?
**A.** I am a chiropractor, Counsel, not a fortune-teller.

**Comment***:* Examiners are better served by conservative statements regarding treatment and recovery. The more definitive the prediction of the future, the more difficult the statement is to defend. A more defensible statement would be:

> In my opinion, the examinee has mechanical spinal dysfunction that would most likely respond to appropriate chiropractic treatment.

**Defending the Report As Written:** When faced with a direct frontal attack by opposing counsel on cross-examination, the examiner can consider being direct himself.

**Q.** You guarantee that the examinee would get better if she had chiropractic care, Doctor?
**A.** Counsel, you are mischaracterizing what I said. I said, "respond favorably to appropriate chiropractic treatment." That is my opinion based on 27 years as a practicing chiropractor and based upon having seen hundreds of people with similar conditions respond favorably to appropriate chiropractic care.

**Example 10.114: Work hardening program recommended**
*Report States:*

> He should have an intensive work hardening program following which he could return to full work.

*Resulting Cross-examination:*
**Q.** Doctor, would you agree that an intensive work hardening program could make the examinee's back condition worse?
**A.** It's possible, but not likely.
**Q.** Success would depend on work tolerance, work rate, mastery of pain, and improved productivity?
**A.** Generally, yes.
**Q.** Are all claimants who undergo an intensive work hardening program successful?
**A.** Many are, not all.
**Q.** You said in your IME report, "He should have an intensive work hardening program following which he could return to full work." You are not sure that will actually occur, are you?
**A.** That's my opinion.
**Q.** So, that's not a fact, is it?

**A.** No, it's my opinion.
**Q.** You would, of course, want to examine the claimant before releasing him to full duty, correct?
**A.** Yes.
**Q.** That would be prudent?
**A.** Yes.
**Q.** To make sure he was ready to return to work at that time without undue risk of re-injury?

**Comment:** Examiners are often called upon to comment on prognosis, the probability and predicted time of recovery. An examiner is in a strong position to defend his opinion when it is expressed as an opinion and not as a guess about possible future recoveries.

> In my opinion, the examinee would benefit from an intensive work hardening program. After the completion of the program, he should be re-evaluated to determine work capacity and the ability to resume his full employment duties.

**Defending the Report As Written:** A prognosis based upon the physician's thorough clinical assessment can be successfully defended.

**Q.** Doctor, would you agree that an intensive work hardening program introduces progressive work-related activities? Patients are reconditioned both in strength and endurance while their capacity is monitored in lifting, pushing, pulling, etc.
**A.** It is my medical opinion, based upon my experience with thousands of back patients, that it is more likely than not that the examinee will benefit from the program and be returned to full work.

**Example 10.115: Prognosis supported by reasons**
*Report States:*

> Ms. Duffy is approximately one year, four months post-injury. She experiences some persistent right shoulder symptoms that are predominantly activity related. Overall, her condition has not changed significantly in some months (particularly based on the information contained in the medical records), and medical conditions unrelated to the 9/6/01 injury preclude more aggressive treatment of her right shoulder condition. Considering this data, the current pattern of symptoms will likely continue.

**Comment:** This is a well-written prognosis section because it is supported by the examiner's reasons for the opinion.

**Example 10.116: Prognosis supported by reasons**
*Report States:*

> **Prognosis:** It is difficult to understand the plaintiff's claim she is presently getting worse, which is inconsistent with the natural history of the vast majority of trauma. In other words, injuries tend to gradually improve, if

> not resolve, over time as a result of the body's natural healing processes, even in the absence of treatment. The examiner suspects her current neck-left shoulder and bilateral knee pain will improve (but not resolve completely) over the subsequent months and years, barring recurrent injury. The improvement will likely be expedited if she exercises regularly, including performance of short-arc and isometric quadriceps strengthening. Weight reduction will likely also improve her general well-being and diminish the loads on her knees.

**Comment:** This is a well-written prognosis section because it is supported by the examiner's reasons for the opinion.

**Example 10.117: Prognosis opinion**
*Report States:*

> In response to the questions posed in the cover letter of April 15, 2002:
>
> *1. What is your current diagnosis and prognosis for Ms. Johnson? Please list any preexisting factors.*
> Ms. Johnson most probably has symptomatic multi-level lumbar degenerative disc disease. Her prognosis is guarded. That is, she is at significant risk to remain symptomatic or to have an aggravation of symptoms if she engages in heavy physical labor. She has preexisting factors in that she injured her back in June of 1998 and gives the impression that she never fully recovered from this.

**Comment:** The examiner here supports his opinion regarding prognosis.

## 10.12 Maximum Medical Improvement

The examiner may be asked to opine regarding maximum medical improvement. Maximum medical improvement (MMI) is a term used to indicate that further recovery and restoration of function can no longer be anticipated to a reasonable degree of medical certainty. Examiners need to know exactly what the term means in the jurisdiction in question.

The American Medical Association's *Guides to the Evaluation of Permanent Impairment,* 5th edition, defines maximum medical improvement as follows:

> Maximal medical improvement (MMI) occurs when a condition or state that is well stabilized and unlikely to change substantially in the next year, with or without medical treatment. Over time, there may be some change; however, further recovery or deterioration is not anticipated.[5]

This assessment implies that a condition is permanent and static. The examiner may be asked to opine when MMI occurred or when it is expected to occur. In determining whether an examinee is at MMI, the examiner should consider, among other factors, whether the current or proposed

---

[5] Page 601.

treatment will result in functional improvement, if surgery has recently occurred, and whether enough time has passed for the process to be stable. The factors considered in making the MMI determination should be explicitly stated in the written report.

The date the examinee reaches maximum medical improvement is significant for several reasons. Examinees are not rated for permanent impairment until they have reached MMI. Secondly, reaching MMI may affect the decision as to whether further medical care is reasonable and necessary.

**Example 10.121: Reasons for not finding MMI stated**

*Report States:*

> Maximum medical improvement (MMI) is defined as the date after which further recovery and restoration of function can no longer be anticipated, based upon reasonable medical probability. She has not attained MMI in that she is actively involved in treatment and reports that she is improving.

**Comment:** This opinion is easily defensible because it states the reasons why the examinee has not reached maximum medical improvement.

**Example 10.122: Opinion inconsistent with definition of MMI**

*Report States:*

> Maximum medical improvement (MMI) is defined as the date after which further recovery and restoration of function can no longer be anticipated, based upon reasonable medical probability. He is at MMI. Mr. Sample may benefit from changes in his treatment program, although it appears unlikely he would seek such treatment. It is estimated that he achieved MMI on December 24, 1992, one year post-surgery.

*Resulting Cross-examination:*

**Q.** Mr. Sample may in fact benefit from changes in his treatment program, correct?
**A.** Yes.
**Q.** What treatment are you referring to?
**A.** Work hardening and physical therapy.
**Q.** If he in fact underwent an aggressive physical therapy and work hardening program, how much recovery could he make?
**A.** That would be difficult to predict.
**Q.** Could he make a substantial recovery?
**A.** He might.
**Q.** If you can't say how much of a recovery he might make and can't say if the recovery may be substantial, then by definition, he has not in fact reached MMI, correct?

**Comment:** When questioned about MMI, the examiner should either have the definition of MMI committed to memory or have it at hand. The examiner can anticipate that counsel will utilize the words and concepts in the MMI definition in his cross-examination. This report was not consistent with the examiner's own definition of MMI.

**Example 10.123: "Probably" reached maximum medical improvement by September 3rd**

*Report States:*

> **Medical Stability:** Ms. Mant probably reached the point of maximum medical improvement with respect to the February 1997 collision by September 3rd of that year, seven months later, when she discontinued treatment.

*Resulting Cross-examination:*

**Q.** Doctor, you selected the date of September 3, 1997 as the date the examinee reached MMI?
**A.** Yes.
**Q.** You selected this date because this was when she discontinued treatment?
**A.** Yes.
**Q.** You were not sure, so you said it was "probably" September 3, 1997?
**A.** That's the date I selected.
**Q.** Even though continued medical treatment has no relationship to MMI?

**Comment:** Examiners should be prepared to explain any "arbitrary" dates they select for MMI. If MMI can be tied into a specific event that corresponds to stabilization of the condition (e.g., return to work), that will strengthen the report.

**Defending the Report As Written:** Examiners commenting on MMI should be able to tie the date into objective facts.

**Q.** Even though continued medical treatment has no relationship to MMI?
**A.** The examinee voluntarily discontinued her medical treatment, medication, and returned to work on September 3, 1997. That is why I selected it for the MMI date.

## 10.13 Permanent Impairment Rating

The examiner may be asked to provide a permanent impairment rating. To make this rating as persuasive as possible, the examiner should do the following.

1. Use the appropriate guidelines. In workers' compensation cases, different states mandate that different rating systems be used.
2. Use the correct edition of the appropriate guidelines. For example, to date, the AMA has published five editions of *The Guides to the Evaluation of Permanent Impairment*. Some states require the latest edition, some older editions.
3. Correctly follow the applicable impairment rating guidelines.
4. Specifically cite the applicable tables and charts used in the permanent impairment calculation.

5. Make sure he has the training he needs to properly perform and document permanent impairment ratings.

Please consider the following examples.

**Example 10.131: Unsubstantiated rating**
*Report States:*
This patient is 17.3% impaired.

*Resulting Cross-examination:*
**Q.** Your IME report indicates that you found the examinee to be 17.3% impaired, correct?
**A.** Yes, that's correct.
**Q.** What rating method did you employ to arrive at the 17.3%?
**A.** I based it on my examination and my 24 years of experience.
**Q.** Did you obtain the history of the medical condition?
**A.** No, not specifically.
**Q.** What about findings from your physical examination?
**A.** That's how I arrived at the 17.3%.
**Q.** Do you list in your IME report the positive and pertinent negative clinical findings?
**A.** No.
**Q.** Did you make a determination about the impact on life activities of the examinee?
**A.** I did not.
**Q.** Do you identify the impairment rating system you used?
**A.** Not in so many words.
**Q.** You just used your experience to come up with the 17.3%?
**A.** My substantial experience, yes.
**Q.** Could you please go to the board and demonstrate how you, based on a reasonable degree of medical certainty, arrived at the 17.3% impairment?

**Comment:** IME examiners who come up with unsubstantiated impairment ratings should expect to have their conclusions vigorously attacked by counsel. When the examiners cannot provide detailed, specific, and scientific explanations for their opinions, the opinions may be discounted, disregarded, or stricken as legally insufficient.

**Defending the Report As Written:** Defending an unsubstantiated impairment rating is difficult if not impossible. The only defense is a frontal assault.

**Q.** What rating method did you employ to arrive at the 17.3%?
**A.** I did not use some artificial number provided in a book, if that's what you are asking. I used the results of my experience in evaluating impairment and the results of my examination. Counsel, if you can explain where the numbers come from in the *Guides to Rating Permanent Impairment*, I would be happy to consider using the text.

**Example 10.132: Edition**

*Report States:*

> This examinee is rated at 5% whole person impairment pursuant to the AMA *Guides.*

*Resulting Cross-examination:*

**Q.** You rated the examinee at 5% whole person impairment pursuant to the AMA *Guides*, correct?
**A.** Yes.
**Q.** That was for his latex allergy?
**A.** Correct.
**Q.** You utilized the 4th edition of the *Guides*, correct?
**A.** Yes, I did.
**Q.** Are you aware that you used the wrong edition to perform the rating as the 5th edition was adopted two years ago by your state legislature?

**Comment:** Before performing an IME, the examiner should know which one of the editions of the AMA *Guides* is the correct one to use. This will vary from state to state and from forum to forum. When there is a question, the examiner should consult the party requesting the exam or counsel familiar with the issue. In addition, the examiner should specify in his report which edition of the *Guides* he used when performing his examination and writing his report.

> This examinee is rated at 5% whole person impairment pursuant to the AMA *Guides*, 5th edition.

**Defending the Report As Written:** Just because the examiner may have used the incorrect or outdated edition of the *Guides* does not necessarily make his impairment rating incorrect.

**Q.** Are you aware that you used the wrong edition to perform the rating as the 5th edition was adopted two years ago by your state legislature?
**A.** Counsel, perhaps you are unaware that the 5th edition and the 4th edition are almost exactly the same in this instance. The examinee falls into class #1 because his signs and symptoms are intermittently present and he has no limitations in the performance of his activities of daily living. The 5% impairment is correct under the 4th and 5th editions since he has demonstrated a true allergic contact dermatitis caused by a substance that might lead to more serious problems.

**Example 10.133: Well-substantiated impairment rating**

*Report States:*

> A permanent impairment rating was performed in accordance with the fourth edition of the *Guides to the Evaluation of Permanent Impairment* (American Medical Association, Chicago, 1993). Impairment is defined as an alteration of an individual's health status, i.e., a deviation from normal in a body part or organ system and its functioning. The *Guides* defines permanent impairment as impairment that has become static or stabilized during a period of time sufficient to allow optimal tissue repair, and that is unlikely to change in spite

> of further medical or surgical therapy. The assessment process includes medical evaluation, analysis of the findings, and comparison of the results of analysis with the impairment criteria. Chapter 3, "The Musculoskeletal System," was used for this evaluation.
>
> The fourth edition utilizes an injury or "Diagnosis-Related Estimates" (DRE) model for spinal impairment. This individual was evaluated for cervicothoracic spine impairment. According to Table 73, page 110, he is classified as category IV for "loss of motion segment integrity or multilevel neurologic compromise." There is a 25% whole-person impairment. According to Section 3.3b, page 95, the cervicothoracic spine comprises 35% of total body function; therefore a 25% whole-person impairment is equal to 71% of the cervicothoracic spine, or "neck."
>
> The examinee has clear-cut multi-level neurologic compromise, including strength deficits in the upper extremities, impotence, lower extremity spasticity, and reported loss of temperature sensation in the lower extremities. However, he does not have severe upper extremity neurologic compromise in that upper extremity function is relatively intact. Likewise, he does not have signs of cauda equina syndrome. Therefore, he clearly falls within cervicothoracic DRE category IV. I would add 5% whole person impairment for his ongoing lower extremity spasticity and impotence, for a total whole body impairment of 30%.

**Comment:** This is a well-written, well-reasoned impairment rating regarding permanent impairment.

**Example 10.134: Misuse of impairment rating guide**

*Report States:*

> Impairment: In accordance with the AMA *Guidelines of Impairment* (5th edition), this patient is partially impaired predominantly by reason of her degenerative disc and joint disease. She has not reached maximum medical improvement.

*Resulting Cross-examination:*

**Q.** Doctor, have you had any formal training in the use of the AMA *Guides to the Evaluation of Permanent Impairment?*

**A.** No.

**Q.** Your IME report states that the examinee has not yet reached maximum medical improvement, correct?

**A.** That's correct. She has not reached a medical end point.

**Q.** Doctor, could you turn to page 19 of the *Guides?* What is the heading of Section 2.4?

**A.** "When are impairment ratings performed?"

**Q.** The fourth sentence of Section 2.4 reads as follows: "Once an impairment has reached MMI, a permanent impairment may be performed." Am I reading that correctly?

**A.** You are.

**Q.** So your permanent impairment rating in this case was premature because

MMI had not yet been reached when you did the rating, correct?
**A.** Apparently so.
**Q.** You rated the examinee's impairment as "partially impaired" in your IME report?
**A.** Yes, I did.
**Q.** Were you aware that the AMA *Guides* rates impairment in percentages and not in terms of partial or total impairment?
**A.** Well, partial impairment would be less than 100% impairment.
**Q.** What percentage impairment does this examinee have?
**A.** I can't say.
**Q.** Doctor, you really didn't rate the impairment in accordance with the 5th edition of the AMA *Guides*, correct?

**Comment:** Examiners who are not trained in the use of the AMA *Guides* should either obtain the proper training or refrain from doing impairment ratings. Due to the complexity and size (over 600 pages) of the 5th edition, it is very difficult for the untrained physician to do a proper and technically correct impairment rating.

**Defending the Report As Written:** It may be possible to defend what look like obvious mistakes.

**Q.** Doctor, you really didn't rate the impairment in accordance with the 5th edition of the AMA *Guides*, correct?
**A.** I was waiting for maximum medical improvement before I performed a precise evaluation and assigned a percentage of impairment according to the book.

**Example 10.135: Substantiated impairment rating**
*Report States:*

> Ms. Johnson is stable for rating purposes. She will be rated using the *Guides to the Evaluation of Permanent Impairment*, fifth edition, published by the American Medical Association.
>
> Referring to Figure 16-40, on page 476, limitation of right shoulder flexion to 150 degrees represents 2% impairment of the upper extremity. Limitation of extension to 45 degrees represents 1% impairment of the upper extremity (with rounding).
>
> Referring to Figure 16-43, on page 477, limitation of abduction to 120 degrees represents 3% impairment of the upper extremity. Limitation of adduction to 30 degrees represents 1% impairment of the upper extremity.
>
> Referring to Figure 16-46, on page 479, limitation of internal rotation to 30 degrees represents 2% impairment of the upper extremity.
>
> These impairment values are additive, for a total of 8% impairment of the upper extremity.

**Comment:** This is a concise, straightforward, and effective presentation of the examiner's permanent impairment opinions. The edition of the *Guides* used was identified, as were the figures and pages of the book. In addition, the report noted that the rater added, as opposed to combined, the ratings.

## 10.14 Work Capacity and Disability

Referral sources may request an examiner's opinions in the areas of work capacity and disability. Such opinions, when provided, should be precisely stated and objectively supported. If an examiner cannot objectively support an opinion regarding work capacity or disability, it is best to inform the referral source that the examiner is not prepared to opine in these areas.

Work capacity and disability opinions contain many potential serious pitfalls. These include the following.

1. The examiner commenting on what jobs the examinee can and cannot perform without the examiner having a thorough understanding of what is required of the jobs in question.
2. The examiner conducting or ordering functional capacity evaluations that may injure the examinee, thus subjecting the examiner to potential liability.
3. The examiner commenting on work capacity or disability despite not being truly qualified to do so.
4. The written job description provided to the examiner is not likely to be 100% accurate.
5. The examiner misusing definitions from the U.S. Department of Labor's *Dictionary of Occupational Titles.*
6. Not having a sufficient understanding of the examinee's activities of daily living.

A defensible opinion regarding work capacity is an informed decision. Opinions based on a substantial amount of high quality information will be the easiest to defend during cross-examination. Opinions based on suspect or incomplete information and opinions that the examiner may not have been truly qualified to provide will be most vulnerable to cross-examination. A detailed interview with the examinee is one potential way to make up for a lack of documentary and other evidence.

**Example 10.141: Light work capacity**

*Report States:*

This examinee has at least a light work capacity as defined in the *Dictionary of Occupational Titles,* United States Department of Labor. Light work is defined as exerting up to 20 lbs. of force occasionally and/or up to 10 lbs. of force frequently and/or a negligible amount of force constantly to move objects. Physical demands are in excess of those for sedentary work. Light work usually requires a substantial amount of walking or standing. However, if the worker sits most of the time but the use of arm and/or leg controls requires exertion of forces greater than those for sedentary work, the job is rated as light work.

He can work full time. The return-to-work process may be facilitated by starting with less than a full day and slowly increasing the number of hours per day. He should alternate between sitting and standing based upon comfort. He can lift up to 25 lbs. occasionally and up to 10 lbs. frequently, depending upon the circumstances. Factors include the height of the lift, the distance from the body, and the bulk. He may have greater capabilities, particularly with conditioning. He can occasionally bend and twist. If the examinee has no pain into the legs, there are no restrictions on operating foot controls. Prolonged whole-body vibrations should be avoided.

The above restrictions should remain in effect until performance of a functional capacity assessment. His current work status is indicated on the enclosed Functional Capacities Evaluation form. The recommendations are based on the examinee's own report and on my clinical assessment. A formal functional capacities evaluation by a physical therapist skilled in these assessments is recommended. This would best be performed utilizing a standardized, validated protocol such as the Key Functional Assessment.

He is capable of performing other work within the above guidelines.

I would be pleased to review any written functional job descriptions or videotapes of jobs, to make arrangements to view work being considered, and/or to discuss any issues concerning work capability or the return-to-work process.

*Resulting Cross-examination:*

**Q.** You stated your opinion on work capacity on page 3 of your IME report, correct?

**A.** Yes.

**Q.** Are you aware of the examinee's pre-injury capabilities?

**A.** Only to the extent that he was able to do his job.

**Q.** So, you can't say how the injury changed his capabilities?

**A.** That's correct.

**Q.** You didn't actually measure his functional capabilities, correct?

**A.** That's correct. I indicated that he should be sent for a functional capacity evaluation.

**Q.** That's because they would in a functional capacity evaluation actually test and determine the examinee's capacity to perform labor whether sustained, peak, or intermittent, correct?

**A.** That's correct.

**Q.** You also were not provided with written functional job descriptions, correct?

**A.** That's correct.

**Q.** Before you actually determine work capability, work capacity, and the return-to-work process, you would need to see the results of the functional capacity evaluation and the functional job description, correct?

**A.** Yes, that's true.
**Q.** So, your comment on work capacity is not based on all the facts you need to make a fair, accurate, and safe determination, correct?

**Comment:** The fundamental problem with this opinion is the lack of a detailed job description and the lack of a functional capacity evaluation.

**Defending the Report As Written:** Frequently, the examiner is provided with neither a functional capacity evaluation nor a functional job description before he opines on work capacity. While this makes it more difficult, the examiner can still vigorously defend his opinion.

**Q.** So, your comment on work capacity is not based on all the facts you need to make a fair, accurate, and safe determination, correct?
**A.** No. I examined the examinee and determined how much he could lift, stand, sit, bend, and twist. I stated that he should start out at less than a full day and slowly increase the number of hours he works each day. My opinion is fair, accurate, and safe.

**Example 10.142: Not understanding "real world" job requirements**
*Report States:*

> In my opinion, based upon a reasonable degree of medical certainty, this examinee can return immediately to her full-time job as a file clerk. She is clearly capable of such light duty work and her knee injury only affects her ability to bend and squat, not to walk.

*Resulting Cross-examination:*
**Q.** Your IME report indicated that the examinee can return to her full-time job as a file clerk, correct?
**A.** Yes, that's what I said.
**Q.** Did you have a functional job description available when you formed that opinion?
**A.** No, but I know what a file clerk does, Counsel.
**Q.** Do many of them wear sneakers or running shoes to work?
**A.** Some do.
**Q.** When a "stat" order is placed for medical and hospital records, does the file clerk walk to the elevator and wait for it to come?
**A.** No, not usually.
**Q.** The file clerk grabs the records and runs down or up the stairs with the records, don't they?
**A.** Yes, sometimes they do.
**Q.** That's why they wear running shoes?
**A.** I suppose.
**Q.** Sometimes these records can be voluminous and heavy?
**A.** Yes.
**Q.** Can they sometimes be 30-40 or more pounds?
**A.** In some cases.
**Q.** Sometimes the records are so large they push them around in carts, don't they?

**A.** Yes, I have seen that.
**Q.** Are you aware that the file cabinets go right to the floor so that the clerks have to kneel down to pull them out of the bottom drawer?
**A.** I was unaware of that.
**Q.** Did you ask the examinee about her specific duties, how much she has to lift, bend, run, carry, or kneel at work before you said she could return full time to her job?
**A.** No, I did not.
**Q.** Did you consult the *Dictionary of Occupational Titles* to determine what a file clerk in a hospital actually does?
**A.** No.
**Q.** Did you view a videotape of someone actually performing the job?
**A.** No, I did not.
**Q.** As you sit here today under oath, can you testify that this examinee can return to a job you knew little about without the serious risk of re-injury?

**Comment:** Examiners who are not familiar with the essential tasks of a job are in a very poor position to opine about the examinee's ability to return to work at that job. At a minimum, the examiner should review a written job description before offering an opinion. Because many job descriptions are outdated, incomplete, or inconsistent with the realities of the workplace, the examiner who reviews the actual job duties with the examinee is in the strongest position to defend his opinion and report.

**Defending the Report As Written:** Examiners will not always be provided with all the information necessary to write a bulletproof IME report. Many times they will be given a pre-made, generic return-to-work form to complete. These examiners have the option of obtaining additional information from the client or from the examinee. When this is not practical, they will have to do the best with what is available.

**Q.** Did you have a functional job description available when you formed that opinion?
**A.** No, but I am familiar with the duties of a file clerk in a hospital setting and I asked the examinee about her day-to-day actual duties. After I considered these duties, I expressed my opinion concerning her ability to return to work. Your client wants to return to work as soon as possible and I commend her for her attitude.

**Example 10.143: Vague opinion on disability**
*Report States:*
The examinee is limited to part-time work.

*Resulting Cross-examination:*
**Q.** Doctor, in your IME report, page 4, under the heading "Disability," you stated, "The examinee is limited to part-time work," correct?
**A.** That is correct.
**Q.** Do you know what the physical requirements of his job are?
**A.** He told me he was an exercise physiologist and sports trainer.

**Q.** What are the physical requirements of his job?
**A.** I was not given that information.
**Q.** Did you ask him?
**A.** No.
**Q.** Can the examinee lift 50-100 pounds?
**A.** Because of his thoracic disc disorder, I would not recommend it.
**Q.** Did you place any limitations on his return to part-time work in your IME report?
**A.** No.
**Q.** Was that an oversight or was that intentional on your part?
**A.** It…was…an…intentional.
**Q.** Why was that, Doctor?
**A.** Well, I didn't perform a functional capacity exam, just an IME, Counsel.
**Q.** So you intentionally didn't say in your IME report how much he could bend, stretch, or lift at work?
**A.** Correct.
**Q.** But you did release him to return to work part-time at his job without knowing the physical requirements of the job?
**A.** I found him able to return to part-time work.
**Q.** Can he work 35 hours a week?
**A.** No.
**Q.** Can he work 33 hours a week?
**A.** No.
**Q.** What about 31 hours?
**A.** I don't think so.
**Q.** Can you tell us, Doctor, under oath, how many hours this examinee can work at his old position without risking serious re-injury?

**Comment:** Before commenting on disability in an IME report, the examiner should first have a good working knowledge of the physical requirements of the job. In the above example, this would have assisted the examiner when he was writing his report. For example, the American Medical Association's *Guides to the Evaluation of Permanent Impairment* (5th edition, 2001) states:

> An individual can have a disability in performing a specific work activity, but not have a disability in any other social role…If the physician has the expertise and is well acquainted with the individual's activities and needs, the physician may also express an opinion about the presence or absence of a specific disability.[6]

The examiner in the above example would have been better served by a more specific statement.

> The examinee has residual exercise and work intolerance due to his ongoing problem with a thoracic disc disorder. He can return to work on a part-time basis no more than 20 hours per week as tolerated. He should not lift more than 25 lbs. occasionally and should not be required to stretch or bend more than occasionally.

[6] Sec. 1-2B, p. 8.

**Defending the Report As Written:** When faced with a vague comment on disability in an IME report, the physician should be prepared to explain it.

**Q.** Did you place any limitations on his return to part-time work in your IME report?
**A.** Yes. I stated he is limited to part-time work and I should have added "as tolerated."

**Example 10.144: "Can resume his employment"**
*Report States:*

He can resume his employment as a salesman of medical products.

*Resulting Cross-examination:*
**Q.** Under "Disability Status" in your IME report, you concluded that the examinee "can resume his employment as a salesman of medical products," correct?
**A.** Yes.
**Q.** Do you have a job description for the position you found the examinee could resume?
**A.** No, I was not furnished one.
**Q.** Did you ask for one, Doctor?
**A.** No.
**Q.** Did you check the *Dictionary of Occupational Titles* to see what the duties of a salesman of medical products actually are?
**A.** No, Counsel, I did not.
**Q.** You did, of course, at least ask the examinee what his job duties were before you medically cleared him to return to work?
**A.** Well, I have no information on his duties in the occupational status portion of my report.
**Q.** Is that a no, Doctor?
**A.** It appears to be.
**Q.** You don't know how far the examinee had to drive each day, what he had to lift and how often he had to lift it, and what medical products he had to demonstrate. Is that correct?
**A.** Yes.
**Q.** If this was a patient of yours who you were treating for neck and back problems, would you want to know his job duties before you medically cleared him to return to work, Doctor?

**Comment:** When a physician deals directly with disability in his IME report and clears the examinee to return to work, the physician needs to understand the examinee's job duties.

> The examinee is a salesman of medical products consisting primarily of pillow cases and sheets. He informs me that he has a small territory of 25 miles requiring driving of no more than 30 minutes per day. The examinee informs me that he is required to lift no more than 10 pounds occasionally. The examinee can resume his employment as a salesman of medical products.

**Defending the Report As Written:** IME physicians need to be able to look beyond the precise question to the total information on hand to best defend their reports. In addition, they might want to push back at counsel every once in a while.

**Q.** If this was a patient of yours who you were treating for neck and back problems, would you want to know his job duties before you medically cleared him to return to work, Doctor?
**A.** I am not a treating physician and was asked to do an IME only. If this was my patient, however, he would have been back to work a long time ago, Counsel, assuming he didn't want to stay out to maximize his legal recovery.

**Example 10.145: Work restrictions without benefit of job description**
*Report States:*

> Examinee can return to a light duty position with restrictions regarding bending, stooping, and squatting, as well as allowing for frequent breaks.

*Resulting Cross-examination:*
**Q.** Doctor, your April 20, 2000 IME report found that the examinee could "return to a light duty position with restrictions regarding bending, stooping, and squatting, as well as allowing for frequent breaks." You specified the restrictions as follows:

> "LIGHT WORK: Lifting 20 pounds maximum with frequent lifting and/or carrying of objects weighting up to 10 pounds. Even though the weight lifted may be only a negotiable amount, a job is in this category when it involves sitting most of the time with a degree of pushing/pulling of arm and/or leg controls. Limited use of affected extremity—limited bending, squatting, climbing, and lifting."
> Is that correct?

**A.** Yes.
**Q.** Did you examine the examinee subsequent to April 19, 2000, Doctor?
**A.** No.
**Q.** You then sent a letter to the Office of Workers' Compensation dated September 13, 2000, stating that the examinee could resume her employment as a service operator?
**A.** Yes.
**Q.** Before you stated the examinee could resume her employment, were you provided with the job description, which provides the physical requirements of the job as follows:

> "PHYSICAL REQUIREMENTS: Due to the duties required of the Environmental Services Department you must be capable of lifting objects properly/capable of bending, stooping, kneeling/reaching with no problems/lifting, carrying objects for short distances/capable of standing and walking for up to seven to eight hours per shift/able to climb a ladder and complete cleaning duties from a ladder/able to use hands and fingers while performing duties from the ladder/able to use hands and fingers while performing duties for seven to eight hours per day repetitively/capable of pushing/pulling carts by utilizing both hands and legs/able to lift object such as mop buckets 15 to 20 times per shift. Reaching and handling objects at

> chest level/above the shoulders. Capable of lifting objects up to 25 pounds and capable of pushing and pulling wheeled carts with empty boxes and office/exam room trash. Able to use body when dust mopping, wet mopping, vacuuming, and daily cleaning duties."

**A.** No, I was not.
**Q.** Is the job description consistent with the restrictions in your April 20, 2000 IME report?

**Comment:** An examiner who releases an examinee to "return to work" without first knowing the precise nature and duties of the position is in a weak position to defend his IME report. Examiners who are asked to opine about disability status and/or return to work, but who are not first provided with job descriptions should refuse to do so.

**Defending the Report As Written:** Examiners who are familiar with the realities of the workplace are in the best position to defend work restrictions in their IME reports. These examiners may be able to "turn the tables" on opposing counsel.

**Q.** Is the job description consistent with the restrictions in your April 20, 2000 IME report?
**A.** It is consistent with what the examinee told me she actually did on the job. As you know, Counsel, many job descriptions are written by HR people who have little or no idea about what is really going on outside of their ivory towers.

**Example 10.146: Misuse of *Dictionary of Occupational Titles* term**
*Report States:*

> He is medically capable of light lifting of no more than 10 pounds maximum.

*Resulting Cross-examination:*
**Q.** Doctor, you found the examinee capable of light work, correct?
**A.** Yes. I stated in my report, "He is medically capable of light lifting of no more than 10 pounds maximum."
**Q.** You used the standard definition of light work found in the *Dictionary of Occupational Titles?*
**A.** Yes.
**Q.** Are you aware that the *Dictionary of Occupational Titles* defines light work as "exerting up to 20 lbs. of force occasionally"?
**A.** No, I was not aware of that.
**Q.** Would it be more accurate to say, Doctor, that the claimant has only the capacity to do sedentary work, defined as being able to lift 5-10 lbs?

**Comment:** It is customary for examiners to express work capacity in accordance with the definitions used in the *Dictionary of Occupational Titles*, United States Department of Labor. In addition to being familiar with the definitions, the examiner should also consider discussing endurance, tolerance for sitting, standing, and walking, and the frequencies for lifting and carrying.

> The examinee has a sedentary work capacity as defined in the *Dictionary of Occupational Titles*. He can lift 5 lbs. frequently and up to 10 lbs. occasionally. He should be permitted to return to work gradually. He should limit his standing, bending, and twisting based upon his comfort.

**Defending the Report As Written:** When faced with an alleged improper use of a definition in describing work capacity, the examiner should clarify his meaning and not necessarily accept counsel's characterizations.

**Q.** Are you aware that the *Dictionary of Occupational Titles* defines light work as "exerting up to 20 lbs. of force"?
**A.** What I meant, Counsel, was that the examinee can lift no more than 10 lbs. maximum on a <u>frequent basis</u>, but up to 20 lbs. occasionally. This would still place him in the light work category. You intentionally or unintentionally misquoted the *Dictionary of Occupational Titles,* which states, "Light work is defined as exerting up to 20 lbs. of force occasionally and/or up to 10 lbs. of force frequently."

**Example 10.147: "Not disabled from any activities of daily living that a normal 63-year-old male would participate in"**
*Report States:*

> The examinee is not disabled from any activities of daily living that a normal 63-year-old male would participate in.

*Resulting Cross-examination:*
**Q.** Doctor, do some normal 63-year-old males run marathons?
**A.** Yes, I suppose.
**Q.** Can this examinee run a marathon?
**A.** I don't know.
**Q.** Can he play tennis or squash?
**A.** I am not sure.
**Q.** So, when you said in your IME report under the "Disability" heading, "The examinee is not disabled from any activity of daily living that a normal 63-year-old male would participate in," you misspoke?

**Comment:** IME physicians should be as precise as possible when commenting on disability. Vague generalities will result in unnecessary cross-examination.

> The examinee is not disabled from his activities of daily living.

**Defending the Report As Written:** When faced with his own poor choice of a word or phrase in an IME report, the physician should correct the problem at the first opportunity.

**Q.** Doctor, do some normal 63-year-old males run marathons?
**A.** I should have been more specific in my report. I meant "average," not "normal." So, while certainly some normal 63-year-old males run marathons, the average 63-year old is not able to do so.

**Example 10.148: Work capacity: vague opinion**

*Report States:*

> At this point in time, the examinee has sedentary capabilities. He could, however, not spend any major time on his right foot.

*Resulting Cross-examination:*

**Q.** Doctor, is your opinion on this examinee's work capacity based upon a reasonable degree of medical certainty?
**A.** Yes, it is.
**Q.** Your opinion is that the examinee could not spend any major time on his right foot?
**A.** Yes, that's correct.
**Q.** By "on the foot" you mean standing on the foot?
**A.** Yes.
**Q.** Would the type of floor he spent time on be a significant factor?
**A.** It could.
**Q.** So he could spend less time on concrete flooring than carpeting?
**A.** Yes.
**Q.** What about inclines—would those impact his foot?
**A.** It could.
**Q.** What about temperature—working outside in cold weather—would that affect the time on his foot?
**A.** Yes.
**Q.** The same for uneven flooring?
**A.** Yes.
**Q.** How much time on the foot would be too much?
**A.** That's hard to say.
**Q.** Would three hours a day be too much?
**A.** Probably, yes.
**Q.** What about just five minutes, would that be OK?
**A.** Yes.
**Q.** So somewhere between five minutes and three hours a day. That is your opinion on his work capacity?

**Comment:** When examiners put work restrictions or limitation on examinees, they should be specific. Vague comments, as in the above example, will lead to unnecessary cross-examination and uncertainty.

> The examinee can work four hours a day, five days a week. He should be able to sit and stand based on comfort. He can tolerate walking or standing on his right foot only occasionally. He should not walk or stand on hard flooring, uneven ground, or be exposed to extreme cold.

**Defending the Report As Written:** Examiners can defend vague comments by explaining what they meant when given the opportunity.

**Q.** How much time on the foot would be too much?
**A.** No more than is comfortable for the examinee. He needs to be able to sit and stand based on his comfort level. Remember, this is a young man who had

his foot run over by a bulldozer.

**Example 10.149: Work capacity: left-handed-only work**

*Report States:*

> Work Capacity: On the basis of this exam, I feel that he is unable to perform any manual work with his right hand. He could perform left-handed-only work at this time.

*Resulting Cross-examination:*

**Q.** Doctor, you reviewed no x-rays or medical records prior to writing your IME report, correct?

**A.** Yes. That's correct. None were provided to me.

**Q.** But you did a careful exam and report nonetheless?

**A.** I did my best, Counsel.

**Q.** Do you have any independent memory of this examinee?

**A.** Not really. Just what is in my report.

**Q.** Where in your report, Doctor, do you state whether the examinee is left-handed or right-handed?

**A.** Well, give me a moment. . . .It's not in here.

**Q.** As you sit here today, you don't know whether this examinee was right-handed or left-handed, correct?

**A.** That is correct.

**Q.** Would that be important to know before you offered an opinion on his work capacity?

**A.** Yes.

**Q.** That's because if it is his major hand that was injured, it would be difficult for him to work with his minor hand, correct?

**A.** That's true.

**Q.** This man cannot return to work as a carpenter, correct?

**A.** No, not at this time.

**Q.** Could you tell me, Doctor, what is his educational background?

**A.** I don't have that information.

**Q.** Did you ask him if he can read and write or graduated from high school?

**A.** I did not.

**Q.** You limited your examination to his upper extremities, correct?

**A.** Yes, that's correct.

**Q.** You didn't ask him if he has any other physical problems or limitations?

**A.** Correct.

**Q.** Would you agree, Doctor, that as you don't know if this examinee's major or minor hand was injured, you don't know his educational background, and don't know if he has any other physical problems or limitations, you are not in a position to offer an informed opinion on work capacity?

**Comment:** Examiners who comment on work capacity in their reports should be familiar with the examinee's injury, his educational background, and any other medical limitations.

**Defending the Report As Written:** The report as written would be difficult to defend. The best the examiner could do would be to be more candid as to the examinee's true work capacity.

**Q.** This man cannot return to work as a carpenter, correct?
**A.** Yes, that's correct. In fact, he is facing additional surgery and extensive physical therapy. Any comments about return to work or work capacity would be premature at this time.

**Example 10.1410: Functional capacity**
*Lindsey v. Metropolitan Life Insurance Company,* 909 F.Supp. 1408 (1995)
IME physicians who do not have a full understanding of the examinee's job duties are at a serious disadvantage when attempting to assess functional capacity.

In the case *Lindsey v. Metropolitan Life Insurance Company,* a physician tried to offer the explanation that knowledge of the claimant's job duties is not really necessary to opine on functional capacity. During his deposition, he described functional capacity analysis as:

> an analysis of the expected level of physical or mental activity of the individual as described in the medical records provided as it is—in our analysis we also use a worse case scenario.
>
> In other words, we assume all worse case findings or diagnoses that we possibly can, that it represents a least possible function rather than a greater, maximum capacity. Basically to the insurance company in comparing it to the requirements of either the person's past work or any work, they can make their own decisions whether the person is or is not disabled, or any other decision they need to make.

He went on in that deposition to state the following:

> **Q.** Okay. Do you require, when you do one of these functional capacity analyses, do you require that you be furnished with a specific list of the claimant's job duties before rendering an opinion?
> **A.** No, because the two are independent. In other words, the functional capacity analysis is done independent of what the job duties are. The functional capacity analysis is based on the medical information coming in.
> **Q.** So you don't really care what the—what a specific claimant's job duties are when you render a functional capacity analysis; is that correct?
> **A.** Correct. And in some cases we don't even know what it is either, because the specific job duties are not even in question for the insurance company examiner's own occupation disability question that they are looking at.
> **Q.** So how do you come up with a functional capacity analysis that would inform an insurance company whether or not there are limitations on a claimant's ability to work if you don't know what the claimant's work is?
> **A.** We give them a fairly comprehensive statement of what the person can or can't do and hopefully in the initial information the insurance examiner has had enough experience to ask us about any specific questions that might arise that go beyond the usual general responses. If the insurance examiner has questions that we have not answered because the questions weren't asked or our answer in summary was incomplete, they can ask us to address that issue specifically.
> **Q.** How often does that occur?
> **A.** It's not very common.

**Q.** It's in fact very rare, is it not?
**A.** Yeah, fairly rare. At 1418, 1419.

As one might expect, the Court was not impressed with the physician's assessment of functional capacity in this fashion.

## 10.15 Past and Future Care

The examiner may be asked to opine on the medical appropriateness of past care and what care will be needed in the future. As always, the most defensible opinions will be those supported by objective reasons that are clearly documented in the report. There are many potential pitfalls in opining in these areas. The following are some potential problem areas.

1. The temptation to use the IME report as a vehicle to take pot shots at different schools of medicine, different specialties, or specific individual providers. This can be used against the examiner to show bias and should be avoided.
2. Estimating costs of future medical care. This may not be within the examiner's true area of expertise and should, generally, be avoided.
3. Potentially giving an opinion that other providers have unnecessarily or fraudulently treated the examinee. This could potentially ignite a firestorm. It is better practice to objectively state the facts regarding treatment and leave the issue of potential wrongdoing to others.
4. Second-guessing a colleague, despite the fact that the examiner was not present during the alleged over-treatment and may not even be of the same specialty or profession as the colleague.

**Example 10.151: Unqualified to comment on standard of care of chiropractor**

*Report States:*

Her chiropractic care has been consistent with the usual standards of care for this injury.

*Resulting Cross-examination:*

**Q.** Your IME report indicates that you feel that the examinee's chiropractic care has been consistent with the usual standards of care for this injury, correct?
**A.** Yes, it does.
**Q.** Are you a chiropractic doctor?
**A.** No, I am a neurologist.
**Q.** Have you had chiropractic training?
**A.** No, but I see many chiropractic reports.
**Q.** Do you attend chiropractic continuing education courses?
**A.** No.
**Q.** Do you perform chiropractic manipulations?
**A.** No.

**Q.** If a member of your family needed a chiropractic manipulation, would you do that yourself or refer them to a chiropractor?
**A.** Refer them to a chiropractor.
**Q.** That's because you are not qualified to render chiropractic care?
**A.** That's correct.
**Q.** Are you familiar with the standards of appropriate care for chiropractors?
**A.** Somewhat.
**Q.** Are you familiar with the criteria outlined in the RAND study entitled "The Appropriateness of Spinal Manipulation for Low Back Pain"?
**A.** I am generally familiar with the study.
**Q.** The study concluded that up to 16 adjustments were appropriate, but chiropractic beyond that point was not and that the number of manipulations needed for the average patient to achieve a substantial clinical response in a case of low back pain was 5 and the number of subsequent manipulations was 11, isn't that correct?
**A.** I don't know.
**Q.** If we were to assume that to be true, the examinee's 37 manipulations are not consistent with "the usual standards of care for this injury," correct, Doctor?

**Comment:** When an examiner leaves his field of expertise to comment on the appropriateness of care in another discipline, he should do so with caution. When, and only when, the examiner familiarizes himself with the applicable standards, will he be in a position to properly defend his opinion and report.

**Defending the Report As Written:** When questioned about standards of appropriateness of care by opposing counsel, the experienced examiner asks to see the standards. He does this to:

1. make sure counsel is not mischaracterizing them, and
2. to ensure that counsel is not leaving anything out.

**Q.** If we were to assume that to be true, the examinee's 37 manipulations are not consistent with the "usual standards of care for this injury," correct, Doctor?
**A.** Counsel, may I please see the Rand Study you are waving around? Actually, you left out a crucial part of two sentences. It states, "The number of manipulations needed for the *average* patient to achieve a substantial clinical response in a case of low back pain *without neurologic findings or disc herniation was 5* while the number of subsequent manipulations, if any, needed for the *average* patient to reach maximal therapeutic benefit was 11."

Here the examinee had *both neurologic findings and disc herniation.* She was not an average patient. In addition, the orthopedic specialists gave up on her and said that she had no other alternatives. That is why, in my opinion, the 37 manipulations were appropriate and consistent with the standards of care.

**Example 10.152: Accusing colleague of malpractice**
*Report States:*

> His care has not been consistent with the usual standard of care for this condition.

*Resulting Cross-examination:*
**Q.** Your report indicates that the examinee's care has not been consistent with the standard of care for this problem, correct?
**A.** Yes.
**Q.** So you are accusing the treating physician of malpractice or incompetence?
**A.** The examinee received substandard care that resulted in his prolonged disability and permanent harm.
**Q.** Did you report the physician to the medical society or anyone else for the sub-standard care he rendered?

**Comment:** IME examiners should exercise extreme caution when opining on the malpractice or incompetence of a physician. The physician can be expected to "fight back" with ethical complaints and, in extreme cases, take action for libel. The cautious examiner states objective facts and lets the reader draw his own conclusions.

> Dr. Jones performed four back surgeries on the examinee, including two discectomies, a fusion, and a second fusion. The examinee states the surgeries were unsuccessful and left him in constant pain. The examinee refused a proposed fifth surgical procedure by Dr. Jones.

**Defending the Report As Written:** Examiners who choose to comment on the treating physician's lack of skill or on failed procedures need to be able to back up their reports with objective facts.

**Q.** So you are accusing the treating physician of malpractice or incompetence?
**A.** Dr. Jones's track record speaks for itself—four failed back surgeries on an examinee with arachnoiditis.

**Example 10.153: List of recommendations for future care**
*Report States:*

> I recommend that future therapeutic and diagnostic health care needs will be required for Mr. Babitsky's maintenance and stability of his pathology:
>
> a) Implantable pain device for lumbar spine pain as his condition progresses or deteriorates.
>
> b) Pharmacological pain management approaches with possible injections for lumbar spine pain as his condition progresses or deteriorates.
>
> c) He will require orthopedic surgical evaluations on an as-needed basis or for flares of the lumbar spine as his condition progresses or deteriorates.
>
> d) He will require a drug supply depending on the providers' recommendations and his progressive pathologies as his condition progresses or deteriorates.

e) He will require a psychiatric evaluation and pharmacological intervention to address the chronic behavioral impairments that he has been unable to manage on his own.

f) Given the significant degree of work restriction, a functional work capacity evaluation is indicated to more accurately determine the examinee's work capacity.

**Comment:** This is an easy-to-read format and the recommendations are supported by the examiner's reasons.

**Example 10.154: Past and future care**
*Report States:*

*Past:* The evaluation and treatment rendered in the ER at General Hospital by Dr. Allara and at Southern Health Care Co. through September 3, 1997, probably were necessary for injuries sustained in the February 1997 collision. However, no further diagnostic or therapeutic endeavors were necessary for effects of that collision.

*Future:* No further formal treatment appears warranted at present for the plaintiff's neck-upper-back-left shoulder or bilateral anterior knee pains. However, as repeatedly advised by others, she would be well advised to continue a self-directed program of stretching, strengthening, and aerobic conditioning exercises. Weight reduction is also recommended. Ms. Mant may also wish to take an over-the-counter analgesic on an as-needed basis provided no untoward side-effect results.

**Comment:** This is a concise and well-written section that features objective, non-inflammatory language.

**Example 10.155: Well-supported recommendations for future care**
*Report States:*

*What are your recommendations for future medical care? Please be specific with regard to the frequency and duration of this care. Is this care needed as a direct result of the accident of 08/13/01?*

There are certainly no curative therapies for her condition. She has a chronic multi-level lumbar degenerative disc condition. She needs to understand that self-care will be the key to management of this problem. Since there has been some uncertainty about future options for her, I think it would be reasonable for her to have one additional brief trial of physical therapy that focuses on teaching her a self-directed exercise program. Additional pharmacologic management might also be appropriate as long as her response is carefully monitored and it is clear that the pharmacologic interventions are helping. One possibility would be to modify her opiate regimen. More importantly, I think that she could benefit from anti-depressant medication to help her deal with emotional distress related to her ongoing back pain and disability. This care would be appropriate to help her return to the functional status that she had prior to 08/13/01. Her need

> for treatment appears to be a direct result of her injury of 8/13/01, as noted above.

**Comment:** This opinion is clearly written, informative, and supported by objective evidence.

**Example 10.156: Care was appropriate**
*Report States:*

> **Appropriateness of Care**
> The client has asked that I specifically address the issue of appropriateness of medical care. Based on the specifics of this care, it is my professional opinion that care has been consistent with the usual standards of care for this problem.

**Comment:** This examiner addressed the issue of appropriateness of care clearly and concisely.

**Example 10.157: Exaggerated/sloppy comments on appropriateness of care**
*Report States:*

> All of her treatment appears to have been quite excessive.

*Resulting Cross-examination:*
**Q.** The examinee was hit from behind in a motor vehicle accident, felt immediate neck and back pain, and was transported by the emergency squad to the local hospital emergency room for evaluation and treatment, correct?
**A.** Yes, that is the history I have.
**Q.** Were the evaluation and treatment at the hospital emergency room quite excessive?
**A.** No.
**Q.** She was then referred to her family physician for an office visit. Was this one office visit quite excessive?
**A.** No.
**Q.** She was referred by her family doctor to see an orthopedic specialist, whom she saw on one occasion. Was this one office visit with the orthopedic specialist quite excessive?
**A.** No.
**Q.** So, Doctor, when you said in your IME report, page 3, "All of her treatment appears to have been quite excessive," were you exaggerating or mistaken?

**Comment:** When the examiner in the above example exaggerated the extent of excessive treatment, he made himself vulnerable to cross-examination. The physician would have been in a stronger position had he limited his comments on the appropriateness of care.

> It is my opinion that there are no objective findings to support an ongoing need for manipulation.

**Defending the Report As Written:** When the examiner prepares to testify at deposition, hearing, or trial, he should carefully review his IME report. The examiner should flag any comments he made in the report that were exaggerations. At the first opportunity during his testimony, he should set the record straight.

**Q.** Were the evaluation and treatment at the hospital emergency room quite excessive?
**A.** When I said in my report that all of the treatment appears to be quite excessive, I was referring to the manipulation only. The manipulation has been going on for one-and-one-half years, three times per week. The emergency room treatment was not excessive.

**Example 10.158: Tirade against chiropractors**
*Report States:*

> I never cease to be amazed at the number of chiropractors who seem totally oblivious to the existence of mental health problems and their influence upon somatic complaints, inevitably attributing whatever symptoms in whatever distribution to one, or more often multiple, physical diagnoses, generally "subluxations."

*Resulting Cross-examination:*
**Q.** Doctor, you have an axe to grind with chiropractors, don't you?
**A.** That's not true.
**Q.** Your IME report says on page 3, "I never cease to be amazed at the number of chiropractors who seem totally oblivious to the existence of mental health problems and their influence upon somatic complaints, inevitably attributing whatever symptoms in whatever distribution to one or more multiple physical diagnoses, generally 'subluxations'"?
**A.** Yes, that's what it says.
**Q.** You also said that the chiropractic treatment was counterproductive, promoted patient dependency, and enabled the examinee's symptoms?
**A.** Yes, I did.
**Q.** You question the appropriateness of manipulations for neck pain in any case, didn't you?
**A.** Yes.
**Q.** This despite the fact that almost every chiropractor performs manipulations for neck pain?
**A.** That doesn't make it right, Counsel.
**Q.** So you are saying that every chiropractor is doing something wrong, but you don't have an axe to grind with chiropractors?

**Comment:** Physicians drafting IME reports should be careful not to evidence a bias against a certain discipline or category of caregivers. Even when the physician does not have a true bias, the physician should still be cautious. There is no need to help opposing counsel imply or demonstrate real or imagined bias against any discipline.

**Defending the Report As Written:** IME physicians who comment on the effectiveness of another discipline need to be able to back up their comments.

**Q.** Doctor, you have an axe to grind with chiropractors, don't you?
**A.** Not generally, but in this case I do. The criteria outlined in the RAND study *The Appropriateness of Spinal Manipulation for Low Back Pain* found 5-11 manipulations optimal to reach maximal therapeutic benefit. In this case, the chiropractor performed 75 manipulations over 3 months. This is not appropriate care and I do have a serious problem about what was done to this examinee.

**Example 10.159: Patient will not undergo further treatment, therefore, patient desires to remain disabled**
*Report States:*

> I feel that the patient's desire not to proceed with other treatments but rather is satisfied with his present status and desires to remain like that, is consistent with a patient who desires to remain in a disabled status.

*Resulting Cross-examination:*
**Q.** Doctor, this examinee injured his back in 1991, 1995, 1996, and 2001 and each time returned to work?
**A.** Yes, that's the history I have.
**Q.** Is returning to work four times after injury consistent with a patient who desires to remain disabled?
**A.** No, but he did eventually stop working.
**Q.** He stopped when the back and radiating leg pain were so bad he had trouble sitting, standing, and walking?
**A.** That's correct.
**Q.** You found that the examinee suffers from chronic lower back arthritis, correct?
**A.** Yes.
**Q.** Did you review the x-rays from 1991, 1995, 1996, and 2001, Doctor?
**A.** No.
**Q.** Do you know why they were not provided to you?
**A.** No, I don't.
**Q.** Did you ask for them?
**A.** No, I didn't.
**Q.** Would x-rays have been of assistance in helping diagnose osteoarthritis?
**A.** Not necessarily.
**Q.** You feel that the patient would benefit from back surgery, correct?
**A.** Yes, definitely.
**Q.** The examinee, of course, is not your patient, correct?
**A.** Yes.
**Q.** He was the patient of Dr. Adler, the orthopedic surgeon, correct?
**A.** Yes.
**Q.** What did the treating physician recommend to his patient?
**A.** Not to have surgery.
**Q.** Would you be willing to guarantee what the results of the surgery would be?
**A.** No.
**Q.** The failure of the examinee to go forward with the surgery that was not recommended by his treating orthopedic surgeon makes you conclude the examinee wants to remain disabled?

**Comment:** Examiners who express their opinions about the examinee's failure to undergo surgery are opening themselves up to cross-examination. The examiner who tries too hard to make the case for lack of motivation runs the substantial risk of being perceived as biased and an advocate.

**Defending the Report As Written:** When undergoing cross-examination, the IME physician can "fight back" when it is appropriate.

**Q.** Would you be willing to guarantee what the results of the surgery would be?
**A.** I guarantee you that if I was in constant pain and spent my day sitting around the house unable to do anything, I would have the surgery.

**Example 10.1510: Estimating cost of future care**
*Report States:*

> This lumbar strain/sprain can be expected to never fully resolve. It is likely that the examinee will need continuing manipulation and physical therapy and potentially analgesic intervention. Her future medical costs from this injury could be $50,000 plus.

*Resulting Cross-examination:*
**Q.** Doctor, do you agree with Dr. Sheldon Jellinek that 90% of examinees with lumbar strains recover within one to two months?
**A.** Most do, but I am not sure about the statistics.
**Q.** This examinee, in your opinion, will never recover?
**A.** That's my opinion.
**Q.** Of course, she could wake up tomorrow and be all better, correct?
**A.** It's possible, not likely.
**Q.** She will need manipulation for the rest of her life?
**A.** Yes.
**Q.** Even though it will not help to cure her?
**A.** It will provide temporary relief.
**Q.** Until the next chiropractic visit?
**A.** Yes.
**Q.** What is the examinee's life expectancy, Doctor?
**A.** I don't know precisely. . . maybe 20 years?
**Q.** Are you an expert on chiropractic manipulation?
**A.** No.
**Q.** As you sit here today, can you say with a reasonable degree of medical certainty how often she will go to a chiropractor one or two years from now?
**A.** No. I just assumed two times a week.
**Q.** That certainly could change in the future?
**A.** Yes.
**Q.** Are you an expert on accurately projecting future medical costs?
**A.** No.
**Q.** So, despite the fact that you don't know the examinee's life expectancy, are not an expert on chiropractic manipulation, and are not an expert on projecting

future medical expenses, you are willing to offer an opinion under oath about this examinee's future medical expenses?

**Comment:** Examiners who offer ballpark projections of future medical expenses are vulnerable to the above type of cross-examination. Most examiners are better served by not speculating about future medical costs and expenses.

**Defending the Report As Written:** Examiners who estimate future medical costs need to be able to explain and support their opinions.

**Q.** Are you an expert on chiropractic manipulation?
**A.** I relied on the treating chiropractor, who stated the examinee would need once-a-week treatment for the rest of her life. This is what I based my opinion on for future medical costs.

## 10.16 Symptom Magnification, Fraud, Malingering, and Objective Support for Subjective Findings

Examiners should be very careful when opining in the areas of symptom magnification, fraud, malingering, and whether the subjective complaints of the examinee are supported by objective findings. These areas can be extremely challenging for a number of reasons, including the following.

1. "Fraud" is a technical *legal* term. It should not be used by independent medical examiners.
2. "Malingering" is a technical psychiatric diagnosis contained in DSM-IV. Using the term "malingering" raises the question as to whether the examiner is qualified to give a psychiatric opinion. Examiners who use the term "malingering" should know the DSM-IV definition of this condition.
3. It is impossible to know for certain how much pain another person is in. In addition, pain is a subjective phenomenon. Different individuals experience different levels of pain for the same condition and have different tolerances for pain. There is no way around the fact that the person who is in the best position to determine the extent of the examinee's pain is the examinee, not the examiner.
4. The examiner may be accused during cross-examination of trying to trick the examinee through distraction and other tests.

When expressing opinions in these areas, examiners should remember to not state more than they have to. This usually means limiting the opinion to the fact that the examinee's subjective complaints are not supported by objective findings. Non-inflammatory language should be used. Examiners should be well-prepared to respond to counsel's questions regarding evaluating pain and any distraction tests used by the examiner.

**Example 10.161: Lengthy discussion of and opinions regarding symptom magnification and non-organic findings**

*Report States:*

Symptom magnification (SM) is exaggeration of pain or other complaints, often precipitated by an injury or illness. While physical effects of the trauma or disease improve and perhaps resolve, the symptoms persist, and may increase in severity and/or distribution over time. The magnification may be conscious or unconscious.

The severity of pain is commonly exaggerated in SM, e.g., 9, 10, or even greater on a 0-10 scale. Ms. Mant was asked today to quantify her discomfort from 0 (none) to 10 (the worst pain imaginable). While the reader may have another mental picture, the examiner envisions an individual with discomfort of 10 in severity writhing in agony on the ground, floor, or bed while awaiting ambulance transportation to an emergency room. In other words, someone with 10/10 pain is, or should be, hospitalized.[7] Whether the plaintiff was actually having pain of 10 in severity after the February 1997 collision as claimed cannot be confirmed or denied, but she was not hospitalized. A rating of 7 implies moderately severe pain for which one needs to see a doctor now. Notwithstanding her comfortable appearance during the interview, Ms. Mant reported having neck pain of 6-7 in severity at present.

While few musculoskeletal conditions produce constant pain, the most notable examples being infection and tumor, symptom magnifiers often claim omnipresent discomfort. Pain due to physical injuries or degenerative disease is usually mechanical, precipitated by activity or prolonged maintenance of one position, persists for a period of time thereafter, then resolves with cessation of the offending activity and rest, or a change in position. Today Ms. Mant claimed to have constant neck pain.

Sometimes discomfort is hyperbolically characterized, e.g., horrible, unbearable, or devastating. The plaintiff did not use these emotionally laden descriptors. Persons exaggerating their pain or other complaints may also employ "polycharacterization." For example, Ms. Mant characterized her neck pain as aching, burning, and tightness; and bilateral anterior knee pain as aching, stabbing, and/or throbbing.

Symptoms may also be magnified into implausibly widespread or nonanatomical distributions, for example, "everything hurts," numbness "from the elbow down" or weakness "of the whole leg." Sometimes complaints migrate from one side or area to another, or "metastasize," involving progressively more body parts over time. By contrast, Ms. Mant's complaints have been fairly well localized and reasonably consistent in distribution.

---

[7] Dorto, AJ. "Symptom Magnification and the Role of the Disability Evaluating Physician." *ABIME Perspective,* Summer 1999, 1-13.

Physical examination findings (signs) that do not fit known patterns of injury or illness are labeled nonorganic. In contradistinction to objective findings such as scars, masses, reflexes, or limb circumferences that can be observed, felt, tested, or measured respectively, most signs are subjective, dependent upon the behavior or responses of the patient or examinee. As implied, nonorganic physical findings are not consistent with anatomical or physiological derangement due to trauma or disease. Related terms, sometimes used interchangeably with NPF (non physiologic findings), are abnormal pain behavior, illness behavior, or functional overlay. However, the latter may be a confusing misnomer, since these signs are almost always associated with some degree of (at least claimed) dysfunction.

Ms. Mant did not put forth good effort upon some left shoulder motions. For instance, abduction was initially limited to 55°. However, shortly thereafter, when beginning upper extremity strength testing, the examiner demonstrated 90° of shoulder abduction bilaterally, with elbows flexed, as the position to maintain while he pushed down on her lateral arms to assess strength of shoulder abductor muscles. Ms. Mant easily adopted the position, nearly doubling her allegedly maximum active shoulder abduction.

The examiner cannot definitively confirm or deny validity of the grade 4/5 weakness demonstrated on left shoulder external rotation, flexion, and abduction. However, suboptimal effort thereon seems probable, perhaps due to the plaintiff's concern about possibly causing pain.

The examiner is unaware of any plausible explanation for the initial weakness of finger abduction bilaterally apart from suboptimal effort. Normal strength was eventually achieved, but only after repeated encouragement.

The instructions regarding grip strength assessment on page 508 of the AMA *Guides to the Evaluation of Permanent Impairment*, Fifth Edition, state, "Tests repeated at intervals during an examination are considered…reliable if there is less than 20% variation in the readings. If there is more than 20% variation…one may assume the individual is not exerting full effort." As indicated, Ms. Mant's grip strength was measured with a Jamar dynamometer in three temporally separate trials. The measurements of 10, 6, and 4 kg on left and 25, 16, and 14 kg on right far exceed the 20% variation cutoff for reliability.

SM and NPF are 3 to 4 times more common in the setting of a compensable injury or illness[8]; suggesting claimants or plaintiffs believe they will derive greater monetary or other benefit by inflating the duration, distribution, and/or severity of their complaints and findings. Indeed the most obvious external incentives for these behaviors are tangible. While often financial, e.g., an impairment award, time loss compensation, reimbursement for

[8] Snider, RK, ed. *Essentials of Musculoskeletal Care*. (Rosemont, IL: American Academy of Orthopaedic Surgeons, 1997) 43-45.

treatment costs, or judgment for pain and suffering; the tangible motive may be non-pecuniary, e.g., obtaining vocational retraining or drugs such as narcotics. Secondary gain may also be intangible. e.g., avoidance of undesirable occupational or home duties, sympathy from friends and relatives, nuturing from caregivers, etc.

However, because SM and NPF can occur unconsciously, and the individual exaggerating or fabricating the complaints and subjective findings may be unaware of the motivation, one should not necessarily equate their presence with malingering. Nonanatomical-nonphysiological symptoms and signs commonly reflect an individual's psychosocial makeup, including upbringing, cultural background, educational level, family situation, employment or lack thereof, etc.

Persons with pre-existing mental health problems, particularly a prior history of physical, emotional, and/or sexual abuse are prone to develop disproportionate somatic complaints subsequently. However, Ms. Mant did not report any prior or current abuse on today's questionnaire.

Rather than conscious magnification or fabrication of symptoms and signs for external gain (malingering), SM and NPF are commonly a means to communicate distress: "See how bad I am" or "I'm not getting the help I need." Furthermore, the presence of nonorganic complaints and findings does not rule out organic (physical) pathology. There may be significant underlying injury or illness, masked by the "functional overlay."

SM and NPF are often noted by independent medical examiners, but rarely by treating doctors, therapists, etc. There several possible reasons for the discrepancy. Health care providers often fail to identify SM or NPF because they have not been trained to recognize same. On the other hand, assessment of the validity of symptoms and signs is an integral part of any quality independent medical examination (IME).

The discrepancy in notation may also reflect bias. The attending physician may be a patient and/or personal advocate, perhaps recognizing "there's something wrong with this picture," but fail to report the suspicion fearing it would diminish their patient's credibility and the value of their claim or lawsuit. Notation of SM or NPF might also prompt a third party to conclude diagnostic studies and/or treatment were unnecessary, and deny payment for services rendered, thereby diminishing the provider's income. The examiner may also become an advocate, but for their client, inflating the importance of nonorganic symptoms or signs which are few in number or marginal in significance.

Lastly, patients often behave differently than examinees. To please, and avoid offending, their treating doctor, therapist, etc., patients frequently report more favorable treatment outcomes (lesser symptoms) than they would to an examiner or new health care provider.

> By virtue of prior experience or conversation with a coworker, union steward, or attorney, claimants and plaintiffs may also view an IME in an adversarial light, and exaggerate or fabricate complaints and findings in an attempt to avoid cessation of time loss compensation, denial of further treatment, diminution in an impairment award or settlement for pain and suffering, etc.
>
> In summary, there was evidence of symptom magnification and were some nonorganic findings during today's history and examination, respectively. However, neither was flagrant.

*Resulting Cross-examination:*
**Q.** Doctor, are you saying that Ms. Mant is lying about her pain?
**A.** I never said she was lying.
**Q.** You said that when you saw her she didn't look like she was in that much pain?
**A.** She had a comfortable appearance is what I said.
**Q.** Are you saying that you can look at an examinee and see how much pain they are in?
**A.** Well, there are signs trained evaluators like me can spot.
**Q.** Did she hyperbolically characterize her pain?
**A.** No, she did not.
**Q.** Is that an indication that she was telling the truth?
**A.** Yes.
**Q.** Were Ms. Mant's complaints fairly well localized and reasonably consistent in distribution?
**A.** Yes.
**Q.** Is that an indication she was telling the truth?
**A.** Yes.
**Q.** Did she achieve normal strength in finger abduction?
**A.** Yes, after encouragement.
**Q.** Doctor, do you consider Demeter's *Disability Evaluation* an authoritative text in the field of disability evaluation?
**A.** Yes, I do.
**Q.** Do you agree with Demeter who states on page 592, "symptom magnification is a term (not a diagnosis)…."?
**A.** Well, it's commonly used.
**Q.** Doctor, here is DSM-IV. Please show me where the diagnosis "symptom magnification" appears.
**A.** Well, it is not in there as such.
**Q.** Isn't it a fact that it is not in there at all?
**A.** That's correct.
**Q.** Do you agree with Demeter when he states on page 592, "There is often disagreement between examiners as to whether symptom magnification is present and concerning its significance"?

**Comment:** Examiners who use the terms "symptom magnification," "malingering," "factitious disorder," "somatization disorder," etc., should have a full and complete understanding of the terms, their medical definitions, and their medical-legal significance.

**Defending the Report As Written:** When faced with counsel who is taking words, phrases, or sentences from a text for cross-examination, the examiner should ask to see the entire page or section. Counsel may selectively excerpt the helpful portions and leave out the less-than-helpful portions of the text.

**Q.** Do you agree with Demeter, who states on page 592, "symptom magnification is a term (not a diagnosis)…."?
**A.** Yes, but you are taking the sentence out of context. The section also states on page 592:

> "Whether the component of symptom magnification is to be considered part of the permanent impairment will vary with the specific situation. In an individual with histrionic traits, the tendency to magnify symptoms stems from the pre-existing personality and may be permanent. If the symptom magnification stems from a desire for secondary gain, such as to avoid an unpleasant work situation, to be vindicated, or to obtain financial reward, the magnified component may be expected to diminish or disappear after the litigation is over."

**Example 10.162: Non-opinion on objective support for subjective findings**
*Report States:*

> *Are Ms. X's subjective complaints supported by objective findings? How do the findings relate to the injury of 08/13/01?*
>
> The examinee appears to have more disability than one usually sees in an individual with multi-level degenerative disc disease. I have no explanation for this. She reports a marked aggravation of her symptoms on 08/13/01. There is no medical basis on which I can either confirm or disconfirm this report. It is worth noting, though, that many individuals with vulnerable low backs will report marked aggravations of their symptoms in response to relatively modest trauma.

*Resulting Cross-examination:*
**Q.** The examinee has more disability than the average person with multi-level disc degeneration, correct?
**A.** Yes, she does.
**Q.** Of course, using an average-person test, some would have more disability and some less than the average, correct?
**A.** Yes.
**Q.** Do you know this examinee's prior employment history, Doctor?
**A.** No. Just that she was working as a cable installer when injured.
**Q.** She could have been predisposed to degenerative disc disease due to heavy lifting, exposure to vibration, or sitting for long periods, correct?
**A.** Yes, those can lead to early degeneration.
**Q.** You don't know why she has the disability, correct?
**A.** Yes.
**Q.** It may be from the injury?

**A.** Yes.
**Q.** Thank you, Doctor.

**Comment:** The examiner here expresses no legally sufficient opinion on the cause of the increased disability. This report would carry little, if any, weight on the issues and thus counsel did not pursue the matter further.

**Defending the Report As Written:** The examiner can "fill-in" the incomplete report during cross-examination.

**Q.** You don't know why she has the disability, correct?
**A.** Other than her stated desire to retire and move to Florida, no.

**Example 10.163: Examiner finds objective support for examinee's complaints**

*Report States:*

> In response to questions outlined in your letter:
>
> 1. Objective versus subjective complaints: As outlined above, this individual does have objective findings for cervical radiculopathy and possibly left ulnar nerve elbow entrapment.

**Comment:** The highest compliment that can be given to an expert is that the expert "calls them as he sees them." That's exactly what happened here where the examiner stated that there was indeed objective evidence for the subjective complaints.

**Example 10.164: Distraction tests: Tricking the examinee?**

*Report States:*

> I performed axial loading and the Burns bench test. The results of these indicated symptom magnification.

*Resulting Cross-examination:*

**Q.** Doctor, you performed a series of tests to try to trap the examinee, correct?
**A.** That's not true.
**Q.** You used the Burns bench test to try to trap the examinee into claiming that he couldn't perform the test on overbalancing so you could build a case for symptom magnification?
**A.** I asked him to perform the test and he said he could not.
**Q.** Then you pressed on his head and asked him if this made his back worse?
**A.** That is axial loading.
**Q.** You knew that this should not make the back worse?
**A.** Yes.
**Q.** Then you sprung the trap on the examinee and reported symptom magnification?
**A.** I reported what he said.
**Q.** Let's go over the other distraction tests you tried unsuccessfully to trap the examinee with but didn't list in your IME report.

**Comment:** Examiners who use distraction tests should be prepared to meet the trying-to-trap-the-examinee line of questioning. The more objective the tests and results, the more difficult the cross-examination.

**Defending the Report As Written:** When faced with a direct assault, the examiner should consider fighting back.

**Q.** Then you sprung the trap on the examinee and reported symptom magnification?
**A.** Counsel, your client didn't have to lie. He could have told the truth.

**Example 10.165: Use of words "malingering" and "fraud" without knowing their definitions**
*Report States:*
This examinee is clearly malingering and defrauding the system.

*Resulting Cross-examination:*
**Q.** Doctor, you said in your IME report that the examinee is clearly malingering and defrauding the system?
**A.** You read well, Counsel.
**Q.** What is the legal definition of fraud, Doctor?
**A.** I am not a lawyer.
**Q.** So, although you don't know what fraud is, this examinee is guilty of it?
**A.** Exactly.
**Q.** What are the four criteria for malingering set forth in DSM-IV, Doctor?
**A.** I don't know them off the top of my head.
**Q.** Is malingering different than factitious disorder, Doctor?
**A.** Yes.
**Q.** What is the difference?
**A.** I don't know.
**Q.** So, although you don't know what fraud and malingering are, this examinee is *clearly* involved in malingering and defrauding the system?

**Defending the Report As Written:** Examiners need not memorize each and every definition before they use them in their IME reports.

**Q.** What are the four criteria for malingering set forth in DSM-IV, Doctor?
**A.** (Doctor pulls book off the shelf.) They are, and I quote:
"Malingering should be strongly suspected if any combination of the following is noted:
1. Medicolegal context of presentation (e.g., the person is referred by an attorney to the clinician for examination)
2. Marked discrepancy between the person's claimed stress or disability and the objective findings
3. Lack of cooperation during the diagnostic evaluation and in complying with the prescribed treatment regimen
4. The presence of Antisocial Personality Disorder."

**Example 10.166: Stating opinion regarding level of examinee's pain**
*Report States:*

> It is my opinion, based on a reasonable degree of medical certainty, that the examinee is over-reporting her alleged pain.

*Resulting Cross-examination:*
**Q.** Are you stating that the examinee is lying about her pain?
**A.** No, just over-reporting her pain.
**Q.** Is she exaggerating her pain?
**A.** Yes.
**Q.** Is there any objective way to measure pain, Doctor?
**A.** No.
**Q.** Who is the only person who truly knows how much pain the examinee is in?

**Comment:** Examiners who make subjective comments about examinees in their IME reports are best served if they are able to support the comments with objective facts.

**Defending the Report As Written:** Examiners can push back during cross-examination.

**Q.** Is she exaggerating her pain?
**A.** She is over-reporting it. When asked to rate her pain from 0-10, she stated her pain was 10 all the time. This is after it was explained to her that 10 was excruciating, horrible pain. I examined her for two hours. She is not in excruciating, horrible pain all the time.

# Chapter 11 Making Your Report Powerful, Persuasive, and Understandable

## 11.1 Executive Summary

There are numerous techniques that can make an IME report powerful, persuasive, and understandable. The authors recommend the following.

- State things clearly and directly.
- Do not speculate or guess.
- Document all reasons that support findings and conclusions.
- Take extra care when opining on future medical costs.
- Avoid, or at least minimize, the use of boilerplate language.
- If boilerplate language is used, carefully proof the report for internal inconsistencies before signing off on it.
- Avoid the use of absolute words, such as "always" and "never."
- Make sure the report is not vague, equivocal, or uncertain.
- Avoid emphatic language, exclamation points, bolding, italics, and capital letters to emphasize findings, conclusions, and other information.
- Use the active voice rather than the passive voice.
- Use precise language.
- Use the first person when referring to oneself in the report.
- Write with confident language and avoid hedge words, such as "it seems," "could," "apparently," and "I believe."
- Define all technical medical terms and jargon.
- Use objective language and avoid subjective characterizations to describe the examination, findings, and conclusions.
- Explain the meaning of any medical abbreviations used.
- Avoid argumentative language.
- Document all inconsistencies, but avoid opining on the credibility of the examinee.
- Make sure the report is internally consistent and consistent with any previous reports in this case or other cases.
- Avoid any appearance of bias in the report.
- Be very careful when using computer-generated standard language or report templates in the IME reports.

## 11.2 State Things Clearly and Directly

The examiner should use clear language and state things directly. An examiner's role is to state and provide an opinion, not to hide one.

**Example 11.21: Opinion not stated directly**
*Report States:*

> The examinee was involved in a motor vehicle accident on 7/19/2001 for which he was treated. As a result of this, the examinee claims neck, shoulder, and back pain. All of the examinee's symptoms, according to the examinee, pre-dated the second motor vehicle accident of 4/15/2002. The motor vehicle accident of 4/15/2002 just exacerbated his symptomatology but did not cause it. His physical therapy helped the exacerbation of symptoms but did not return the exacerbation of symptoms to the pre-4/15/2002 level. The pain in his back pre-dates the motor vehicle accident of 4/15/2002 and has nothing to do with it as it was apparently caused by the accident of 7/19/2001 and was not substantially exacerbated by the 4/15/2002 accident. I trust this clarifies the medical picture in this claim.

**Comment:** This opinion would have been easier to read and more persuasive had the opinion been stated clearly and directly.

> My opinion, based on a reasonable degree of medical certainty, is that the examinee injured his neck, shoulder, and back in a 7/19/2001 motor vehicle accident. The examinee's second motor vehicle accident on 4/15/2002 exacerbated his symptomatology in his neck and shoulders. The examinee's symptomatology has not returned to his pre-4/15/2002 state at the date of this report.

**Example 11.22: Opinion could have been written more clearly**
*Report States:*

> Having reviewed the available collateral sources of information; having administered and reviewed the results of various psychological tests; and having interviewed Mr. Plaintiff 2, I offer the following conclusion:
>
> [1] Mr. Plaintiff 2's alleged complaints cannot reliably be understood to have arisen solely, if at all, as a result of the actions which he alleges occurred in his workplace [i.e., Mr. Plaintiff 2's current emotional state is <u>not</u> consistent with the possibility that the alleged workplace events produced the current claimed intense symptom pattern].
>
> [2] There is abundant empirical evidence of Mr. Plaintiff 2's direct, intentional effort to malinger.

**Comment:** A clearer wording of this opinion follows.

> It is my opinion, based on a reasonable degree of psychological certainty that:
>
> 1) Mr. Plaintiff 2's alleged complaints are not a result of the alleged workplace events.
>
> 2) Mr. Plaintiff 2 is malingering.

> The above opinions are based upon my review of the above-listed collateral information, my interviews with Mr. Plaintiff 2, and the various psychological tests that I administered to Mr. Plaintiff 2.

## 11.3 Do Not Speculate or Guess

Examiners should not guess in their IME reports. Guesses undermine the credibility of the examiner and her entire report. Counsel will use an expert's guesses against the examiner by attempting to show that the examiner's opinion is guesswork or is based on guesswork. It is best to avoid qualifying phrases like "I suspect," "I believe," and "I would imagine" that suggest guessing. The examiner should state reasons that support her opinions. (See Section 10.3.)

**Example 11.31: "In the arbitrary opinion of the undersigned"**

*Report States:*

> In the arbitrary opinion of the undersigned, a fair and accurate permanent impairment rating for the whole person would be 3%.

*Resulting Cross-examination:*

**Q.** Sir, as I understand it, you offer two kinds of opinions—regular opinions and arbitrary opinions, correct?
**A.** No, that's not true.
**Q.** Sometimes you conclude your reports with the phrase, "In the opinion of the undersigned" and sometimes you say, "In the arbitrary opinion of the undersigned."
**A.** That's true for what it's worth, Counselor.
**Q.** Do you know the definition of the word "arbitrary"?
**A.** No, not really.
**Q.** Could you read the definition from this American Heritage Dictionary?
**A.** "Determined by whim or caprice."
**Q.** This opinion you are offering to the jury is one of your arbitrary ones, is it not?
**A.** If you say so.
**Q.** It's not what I say, sir, it's what you said. Could you read the final line of your report?
**A.** "In the arbitrary opinion of the undersigned, a fair and accurate permanent impairment rating for the whole person would be 3%."

**Comment:** Making arbitrary conclusions can be fatal to an examiner's credibility. Any estimates an examiner is forced to make should be based upon as much objective data as possible. This objective data should be stated explicitly in the report.

> It is my opinion, based upon a reasonable degree of medical certainty, that the examinee has a 3% impairment of the whole person. This is based upon the 5th edition of the American Medical Association's *Guides to the Evaluation of Permanent Impairment,* Section 8.5 (5th ed., p. 177), Section

8.1 (5th ed., pp. 174-175), Section 8.7 (5th ed., pp. 178-187), Table 8-2 (5th ed., p. 178).

**Example 11.32: "I suspect"**
*Report States:*

I have not seen the chiropractic records. I suspect multiple and prolonged manipulations without positive effect may be found there.

*Resulting Cross-examination:*
**Q.** You do not know what is contained in the chiropractic records, correct?
**A.** Yes.
**Q.** That's because you weren't provided them, correct?
**A.** Yes.
**Q.** You never even had an opportunity to read them, did you?
**A.** I did not.
**Q.** So your suspicions are just educated guesses?

**Comment:** The use of the term "I suspect" is counterproductive in an examiner's report. It connotes guessing.

**Defending the Report As Written:** If the examiner's suspicion has a basis in fact, the examiner should be prepared to state this during cross-examination.

**Q.** So your suspicions are just educated guesses?
**A.** Not at all. My suspicion was based upon the fact that the examinee told me that he went to the chiropractor approximately three times per week for a year and that he didn't improve.

**Example 11.33: "I believe"**
*Report States:*

He is presently taking Prozac and Percocet and takes both of these more or less on a p.r.n. basis. I believe that he had one of each today prior to me examining him.

*Resulting Cross-examination:*
**Q.** Doctor, you said you "believe" that he had one of each pill today prior to your examination.
**A.** Yes.
**Q.** You said "believe" because you wanted to be fair and accurate in your report, correct?
**A.** That's correct.
**Q.** And, also, because you were not sure he actually had two pills?
**A.** That's correct.

**Comment:** Guessing will negatively affect the examiner's credibility. Examiners should objectively base their assumptions and never guess.

> He is presently taking Prozac and Percocet and takes both of these more or less on a p.r.n. basis. He stated to me that he had one of each today prior to me examining him.

**Defending the Report As Written:** If given an opening by counsel, the examiner should use it.

**Q.** You said "believe" because you wanted to be fair and accurate in your report, correct?
**A.** It's a figure of speech. I "believed" he had one of each because that's what he told me. Are you suggesting that your client shouldn't be believed?

**Example 11.34: Speculating on results of calculation examiner can't perform**

*Report States:*

> The effect of carrying a heavy manual could be estimated on the basis of the ratio between the weight of the manual and the weight of her body and the distance walked carrying the manual compared with the distance walked and time spent standing without the manual. Such a calculation would demonstrate a negligible effect of the manual upon the overall time and extent of weight borne by the joint.

*Resulting Cross-examination:*
**Q.** To do the calculation you mention in your IME report, you would need to know how much the claimant weighed, correct?
**A.** Yes.
**Q.** How much did she weigh?
**A.** I don't know.
**Q.** You would also need to know how much the manual weighed, correct?
**A.** Yes.
**Q.** How much did it weigh?
**A.** I was not told that information.
**Q.** You were told by the insurer it was a very heavy manual, correct?
**A.** Yes.
**Q.** So, you put in your report it was a heavy manual?
**A.** Yes.
**Q.** Do you know the distance walked carrying the manual as opposed to the distance walked without the manual?
**A.** No.
**Q.** So you don't know any of the four variables that you need to perform your so-called calculation, but you still stated in your report, "such a calculation would demonstrate a negligible effect of the manual upon the overall time and extent of weight borne by the joint"?

**Comment:** In the above example, the examiner moved beyond expressing an opinion based upon a reasonable degree of medical probability. When an examiner starts to speculate in his report, he should expect to be cross-examined about this speculation. Suspicions and speculation have no place in IME reports.

**Defending the Report As Written:** It would be very difficult to defend the above report as written. An aggressive examiner might want to attempt to go for the jugular. He would run the risk, however, of appearing to be an advocate, partisan, or biased.

**Q.** You were told by the insurer it was a very heavy manual, correct?
**A.** No, that's not correct. That is how the claimant characterized the manual. During this three years of litigation, she just kept referring to it as "very heavy" without any mention of how much it actually weighted. She has degenerative disease of the hip. By her own account, she was advised not to walk and bear weight on that joint but she continued to do so. Once the degenerative arthritis had set in, bearing weight could be an aggravating factor, however. The principal weight that the diseased joint was bearing was the weight of her body, not some manual.

## 11.4 Guessing About Future Medical Costs

Predicting future medical costs can be problematic. Examiners are best served when they have objective and substantial justification for their predictions. Examiners should not opine on future medical costs unless they are qualified to do so. (Please see Section 10.15.) Guessing, or what amounts to guessing, regarding future medical costs should be avoided.

**Example 11.41: Cost estimate unsupported by objective information**
*Report States:*

> The permanent injuries described above will most likely require physician-directed supportive care conservatively estimated at an ongoing cost of $1,200.00 to $1,500.00 per year for a minimum of two years and on a possible lifetime basis.

*Resulting Cross-examination:*
**Q.** Your estimate is that the future medical expenses could be $2,400, or $3,000, or $95,000 for this 25-year old?
**A.** Yes.
**Q.** Can you tell us if he will need this medical care for 1 year or 2 years or 50 years?
**A.** No.
**Q.** Could you explain on what you based your $1,200 to $1,500 per year estimate?
**A.** My years of training and experience.
**Q.** What training do you have in the accurate projection of future medical expenses?
**A.** None.
**Q.** Did you consult with an expert in the field before you came up with your estimate?
**A.** No.
**Q.** So, in fact, you have no objective guidelines or support for your figures, is that correct?

**Comment:** This examiner's cost estimate is on extremely shaky ground. He did not provide objective justification for the cost estimates. In addition, this examiner didn't even appear to be qualified to comment in this area. This examiner should have either refrained from offering an opinion in this area or provided an objective justification for his cost estimates.

**Defending the Report As Written:** Medicine is not an exact science. When examiners opine about future medical care and expenses, they need to be able to articulate the rationale behind their opinions.

**Q.** Can you tell us if he will need this medical care for 1 year or 2 years or 50 years?
**A.** Counselor, medicine is not an exact science. Based on his recovery to date, the minimum amount of care he will need is 1 to 2 years. If he does not make a recovery, which is looking less and less likely as time goes on, he will need the care for the rest of his life. Nobody can say how long he will actually live, but according to the latest federal government tables, his life expectancy is 50 years.

## 11.5 Avoid Boilerplate Language

Most examiners produce many IME reports each year. Computer-generated, boilerplate, or standard language is often used in IME reports. Examiners use boilerplate or standard language for various reasons.

1. It is a way of using tried and tested language.
2. It helps to cover standard issues that arise frequently.
3. It makes the report longer and appear more detailed.
4. It is simple and easy to use.

Boilerplate language in IME reports commonly includes the following.

1. Disclaimers of liability on the part of the examiner.
2. The reservation of the right of the examiner to change the report, usually because of new information.
3. Extraneous "friendly" language, such as thanking the referral source.
4. Standard language dealing with work capacity, symptom magnification, pain inventories, pain drawings, and other common IME issues.

There are many potential pitfalls associated with the use of boilerplate language in IME reports.

1. Boilerplate language can make the examiner's reports all look the same.
2. It is easy to forget or fail to remove the language when it is

inconsistent with other phrases or findings or when it is inappropriate for the report at hand.

3. Boilerplate language can be exceptionally fertile grounds for cross-examination.
4. It is easy to overuse boilerplate language. This exacerbates the above three problems.

The authors recommend that examiners avoid, or at least minimize, the use of boilerplate language. If boilerplate language is used, the examiner needs to carefully proof each report to ensure that the boilerplate language is not internally inconsistent.

**Example 11.51: Warranty**
*Report States:*
No warranty or guarantee, express or implied, is made.

*Resulting Cross-examination:*
**Q.** Is your five-page IME report accurate?
**A.** Yes.
**Q.** Is your five-page IME report truthful?
**A.** Yes.
**Q.** Can you guarantee for the jury the report's accuracy and truthfulness?
**A.** Yes.
**Q.** When you said on page five, last paragraph of your report, "no warranty or guarantee, express or implied, is made," that's not true, is it?
**A.** No.
**Q.** That last statement was not accurate, was it?
**A.** It was not.
**Q.** Was it truthful?
**A.** No.
**Q.** Is the rest of your report filled with similar inaccuracies and untruths?

**Comment:** Kitchen knives sold on TV infomercials come with a warranty, but IME reports should not. This type of boilerplate "lawyer" language is distracting, cheapens the examiner, and should not be included in the report.

**Defending the Report As Written:** Examiners who use boilerplate language need to be able to explain its meaning when they are cross-examined.

**Q.** When you said on page five, last paragraph of your report, "no warranty or guarantee, express or implied, is made," that's not true, is it?
**A.** Yes, it is. My report is accurate and truthful, however, I cannot guarantee that the statements made by others to me are accurate.

**Example 11.52: Not responsible for the accuracy of information provided**
*Report States:*
The examiner is not responsible for the accuracy of any information that was provided to him.

*Resulting Cross-examination:*

**Q.** You are not responsible for the accuracy of information provided?
**A.** That's correct.
**Q.** That includes only parts of your seven-page report, correct?
**A.** No, Counselor, that's for the entire report.
**Q.** So that includes your factual assumptions?
**A.** Yes.
**Q.** Your analysis?
**A.** Yes.
**Q.** Your examination?
**A.** Yes.
**Q.** Your opinions?
**A.** Yes.
**Q.** And your conclusions?
**A.** Yes.
**Q.** So, if there is anything at all wrong with this seven-page IME report, it's not your fault, correct?
**A.** That's correct.
**Q.** Who signed this report?
**A.** I did.
**Q.** As I understand it, the same person who wrote the report, signed it, and got paid for it is not responsible for the accuracy of the information provided?

**Comment:** Examiners who attempt to abdicate responsibility for their own reports reduce the weight the fact finder will give to these reports. If the examiner will not stand behind the report, why should anyone believe it?

**Defending the Report As Written:** Examiners who attempt to disclaim responsibility for the information provided by others need to be able to articulate their position.

**Q.** You are not responsible for the accuracy of information provided?
**A.** I am not responsible for the accuracy of the information that was provided to me by others. For example, I am not responsible for the accuracy of the history your client gave to me. I am responsible for the accuracy of my analysis, opinions, and conclusions expressed in my report.

**Example 11.53: Reserve the right to amend**

*Report States:*

> This report does not necessarily embody the details of all of my opinions. I reserve the right to amend and add to my opinions upon further review of records.

*Resulting Cross-examination:*

**Q.** Which opinions did you leave out of your nine-page IME report?
**A.** None.
**Q.** Which details of your opinions did you leave out?
**A.** The unimportant ones.
**Q.** The ones that were so unimportant that you specifically and in writing

reserved the right to amend them?
**A.** That's just a phrase I use in all my reports.
**Q.** In other words, boilerplate language?
**A.** Standard language.
**Q.** You use it sometimes when it really doesn't apply to the report?
**A.** It's always in there.
**Q.** Do you have other standard language in your reports?
**A.** Yes, some.
**Q.** Could you go through this nine-page report and highlight with this yellow marker all of the standard language?
**A.** That would be difficult to do.
**Q.** Would it help you if I provided you with six other reports you issued with paragraph after paragraph of boilerplate language?

**Comment:** This example shows how boilerplate language most often does more harm than good. It would have been better to leave this language out of the report.

**Defending the Report As Written:** Examiners should not be defensive when replying to questions about standard or boilerplate language in their reports. The more they protest or justify, the more it looks like they did something wrong.

**Q.** Could you go through this nine-page report and highlight with this yellow marker all of the standard language?
**A.** With pleasure.

**Example 11.54: Inconsistent boilerplate language**
*Report States:*

> Thank you very much for the opportunity to participate in the care of this claimant's interesting problem.

*Resulting Cross-examination:*
**Q.** Doctor, did you or did you not render medical care in this case?
**A.** I absolutely did not.
**Q.** So, when you say in your report, "Thank you very much for the opportunity to participate in the care of this claimant's interesting problem," are you not saying you were rendering medical care?
**A.** No, that's just a standard phrase I add to the end of many of my IME reports.
**Q.** Just boilerplate?
**A.** Standard language.
**Q.** The phrase in your report, "no treatment was given or suggested," did you mean that, Doctor, or was that more boilerplate?
**A.** Yes, I meant it and yes, it is also standard language.
**Q.** Was it standard language when you said on page 3 of your IME report, "I recommend prompt removal of all implants"?
**A.** No, that's my recommendation.
**Q.** Recommendation for treatment, Doctor?

**A.** Absolutely not.
**Q.** What is the paragraph heading under which you wrote, "I recommend prompt removal of all implants"?
**A.** "Recommended Treatment."
**Q.** You also wrote on page 3 of your IME report, "I recommend in-patient drug detoxification and a twelve-step program." That was your recommendation for medical treatment, was it not, Doctor?
**A.** No.
**Q.** What heading is that phrase under in your IME report?
**A.** "Recommended Treatment."
**Q.** So, you:

1. thanked the insurance company for the "opportunity to participate in the care of the claimant's interesting problem,"
2. recommended prompt removal of all implants, and
3. recommended in-patient drug detoxification and a twelve-step program.

But treatment was not suggested, Doctor?

**Comment:** In the above case, the examiner would have been better served had he not used this extraneous boilerplate language.

**Defending the Report As Written:** The examiner may be best served by clearing up any misimpressions opposing counsel is leaving with the jury.

**Q.** Doctor, did you or did you not render medical care in this case?
**A.** The claimant was examined in accordance with the rules concerning an independent medical examination. I informed the claimant that no doctor/patient relationship exists or is implied by the examination. I gave no treatment to the claimant nor did I discuss my findings or my recommendations in this case with the claimant. I did not render medical care in this case.

**Example 11.55: Inapplicable boilerplate left in report**
*Report States:*

> In formulating these opinions and recommendations, only the allowed condition of record is considered.

*Resulting Cross-examination:*
**Q.** Doctor, the issue in this claim was whether the examinee's hip pain was related to her fall at work?
**A.** Yes, that's correct.
**Q.** What was the "allowed condition" prior to your exam and report?
**A.** There was none, Counsel.
**Q.** Your report says in the final paragraph, "In formulating these opinions and recommendations, only the allowed condition of record is considered," correct?
**A.** That is what it says.
**Q.** Can you explain how, if there were no "allowed conditions," and you only considered allowed conditions, you offered an opinion on the hip condition?

**Comment:** Examiners should proofread for inconsistent statements before signing off on their reports. In the above example, the standard language should not have been left in the report.

**Defending the Report As Written:** When faced with inconsistent statements in their reports, examiners should attempt to clarify the inconsistencies. This does not mean, however, that they will necessarily need to change their opinions.

**Q.** Can you explain how, if there were no "allowed conditions" and you only considered allowed conditions, you offered an opinion on the hip condition?
**A.** The hip condition was contested and I offered an opinion on causal relationship. The statement at the end of my report is poorly worded and I will correct it in the future.

**Example 11.56: Inconsistent boilerplate language**
*Report States:*

> The opinions on work capacity are to facilitate job placement and do not necessarily reflect an in-depth, direct-threat analysis.

*Resulting Cross-examination:*
**Q.** Doctor, where in your IME report do you express an opinion on work capacity?
**A.** In this report….I didn't express an opinion on work capacity.
**Q.** Why then does your report state on page number 4, "The opinions on work capacity are to facilitate job placement and do not necessarily reflect an in-depth, direct-threat analysis"?
**A.** That is part of a form—standard language I use because I usually do include an opinion on work capacity.
**Q.** Your reports are so similar that you just plug in paragraphs, report after report, even when they do not apply?
**A.** Counsel, that's not fair. It's just a few lines in a four-page report. To generalize from that one oversight is just a typical, cheap lawyer trick.
**Q.** Well, Doctor, how do you then explain the rest of the paragraph on page number 4 on appropriateness of care when you also don't have an opinion on appropriateness of care?

**Comment:** Examiners who use standard boilerplate language or templates should take great care to remove language that is inconsistent with the rest of the report. For example, saying in one part of an IME report that the pain drawings show XYZ, and in another part saying the examinee refused to complete *any* pain drawings, is a very serious drafting mistake.

**Defending the Report As Written:** When faced with an obvious mistake, the examiner is best served by taking responsibility and admitting the error and forcing counsel to move on. The examiner who thoroughly prepares for her testimony will catch many of these mistakes and will not be taken by surprise during cross-examination.

**Q.** Doctor, where in your report do you express an opinion on work capacity?
**A.** There's an error on page 4 of my report. The paragraphs discussing work capacity and appropriateness of care should not have been included in the report because I do not express opinions on these issues. That is my mistake.

**Example 11.57: Overuse of boilerplate language**

*Report States:*

> This individual reports symptoms that are essentially nonnegotiable, serve to control the environment, and result in significant amplification of perceived and expressed functional limitations. This should not be interpreted to suggest an intentional misrepresentation of pain and disability, but more likely represents a leaned pattern of illness behavior.

*Resulting Cross-examination:*

**Q.** Doctor, your 7/14/2001 IME report is replete with boilerplate language that you just copied out of a book, isn't that true?
**A.** No, that's not true and I resent the implication.
**Q.** Your IME report does state on page 3, "This individual reports symptoms that are essentially nonnegotiable, serve to control the environment, and result in significant amplification of perceived and expressed functional limitations. This should not be interpreted to suggest an intentional misrepresentation of pain and disability, but more likely represents a leaned pattern of illness behavior," does it not?
**A.** That's correct. That's what I dictated after my examination of the claimant.
**Q.** That was not just copied from a textbook?
**A.** No. Absolutely not.
**Q.** Doctor, I show you a textbook entitled *How to Make More Money from Performing IMEs*, copyrighted 1999, and ask you if the paragraph you dictated is found on page 23 of the book under "Symptom Magnification"?
**A.** Well, yes. But that doesn't mean that I copied it. I may have read it and just remembered it.
**Q.** Word for word?
**A.** I have a good memory.
**Q.** What about your spelling, Doctor?
**A.** Excuse me?
**Q.** Are you aware that you misspelled the same word "leaned" instead of "learned" in your report as was done in the text, Doctor?
**A.** Even if that is true, it is only one paragraph out of a four-page report. It's inconsequential.
**Q.** Please turn to the last page of your IME report. Isn't the entire page also copied out of the same book, Doctor?

**Comment:** IME examiners can and do use boilerplate language that they find in textbooks and in the reports of experienced colleagues. Physicians who overuse boilerplate language run the risk of the "cookie-cutter" cross-examination. In this cross-examination, counsel will show that because all of the physician's reports look the same, they are of a cookie-cutter type and are not to be trusted. Examiners are better served by avoiding or at least judiciously using boilerplate language.

**Defending the Report As Written:** Examiners who use standard/boilerplate language in their reports need to be able to defend their use when this issue is raised during cross-examination.

**Q.** This was not just copied from a textbook?
**A.** In fact, I used the templates found in the best book written on IMEs to help me dictate my report. In this report, I used it twice; first on page 1 and then on the last page. It is mostly standard definitions. The rest of the 7-page report, including the history, injury, clinical chronology, summary of diagnostic studies, current status, etc., was dictated by me with reference to no texts.

**Example 11.58: Boilerplate language inconsistent with report**
*Report States:*

> The opinions expressed do not constitute a recommendation that specific claims or administrative actions be taken or enforced.

*Resulting Cross-examination:*
**Q.** You stated in the final paragraph of your IME report that, "The opinions expressed do not constitute a recommendation that specific claims or administrative actions be taken or enforced," correct?
**A.** Yes.
**Q.** This is standard language that you put in your IME reports?
**A.** Sometimes I put it in IME reports.
**Q.** I show you 27 of your IME reports and ask you to look at the final page of the reports. How many of these have that phrase?
**A.** All of them.
**Q.** In this case, your IME report does make specific recommendations about what actions should be taken, correct?
**A.** No, it does not.
**Q.** On page 14 of your report, what is the heading on the top of the page?
**A.** "Recommendations."
**Q.** Under the "Recommendation" heading you say:

> **"DIAGNOSTIC:** Additional diagnostic testing is neither medically necessary nor reasonable for the cure, relief, or evaluation of the claimant's symptoms, complaints, or condition.
> **THERAPEUTIC:** Additional treatment is neither medically necessary nor reasonable for the cure or relief of the claimant's symptoms, complaints, or condition. The claimant will require no future medical treatment as a consequence of his injury of record.
> The claimant is specifically not a candidate for ongoing treatment with oral addictive narcotic pain medications. The claimant is not a candidate for maintenance on any narcotic medications nor oral addictive narcotics."
> Correct?

**A.** Yes, that is what it says.
**Q.** These are your recommendations you made at the same time your report states the opinions expressed do not constitute recommendations?

**Comment:** Examiners should pay particularly careful attention to standard/boilerplate language to make sure it is consistent with the rest of the report. While standard language does have its usefulness, it should not be used indiscriminately. Care should be taken to delete any standard language that is inconsistent with the rest of the IME report.

**Defending the Report As Written:** When faced with challenges to an IME report, the examiner needs to examine the report to see if true inconsistencies exist.

**Q.** In this case your IME report does make specific recommendations about what actions should be taken, correct?
**A.** You are intentionally or unintentionally mixing up two separate and distinct concepts, Counsel. In the final paragraph, I wrote that my "opinions do not constitute a recommendation that specific claims or administrative actions be taken or enforced." On page 14 of the report, I am expressing my medical opinion as to the clinical management of the examinee's medical care. I do not make any recommendations about claims action.

**Example 11.59: Boilerplate inconsistency**
*Report States:*

> No consideration is given to any psychiatric problems that the examinee might have.

*Resulting Cross-examination:*
**Q.** Doctor, you performed a very detailed interview and examination in this case, correct?
**A.** I am not sure what you mean by very detailed, Counsel.
**Q.** The examinee was in your office for over six hours, correct?
**A.** Yes, that's correct.
**Q.** You wrote an extensive and detailed IME report as well?
**A.** Again, Counsel…
**Q.** Your IME report is 24 pages single-spaced?
**A.** Yes, it is.
**Q.** You billed the insurer for 17 hours of your time on this IME?
**A.** Actually, I only billed for 16.5 hours.
**Q.** You stated in your IME on page 14 that this IME was complex due to the fact that the examinee has a psychiatric disease as the cause of her complaints?
**A.** Yes, I did.
**Q.** On page 16 of your IME report you state:

> "After reviewing the available data at great length, within reasonable medical probability, the cause for her progressive complaints is actually a psychiatric disease which is not related to the motor vehicle accident at all. She has not had a psychiatric IME with psychometric testing to determine the exact diagnoses present as the cause of her complaints. The data available at this time suggest an Axis II personality disorder as well as other possible disorders such as Factitious Disorder (a psychiatric diagnosis that should not be confused with malingering)."
> Correct?

**A.** Yes, that's correct. Is there a point to this, Counsel?
**Q.** Yes, Doctor. You state in your final paragraph of your IME report, "No

consideration is given to any psychiatric problems that the examinee might have." Am I reading that correctly?
**A.** Well, yes.
**Q.** Doctor, can you explain how you can diagnose psychiatric disease when you gave no consideration to psychiatric problems?

**Comment:** The above is a classic example of the potential ruin of an excellent IME report by inappropriate boilerplate language. Examiners should carefully scrutinize standard language to make sure it is consistent with the rest of their IME reports. Failure to do so is often a very damaging mistake.

**Defending the Report As Written:** The only way to deal with an obvious error, as in the above example, is to admit it as graciously as possible and force counsel to move on.

**Q.** Yes, Doctor. You state in your final paragraph of your IME report, "No consideration is given to any psychiatric problems that the examinee might have." Am I reading that correctly?
**A.** Unfortunately, you are reading it correctly. That is an obvious mistake that I should have caught. I apologize for the confusion. I did, of course, give detailed consideration to the examinee's psychiatric condition.

**Example 11.510: Inconsistency**
*Report States:*

> The pain drawings completed by the examinee are consistent with my findings of symptom magnification.

*Resulting Cross-examination:*
**Q.** Doctor, on page 7, the last page of your report, you state, "The pain drawings completed by the examinee are consistent with my findings of symptom magnification," correct?
**A.** That's what it says.
**Q.** On page 1 of your IME report, you indicate that the examinee refused to fill out the pain inventories. Is that what it says?
**A.** There must be some mistake.
**Q.** On that we can agree, Doctor.

**Comment:** This is the risk of boilerplate language and why, in the opinion of the authors, it is best to avoid, or at least to minimize, the use of boilerplate language.

**Defending the Report As Written:** Obvious mistakes should be admitted.

**Q.** On page 1 of your IME report, you indicate that the examinee refused to fill out the pain inventories. Is that what it says?
**A.** Yes, that was my mistake. The examinee did fill out the pain drawings.

## 11.6 Avoid Absolute Words

Examiners should avoid absolute language, such as "always" or "never," in an IME report. Use of absolute language leaves the examiner wide open to damaging cross-examination. When absolute language is used, all the cross-examiner has to do is to present the examiner with a single counterexample where the examiner's statement is not correct. It will then be established that the examiner was either exaggerating or flat out wrong when the absolute language was used. In either event, the examiner will lose credibility.

**Example 11.61: Stress never causes heart attacks**

*Report States:*

Stress can never cause heart attacks.

*Resulting Cross-examination:*

**Q.** Your IME report states that stress can never cause heart attacks?
**A.** That's correct.
**Q.** If the examinee's bank was taken over by armed terrorists who were demanding $10 million and they were shooting bank employees in the head every hour and as the gun was put to the examinee's head, she suffered a massive heart attack, would you still maintain that the heart attack was unrelated to the stress?

**Comment:** Using absolute words in medical situations can lead to this type of cross-examination. The examiner is either forced to change her opinion and admit that stress can sometimes cause heart attacks or take the absurd position that the heart attack was just a coincidence. Examiners who avoid the use of absolute words are best positioned to defend their opinions and their reports.

It is extremely rare for stress to cause heart attacks. Stress was not the cause in this case.

**Defending the Report As Written:** Examiners who are faced with outlandish hypothetical questions should not let themselves be bullied into changing their opinions.

**Q.** If the examinee's bank was taken over by armed terrorists who were demanding $10 million and then were shooting bank employees in the head every hour and as the gun was put to the examinee's head, she suffered a massive heart attack, would you still maintain that the heart attack was unrelated to the stress?
**A.** I think I saw that movie, Counsel. That is a hypothetical question that bears no relationship to this case in which the examinee, who was morbidly obese, had sky-high cholesterol, and who has a long family history of heart disease, suffered a nervous breakdown when her boss asked her to drive one mile and pick up the office mail from the post office.

**Example 11.62: "All…without limits…complete recovery"**
*Report States:*

> He is capable of return to full and unrestricted employment in his position of truck driving. He can pursue all vocational and avocational activity at this time without restriction as a result of the completion of this examination which was entirely within normal limits. He has recovered completely and it was exhibited throughout this examination.

*Resulting Cross-examination:*
**Q.** In your opinion, the employee can pursue all vocational and avocational activities at this time?
**A.** Well, yes, as a truck driver.
**Q.** You didn't limit him to that restriction in your report, did you?
**A.** Well, no, not in those words.
**Q.** You didn't do it in any words, did you?
**A.** No.
**Q.** Did you intend to release him for *all* vocational activities from airplane pilot to x-ray technician?
**A.** No.
**Q.** Did you intend to release him to pursue all avocational activities from bungee jumping to skydiving?
**A.** No.
**Q.** Why don't you tell us what you really meant, Doctor?

**Comment:** It's easy to poke holes in absolute language. The examiner would have been better off toning down the absolute language in the report to refer to only the examinee's prior usual and customary activities.

> He is capable of return to full and unrestricted employment in his position of truck driving. He can pursue his prior usual and customary vocational and avocational activity at this time without restriction as a result of the completion of this examination, which was entirely within normal limits. He has recovered completely as exhibited throughout this examination.

**Defending the Report As Written:** Examiners should be prepared to clarify any absolute language used in their reports.

**Q.** Did you intend to release him for *all* vocational activities from airplane pilot to x-ray technician?
**A.** No, of course not. I wasn't clearing him to be an NFL linebacker. What I meant was his usual and customary job as a truck driver.

**Example 11.63: Absolute confidence in opinion: "There is no question"**
*Report States:*

> There is no question but that the arthritis at the base of the thumb is an aging phenomenon. I do not really think that the use of the thumb as a bank teller caused this.

*Resulting Cross-examination:*
**Q.** One of the issues in this case was the etiology of the arthritis at the base of the thumb, correct?
**A.** Yes.
**Q.** That was one of the questions disputed by the medical experts?
**A.** Yes.
**Q.** It was your opinion that it did not result from the use of the thumb as a bank teller?
**A.** That's correct.
**Q.** Did you review the job description for a bank teller?
**A.** No.
**Q.** Did you review the *Dictionary of Occupational Titles* for the duties of this position?
**A.** No.
**Q.** If you do not know what the job consisted of, are you in the best position to express an opinion as to whether the arthritis resulted from her work as a bank teller?

**Comment:** This expression of absolute certainty can be used to make the examiner appear closed minded. This will lessen the examiner's credibility. The IME report would have been better had it avoided the absolute language.

> It is my opinion, based on a reasonable degree of medical certainty, that the arthritis at the base of the thumb is an aging phenomenon. It is my opinion, based on a reasonable degree of medical certainty, that the use of the thumb as a bank teller did not cause the arthritis.

**Defending the Report As Written:** Examiners should be prepared to clarify any absolute language used in their reports.

**Q.** It was your opinion that it did not result from the use of the thumb as a bank teller?
**A.** Yes, based upon the history provided and the medical records, which showed complaints at the base of the thumb at least five years prior to the three months she worked as a bank teller.

## 11.7 Avoid Vague, Equivocal, and Uncertain Reports

The courts continue to reject reports where the expert's opinion is expressed vaguely, equivocally, or with insufficient certainty. (Please see Section 10.2.)

## 11.8 Do Not Use Emphasis When Expressing Findings or Conclusions

Examiners often use emphatic language, exclamation points, bolding, italics, and capital letters to emphasize their findings, conclusions, or other information in their reports. A well-written IME report will not need such emphasis. A seasoned trial attorney will use an examiner's use of emphasis against that examiner. The trial attorney may attempt to show that the examiner's use of emphasis is a sign of bias.

**Example 11.81: "THIS IS NOT TRUE"**

*Report States:*

> I saw the claimant for purposes of his 8/17/01 back injury. He denied episodes of back pain prior to 8/17/01. **THIS IS NOT TRUE.**

*Resulting Cross-examination:*

**Q.** Your 14-page IME report only has four words in bold capital letters, correct?
**A.** Yes.
**Q.** These four words are **"THIS IS NOT TRUE,"** correct?
**A.** Yes, those are the words.
**Q.** You wanted to make sure the workers' compensation insurer did not miss these four words?
**A.** Yes.
**Q.** That's because these words were the most important words in your 14-page IME report?
**A.** They are important.
**Q.** By showing the claimant was not truthful, you succeeded in casting doubt on his credibility, correct?
**A.** Yes, I did.
**Q.** You tried everything you could to cast doubt on the claimant's veracity, did you not?
**A.** I took a history and examined him.
**Q.** You asked him to respond to the statement, "Nothing makes me feel better," and when he answered "True," you found this to be disingenuous, correct?
**A.** Yes, I did.
**Q.** If he answered "False," you would then have him list the things that make him feel better?
**A.** Yes, I would.
**Q.** You surreptitiously observed him exiting his vehicle and interpreted his ability to do so as another sign he was exaggerating his symptoms?
**A.** Yes, I did.
**Q.** You stated in your IME report that he presented with a cane for balance but did not use it in your presence. You took this to mean he didn't need or use the cane?
**A.** That's correct.
**Q.** You didn't boldface any of these findings in your report?
**A.** That's correct.
**Q.** The reason you bolded the four words **"THIS IS NOT TRUE"** is so that the fact finder and insurer would not miss them. That's because you didn't think that they were smart enough or diligent enough to find and understand these four words themselves?

**Comment:** IME physicians are best served by not bolding, capitalizing, underlining, or italicizing words. Such emphasis can imply that the examiner was biased or acted as an advocate. This also diminishes the remainder of the report.

**Defending the Report As Written:** When faced with a challenge to explain why they emphasized certain words, IME examiners should look at it as an opportunity.

**Q.** You tried everything you could to cast doubt on the claimant's veracity, did you not?
**A.** The claimant told a boldface lie when asked about a prior back injury. This was five minutes into the interview. This is an objective fact borne out by the prior medial records. This was just the start of two hours of symptom exaggeration, inappropriate illness behavior, and malingering. I did not need to cast doubt on his veracity. He did that himself.

**Example 11.82: Underlining**
*Report States:*

> However, again, <u>there is not the slightest appearance of any objective findings to support this examinee's subjective complaints.</u>

*Resulting Cross-examination:*
**Q.** You underlined parts of your conclusion to make sure that the reader would not miss these words, correct?
**A.** Yes.
**Q.** You selected only the key words?
**A.** The important ones.
**Q.** So you didn't feel the rest of your three-page, single-spaced report was important, or was it that you didn't feel the judge and jury were smart enough to figure out what was important for themselves?

**Comment:** A well-written report does not need emphasis of this type. This report would have been far more effective without the emphasis.

> The examinee's subjective complaints were not supported by objective findings.

**Defending the Report As Written:** When faced with such a challenge, the examiner should look at it as an opportunity.

**Q.** So you didn't feel the rest of your three-page, single-spaced report was important, or was it that you didn't feel the judge and jury were smart enough to figure out what was important for themselves?
**A.** It was the key reason for my opinion, so I underlined it. As for the jury, my guess is that they'd much rather hear about the facts of this case as opposed to the punctuation in my report.

## 11.9 Use the Active Voice

Examiners should write their reports in the active voice. Sentences that use the passive voice are more likely to be ambiguous. Sentences that use the passive voice also tend to sound awkward. Active-voice sentences are clearer and more persuasive.

**Example 11.91: Passive voice creates ambiguity**
*Report States:*

> After being examined by both Dr. Lang and Dr. Gerald and discussion with Dr. O'Neill, a decision was made to admit Mrs. Elderly.

*Resulting Cross-examination:*
**Q.** Your report indicates, page 5, paragraph 3 that, "After being examined by both Dr. Lang and Dr. Gerald and discussion with Dr. O'Neill, a decision was made to admit Mrs. Elderly." Is that correct?
**A.** Yes, that's right.
**Q.** Who, in your opinion, made the decision? Was it Dr. Lang, Dr. Gerald, or Dr. O'Neill?
**A.** Dr. O'Neill made the decision because he was her treating physician.
**Q.** Does your report indicate what time Mrs. Elderly arrived at the emergency room of the Memorial Hospital?
**A.** Yes. "By 9:55 P.M."
**Q.** Doctor, was that at 8:00 P.M., 8:30 P.M., 9:00 P.M., or 9:55 P.M.?
**A.** Sorry. It was at 9:55 P.M.
**Q.** Does your report indicate whether a chest x-ray should have been performed and laboratory data collected?
**A.** Yes, it does.
**Q.** What does your report indicate?
**A.** "I see no reason for a chest x-ray or laboratory data to be collected in this patient. No indication existed."
**Q.** Doctor, can you explain or clarify that?
**A.** Sure. What I meant to say was that there was no reason for a chest x-ray or laboratory data to be collected in this patient, no indication existed. The standard of care in emergency room medicine does not call for testing to be performed without a clear indication.
**Q.** Thank you, Doctor.

**Comment:** Rewriting this report segment in an active voice makes the report clearer and more persuasive.

> Dr. Lang and Dr. Gerald examined Mrs. Elderly. Immediately following these examinations, Dr. O'Neill consulted with Drs. Lang and Gerald. Dr. O'Neill then decided to admit Mrs. Elderly. Mrs. Elderly was admitted at 9:55 P.M.

**Defending the Report As Written:** An examiner need not sit in the witness box like a potted plant while counsel picks her and her report apart.

**Q.** Doctor, was that at 8:00 P.M., 8:30 P.M., 9:00 P.M., or 9:55 P.M.?
**A.** Counsel, I was told a long time ago that lawyers who have no case and are desperate start picking on witnesses and their reports. To be more precise, it was at 9:55 P.M.

**Example 11.92: Passive voice is awkward**
*Report States:*

> The impression was that Mr. Miller had some discomfort and pain from his original surgery, markedly improved from when last seen on March 6, 2002.

**Comment:** The passive voice in this example makes the report sound awkward. Rewriting this report segment in an active voice makes the report more clear and, therefore, more persuasive.

> Mr. Miller stated that he still has some pain and discomfort from his original surgery. Dr. Green last saw him for follow up on March 6, 2002. Mr. Miller stated that his pain and discomfort have improved markedly since then.

## 11.10 Use Precise Language

Precise language should be used in IME reports where possible. The use of precise language will make the IME report more persuasive. On the other hand, the use of imprecise language will make the IME report less persuasive.

**Example 11.101: Imprecise language**[1]
*Report States:*

> A review of the medical literature will find fundamental agreement with the following principles.

**Comment:** More precise language would make this report more credible.

> My opinions are supported by the following medical literature, which I reviewed prior to drafting my report.
>
> 1. Krasinski, Keith, Riata LaCouture and Robert S. Holzman, "Effect of Changing Needle Disposal Systems on Needle Puncture Injuries," *Infection Control,* v. 8 #2 (1987): 59-62.
> 2. Jacobson, Julie T., John P. Burke and Marlyn T. Conti, "Injuries of Hospital Employees From Needles and Sharp Objects," *Infection Control* v. 4 #2 (1983): 100-102.
> 3. *Selecting, Evaluating, and Using Sharps Disposal Containers.* Atlanta, GA: National Institute for Occupational Safety and Health, January 1998.
> 4. Sanborn, Cindi, Nancy Luttrell and Karen Hoffmann, "Creating a Safer Environment for Health Care Workers: Implementing a Point-of-Use Sharps Disposal System," *Nursing Administration Quarterly,* v. 12 #2 Winter 1988): 24-31.

[1] For more information on how to best cite supporting authority, please see Section 9.2.

**Example 11.102: Imprecise language, missing object**

*Report States:*

> Thank you for referring the above examinee for plaintiff medical evaluation. I explained that I was a certified independent medical examiner. I also explained that this evaluation did not constitute a doctor/patient relationship, and that I would not be a treating physician.

*Resulting Cross-examination:*

**Q.** Your report indicates, page 1, paragraph 1, that, "I explained that I was a certified independent medical examiner." Is that correct?
**A.** Yes, that's right.
**Q.** I'm confused. It is unclear to me who this is being addressed to. Is it the reader or did you say this to the plaintiff?
**A.** The plaintiff.
**Q.** OK. Now, just to clear up some more confusion, when you say in the very next sentence, "I also explained that this evaluation did not constitute a doctor/patient relationship, and that I would not be a treating physician," you were again reporting something you said to the plaintiff?
**A.** Yes.

**Comment:** This type of "I'm confused" cross-examination is not earth-shattering, but it can be effective in eroding an examiner's credibility. The examiner would have been better off using more precise language.

> Upon meeting the plaintiff, I introduced myself and explained to him that I was a certified independent medical examiner. I also explained to the plaintiff that the evaluation I was about to conduct did not create a doctor/patient relationship, and that I would not be giving him any treatment or advice.

**Defending the Report As Written:** Examiners are normally best served by just truthfully and artfully replying to counsel's cross-examination questions. When counsel is sarcastic or acts like a jerk, the examiner may be tempted to put him in his place.

**Q.** I'm confused. It is unclear to me who this is being addressed to. Is it the reader or did you say this to the plaintiff?
**A.** Counsel, perhaps you have the time to play these lawyer games. I don't appreciate them, nor, I suspect, does the judge. My comments were obviously addressed to the plaintiff.

**Example 11.103: "Normal rear-end accident"**

*Report States:*

> In a normal rear-end accident there is no abnormal stress to the TMJ joint.

*Resulting Cross-examination:*

**Q.** You based your opinion in part on the fact that "in a normal rear-end accident there is no abnormal stress to the TMJ joint." Is that correct?
**A.** Yes, that's correct.

**Q.** How do you define "normal rear-end accident," Doctor?
**A.** Well, you know…an accident where one vehicle is struck from the rear by another vehicle.
**Q.** Would this include a passenger car being struck by a truck?
**A.** Yes, it would.
**Q.** A truck being struck by a car?
**A.** Well, yes.
**Q.** Would it include the situation where both vehicles were moving?
**A.** Yes, it could.
**Q.** What about if one was stopped and struck by a moving vehicle?
**A.** That would be included.
**Q.** If the victim was wearing or not wearing seatbelts, would that make any difference whether you would include it in your "normal rear-end accident"?
**A.** I don't think so.
**Q.** Would the presence or absence of airbags make a difference for your "normal rear-end accident" definition?
**A.** It might.
**Q.** If one vehicle was speeding and struck a stopped vehicle, would that be a "normal rear-end accident"?
**A.** It would depend on how fast the vehicle was going.
**Q.** What about 30 in a 20 m.p.h. zone?
**A.** No, I don't think so.
**Q.** Tell me, Doctor, what speed would make it an abnormal rear-end accident?
**A.** I really couldn't say with precision.
**Q.** That's because you don't know, Doctor?
**A.** That's correct.
**Q.** If the vehicle struck burst into flames, would that be a "normal rear-end accident"?
**A.** No.
**Q.** So, the amount of damage done to the stationary vehicle would be a factor in your mind?
**A.** Yes.
**Q.** Doctor, in this case, do you know how fast the vehicle was going when it struck the plaintiff's stopped vehicle?
**A.** No.
**Q.** Do you know how much damage was done to the plaintiff's vehicle?
**A.** I don't know.
**Q.** Do you know if the plaintiff's vehicle had airbags and whether they were deployed?
**A.** I was not provided that information.
**Q.** So, you can't honestly say if the accident in this case was one of your so-called "normal rear-end accidents," can you, Doctor?

**Comment:** When the IME physician uses a vague or imprecise term in his report, he should expect to be questioned about its definition and meaning. In the above example, note how the physician ended up testifying about vehicles, seatbelts, airbags, and speeding. The physician could have avoided this with a more precise IME report.

> The examinee's stopped vehicle was struck by a slow-moving (5 m.p.h. to 10 m.p.h.) Toyota Camry in the rear. The examinee did not sustain a direct blow to his jaw and the damage to his vehicle was under $250.00.

**Defending the Report As Written:** When faced with a vague term in an IME report, a successful physician prepares to deal with this issue on cross-examination.

**Q.** How do you define "normal rear-end accident," Doctor?
**A.** I mean a standard, typical collision like this one where the examinee's vehicle was struck by a slow moving vehicle, which did very minimal damage. In normal accidents like these, the driver of the struck vehicle doesn't normally receive extensive, debilitating injuries as are alleged by the plaintiff in this case.

**Example 11.104: Rounded-off times**
*Report States:*

> The examination commenced at 10:00 A.M. and lasted 90 minutes.

**Comment:** More precise times would make the report seem more credible.

> The examination commenced at 10:04 A.M. and concluded at 11:27 A.M.

**Example 11.105: Rounded measurements, "slightly" better passive range of motion**
*Report States:*

| | Right | Left |
|---|---|---|
| Flexion | 150 | 180 |
| Extension | 45 | 50 |
| Abduction | 120 | 180 |
| Adduction | 30 | 40 |
| External Rotation | 70 | 90 |
| Internal Rotation | 30 | 80 |

> There was a slightly greater passive range of motion than active range of motion about the right shoulder.

**Comment:** This report would have been more persuasive had it been more precise.

| | Right | Left |
|---|---|---|
| Flexion | 152 | 179 |
| Extension | 45 | 48 |
| Abduction | 122 | 178 |
| Adduction | 30 | 41 |
| External Rotation | 67 | 88 |
| Internal Rotation | 29 | 81 |

> There was on average a 5% greater passive range of motion than active range of motion about the right shoulder.

## 11.11 Use First-person Singular

Examiners should use the first-person singular when referring to themselves. Some examiners use the third person when describing their qualifications in a report. This is awkward, can be used to make the examiner sound pompous or silly, and should be avoided. Jurors do not commonly refer to themselves in the third person and may not relate well to someone who does.

**Example 11.111: Use of third person to describe qualifications**
*Report States:*

> Dr. Thompson has been board certified in orthopedic surgery since 1979 (CV attached).

*Resulting Cross-examination:*
**Q.** Is this a copy of your report, sir?
**A.** Yes.
**Q.** Are you the author of this report?
**A.** Yes.
**Q.** The only author?
**A.** Yes.
**Q.** I refer you to page 1 of your report, paragraph 3, line 1. It states, "Dr. Thompson has been board certified in orthopedic surgery since 1979." Am I reading that correctly?
**A.** Yes.
**Q.** Who wrote that description of you?
**A.** I did.
**Q.** Do you normally refer to yourself in the third person?
**A.** No.
**Q.** Did you think your qualifications would sound better that way?
**A.** I guess so.

**Comment:** The examiner's use of the third person when referring to himself is a needless distraction that may make the report seem as though it was at least partially written by someone else. It may also make the examiner look pompous. Examiners should instead use the first person when referring to themselves.

> I have been board certified in orthopedic surgery since 1979.

**Defending the Report As Written:** Examiners may choose to put counsel on the defensive.

**Q.** Did you think your qualifications would sound better that way?
**A.** It's an accepted use of language. Any time you want to talk about the facts of the case, I'm ready. I'm sure the jury will be more interested in the case than in your grammatical critique.

## 11.12 Use Confident Language and Avoid Hedge Words

The main purpose of an IME report is to communicate the examiner's findings and opinions. These findings and opinions should be stated in a clear, confident manner. Hedge words, such as "it seems," "could," "apparently," and "I believe," indicate that the examiner does not have confidence in her findings and opinions. They may even make an expert's report insufficient as a matter of law.[2] Use of such hedge words will decrease the persuasiveness of the IME report and should be avoided.

**Example 11.121: "I believe"**
*Report States:*

> Consequently, I believe that the examinee's current condition is causally related to the March 6, 2003 workplace injury.

*Resulting Cross-examination:*
**Q.** Do you believe in God, sir?
**A.** Yes.
**Q.** Have you ever seen God?
**A.** Of course not.
**Q.** Do you know of any objective or scientific proof supporting the existence of God?
**A.** No. I have faith.
**Q.** You use the words "I believe" in your report to describe your feeling that the injury was work related, don't you?
**A.** I'm not sure what exact words I used.
**Q.** You state on page 3, and I quote, "Consequently, I believe that the examinee's current condition is causally related to the March 6, 2003 workplace injury." Am I reading that correctly?
**A.** That's what I wrote.

**Comment:** The careless use of "I believe" will lessen the weight given to the examiner's report and opinion. This hedge term should have been omitted.

> It is my opinion, based on a reasonable degree of medical certainty, that the examinee's current condition is causally related to the March 6, 2003 workplace injury.

**Defending the Report As Written:** Examiners are occasionally given an opportunity by opposing counsel to "stick the knife in" and turn the tables on counsel. While this should not be done too often, certain situations cry out for this type of action.

**Q.** Have you ever seen God?
**A.** Counsel, questioning a person's religious beliefs and making a mockery of them is beneath contempt. If you have any decency, you would apologize for what you have just done.

---

[2] See *Samos Imex Corporation v. Nextel Communications* 194F.3rd 301 (1999).

**Example 11.122: "Apparently"**
*Report States:*
Now, apparently, an infusion of urokinase was started at 05:30 on 8/12/99.

*Resulting Cross-examination:*
**Q.** When you say, "apparently," you are indicating you are not certain of that fact. Correct?
**A.** That's what it says in the records.
**Q.** Are you 100% certain that an infusion of urokinase was started at 05:30 on 8/12/99?
**A.** No. I wasn't there, Counselor.
**Q.** Are you 95% certain?
**A.** No.
**Q.** Are you 85% certain?
**A.** No.
**Q.** So you really don't know if in fact an infusion of urokinase was started at 05:30 on 8/12/99?
**A.** That's correct, but it does say that in the records.

**Comment:** The term "apparently" implies to the reader that the examiner was not sure of the facts. This is unnecessary. Consider how this could have been expressed in more confident language.

According to the records, an infusion of urokinase was started at 05:30 on 8/12/99.

**Defending the Report As Written:** This examiner did a fairly good job of defending the report as written.

**Q.** So you really don't know if in fact an infusion of urokinase was started at 05:30 on 8/12/99?
**A.** That's correct, but it does say that in the records and I have no reason to doubt that this did in fact occur as documented.

**Example 11.123: "Appears...should probably"**
*Report States:*
Clinically, her difficulty appears to represent a carpal tunnel syndrome at this point for which a cortisone injection should probably be considered.

*Resulting Cross-examination:*
**Q.** Does the patient's difficulty represent a carpal tunnel syndrome?
**A.** Yes, that's what I said in my report.
**Q.** You said it "appears" to represent, didn't you?
**A.** That's what I meant.
**Q.** That it seems possible that the difficulty represented a carpal tunnel syndrome?
**A.** No...No...more than possible.
**Q.** But less than absolute certainty?
**A.** Yes.

**Q.** Did you say in your report who should consider the cortisone injection?
**A.** Yes.
**Q.** Where is that? What line?
**A.** It's clearly implicit in my report.
**Q.** Just to make it a little easier for the fact finder, could you be more specific?
**A.** The patient…and I guess the doctor also.
**Q.** The injection should presumably be considered?
**A.** No, I said probably be considered.
**Q.** The difference being, just a matter of wording?
**A.** If you say so.

**Comment:** The language in this report makes it sound as if the examiner is not at all sure of herself. If the expert is not confident in her opinion, why should the reader be? Consider a better way to write this.

> It is my opinion, based on a reasonable degree of medical certainty, that Ms. Smith's impairment is caused by a carpal tunnel syndrome. It is my opinion, based on a reasonable degree of medical certainty, that a cortisone injection should be given to Ms. Smith to treat this condition.

**Defending the Report As Written:** Examiners who are familiar with their reports should be able to clear up any apparent ambiguities quickly.

**Q.** Did you say in your report who should consider the cortisone injection?
**A.** I don't remember the exact language used. The injection should be considered by the examinee and her treating physician.

**Example 11.124: "I don't believe so"**
*Report States:*

> I don't believe so.

*Resulting Cross-examination:*
**Q.** In your IME report, how did you answer the question, "Does the claimant have any continuing disability as a result of his 10/1/2001 work-related injury"?
**A.** I stated, "I don't believe so."
**Q.** How much were you paid for this IME, Doctor?
**A.** $750.00.
**Q.** You're positive about the $750.00?
**A.** Yes.
**Q.** As to the question of the claimant's continuing disability, however, you are not as certain of that as you are of the amount of your fee?
**A.** That's correct.
**Q.** How much less certain are you, Doctor?
**A.** That's hard for me to say.
**Q.** You believe that is the case but are not sure?

**Comment:** When examiners use hedge words (for example, "I believe" and "I think") in their IME reports, it weakens their opinions and opens them to unnecessary cross-examination. Examiners are better served by a direct answer.

**Q.** Does the claimant have any continuing disability as a result of his 10/1/2001 work-related injury?
**A.** To a reasonable degree of medical certainty, no.

**Defending the Report As Written:** When the examiner inadvertently uses a hedge word or is faced with one from an old report, he can still truthfully and artfully defend his report.

**Q.** As to the question of the claimant's continuing disability, however, you are not as certain of that as you are of the amount of your fee?
**A.** Counsel, I am not here to play word games. That's apparently your job. How much I was paid is a fact. Whether the claimant has continuing disability is an opinion. In my opinion, based upon a reasonable degree of certainty, he has no continuing disability from his 10/1/2001 work-related injury.

**Example 11.125: Degree of certainty: "I believe"**
*Report States:*

> I believe the examinee's symptoms are attributable to her motor vehicle accident of 6/4/02.

*Resulting Cross-examination:*
**Q.** Doctor, when you say in your IME report, "<u>I believe</u> the examinee's symptoms are attributable to her motor vehicle accident of 6/4/02," that's because you are uncertain of that?
**A.** No. That's what I believe.
**Q.** Are you stating that you are 100% certain about this?
**A.** Well, not 100%. But that's what I believe.
**Q.** Well, how certain are you expressed in a percentage form?
**A.** That's hard to say.
**Q.** Are you 76% certain?

**Comment:** When examiners use equivocal words or phrases when expressing their opinions, they open themselves up to unnecessary cross-examination. The examiner is best served by stating his opinion clearly and in a legally sufficient manner. The examiner should avoid getting into a numbers game with counsel.

> It is my opinion, based upon a reasonable degree of medical certainty, that the examinee's symptoms are attributable to her motor vehicle accident of 6/4/02.

**Defending the Report As Written:** When confronted with an equivocal statement in expressing his opinion, the examiner should, without prompting from retaining counsel, clarify the statement.

**Q.** Doctor, when you say in your IME report, "I believe the examinee's symptoms are attributable to her motor vehicle accident of 6/4/02," that's because you are uncertain of that?
**A.** No, Counsel. I am quite certain and my opinion is based upon a reasonable degree of medical certainty.

## 11.13 Define Technical Medical Terms and Medical Jargon

IME reports are designed for a non-medical audience. To make IME reports easy to understand, clear, and as persuasive as possible, examiners should define technical medical terms, tests, and procedures that the non-medical reader may not be familiar with. This will make the report much more valuable and bolster the report's effectiveness. Consider the following examples.

**Example 11.131: Defining a technical medical term**
*Report States:*

> Bone marrow examination revealed aplastic anemia (failure of bone marrow to make blood cells)...This showed a "dyplastic marrow with excess blasts consistent with conversion to acute leukemia." (Blasts are the earliest blood cells in the bone marrow and may normally be up to 5% of the marrow cells. An excess of blasts is a sign of acute leukemia or a related disorder.)

**Comment:** The medical expert in this case did an excellent job explaining technical medical terms. His report is understandable and, therefore, more likely to persuade the reader.

**Example 11.132: Defining a medical term**
*Report States:*

> The examinee complained of and has well-documented tinnitus, which is a ringing or roaring in the ear.

**Comment:** The lay reader of the IME report may not have been completely familiar with the medical term.

**Example 11.133: Explaining a medical test**
*Report States:*

> I performed the Fitzgerald Compression Test on the examinee, which was negative. In the Fitzgerald Compression Test, the doctor stands behind the patient or at his side. The doctor places his hand at the top of the patient's head and has the patient bend his neck on both sides. The patient is then instructed to rotate his chin toward his shoulder. The doctor compresses to determine any joint swelling or instability of the articular facets. An increase in pain is indicative of facet inflammation, misalignment, or injury.

**Comment:** The examiner in the above example explains the test she performed on the examinee. This simple explanation permits the reader to better understand what the examiner did.

**Example 11.134: Explaining a technical term**
*Report States:*

> He arrived early for his testing and interview sessions and at each appeared initially put out or impatient that he was here at all. Throughout, he spoke in a *soto voce* [soft voice] that was at times difficult to hear at first listening.

**Comment:** A report (like the above) that explains technical terms is more valuable to the reader.

## 11.14 Use Objective Language

IME reports should be written using language that is as objective as possible. Subjective characterizations should be avoided. Subjective characterizations seldom add anything of substance to the report and make the report less, as opposed to more, credible. Subjective characterizations provide fertile grounds for cross-examination. Consider the following examples.

**Example 11.141: "Complete absence" and "egregious"**
*Report States:*

> The complete absence of any objective findings supports the diagnosis of egregious malingering.

*Resulting Cross-examination:*
**Q.** Doctor, can you explain the difference between "absence of any objective findings" and "complete absence of any objective findings" in your report?
**A.** There is no difference, Counselor. I was just trying to emphasize the point.
**Q.** Malingering is your diagnosis in this case, correct?
**A.** Yes.
**Q.** So, you added the modifier "egregious" in your report for what reason, Doctor?
**A.** To explain the malingering.
**Q.** Can you quantify "egregious" malingering?
**A.** Well, no. It's just apparent.
**Q.** How does "egregious malingering" differ from just plain malingering?
**A.** That's hard to quantify.
**Q.** To whom, Doctor?
**A.** To me.
**Q.** If ten different doctors looked at this case, how many would diagnose the examinee with "egregious malingering"?
**A.** I don't know.
**Q.** That's because they would all describe it in a different way, or in their own way?
**A.** Yes.
**Q.** We would have ten different doctors with ten different diagnoses?
**A.** Yes, right.
**Q.** So, in fact, your diagnosis is your subjective characterization of the plaintiff?
**A.** It doesn't change my opinion, Counselor.
**Q.** So, your opinion is engraved in stone?
**A.** Yes, absolutely.

**Comment:** The "egregious" characterization used by the author of this report commits the examiner and retaining counsel to proving more than the law requires. This characterization may also be used to suggest that the examiner is a hired gun who is making any statements necessary to help "his" team win. In either case, these characterizations make defending the IME report on cross-examination much more difficult. This examiner would have been better served by leaving the characterization out of his report.

> In my opinion, based on a reasonable degree of medical certainty, the absence of objective findings supports the diagnosis of malingering.

**Defending the Report As Written:** When given an opening by counsel, the experienced IME examiner sometimes uses it to drive home his point.

**Q.** Can you quantify "egregious" malingering?
**A.** When an examinee like your client cuts her finger with an apple corer and ends up out of work for seven months, that is egregious malingering.

**Example 11.142: "Complete and thorough"**
*Report States:*

> Examination of the plaintiff involved the following interview and clinical diagnostic procedures:
> ~ Complete and thorough intraoral and extraoral dental examinations

*Resulting Cross-examination:*
**Q.** This examination was no different from any other of your examinations, correct?
**A.** I don't follow.
**Q.** This exam "was complete and thorough," was it not?
**A.** Yes.
**Q.** As are all of your examinations, correct?
**A.** Yes.
**Q.** So, in fact, the exam was no different from any of your examinations, correct?
**A.** Yes, that's correct.

**Comment:** This examiner has set a very high standard for her examinations. She then must defend this standard on cross-examination. She would have been better served by not including the self-serving characterization of her own investigation.

> Examination of the plaintiff involved the following interview and clinical diagnostic procedures:
> ~ intraoral and extraoral dental examinations

**Defending the Report As Written:** Examiners can push back when counsel pushes them on cross-examination.

**Q.** So, in fact, the exam was no different from any of your examinations, correct?
**A.** It was the results of the exam that were different and, in fact, extraordinary. May I explain?

**Example 11.143: "Fairly detailed history"**

*Report States:*

> I took a fairly detailed history of what the claimant did while working at ABC Homes.

*Resulting Cross-examination:*

**Q.** Doctor, in your IME report you indicate you "took a fairly detailed history of what the claimant did while working at ABC Homes," correct?

**A.** Yes, that's correct.

**Q.** Sometimes you take a detailed history of what the claimant did while working?

**A.** Yes, I do.

**Q.** And sometimes you just take a history of what the claimant did at work?

**A.** Yes.

**Q.** Could you explain the difference between a fairly detailed history, a history, and a detailed history, Doctor?

**Comment:** The examiner in the above example opened himself up to cross-examination when he used the term "fairly detailed history" in his report. His equivocal, subjective statement made him vulnerable to cross-examination. He would have been better served with a simple, direct statement.

> I took a history of what the claimant did while working at ABC Homes.

**Defending the Report As Written:** When faced with questioning during cross-examination about an inadvertent, equivocal statement, the IME doctor can take the offensive when answering instead of being led down the primrose path. The physician can give his explanation first and then answer questions. This technique will make it more difficult for opposing counsel to cut him off.

**Q.** Doctor, in your IME report you indicate you "took a fairly detailed history of what the claimant did while working at ABC Homes," correct?

**A.** I determined his dates of employment, the type of work he did, and the lifting involved. For example, page 2 of my report indicates:

> "This gentleman was involved in all modes of construction of the mobile and modular homes. The gentleman did extremely heavy lifting involving decking, carpeting, and steel. When he was working as a welder, he would take 10- to 12-foot sections of I beams. He would use a tommy bar to flip it onto a roller and toll it inside and then would weld pieces together to get the length of the house they were doing, whether it was 40, 50, or 60 feet. After he welded it, he again used a tommy bar to flip this so he could weld the other side.
>
> He also worked with 4-inch steel, what are called junior I beams, made out of ¼-inch steel that are very heavy. He would take a 40-foot piece of this, again flip it onto the rollers and take it to a saw where he cut it to the proper length. Then it was put into a jig. He used a forklift to help lift the 40-foot I beams that weighed 500 pounds, plus/minus. He had to use the forklift to move it and settle it down into a jig. It was actually a one-person job. Sometimes one to two people would weld and then he would pick

> these up and put it in the jig and he would actually have to lift the pieces into the jig, one end and then the other until it settles properly. He said his quota was 7 to 8 frames per day and sometimes they would do as many as 10. In doing this, he never had any help with the lifting."
> So, yes, Counsel, I took a fairly detailed history. As a matter of fact,

looking back at it, I actually took a very detailed work history.

**Example 11.144: "Lengthy, careful, and objective"**
*Report States:*

> A lengthy, careful, and objective physical examination was performed.

*Resulting Cross-examination:*

**Q.** What percentage of your examinations are done carefully?
**A.** 100% of the time.
**Q.** How often do you do them objectively?
**A.** 100% of the time.
**Q.** I have six of your prior IME reports. Can you explain why in none of the six reports do you say the exam was done "carefully and objectively"?
**A.** Well, not really. Just to…save time, I guess.
**Q.** Talking about time…how much do you charge per hour?
**A.** $350.00 an hour.
**Q.** So, the longer the examination, the more money you charge, correct?
**A.** Yes.
**Q.** And in this case you were able to charge for how many hours?
**A.** 50.
**Q.** So, your "lengthy examination" has resulted in payment of fees of $15,000?
**A.** Well, I have been only paid $12,500 to date.
**Q.** You will get additional fees after you testify objectively here today?
**A.** Yes.

**Comment:** This IME report would have been stronger and more defensible had the examiner described his examination in objective, rather than subjective, terms.

> A physical examination was performed. This examination started at 10:57 and concluded at 12:17. The examination consisted of the following elements:
> 1. Measurement of vital signs
> 2. Height and weight measurement
> 3. Neurological examination….

**Defending the Report As Written:** Examiners who charge by the hour need not be defensive about their fees or charges.

**Q.** Talking about time…how much do you charge per hour?
**A.** About $100 an hour less than you do—$350 an hour.

**Example 11.145: "Unjustifiable"**
*Report States:*

> The amount of physical therapy performed to date is unjustifiable.

**Comment:** The use of objective terms in stating the examiner's opinion would make this report more credible and persuasive.

> It is my opinion, based upon a reasonable degree of medical certainty, that the plaintiff's course of physical therapy was not medically reasonable, necessary, or appropriate.

**Example 11.146: "Unconscionable"**
*Report States:*

> For a chiropractic provider to treat this patient 83 times over a course of 10 months without any improvement is unconscionable in this examiner's opinion.

**Comment:** Objective language would make this expert's opinion sound less like it was a bought-and-paid-for commodity.

> It is my opinion, based on a reasonable degree of medical certainty, that the care provided by Doctor X., DC, was excessive. I base this opinion on the following:
>
> 1….

**Example 11.147: "Carefully reviewed"**
*Report States:*

> I have carefully reviewed all of the medical records in this case.

**Comment:** This examiner has set himself up to be cross-examined on the contents of all of the lengthy medical records in the case. She would have been better off removing the self-serving "carefully" characterization.

> I have reviewed the medical records in this case.

**Example 11.148: "Ridiculous"**
*Report States:*

> The plaintiff's subjective complaints have no objectively verifiable basis, and are, quite frankly, ridiculous.

**Comment:** More objective language that does not include taking a gratuitous shot at the examinee would be more persuasive.

> The plaintiff's subjective complaints are not supported by objective findings.

**Example 11.149: "Conscious indifference"**
*Report States:*

> The staff at Manor Nursing Home displayed a conscious indifference to Mr. Lee's safety by failing to take action when it was apparent that he was severely nutritionally compromised.

*Resulting Cross-examination:*
**Q.** Is it your testimony that the staff intentionally tried to starve Mr. Lee?
**A.** No, but they should have been more careful.
**Q.** When you say "apparent," apparent to whom?
**A.** To the staff.
**Q.** So they should have noticed this?
**A.** Exactly.
**Q.** But they didn't?
**A.** Correct.
**Q.** So, it was not apparent to them, correct?
**A.** It should have been.
**Q.** But it wasn't?
**A.** Correct.
**Q.** If they were unaware of the problem, they could not be "consciously" indifferent to it, could they?
**A.** They should have noticed it.
**Q.** But they didn't, did they?
**A.** Yes. But that's not an excuse. You're twisting my words.
**Q.** You did use the words "apparent," "conscious," and "indifference" in your report?
**A.** Yes. But that's not what I meant…I mean….
**Q.** Would you like to restate your opinion using different words?

**Comment:** This original sentence from the report is full of subjective characterizations that the author would have been better off replacing with more objective language.

> The staff at Manor Nursing Home violated the standard of care by failing to take action after Mr. Lee became nutritionally compromised.

**Defending the Report As Written:** Examiners need not participate in a semantic Olympics with cross-examining counsel.

**Q.** So, it was not apparent to them, correct?
**A.** Counsel, you can play all the word games you want. The fact is, the patient starved to death right before their eyes.

**Example 11.1410: "Independently review," "very complex case"**
*Report States:*

> Thank you for asking me to independently review and opine on this very complex case.

**Comment:** These subjective, extraneous characterizations can and will be used against the examiner. They should not have been included in the examiner's report.

**Example 11.1411: "Extended clinical interview," "grossly overstating"**
*Report States:*

Based upon:

- my extended clinical interview with Mr. Plaintiff 2,
- my review of psychological test data generated by his responses to test questions completed by Mr. Plaintiff 2, and
- my review of collateral material and interviews with collateral informants,

I can state with psychological certainty that:

- Mr. Plaintiff 2 is not suffering from any psychological symptoms that are consistent with, or attributable to, alleged discriminatory actions in his former place of employment.
- Mr. Plaintiff 2 is grossly overstating, if not making up, the presence of any symptoms consistent with his claims of psychological distress for the purpose of gaining compensation in this litigation.

**Comment:** This report would have been more effective had it used precise, objective, defensible language.

Based upon:

- my 256-minute clinical interview with Mr. Plaintiff 2,
- my review of psychological test data generated by his responses to test questions completed by Mr. Plaintiff 2, and
- my review of collateral material and interviews with collateral informants,

I can state to a reasonable degree of psychological certainty that:

- Mr. Plaintiff 2 is not suffering from any psychological symptoms that are consistent with, or attributable to, alleged discriminatory actions in his former place of employment.

**Example 11.1412: "Comprehensive musculoskeletal evaluation"**
*Report States:*

I then performed a comprehensive musculoskeletal evaluation.

**Comment:** This examiner has opened himself up to easy cross-examination by his use of the term "comprehensive" to describe his evaluation. On cross-examination, he can be asked everything that he didn't do as part of his "comprehensive" evaluation.

## 11.15 Explain the Meanings of Medical Abbreviations

An IME report is written to communicate the examiner's findings and conclusions to lay people, such as adjusters, attorneys, judges, jurors, and others. These lay people may not readily understand every medical abbreviation in the report. It is, therefore, recommended that examiners not use an abbreviation in their IME reports without explaining the meaning of the abbreviation the first time it is used in the report. The best practice is to write the term out longhand the first time it is used and to follow this with a parenthetical reference to the abbreviation that the author will use in the remainder of the report.

**Example 11.151: Explanation after abbreviation**

*Report States:*

> ACEP's cost containment committee verifies that chest x-rays and labs that have no clinical indication should not be done....Chest compressions during ACLS treatment lasted for 69 minutes.

*Resulting Cross-examination:*

**Q.** ACEP is an abbreviation for what?
**A.** American College of Emergency Physicians.
**Q.** Why did you abbreviate it?
**A.** Because I assumed everyone would know what it meant.
**Q.** I didn't.
**A.** Sorry.

**Comment:** This report would have been more readily understandable to a lay reader, and thus more persuasive, had the examiner included explanations of the meanings of the abbreviations used.

> The American College of Emergency Physicians (ACEP) cost containment committee verifies that chest x-rays and labs that have no clinical indication should not be done....Chest compressions during Advanced Cardiac Life Support (ACLS) treatment lasted for 69 minutes.

**Example 11.152: Hereinafter parenthetical**

*Report States:*

> All of the above test results were within normal limits (hereinafter "WNL").

**Comment:** If an examiner wants to use abbreviations, it is best to write the term out longhand for its first use followed by a parenthetical reference to the abbreviation that the author will use in the remainder of the report.

**Example 11.153: Abbreviations explained**

*Report States:*

> At the first meeting Mr. Plaintiff 2 was given the following objective test instruments to complete:
>
> - The *Minnesota Multiphasic Personality Inventory - 2 (MMPI-2),*
> - The *Millon Clinical Multiaxial Inventory (MCMI-III),*

- The *Millon Behavioral Health Inventory (MBHI),*
- The *Trauma Symptom Inventory (TSI),*
- The *Malingering Probability Scale (MPS),* and
- The *Validity Indicator Profile (VIP).*

**Comment:** IME reports are more valuable to the reader when medical abbreviations are explicitly defined as in the above example.

## 11.16 Avoid Argumentative Language

The tone of the IME report should always be formal and objective. Argumentative language should be avoided. Argumentative language makes the examiner appear as though she is biased and has an interest in the case. This will result in a loss of credibility.

**Example 11.161: "Makes this issue moot"**
*Report States:*

> The fact that the examinee has a house in Key West that he would probably like to retire to makes the issue of rehabilitation moot.

*Resulting Cross-examination:*
**Q.** You stated in your IME report that because the examinee owns a house in Key West he should not be afforded rehabilitation?
**A.** What's the point if he wants to retire to Florida?
**Q.** Did this 46-year-old examinee tell you he wants to retire to Florida and not return to work?
**A.** Not in so many words.
**Q.** Let's go over how you drew this conclusion you testified to under the pains and penalties of perjury.

**Comment:** The examiner in the above example appears to have jumped to an unwarranted conclusion. This makes him appear biased and makes him look like he is seeking to reach a specific result.

**Defending the Report As Written:** Examinees can defend reports that are "less than perfect" in their formulation.

**Q.** You stated in your IME report that because the examinee owns a house in Key West he should not be afforded rehabilitation?
**A.** He told me, Counsel, that he wants to get this case settled and move to Key West. I'm sure he told you the same thing.

## 11.17 Beware of Commenting on the Credibility of the Examinee and Others

Examiners often make explicit or implicit comments regarding the veracity of the examinee and others involved in the case. This includes witnesses and medical providers. Generally speaking, it is the duty of the hearing officer, jury, or other fact finder, not the examiner, to determine the veracity of the witnesses in the case. Although it is correct and necessary to document inconsistencies and disagreements, examiners are usually best served by not commenting on the veracity of the claimant and others. When examiners comment about the veracity of the examinee and others in a report, they are probably beyond their true area of expertise and may appear to be biased and may thus lose credibility.

**Example 11.171: Treating physician untruthful**

*Report States:*

Plaintiff's treating physician would have us believe that all of the plaintiff's myriad physical and emotional problems are causally related to the alleged 8/1/2003 workplace accident. This couldn't be further from the truth.

*Resulting Cross-examination:*

**Q.** You're accusing the plaintiff's treating physician of lying, correct?
**A.** No. But he is wrong.
**Q.** You said his report's conclusion could not be further from the truth, didn't you?
**A.** Yes.
**Q.** If he is intentionally not telling the truth, he is lying, correct?
**A.** Yes. But I didn't say his error was intentional.
**Q.** It's your opinion that he is wrong?
**A.** Correct.
**Q.** And it is his opinion that you are wrong?
**A.** You would have to ask him that.
**Q.** Counsel who retained you asked you to comment on the opposing expert's veracity, correct?
**A.** Yes.
**Q.** And you accommodated her with this personal attack accusing the physician of lying?

**Comment:** The examiner's comment regarding the treating physician's veracity makes the examiner seem partisan and biased. This comment should have been avoided. The examiner would have been better served with more objective, less inflammatory, language.

> I disagree with plaintiff's treating physician's opinion that all of the plaintiff's myriad physical and emotional problems are causally related to the reported 8/1/2003 workplace accident. This is based on the following:
>
> 1....

**Defending the Report As Written:** When confronted with a direct assault, the examiner can either:

1. just answer the questions, or
2. attack back if given an opportunity.

**Q.** Counsel who retained you asked you to comment on the opposing expert's veracity, correct?
**A.** I felt it was important not to let this type of outrageous and medically suspect conclusion go by without pointing it out. This was my idea, not counsel's.

**Example 11.172: Implicit attack on examinee's credibility**
*Report States:*

> In early 2002 he was operating a charter fishing business and "hurt" his back while working on his boat.

*Resulting Cross-examination:*
**Q.** Doctor, in your four-page, single-spaced IME report, you have only one word in quotes. Is that correct?
**A.** Yes.
**Q.** What is that word?
**A.** "Hurt."
**Q.** You put quotes around this history because you think the claimant is a liar?
**A.** Well, I wouldn't go that far, Counsel.
**Q.** If you were not saying or attempting to imply the claimant was lying, why did you put the word in quotes, Doctor?

**Comment:** An examiner who attempts to call into question the veracity of the claimant by language, punctuation, asides, musings, etc., can damage his own credibility. Opposing counsel will pounce on this and attempt to show that the physician intentionally or unintentionally revealed his bias by the off-hand comment. Examiners are better served by omitting such comments.

**Defending the Report As Written:** When confronted by opposing counsel attempting to show bias, the best defense may be for the IME examiner to take the offensive. This works particularly well when counsel makes the mistake of asking why the examiner did what he did. When asked to explain, the examiner can easily transition from defense to offense.

**Q.** If you were not saying or attempting to imply that the claimant was lying, why did you put the word in quotes, Doctor?
**A.** Counsel, I was given a vague history of your client getting hurt on a fishing boat. There was no specific incident or incidents described. There was no date provided, not even a month provided. I put it in quotes due to the lack of any specific allegation. Just a general comment, "I hurt my back."

**Example 11.173: Ridiculing the veracity of the examinee**
*Report States:*

> The examinee's memory in this area is clearly selective and self-serving.

*Resulting Cross-examination:*
**Q.** Do you have absolute recall, Doctor?
**A.** No.
**Q.** Some things you remember and some things you do not?

**A.** Yes, that's correct.
**Q.** Just like the examinee in this case?
**A.** No. He has a selective memory.
**Q.** So, as an unbiased and impartial expert, it is your testimony here today that you can tell this jury which statements Mr. Smith recalls and which he does not?
**A.** It's just hard for me to believe that is his memory of the situation.
**Q.** Just like it is hard for us to believe that you can, with a reasonable degree of medical certainty under oath, testify as to what another person remembers?

**Comment:** This expert's report sounds more like an attorney's closing argument than it does a forensic report. This type of language should be avoided because it makes the examiner appear biased.

**Defending the Report As Written:** If an examiner comments on an examinee's credibility, he should be well-prepared to back up those comments.

**Q.** So, as an unbiased and impartial expert, it is your testimony here today that you can tell this jury which statements Mr. Smith recalls and which he does not?
**A.** He has an extensive history of prior injuries, Counselor. I am sorry, but it is simply not believable that he doesn't remember any of his years of treatment for these multiple injuries.

**Example 11.174: Opinion based on veracity of the claimant**
*Report States:*

> Based upon the veracity of the claimant and my examination, it is my opinion that the examinee is temporarily and totally disabled due to his right foot industrial injury.

*Resulting Cross-examination:*
**Q.** Doctor, how many times did you meet the examinee?
**A.** Once.
**Q.** How long did your meeting last?
**A.** Approximately one hour.
**Q.** You based your opinion on disability, in part, on the examinee's veracity?
**A.** Yes.
**Q.** Are you always able to tell if people you meet once are telling you the truth?
**A.** Not always, but usually.
**Q.** But sometimes you are mistaken?
**A.** Yes.
**Q.** If you were mistaken about the examinee's veracity, would you then change your opinion on disability?
**A.** I would consider changing it depending on what new information I was provided with.
**Q.** Doctor, have you seen the surveillance tape of the claimant?

**Comment:** An examiner is best served by basing his opinion on reports, studies, results, and an examination, and not on intuitive feelings that the examinee is or is not telling the truth.

> Based on the medical records I have reviewed and my examination, it is my medical opinion that this examinee is temporarily and totally disabled due to his right foot industrial injury.

**Defending the Report As Written:** When faced with defending his opinion, the examiner can and should use his medical knowledge and findings to support the opinion. When given an open-ended question, the experienced examiner will seize the opportunity to explain in detail.

**Q.** You based your opinion on disability, in part, on the examinee's veracity?
**A.** The examinee had a forklift run over his right foot. On examination, there was clear-cut evidence of reflex sympathetic dystrophy of the right foot. There was discoloration with the right foot being hyperemic and darker than the left. The right foot was colder than the left. There was hyperalgesia of the right leg and foot, especially from the ankle distally. Gentle squeezing of the right foot resulted in complaints of severe pain. Neurologic examination revealed hypesthesia in the dorsal aspect of the right foot all the way from the ankle joint to the toes. I found his history and complaints to be completely consistent with the extensive medical records, so I found him to be truthful about his mangled foot.

**Example 11.175: Examinee looked examiner in the eye**
*Report States:*

> He looks me right in the eye when he talks.

*Resulting Cross-examination:*
**Q.** You indicate in your IME report on page 5 that the examinee "Looks me right in the eye when he talks," correct?
**A.** Yes.
**Q.** You noted that in your report because you felt it was unusual or significant?
**A.** Both actually.
**Q.** You felt it was significant because people who look you in the eye generally are telling the truth?
**A.** Yes.
**Q.** Would that be like President Clinton when he looked millions of Americans in the eye and stated, "I didn't have sex with that woman"?
**A.** Not quite the same.
**Q.** How unusual was it for a claimant to look you right in the eye when he talks with you?
**A.** 10% or less of claimants do that.
**Q.** So, your conclusion, Doctor, is that the other 90% or so are lying because they don't look you in the eye?

**Comment:** The examiner in the above example would have been better served had he just omitted the passing comment about the claimant looking him in the eye. These passing comments just serve as red herrings or jumping off points for opposing counsel to cross-examine the examiner. Counsel would often prefer to cross-examine the examiner about ancillary issues as opposed to medical findings, objective test results, etc.

**Defending the Report As Written:** When faced with a passing comment on cross-examination, the examiner does not have to agree with counsel's characterization or interpretation of the comment.

**Q.** You noted that in your report because you felt it was unusual or significant?
**A.** No, actually, I thought it was polite. Where I was raised, you looked people in the eye when you talked to them. It's just a matter of respect and politeness, nothing sinister, Counsel.

**Example 11.176: Dignified, objective treatment of symptom magnification**
*Report States:*

> The subjective complaints are not entirely consistent with the objective findings. Symptom magnification was evident. The examinee's lack of use of her right upper extremity is out of proportion to her physical examination and EMG findings. Her function is not significantly impaired.
>
> The examinee's pain inventories, including the pain diagram, and posturing of the right upper extremity indicate symptom magnification. The diagnosis of symptom magnification syndrome is not intended to discredit the subjective complaint of pain, its possible basis in organic pathology, or the existence of a certain degree of objective disability. This individual reports symptoms that are essentially nonnegotiable, that serve to control the environment, and that result in significant amplification of perceived and expressed functional limitations. This should not be interpreted to suggest an intentional misrepresentation of pain and disability, but more likely represents a learned pattern of illness behavior.
>
> In regards to the examinee's reports of chronic pain of her extremity; pain is an entirely subjective complaint which cannot be verified. In most cases the pain of this type of injury gradually subsides to a very low level. The pain status inventories indicate a magnification of symptoms. There may be some pain present, but in my opinion this condition would not cause a great deal of pain at this time.

**Comment:** This examiner dealt with the issue of the examinee's truthfulness appropriately. That is, he did not directly comment on truthfulness but presented his opinions regarding symptom magnification in an objective, non-inflammatory manner and provided the reasons for his opinion.

## 11.18 Maintain Consistency in and amongst Reports

The IME report needs to be internally consistent. (Please see Section 11.5 regarding the inconsistency problems that can arise when boilerplate language is used.) If the examiner has issued more than one report, these multiple reports need to be consistent. When counsel can point out significant internal inconsistencies or discrepancies between an examiner's own reports, she can cast substantial doubts about the examiner's credibility. The effectiveness of this technique is magnified when counsel can show that the discrepancies may be a result of the use of the examiner's reports in different legal forums to achieve different results or that changes were made after the referral source reviewed the first report. It is more and more likely that counsel will be able to obtain an examiner's reports from other cases to check for inconsistencies; for example, if a physician in one case wrote that fibromyalgia does not exist and in a subsequent case diagnosed an examinee with fibromyalgia.

**Example 11.181: Discrepancies in and amongst reports**
*Sita v. Danek Medical, Inc.*, 43 F.Supp.2d 245 (E.D.N.Y. 1999)
The court closely examined apparent discrepancies in and amongst an examiner's reports.

> Plaintiff has also failed to explain a number of discrepancies within and between Dr. Einhorn's May 1995 and 1997 reports. First, the May 1995 report is internally inconsistent. When asked to examine plaintiff for the purpose of assessing plaintiff's entitlement to Workers' Compensation benefits, Dr. Einhorn diagnosed plaintiff with pseudarthrosis (non-union or failure of the bone to fuse). *See* Einhorn Letter, dated 5/16/95. However, Dr. Einhorn had earlier in the same report observed that he could not tell whether the bone from any of plaintiff's spinal surgeries had fused. *See id.* Thus, Dr. Einhorn's finding that plaintiff suffered from pseudarthrosis is implausible.
>
> There are also several discrepancies between the May 1995 and September 1997 reports. In his September 1997 report, Dr. Einhorn noted that "[his]...[that] one of the lower pedicle screws was broken." Einhorn Report, dated 9/29/97. Dr. Einhorn did not make this finding in his May 1995 report, perhaps because the fact of the broken pedicle screw would not have been important to a Workers' Compensation determination. Nor did Dr. Einhorn then conclude that any of defendant's TSRH screws had caused or contributed to plaintiff's pain, as he did in his 1997 report. Again, this discrepancy might be explained away because in a Workers' Compensation proceeding, medical causation of the type at issue here may not be material. However, Dr. Einhorn did not, in May 1995, indicate, as he did in his September 1997 report, that plaintiff had a fractured pedicle, a fact that might well have been important to a Workers' Compensation determination. These unexplained inconsistencies—the finding of pseudarthrosis without evidence of non-union and the failure to diagnose a fractured pedicle in May 1995—cast a shadow of doubt upon the credibility of Dr. Einhorn's report. At 253.

**Example 11.182: Two reports, two different opinions**
*Cross-examination:*
**Q.** You issued a report dated 9/15/2000 in this case, correct?
**A.** Yes.
**Q.** Your opinion was that the accident plaintiff had a 19% whole person impairment?
**A.** Yes.
**Q.** Prior to formulating this opinion, which documents did you review?
**A.** The complete file including all the medical records.
**Q.** What other work did you perform prior to formulating your opinion expressed in your 9/15/2000 report?
**A.** I examined Mr. Duff.
**Q.** You issued a second report on 1/17/2001, correct?

**A.** Yes. That's correct.
**Q.** In your second report you stated that the plaintiff had a 20% whole person impairment?
**A.** That's correct.
**Q.** What additional examination or record review did you do between 9/15/2000 and 1/17/2001?
**A.** None.
**Q.** Why did you issue a new report?
**A.** Attorney Jones requested me to.
**Q.** He told you at that time that under applicable law, Mr. Duff is not entitled to any compensation for a 19% impairment, but gets substantial compensation if the 20% threshold is met, did he not?
**A.** I don't recall that.

**Comment:** Examiners can expect to be questioned closely about any inconsistencies between their multiple reports. Inconsistencies will result in a loss of credibility, especially if it can be shown that the referral source influenced the findings and conclusions in the newly issued reports.

**Defending the Report As Written:** Examiners need to be prepared to provide plausible explanations for inconsistencies amongst their reports.

**Q.** What additional examination or record review did you do between 9/15/2000 and 1/17/2001?
**A.** I reviewed the applicable impairment rating guidelines and discovered an error in my September rating. This was fixed in the January rating.

**Example 11.183: Cross-examination permitted on discrepancies between reports**
*People v. Gregg,* 732 N.E.2d 1152 (Ill.App.1 Dist. 2000)
In this case, the court permitted the cross-examination of the expert regarding discrepancies between his two reports. The court stated:

> Furthermore, any additional reports that defendant produced from Dr. Schwartz and that contradicted Dr. Schwartz's previous report were properly used by the State for impeachment. The credibility of a witness is put in issue when the witness testifies during trial. *People v. Bull,* 185 Ill.2d 179, 235 Ill.Dec. 641, 705 N.E.2d 824 (1998). Here, Dr. Schwartz prepared two reports, one dated October 1995, and the other, August 1998. The 1998 report included pertinent information not contained in the 1995 report. As such, the State had a right to cross-examine Dr. Schwartz regarding the discrepancies in the two reports, including the omissions in the 1995 report and the new information in the 1998 report which was submitted closer in time to trial.

## 11.19 Avoid Drafting Reports That Appear Biased or Partisan

An IME report that evidences bias, lack of impartiality, or the selective use of data to support a theory will normally be discounted, discredited, or stricken.

**Example 11.191: Cheap shot**

*Report States:*

Treatment for the meralgia paresthetica would normally include the use of tricyclic antidepressants. These are unlikely to work due to the examinee's being an obsessive-compulsive.

*Resulting Cross-examination:*

**Q.** You stated in your IME report that the examinee was obsessive-compulsive, correct?
**A.** Yes, that's correct.
**Q.** You are a psychiatrist, Doctor?
**A.** No, I am a neurologist.
**Q.** Did you perform psychological testing to arrive at this diagnosis, Doctor?
**A.** No, it seemed obvious.
**Q.** Which one of eight diagnostic criteria for obsessive-compulsive disorders under DSM-IV did the examinee exhibit?
**A.** I don't have them committed to memory, Counselor.
**Q.** Let me help you, Doctor. Here are the eight criteria:

(1) Is preoccupied with details, rules, lists, order, organization, or schedules to the extent that the major point of the activity is lost
(2) Shows perfectionism that interferes with task completion (e.g., is unable to complete a project because his or her own overly strict standards are not met)
(3) Is excessively devoted to work and productivity to the exclusion of leisure activities and friendships (not accounted for by obvious economic necessity)
(4) Is over-conscientious, scrupulous, and inflexible about matters of morality, ethics, or values (not accounted for by cultural or religious identification)
(5) Is unable to discard worn-out or worthless objects even when they have no sentimental value
(6) Is reluctant to delegate tasks or to work with others unless they submit to exactly his or her way of doing things
(7) Adopts a miserly spending style toward both self and others; money is viewed as something to be hoarded for future catastrophes
(8) Shows rigidity and stubbornness.

**A.** Well, he exhibited #3.
**Q.** That's the one where he is excessively devoted to work?
**A.** Among other things.
**Q.** Any others?
**A.** Well, yes, #8 as well.
**Q.** Based on these two you diagnosed obsessive-compulsiveness that would interfere with his treatment despite the fact that the diagnostic criteria in DSM-IV calls for four or more of the criteria to be present?

**Comment:** The examiner in the above example tried to diagnose the examinee with a diagnosis that he was not qualified to make and that did not fit the diagnostic criteria for the condition. The fact finder will likely find the examiner was biased and stretched the truth to reach a desired result.

**Defending the Report As Written:** Even when examiners are wrong and make mistakes in their reports, they can still be dangerous witnesses.

**Q.** Based on these two you diagnosed obsessive-compulsiveness that would interfere with his treatment?
**A.** Based on these two traits and the fact that he was working out on his own for three hours a day at a gym and clearly exceeding the physical therapist's recommendations. That's how he got reinjured.

**Example 11.192: Examinee "rewarded for illness behavior"**
*Report States:*

> It is difficult to assess this examinee's pain in this litigated workers' compensation setting where he is rewarded for illness behavior.

**Comment:** This kind of comment may very well be viewed as a cheap shot and an indication of bias by the examiner.

**Example 11.193: Judicial finding of bias**
*Petway v. Ogbonna,* 261 A.D.2d 700, 689 N.Y.S.2d 725 (1999)
An IME physician who develops a reputation for bias may, under certain circumstances, be stopped from performing IMEs. In the case *Petway v. Ogbonna,* the court stated:

> It is apparent from this record, which contains excerpts from medical reports prepared by Altchek and transcripts of trial testimony given by him in other personal injury cases, that he has an unabashed antipathy to those seeking damages for pain and suffering based upon subjective complaints. This predispostion, coupled with the expressed concern by plaintiffs' counsel (not dispelled in the record) that Altchek may well be biased against him because he had previously been involved in litigation directed at the doctor—leads us to conclude Supreme Court did not abuse its discretion in granting plaintiffs the relief sought. At 726.

## 11.20 Computer-assisted Report Templates and Standardized Language

Many examiners use computers to help them create their IME reports efficiently. This practice can generate many potential problems, including inapplicable or inconsistent boilerplate language and the examiner's IME reports appearing to be mass produced. IME reports that use computer-generated standard language should be very carefully reviewed to ensure that all language contained in the report is appropriate for the particular case in question.

Some examiners have created detailed templates that they use in preparing their reports. Other examiners follow the templates of referral sources who require that the IME report use and follow their formats and templates. Such templates certainly speed the report preparation process. However, they are also likely to result in close questioning on cross-examination. Examiners need to be prepared for such questioning and to defend the accuracy of their computer-assisted reports.

**Example 11.201: Report template**

*Report States*:

**Paul Sandhu, M.D.**
Pain Management
***Board Certified, ABPM&R***
*Board Certified, ABPM*
***Q.M.E.***
*www.painsolvers.com*

130 La Casa Via
Bldg. 2 - Suite 106
**Walnut Creek, CA. 94598**
**(925) 933-PAIN**

1600 Broadway
Suite 200
**Oakland, CA 94612**
**[510] 444-PAIN**

**COMPREHENSIVE HISTORY AND PHYSICAL EXAMINATION**
**4050 examination or equivalent**

Referred by:

Date

This report has an attached billing which is an integral component of the report. It is not to be removed or separated from the original report for any reason.

Dear ,

Thank you for asking me to evaluate for ongoing industrial-related complaints and your authorization for this consultation/evaluation per Labor Code 4603.2B.

**CHIEF COMPLAINT:**

HISTORY OF PRESENT ILLNESS:
is a very pleasant year old handed who presented to our clinic for comprehensive pain evaluation.

The patient describes the current pain as , occurring % of the time. The pain quality is described as . The current pain is described as a on a 10-point scale, with 10 being the worst pain in the patient's life. At its best it goes to a , and at its worst a

. The average pain over the last week has been a .

Relieving factors for the patient's pain are .

The pain is aggravated by
The pain is unchanged by

FUNCTIONAL LIMITATIONS:
The patient has avoided over the last month due to the pain.

PAST MEDICAL HISTORY:
[ ] Cancer
[ ] Diabetes
[ ] Coronary Artery Disease/Angina
[ ] Asthma
[ ] Hypertension
[ ] Orthopedic or musculoskeletal trauma:

**ALLERGIES:**

**MEDICATIONS:**

**PRIOR PAIN TREATMENTS:**

**SOCIAL HISTORY:**
Education:
Legal:
Psychological:
Substance abuse:
Employment:
Family life:

**REVIEW OF SYSTEMS:**

| | |
|---|---|
| Constitutional Sx: | No fevers, no unplanned weight loss. |
| Eyes: | No double or blurred vision. |
| ENT: | No loss of hearing or difficulty swallowing. |

| | |
|---|---|
| Heme/Lymph: | No bleeding gums, bruising or low platelet count. |
| Endocrine: | No known thyroid disease or heat/cold intolerance. |
| Skin: | No new rashes or skin lesions. |
| Respiratory: | No dyspnea or wheezing. |
| Cardiovascular: | No chest pain or palpitations. |
| GI: | No constipation, abdominal pain, nausea/vomiting, diarrhea. |
| GU: | No urinary retention, dysuria, sexual dysfunction. |
| Neurological: | No fainting spells, loss of consciousness, blackouts, memory loss, seizures, and dizziness. |
| Musculoskeletal: | |

**PHYSICAL EXAMINATION:**

General:

Blood pressure , pulse , respirations: , and weight: .

Normally developed, no deformities, well groomed.

Oriented to time, person, and place.

Normal attention span and concentration.

Eyes: Sclerae normal, pupils reactive and equal with normal accommodation, extraocular movements intact.

ENT: External inspection of ears and nose reveal no apparent abnormalities.

Lungs: Chest expansion normal, clear to auscultation bilaterally throughout.

Heart: Regular rate and rhythm, normal S1, S2; no murmurs, rubs or gallops.

Abdominal: Non-tender to palpation, no rebound tenderness, non-distended.

Skin: No lesions, new scars, bruises.

Gait/Station:

Assistive Devices:

**LUMBAR EXAMINATION:**

Lumbar range of motion:

The range of motion of the lumbosacral spine was noted in degrees as follows: Flexion 90/90, extension 25/25. Lateral flexion 20/20 bilaterally, rotation 85/85 bilaterally.

| Test | Left | Right |
|---|---|---|
| Gaenslen's | - | - |
| Patrick's | - | - |
| Ober's | - | - |
| Straight leg raise | - | - |
| Pace | - | - |
| Hip hyperextension | - | - |

TENDERNESS:
Facet Joints: Non-tender.
Sacroiliac Joints: Non-tender.
Greater Trochanters: Non-tender.
Paraspinal muscles: Non-tender.

HIP EXAMINATION:

**Hip range of motion:**

Hip flexion
L: 110/110
R: 110/110
External rotation
L: 50/50
R: 50/50
Internal rotation
L: 35/35
R: 35/35
Hip Abduction
L: 50/50

R: 50/50
Hip Adduction
L: 30/30
R: 30/30

Tenderness: No tenderness.

**KNEE EXAMINATION:**

Knee range of motion:
Knee flexion
L: 130/130
R: 130/130
Knee extension
L: 180/180
R: 180/180

| | | Left | Right |
|---|---|---|---|
| Alignment: | | Tibia Vara proximal third bilaterally | |
| Thigh Circumference: | | | |
| Calf Circumference: | | | |
| Effusion: | | - | - |
| Patellofemoral crepitus: | | 0 | 0 |
| Quadriceps angle: | | 10-15 deg. | 10-15 deg. |
| ACL testing: | Anterior Drawer: | - | - |
| | Pivot shift: | nl | nl |
| | Lachman's: | nl | nl |
| PCL testing: | Posterior Drawer: | nl | nl |
| | 'Sag' sign: | nl | nl |
| MCL: | Valgus stress 30° | nl | nl |
| LCL: | Varus stress 30° | nl | nl |
| Special testing: | | | |
| McMurray's | | - | - |
| Apley's Compression test: | | - | - |
| Patellar Compression test: | | - | - |
| Tenderness: | | None | None |

ANKLE EXAMINATION:
Ankle flexion [plantar flexion]
L: 50/50
R: 50/50

Ankle extension [dorsiflexion]
L: 15/15
R: 15/15
Ankle Inversion
L: 35/35
R: 35/35

Ankle Eversion
L: 20/20
R: 20/20

Tenderness: None.

**CERVICAL EXAMINATION:**
Cervical Spine Range of motion:
The range of motion of the cervical spine was noted in degrees as follows: Flexion 50/50, extension 60/60. Lateral flexion 45/45 bilaterally, rotation 85/85 bilaterally.
Palpation: The spinous processes were normally aligned.
Tenderness: None.
Spurling's/foraminal compression test: Normal.
Lhermitte's test: Negative.

SHOULDER EXAMINATION:

| Test | Left | Right |
|---|---|---|
| Flexion | 170/170 | 170/170 |
| Extension | 30/30 | 30/30 |
| Abduction | 170/170 | 170/170 |
| Adduction | 60/60 | 60/60 |
| Internal rotation [90° abd] | 60/60 | 60/60 |
| External rotation [90° abd] | 80/80 | 80/80 |
| Internal rotation [neutral] | T5 | T5 |
| External rotation [neutral] | 80/80 | 80/80 |
| Neer's test | Nl | Nl |
| Hawkins-Kennedy | - | - |
| Jobe's test | - | - |
| Drop-arm test | - | - |
| Speed's test | - | - |
| O'Brien's test | - | - |
| Yergason's test | - | - |
| Instability | - | - |

## WRIST /ELBOW EXAMINATION:

Range of motion [degrees]:

| | Left | Right |
|---|---|---|
| Elbow Flexion | 150/150 | 150/150 |
| Elbow Extension | 180/180 | 180/180 |
| Elbow Supination | 85/85 | 85/85 |
| Elbow Pronation | 85/85 | 85/85 |
| Wrist Extension/Dorsiflexion | 65/65 | 65/65 |
| Wrist Volar/Palmar Flexion | 70/70 | 70/70 |
| Wrist Ulnar Deviation | 35/35 | 35/35 |
| Wrist Radial Deviation | 20/20 | 20/20 |
| Tenderness | | |

## HAND EXAMINATION:

Individual ranges of the digits of the hands:
All within normal limits.

Thumb:
Abduction:
L: 55/55
R: 55/55

Left Hand:

| | | Proximal | Middle | Distal |
|---|---|---|---|---|
| Thumb | Extension | 175/175 | ***** | 200/200 |
| | Flexion | 50/50 | ***** | 75/75 |
| Index | Extension | 180/180 | 180/180 | 180/180 |
| | Flexion | 85/85 | 100/100 | 70/70 |
| Middle | Extension | 180/180 | 180/180 | 180/180 |
| | Flexion | 90/90 | 100/100 | 70/70 |
| Ring | Extension | 180/180 | 180/180 | 180/180 |
| | Flexion | 90/90 | 100/100 | 70/70 |
| Little | Extension | 180/180 | 180/180 | 180/180 |
| | Flexion | 90/90 | 100/100 | 70/70 |

Right Hand:

| | | Proximal | Middle | Distal |
|---|---|---|---|---|
| Thumb | Extension | 175/175 | ***** | 200/200 |
| | Flexion | 50/50 | ***** | 75/75 |
| Index | Extension | 180/180 | 180/180 | 180/180 |
| | Flexion | 85/85 | 100/100 | 70/70 |
| Middle | Extension | 180/180 | 180/180 | 180/180 |

| | Flexion | 90/90 | 100/100 | 70/70 |
|---|---|---|---|---|
| Ring | Extension | 180/180 | 180/180 | 180/180 |
| | Flexion | 90/90 | 100/100 | 70/70 |
| Little | Extension | 180/180 | 180/180 | 180/180 |
| | Flexion | 90/90 | 100/100 | 70/70 |

MCP = METACARPOPHALANGEAL JOINTS
PIP = PROXIMAL INTERPHALANGEAL JOINTS
DIP = DISTAL INTERPHALANGEAL [INTERPHALANGEAL FOR THUMBS] JOINTS

| | Left | Right |
|---|---|---|
| Tinel's | - | - |
| Phalen's | - | - |
| Finkelstein's | - | - |
| Durkin's | - | - |
| Jamar grip testing: | | |

Tenderness: None.

**NEUROLOGICAL DETAILED EXAMINATION:**

Mental status examination:

| | |
|---|---|
| Judgement: | normal |
| Affect: | normal |
| Mood: | normal |
| Insight: | normal |
| Orientation: | Person, place and time |
| Memory: | 3/3 Immediate<br>3/3 Short term<br>3/3 Long term |
| Speech: | Normal rate, affect, tone; no echolalia or tangentiality |

Depression Assessment:

| | |
|---|---|
| Suicidality: | no |
| Lack of interest: | no |
| Feelings of guilt: | no |
| Decreased energy: | no |
| Concentration deficit: | no |
| Impaired appetite: | no |
| Psychomotor retardation: | no |
| Sleep disturbance: | no |

[Greater than 4/8 is highly suggestive of depression]

**Cerebellar:**
[-] Dysmetria
[-] Intention Tremor
[-] Nystagmus
[-] Cerebellar Ataxia

Motor:
Normal; 5/5 bilaterally throughout

Sensory:
Normal pain, proprioception, and joint position sense bilaterally throughout.

Cranial nerves: II-XII grossly intact bilaterally.

**Reflexes:**

| Test | Left | Right |
|---|---|---|
| Biceps [c6] | 2+ | 2+ |
| Triceps [c7] | 2+ | 2+ |
| Brachioradialis [c8] | 2+ | 2+ |
| Quadriceps [L4] | 2+ | 2+ |
| Achilles Tendon [S1] | 2+ | 2+ |
| Plantar Response ['Babinski'] | Down | Down |

REVIEW OF MEDICAL RECORDS:
**Medical Reports**

DIAGNOSTIC IMAGING/LAB/ X-RAY REVIEW:

CT Scans:

X-rays:

MRI:

Labs:

**Electrodiagnostic studies:**

**DIAGNOSES:**

**THERAPEUTIC PLAN:**
*Please consider the following treatment plan as a formal request for pre-authorization of services described therein. In the event that a written denial, authorization or notice of delay is not received by our office within seven business days with a description of the review by a qualified physician with training in Dr. Sandhu's area of expertise [as per the dictates of California Code of Regulations 9792.6] we will assume de facto authorization.*

*If prior pre-authorization has been requested in an earlier report or therapeutic plan, please consider the date of the prior request as applicable for purposes of the formal date of request.*

Periodic muscle strength testing with range of motion analysis and torque curves will be performed on this patient by Dr. Sandhu or one of his assistants. This testing may be separate from evaluation/management and physical therapy services. The frequency of this testing may be as often as once per month depending upon the patient's presentation.

**FUNCTIONAL LIMITATIONS:**

Sitting:
Standing:
Walking:
Lifting:
Reaching:
Postural limitations:
Grasping, fingering, feeling, handling:

One of Dr. Sandhu's allied medical professionals, including a nurse, nurse practitioner, physician's assistant, medical assistant, or physician, hereafter may be attending upon this patient in the context of a medical conference with Dr. Sandhu or another physician designee in order to ensure continuity of care.

**PERMANENT AND STATIONARY:**
The patient is not currently Permanent and Stationary pending treatments recommended above.

Thank you again for allowing me to participate in the treatment of this pleasant individual. Please feel free to call on me if there is any additional information I may be able to provide.

**AFFIRMATIONS AND SIGNATURE:**

Pursuant to 4628(j), I declare under penalty of perjury that the information contained in this report and its attachments, if any, is true and correct to the best of my knowledge and belief, except as information I have indicated I have received from others. As to that information, I declare under penalty of perjury that the information accurately describes the information provided to me and, except as noted herein; I believe it to be true.

I further declare under penalty of perjury that I personally performed the evaluation of the patient or, in the case of a supplemental report, I personally performed the cognitive services necessary to produce the report on , 2003, at in our clinic, , in County, California and that, except as otherwise stated herein, the evaluation was performed and the time spent performing the evaluation was in compliance with the guidelines, if any, established by the Industrial Medical Council or the administrative director pursuant to paragraph (5) of subdivision (j) of Section 139.2 and Section 5307.6 of the California Labor Code.

I further declare under penalty of perjury that I have not violated the provision of California Labor Code section 139.3 with regard to the evaluation of this patient or the preparing of this report.

I further declare under penalty of perjury that the name and qualification of each person who performed any services in connection with the report, including diagnostic studies, other than clerical preparation, are as follows:

| NAME: | QUALIFICATION: |
|---|---|
| None. | None. |

I further declare under penalty of perjury that the total time on the following activities is true and correct:

a. reviewing the records, job analysis, ergonomics status, work limitations work capacity, or communications with other professionals and/or the patient/family
[ ] hours/minutes.

b. face to face time with the patient
[ ] hours/minutes.

c. preparing the report
[ ] hours.

d. any other relevant activities
detailed in report (research)
[ ] hours.

Date of Report:

Paul Sandhu, M.D., Q.M.E.
[Electronic Signature – original on file]
Board Certified, American Board of PM&R

Board Certified, American Board of Pain Medicine

Signed this on day of 2003, at County, California.

Cc:

**Proof of Service by Mail/FAX**

I declare that I am over the age of eighteen [18] years and not a party to the:

Industrial Claim and/or litigation concerning:

My address is:
Painsolvers, Inc.
130 La Casa Via, Bldg. #2, Suite #106
Walnut Creek, CA 94598

On , I served the attached letter by placing a true copy enclosed in a sealed envelope with postage fully prepaid in the United States Mail and/or sent the report via FAX, addressed as follows:

I declare under penalty of perjury that the foregoing is true and correct and that this declaration was executed on in Walnut Creek at the above address in Contra Costa County, California.

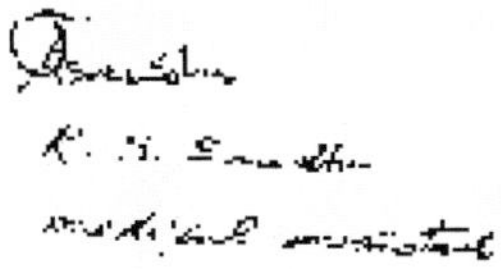

Ranbir S. Sandhu, PhD
[Electronic Signature – original on file]

**BILLING STATEMENT**

**Payment should be made to:**
**Paul Sandhu, M.D./Painsolvers, Inc.**
**P. O. Box #4899**
**Walnut Creek, CA 94596-0899**

Patient:
Claim#:
Date of Injury:
Date of Billing:
Date of Services:

Summary of charges:

| | | |
|---|---|---|
| 99244 | Office Consultation – Moderate Complexity | $220.00 |
| 99354 | Prolonged Service, Face to Face, 60 Minutes | $180.20 |
| 99080 | Report, 1st Page | $39.98 |
| 99080 | Report, Each Additional Pg. ($24.60 Per Page X Pages) | $ |
| 99358 | Prolonged Service, Non Face to Face, Each 15 Min. ($38.25 X - 15 Min. Increm.) | $ |
| TOTAL | | $ |

**Total due: $**

**Provider Information**
**Provider Name: Paul S. Sandhu M.D.**
**License: A72161**

**Commercial PIN: AAA1234**
**SSN or EIN: 123-45-6789**

**Billing Justification:**
[This is an integral component of the report; it is not to be removed]

**Dear Claims Adjuster:**

**Please note the following in reviewing this claim:**

**<u>CPT code 99080 [report] for $162.98</u>**
1] My charge for CPT code #99080 of $162.98 is based on the official medical fee schedule of California [OMFS]. Official Medical Fee Schedule mandates the reimbursement for reports as $39.98 for the first page [6.5 relative value units at $6.15 each] and then each additional page as $24.60 [4 relative value units at $6.15 each] This is in accordance with state law, as described on page 5 of the OMFS. This report exceeds or equals six pages in length. In terms of pages, which are reimbursable, [OMFS page 5, paragraph #3 under the section on reports] indicates that I must be paid for the first 6. Therefore, by the OMFS, the reimbursable amount is exactly $162.98. This is $39.98 for the first page, and $123 for pages 2-6 [@ $24.60 each].
<u>=$162.98</u>

The reason for this added charge is based on the description of separately reimbursable reports in the OMFS:

*Please refer to the OMFS, page #5, first paragraph under the section marked "reports". This states the terms under which a report is separately reimbursable, and this report falls under those criteria as a comprehensive evaluation requested by a party...*

**<u>CPT code #99354 $180.20</u>**
The OMFS stipulates a reimbursement of 21.2 relative value units @ $8.50 each for a total of $180.20 for the additional time spent in this examination face-to-face [OMFS, page #70]. The report has on the last page a breakdown of all time spent reviewing the case and time spent face to face in interview.
<u>=$180.20</u>

**CPT code #99358 [document review/research, etc..., OMFS page 71].**
The last page of my report breaks down the time spent on this initial evaluation and its report. The OMFS stipulates a reimbursement of 4.5 relative value units @ $8.50 each unit for each 15 minute period spent on records review, review of ergonomics, etc... [see pg. 71 OMFS for details]. This is equal to $38.25 for each fifteen-minute period- the number of such fifteen-minute periods is indicated in the last pages of the report [10] =$382.50

**CPT Code #99244 [Office Consultation, New patient - OMFS page #42].**
This E&M code reimburses at 22.3 relative value units at $8.50/unit for a total of = $189.55

**Our fees on the billing statement reflect our usual and customary fees; the minimum amount we will accept is the OMFS stipulated sum listed above.**

**Please remit the balance due plus all other appropriate charges to:**

**Payment should be made to:**
**Paul Sandhu, M.D./Painsolvers, Inc.**
**P. O. Box #4899**
**Walnut Creek, CA 94596-0899**

By sending this letter, in addition to all of the above-mentioned enclosures, via both facsimile and U.S. mail, we have exceeded our obligation to provide all of the information necessary for these charges to be paid in full. ***Please be advised that if we do not receive payment in full within sixty days as required by Labor Code 4603.2, or a proper objection within thirty days, it is our office policy to submit both a complaint to the Audit and Enforcement Unit of the Division of Workers' Compensation and to submit a lien and Declaration of Readiness to Proceed to the Workers' Compensation Appeals Board. If counsel represents the patient, we will request that the attorney file for penalties on the case due to underpayment of billings submitted to cure or relieve the effects of his/her client's industrial injury. If the patient is not represented, we will recommend that he obtain representation by a competent lawyer to protect his/her industrial benefits.***

Thank you. If you have any questions, please call either my billing manager or myself at (925) 933-7246.

**DISCLOSURE**
I personally performed the history, physical examination, and all other above referenced procedures. I have typed this report in its entirety and all of the opinions expressed are my own. I have not violated Labor Code section 139.3. I declare that the information contained in this report and its attachments is true and correct to the best of my knowledge. These disclosures are made under penalty of perjury.

Sincerely,
Paul Sandhu, M.D., Q.M.E.
[Electronic Signature - original on file]
Board Certified, American Board of PM&R
Board Certified, American Board of Pain Medicine

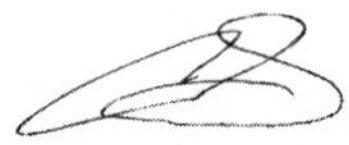

**<u>Entire preceding document copyright Paul Sandhu, M.D., 2003. All reproduction, duplication and other transmission of any logos, text or illustrations in this template is prohibited without the express written permission of Paul Sandhu, M.D.</u>**

*Resulting Cross-examination:*
**Q.** Doctor, you use this template when doing your IME reports, correct?
**A.** Yes.
**Q.** Your reports are impartial and unbiased, correct?
**A.** Correct.
**Q.** You don't prejudge the examinees?
**A.** Absolutely not.
**Q.** Page three of the template indicates that the examinee has no double or blurred vision, no loss of hearing, no new rashes, no constipation, correct?
**A.** Yes.
**Q.** The template is done before the exam, correct?
**A.** Yes. It is used in the exam. I modify it as needed.
**Q.** Page four also has all normal findings programmed into the template?
**A.** Yes.
**Q.** Pages five through nine of the template have all normal findings already programmed in?
**A.** Yes.
**Q.** For example, page eight has no tenderness and page nine a normal mental status exam, correct?
**A.** Yes. It's just a template.
**Q.** Page eleven has a statement that the patient is not currently permanent and stationary programmed into the template?
**A.** Yes.
**Q.** Your testimony under the pains and penalties of perjury is that despite most of the report being filled out <u>before</u> you even see the examinee and the report

stating that the examinee is completely normal, that you are impartial, unbiased, and don't prejudge the examinees?

**Comment:** Examiners use templates to ensure completeness and a thorough examination. The more comprehensive and detailed the template, the more it is subject to the above type of attack.

**Defending the Report As Written:** The well-respected IME examiner in the above example is prepared to defend his template, report, and opinion.

**Q.** Doctor, you use this template when doing your IME report, correct?
**A.** Counselor, this is not a template. This is a detailed checklist I have developed and am very proud of. It is the product of many years of hard work. This permits me and my staff to do a detailed examination and report without recreating the wheel. Each and every abnormal finding is noted and an impartial and comprehensive report is generated. I would be happy to run through it with you if you like.

**Example 11.202: Disclosure statement**
*Report States:*

> **Disclosure Statement**
>
> The above analysis is based upon the available information at this time, including the history given by the examinee, the medical records and tests provided, the results of pain status inventories, and the physical findings. It is assumed that the information provided to me is correct. If more information becomes available at a later date, an additional report may be requested. Such information may or may not change the opinions rendered in this evaluation.
>
> My opinions are based upon reasonable medical certainty. Medicine is both an art and a science, and although an individual may appear to be fit for work activity, there is no guarantee that the person will not be re-injured or suffer additional injury. If applicable, employers should follow the processes established in the Americans with Disabilities Act, Title I. The opinions on work capacity are to facilitate job placement and do not necessarily reflect an in-depth direct threat analysis. Comments on appropriateness of care are professional opinions based upon the specifics of the case and should not be generalized, not necessarily be considered supportive or critical of, the involved providers or disciplines.
>
> Any medical recommendations offered are provided as guidance and not as medical orders. The opinions expressed do not constitute a recommendation that specific claims or administrative action be made or enforced.
>
> I declare under penalty of perjury that the information contained in this report and its attachments is true and correct, to the best of my knowledge and belief, except as to information that I have received from others. As to

> that information, I declare under penalty of perjury that the information accurately describes the information provided to me, and except as noted in this report, that I believe to be true. I further declare under penalty of perjury that to the best of my knowledge and belief, the contents of this report and bill are true and correct. The foregoing was signed in the County of Cumberland, State of State, on the date of this report.
>
> Thank you for asking me to see this examinee in consultation. If you have any further questions, please do not hesitate to contact me.

*Resulting Cross-examination:*

**Q.** You put the Disclosure Statement listed on page 7 of your report in all of your IME reports, correct?

**A.** Not all of them.

**Q.** Doctor, I show you 37 of your IME reports and ask you if all 37 have the statement?

**A.** Well, give me a few minutes to look. Yes, they do.

**Q.** You use this same Disclosure Statement even when it is not true, isn't that a fact?

**A.** That's false.

**Q.** Your Disclosure Statement says your analysis is based on the pain inventories, correct?

**A.** Yes.

**Q.** In fact, there were no pain inventories completed here. The examinee refused to do so, correct?

**A.** Correct, Counsel. That's a minor oversight.

**Q.** Just like when you talk about your comments on the appropriateness of care?

**A.** That's in my report.

**Q.** Page please?

**A.** Well, that's a mistake.

**Q.** That's a minor or major mistake?

**A.** It's a mistake.

**Q.** Just like your lack of comments on work capacity which you swore to under the pains and penalties of perjury?

**A.** Yes.

**Q.** Do you still maintain, Doctor, that you don't use this Disclosure Statement even when it is not true?

**Comment:** Examiners should use boilerplate language in their reports judiciously. Opposing counsel will try to show that all of the examiner's reports are the same (cookie cutter variety) or, even more damaging, that the examiner forgot to customize the language to fit the facts of the case.

**Defending the Report As Written:** When faced with an inconsistency between the boilerplate language and the underlying facts, the examiner should admit his mistake graciously.

**Q.** Your Disclosure Statement says your analysis is based on the pain inventories, correct?
**A.** Counsel, you are correct. This entire Disclosure Statement was erroneously put in the report. It is my mistake and I apologize for the confusion.

**Example 11.203: "Canned" MCS language**
*Report States:*

> *Comments on multiple chemical sensitivity (MCS):* MCS is not recognized as a disease for a number of reasons. The symptoms are widely variable and include fatigue, headaches, memory loss, confusion, skin and mucous membrane irritation, and various other constitutional symptoms. However, there are no significant physical findings in individuals claiming to have MCS that can be used to make the diagnosis and there are no objective and verifiable laboratory tests to diagnose this disorder. The World Health Organization, in fact, has recommended that the name MCS be replaced by "Idiopathic Environmental Intolerance" to signify the fact that environmental chemicals have not been proven to cause these symptoms.
>
> Those who believe MCS postulate that after some type of chemical exposure, a person's immune system is somehow altered so that subsequent very low level exposures to many ubiquitous substances in the environment will trigger symptoms. While this is an attractive hypothesis, useful to explain the symptoms, there is no science available to support it and there have been no well-controlled scientific studies done in humans to substantiate this hypothesis. In fact, this is contrary to our current knowledge about how the immune system functions. Care must be taken not to exclude current scientific knowledge in an attempt to explain a series of unrelated symptoms.

*Resulting Cross-examination:*
**Q.** You have testified in 27 cases involving Multiple Chemical Sensitivity (MCS) for the Maple Street Hospital, Correct?
**A.** Yes.
**Q.** You evaluated each case individually and formed an impartial medical opinion in each case?
**A.** Yes, I did.
**Q.** In each report you included the same comments on Multiple Chemical Sensitivity as are in this report?
**A.** Yes, that's correct.
**Q.** And in each one of the 27 cases you found no MCS, correct?
**A.** That's true.
**Q.** So each time you are hired in the future on an MCS case, the client can expect the same comments on MCS in your report and the same opinion, correct?

**Comment:** The more the same language appears over and over again in an examiner's reports, the more it appears that the reports are not the product of impartial analysis and review. When this is combined with the same or similar opinions, it is devastating.

**Defending the Report As Written:** The IME examiner may use the same or similar language in his report because it is the product of extensive research and is, in fact, correct.

**Q.** In each report you included the same comments on Multiple Chemical Sensitivity as in this report?
**A.** Counsel, I share the opinion of many renowned medical experts that there is no reliable evidence that so-called Multiple Chemical Sensitivity exists. A number of well-controlled studies have shown that when these individuals are exposed to the chemicals which they feel cause or trigger their symptoms, symptoms occur no better than with chance. In one study ("Provocative challenge in patients with Multiple Chemical Sensitivities" published in the *Journal of Allergy and Clinical Immunology* in 1997, pages 438-442), the authors had to stop one placebo challenge because of a patient's severe reaction. In two other challenges to the alleged offending substance, the patient's symptoms abated while re-breathing air from a paper bag, despite continued exposure to the alleged offending substances.

## 11.21 Additional Recommendations

Doctor Stephen Demeter, in his text *Disability Evaluation* (©2003 Mosby) provides the following 17 recommendations to produce a well-written disability report.

**Recommendations to Producing a Well-written Disability Report**[3]
1. Use short paragraphs.
2. Provide space (two or three lines between headings).
3. Avoid surplus words such as compound prepositions and word-wasting idioms when simple, concise words suffice.
4. Employ active verbs. Passive verbs require a supporting verb (was) followed by a preposition (by).
5. Generally, use short sentences, especially when comparing items. Vary sentence length somewhat for variety, which improves readability.
6. Guide your reader. Begin sentences with names and dates. Place new information or important facts at the beginning of a sentence or paragraph.
7. Arrange your words with care, following the normal English word order of placing the subject first followed by the verb and then the object. Avoid wide gaps among the subject, the verb, and the object.
8. Present material in tables when appropriate. Tables present complicated bits of information clearly and concisely.
9. Use commonly understood English phrases and clearly defined terms. For example, instead of using terms like inspection, palpation, percussion, and auscultation, choose verbs (inspect, palpate, percuss, auscultate). Lay language is preferable: I observe, I see, I feel.
10. Avoid language quirks, habits, current catch phrases, and jargon. Maintain neutrality and objectivity.

---

[3] Reprinted from *Disability Evaluation,* 2nd edition, Demeter, p. 123 (©2003 Mosby), with permission from Elsevier.

11. Document all sources of information, both medical and nonmedical. Present these materials chronologically, identifying the date, source, recipient, and subject matter.
12. Carefully proofread and edit your report. Typographical errors and other easily corrected mistakes diminish the impact of the report. Rephrase passages that seem unclear on the second reading. Make sure that your report has successfully translated medical language into good English.
13. Use headings, underlining, and boldface print for emphasis and organization. Strive for a professional format that presents information clearly.
14. Be precise.
15. Be terse in the assessment/conclusion parts of your report.
16. Use phrases such as "within a reasonable degree of medical certainty," "more likely than not," and others where and when appropriate.
17. Provide a list of references as needed. If appropriate, enclose a copy of one or two articles with appropriate passages highlighted. This adds power and credibility to your report.

# Chapter 12 Damaging Extraneous Language and Information that Should Not Be Included in IME Reports

## 12.1 Executive Summary

The only language that should appear in IME reports is language that objectively states or supports an examiner's findings and conclusions or language that is otherwise relevant. All other information is extraneous and should not be included in the report.

Including extraneous language in an IME report is one of the most common mistakes independent medical examiners make. This mistake can cost the examiner's (and the report's) credibility dearly. Superfluous language often provides fertile grounds for cross-examination. The authors recommend the following.

- Avoid "friendly" language to counsel that thanks them for the assignment, invites comments or questions, offers further assistance, or includes personal salutations.
- Do not include speeches in IME reports.
- Make sure the examiner's letterhead does not include references to being an "IME doctor."
- Cover letters accompanying reports should be short and formal. One sentence is ideal.
- Do not document in the IME report discussions with counsel, the adjuster, or the broker unless they are relevant.
- Examiners should self-edit their reports aggressively to remove all other superfluous language, including offers to provide treatment, piling on against a party in the case, the examiner's personal feelings, the name of any third party broker or expert witness service, solicitation of future assignments and snide comments directed at the examinee, opposing counsel, the examinee's providers, or anyone else.

## 12.2 "Friendly" Language Directed at Counsel, Adjusters, or Other Referral Sources

Examiners often make the mistake of including language that thanks the referral source for the assignment, invites comments or questions, offers further assistance, or makes personal salutations. Even seemingly innocuous language can damage an examiner's credibility. It is best to avoid such language.

**Example 12.21: Personal salutation**
*Report States:*
> P.S.: I hope that you, Jean, and the kids have a very Merry Christmas and a Happy New Year!

*Resulting Cross-examination:*
**Q.** You have a professional relationship with counsel who retained you to perform this evaluation, correct?
**A.** Yes.
**Q.** You also have a warm, personal relationship with counsel, his wife, Jean, and their three children?
**A.** Well, I don't know if I would call it a "warm, personal relationship."
**Q.** You meant what you said in your P.S., "I hope you, Jean, and the kids have a very, Merry Christmas and a Happy New Year," didn't you?
**A.** Yes.
**Q.** You don't include a P.S. like that in all of your letters to lawyers, do you?
**A.** No, I don't.
**Q.** The reason being…?
**A.** I don't know them well enough to say something like that.

**Comment:** This language can be used to show that the examiner may be biased in favor of his personal friend, referring counsel. This language should have been omitted from the report.

**Defending the Report As Written:** Examiners do not have to permit counsel to mischaracterize passing comments in IME reports. Nor do examiners have to apologize for having friends.

**Q.** You also have a warm, personal relationship with counsel, his wife, Jean, and their three children?
**A.** Yes, I do. They are great people and I am proud to count them among my friends.

**Example 12.22: "Thank you…please call" with questions**
*Report States:*
> Thank you for the opportunity to prepare this report. If you have any questions regarding the detail and content, please call.

*Resulting Cross-examination:*
**Q.** You are happy to answer questions of Mr. Justin, the adjuster who sent you this examinee, about the preliminary report that you issued?
**A.** Correct.
**Q.** You discuss detail and content?
**A.** Yes.
**Q.** Sometimes you modify your preliminary report when you issue your final report?
**A.** Yes, sometimes.
**Q.** That would take place after you sent them a letter saying, "Thank you for the opportunity to prepare this report. If you have any questions regarding the

detail and content, please call."
**A.** Yes.
**Q.** And after you discuss the report with the adjuster who sent you the case?
**A.** Yes.
**Q.** Then you issue your impartial, unbiased, final report?
**A.** Yes.

**Comment:** Even seemingly innocuous superfluous language can be used against an examiner. This language is unnecessary. No examiner should think that retaining counsel or an adjuster needs a written invitation to call the examiner with a question.

**Defending the Report As Written:** Examiners need not be defensive about common courtesy reflected in their reports.

**Q.** You are happy to answer questions of Mr. Justin, the adjuster who sent you this examinee, about the preliminary report that you issued?
**A.** Yes, I am. It is a matter of common courtesy, something we see too little of today.

**Example 12.23: "I trust this information will be of help"**
*Report States:*
I trust this information will be of help.

*Resulting Cross-examination:*
**Q.** You gave the benefit of the doubt to counsel who retained you when arriving at your opinion, didn't you?
**A.** No, I did not.
**Q.** Did you say in your report, "I trust this information will be of help"?
**A.** Yes.
**Q.** You knew what counsel needed you to say for her to make her case, correct?
**A.** Yes.
**Q.** That's because of the number of times you have testified and the discussion with counsel?
**A.** I talked to counsel.
**Q.** She trusted you to do a good job?
**A.** Yes.
**Q.** And you did not betray her trust?
**A.** I don't understand.
**Q.** You gave her what she wanted and then said, "I trust this information will be of help," correct?

**Comment:** This statement neither supports nor expresses the examiner's findings and conclusions. It should not have been included in the IME report.

**Defending the Report As Written:** When counsel attempts to imply wrongdoing or a conspiracy, it may be proper for the examiner to get upset.

**Q.** Did you say in your report, "I trust this information will be of help"?
**A.** Counsel asked me three questions and I answered them in my report. Trying to imply something improper or sinister smacks of desperation. I didn't think you engaged in this type of gamesmanship, Counsel.

**Example 12.24: Wants to satisfy counsel's needs**
*Report States:*

> I trust the above are sufficient for your needs at this time. If I can be of any further assistance, please do not hesitate to call on me.

*Resulting Cross-examination:*
**Q.** You were retained by counsel to issue a report, correct?
**A.** Yes.
**Q.** And you did so in accordance with the instructions of counsel?
**A.** I answered the questions she asked.
**Q.** You only expressed opinions in the areas she instructed you to do so, correct?
**A.** Yes.
**Q.** You tried to be helpful?
**A.** Yes, within the bounds of professional ethics.
**Q.** You tried to meet counsel's needs?
**A.** Yes.
**Q.** Bottom line—counsel needs to win, correct?
**A.** I guess that's true.
**Q.** And you gave her an opinion sufficient to meet her needs to win?
**A.** You are making it sound sinister, Counselor.
**Q.** Aren't you the one who said in your report, "I trust the above are sufficient for your needs at this time"?
**A.** Yes, I did.

**Comment:** This statement neither supports nor expresses the examiner's findings and conclusions. It should not have been included in the report.

**Defending the Report As Written:** Examiners do not have to sit idly by when counsel impugns their ethics and integrity.

**Q.** And you did so in accordance with the instructions of counsel?
**A.** No. I did so after reviewing and analyzing the records, the history, and examining the claimant. I resent your continuing snide comments and insinuations.

**Example 12.25: "Thank you…urgent basis"**
*Report States:*

> Thank you for asking me to see Mrs. Myers on an urgent basis today.

*Resulting Cross-examination:*
**Q.** You did a rush job for the insurer in this case, correct?
**A.** I did no such thing, Counsel.
**Q.** You saw the examinee on an urgent basis at the request of the insurer?

**A.** Yes, I did.
**Q.** And you rushed to dictate the report as soon as you finished the examination?
**A.** I dictated it the same day.
**Q.** You also reviewed the 200 pages of medical records before you dictated the report, didn't you?
**A.** Yes, I did.
**Q.** You examined the claimant, reviewed 200 pages of medical records, dictated your 12-page IME report, proofed the report, and faxed it to the insurer all in one day due to an urgent request by the insurer, but you maintain under oath that you didn't do a rush job in this case, Doctor?

**Comment:** The examiner in the above example created a potential problem for himself by putting in the passing comment about urgency. Examiners should be mindful of the problems they could create for themselves with seemingly innocent comments. It is not difficult for opposing counsel to make them appear to be sinister. The examiner would have been better served by either omitting the sentence completely or modifying it.

Thank you for asking me to see Mrs. Myers.

**Defending the Report As Written:** While it is normally not a good idea for the examiner to "joust" with opposing counsel, sometimes the lawyer just deserves it.

**Q.** You saw the examinee on an urgent basis at the request of the insurer?
**A.** Actually, it was counsel who waited to the last minute to request the examination. Lawyers for both sides do this all the time, Counsel.

## 12.3 Speeches

An IME report is no place to make speeches espousing the examiner's beliefs. Such speeches are irrelevant, subjective, and will make the examiner appear as though he has interests beyond an objective evaluation of the examinee.

**Example 12.31: Speech on workplace safety**
*Report States:*

> Safety and occupational health professionals and others believe that it is not only morally and ethically responsible to control workplace hazards that could otherwise lead to catastrophic injury and death, it is also good business. That is, we believe that it is much more cost-effective to pay for the added costs to prevent injury and death than it is to cut corners, save safety costs and time, and expose workers to dangers and hope that no injury will occur. When injury does occur, the costs to society are significantly higher than the costs to prevent the injury. Certainly, an "ounce of prevention" is worth a pound of "cure."

*Resulting Cross-examination:*
**Q.** Sir, how many safety and occupational health professionals are there in the United States?
**A.** Well, depending on how you define it, 150,000–200,000.
**Q.** How many "others" are there?
**A.** Others?
**Q.** Yes, as you used the term in your report.
**A.** Well, that would be impossible to say.
**Q.** Have you been elected or selected as a leader or spokesperson for these 200,000 occupational safety and health professionals, and untold others, sir?
**A.** No.
**Q.** So, when you say "we believe" in paragraph one, page 3 of your report, you are just expressing your thoughts, correct?
**A.** Yes.

**Comment:** This language does not support the examiner's findings and conclusions and should not be in the examiner's report.

**Example 12.32: Moral responsibility to pay**
*Report States:*

> There are significant costs associated with workplace injury. But it is much cheaper and it is morally responsible for the entity that creates the hazard, or the company that benefits from not spending the money, to bear all of the costs. These companies should pay the full costs of injury and death because, otherwise, there would be little incentive to prevent injury.

*Resulting Cross-examination:*
**Q.** The company who is legally responsible is always the same as the one who is morally responsible for an injury, correct?
**A.** No, absolutely not.
**Q.** It is your belief that it is not the company who is legally responsible but the company who is morally responsible who should pay for the cost of injury and death?
**A.** No.
**Q.** Didn't you say in your IME report, "…it is morally responsible for the entity that creates the hazard, or the company that benefits from not spending the money, to bear all of the costs"?
**A.** Yes.
**Q.** Who decides who is legally responsible?
**A.** The courts and the judicial system.
**Q.** Who do you propose decides who is morally responsible?

**Comment:** This superfluous language makes the expert appear as though he is a crusader on a mission. This will damage the examiner's credibility because it indicates that the examiner has an agenda of his own to advance. This language has no place in an IME report.

**Defending the Report As Written:** When being cross-examined by counsel, the examiner can sometimes turn the tables on counsel and play directly to the fact finder.

**Q.** Didn't you say in your IME report, "... it is morally responsible for the entity that creates the hazard, or the company that benefits from not spending the money, to bear all of the costs"?
**A.** Don't you agree, Counsel, that the entity that creates the hazard should bear the costs? Isn't that a foundation of our legal system?

**Example 12.33: Carpal tunnel not caused by work**
*Report States:*

> The cause(s) for the development of carpal tunnel syndrome still remains a controversial subject. There are a number of speculations, theories, and hypotheses for the development of carpal tunnel syndrome. The matter is debated in scientific meetings devoted to this subject. However, to this date, not a single well-run scientific research study has proven a direct relationship between the development of this illness and a particular job or vocation.
>
> In my own experience, covering more than 30 years of treating this problem, I have noticed that the majority of my patients have been housewives or retired individuals with no particular job or vocation.

*Resulting Cross-examination:*
**Q.** Doctor, you review workers' compensation carpal tunnel claims for insurance companies, correct?
**A.** Yes. But that's not the only type of case I review.
**Q.** More than 50% of the cases you review are carpal tunnel claims?
**A.** Yes, that's true.
**Q.** The workers' compensation insurance companies use you to review these claims because they know you believe that carpal tunnel syndrome is not related to work, correct?
**A.** That's not true.
**Q.** Why do you find in over 90% of these cases no causal relationship?
**A.** That's my opinion.
**Q.** On page 7 of your IME report just before you find no causation of the carpal tunnel syndrome claim, you state,

> "The cause(s) for the development of carpal tunnel syndrome still remains a controversial subject. There are a number of speculations, theories, and hypotheses for the development of carpal tunnel syndrome. The matter is debated in scientific meetings devoted to this subject. However, to this date, not a single well-run scientific research study has proven a direct relationship between the development of this illness and a particular job or vocation. In my own experience, covering more than 30 years of treating this problem, I have noticed that the majority of my patients have been housewives or retired individuals with no particular job or vocation."

Is that what you said?
**A.** That's what I wrote and that is my opinion.

**Q.** So you don't agree with Dr. Stephen Demeter in his text *Disability Evaluation* when he writes that causes of carpal tunnel syndrome include work-related factors?
**A.** No, I don't.
**Q.** Do you agree with Presley Reed, MD, when he states in the *Medical Disability Advisor*, "Chronic trauma is often related to work that involves repetitive wrist/hand movements, sustained awkward hand positions, prolonged or frequent pressure over the wrist or base of palm, or frequent use of vibrating hand tools"?
**A.** No, I don't.
**Q.** You do keep up with the medical literature on carpal tunnel syndrome?
**A.** Absolutely.
**Q.** Doctor, I show you a list of the latest 120 articles on Medline on carpal tunnel syndrome and ask you to identify the ones that you have read.
**A.** Well, I couldn't say.
**Q.** As you sit here today, under oath, Doctor, can you tell me the names of any medical journal articles you have read in the past year on carpal tunnel syndrome?
**A.** No, I cannot.
**Q.** What about the research studies you allude to in your IME report? Can you name one recent research study on carpal tunnel syndrome that you have read?
**A.** Well, no, I cannot.
**Q.** Doctor, the workers' compensation insurance companies use you on these carpal tunnel cases because your opinion is predetermined and well known and engraved in stone. No causal relationship. Isn't that true?

**Comment:** Examiners who make global statements or speeches in their reports regarding an area of medicine should expect to be closely cross-examined on this issue.

**Defending the Report As Written:** Examiners who want to properly defend their opinions and global statements should be prepared with the research studies and articles they need to answer the anticipated difficult questions.

**Q.** Why do you find in over 90% of these cases no causal relationship?
**A.** First, many healthcare providers over-diagnose carpal tunnel syndrome. Many cases of carpal tunnel syndrome are idiopathic with no clear-cut cause. The National Institute of Neurological Disorders and Stroke (NIDS) has studied carpal tunnel syndrome and found causation a complex issue.

There are many non-occupational causes of carpal tunnel syndrome. Anatomic causes include osteoarthritis, aberrant wrist muscles, small wrist dimension, neoplasms, tubercular granuloma, radial head fracture, and hematoma. Systemic causes include tendonitis, rheumatoid disease, diabetes, collagen-vascular, thyroid disease, gout, renal disease, gynecological disorders, amyloidosis, pregnancy, obesity, alcoholism, dupuytren's disease, hereditary neuropathy with liability to pressure palsies, genetic (trisomy of chromosome 8), endocrinopathies, and medications.

Counsel, I have a 10-page summary of recent medical journal articles on the cause of carpal tunnel syndrome. Would you like to see the list?

## 12.4 Letterhead

Examiners should be careful about what is contained on their letterhead. Their letterhead should not contain any reference to the professional being an "IME doctor." Such references can result in a completely avoidable loss of credibility.

**Example 12.41: "IMEs for…"**
*Report States:*
IMEs for Workers' Compensation, Personal Injury, and Long-term Disability.

*Resulting Cross-examination:*
**Q.** You are a medical doctor, correct?
**A.** Yes.
**Q.** Your degree and license are in medicine, the art of healing?
**A.** Yes.
**Q.** But your letterhead doesn't say anything about healing, does it?
**A.** It speaks for itself.
**Q.** Actually, it speaks for you, sir. It says, "IMEs for Workers' Compensation, Personal Injury, and Long-term Disability," correct?
**A.** Yes.
**Q.** So you promote yourself as an independent medical examiner for hire, correct?
**A.** I do IMEs.
**Q.** You do these IMEs as a business for money, correct?
**A.** Yes.
**Q.** The object in your IME business is to make as much money as possible?
**A.** Yes.
**Q.** Sir, when did you stop being a healer and start being someone who hawks medical-legal reports?

**Comment:** References to IMEs should not be contained on the examiner's letterhead. If such a reference is contained in the letterhead, the examiner is likely to face a line of questioning similar to the above.

**Defending the Report As Written:** Experienced examiners do not permit counsel to get away with half-truths and mischaracterizations.

**Q.** So you promote yourself as an independent medical examiner for hire, correct?
**A.** No. I truthfully list the work I do on my letterhead. I don't have the name of a partner who has been dead for 30 years in my firm name as your firm has, Counsel.

**Example 12.42: "Pro-Witness Forensic Exams and Consulting, Inc."**
*Report States:*
Name of examiner's practice on letterhead is "Pro-Witness Forensic Exams and Consulting, Inc."

*Resulting Cross-examination:*
**Q.** The name of your practice, listed prominently in large block letters on your letterhead, is "Pro-Witness Forensic Exams and Consulting"?
**A.** That's correct.
**Q.** The "Pro" stands for?
**A.** Professional.
**Q.** So you advertise and promote yourself as a "Professional Witness," correct?

**Comment:** This examiner's choice of a name to do business under implies that she is a professional witness. This will damage her credibility. Putting that name on her report will damage it even more.

**Defending the Report As Written:** Examiners who face a grueling cross-examination learn quickly to correct their mistakes.

**Q.** The name of your practice, listed prominently in large block letters on your letterhead, is "Pro-Witness Forensic Exams and Consulting"?
**A.** No, that was changed years ago. Here is my new stationery, Counsel.

## 12.5 Cover Letters

The cover letter accompanying an examiner's report should be short, formal, and contain nothing that can be used against the examiner on cross-examination. For more information on cover letters, please see Section 2.4. If this is not done, the cover letter will itself become a fertile area of contention and provide ammunition for unnecessary cross-examination.

**Example 12.51: Well-written cover letter**
*Cover Letter States:*

Re: *Smith v. Jones*

Dear Attorney Johnson:

Enclosed please find my seven-page written report dated September 28, 2003, in the above-referenced matter.

Very truly yours,
John Q. Examiner, MD

**Comment:** This is a well-written cover letter. It serves its purpose as a cover letter yet provides no ammunition for the cross-examiner to use against the examiner.

**Example 12.52: Extraneous language in cover letter**
*Report States:*

The permanent impairment evaluation is intended as an estimate of the examinee's function.

*Resulting Cross-examination:*
**Q.** Your cover letter of March 6, 2003, states that the permanent impairment evaluation in your report is "intended as an estimate of the examinee's function," correct?
**A.** Correct.
**Q.** So, the figure of 14% whole person impairment you arrived at is not a precise figure?
**A.** It's an estimate.
**Q.** By "estimate," you mean there is a margin of error?
**A.** Yes.
**Q.** What is the margin of error for your entire impairment rating?
**A.** I didn't compute that.
**Q.** Could it be 5%?
**A.** It could be.
**Q.** Could it be 10%?
**A.** Yes.
**Q.** What about 20%?
**A.** Yes.
**Q.** What about 25%?
**A.** No, that's too high.
**Q.** So your rating could be off by as much as 40%?
**A.** No, I said 20%.
**Q.** But that's 20% on the low side or 20% on the high side, so that's a range of up to 40%, correct?
**A.** That's correct.
**Q.** You gave counsel who retained you exactly what she was looking for, correct?
**A.** I gave her my honest opinion.

**Comment:** The examiner would have been better served with a simple cover letter that did not contain any reference to an "estimate."

> My permanent impairment evaluation in the above matter is enclosed.

**Defending the Report As Written:** Examiners should not play the "numbers game" with counsel because it is always a losing proposition.

**Q.** So, the figure of 14% whole person impairment you arrived at is not a precise figure?
**A.** It is my opinion expressed to a reasonable degree of medical certainty.

**Example 12.53: "Glad to be of service" in cover letter**
*Report States:*

> I was glad to be of service to you and if I can assist you in any other way in this case, please do not hesitate to call me.

*Resulting Cross-examination:*
**Q.** Did you not say in your cover letter of March 6, 2003, "I was glad to be of service to you and if I can assist you in any other way in this case, please do not

hesitate to call me"?
**A.** Yes, but I was just being polite.
**Q.** But you do anticipate additional "service" on this matter to counsel, correct?
**A.** I am not sure what you mean.
**Q.** In addition to saying, "If I can assist you in any other way in this case, please let me know," you go on to state, "If I am called upon to testify in this matter, I shall be compensated at my standard fee," correct?
**A.** Yes.
**Q.** You would normally only be called upon to testify if counsel was pleased with the report you furnished her?
**A.** Well…I guess that's true.
**Q.** And when you don't give counsel what they want, they normally do not call upon you to testify?
**A.** Well…ah, I am not sure.
**Q.** So you have a direct pecuniary interest in pleasing counsel with your impairment estimate?
**A.** I am not sure how to answer that.
**Q.** You just did. Thank you.

**Comment:** This examiner could have avoided this entire damaging cross-examination by writing a simple, one-sentence cover letter. In the case of cover letters, less is more.

**Defending the Report As Written:** Examiners need not sit back and let themselves be crucified by cross-examining counsel.

**Q.** So you have a direct pecuniary interest in pleasing counsel with your impairment estimate?
**A.** No. I have an interest in telling the truth, maintaining my reputation, credibility, and integrity, and having a long career as an expert who is known for calling them as he sees them.

**Example 12.54: Overly cooperative examiner**
*Report States:*
I hope this IME report will be useful to you. . .

*Resulting Cross-examination:*
**Q.** Doctor, you tried to cooperate with the insurance company who retained you to perform an IME in this case, correct?
**A.** Yes, I did.
**Q.** In fact, you tried to write your report so the insurer would find it useful, isn't that the case?
**A.** I wrote what I found.
**Q.** You knew from the two questions asked by the insurer that they were attempting to discontinue the temporary total compensation of the claimant and you gave them a report they used to file for the discontinuance, correct?
**A.** I issued my IME report based upon the results of my examination.
**Q.** After you knew they were attempting to discontinue the weekly

compensation of the claimant, you wrote in your report, "I hope this IME report will be useful to you," correct?
**A.** I didn't mean anything by the comment.
**Q.** Could you explain under oath, Doctor, what you did mean by, "I hope this IME report will be useful to you"?

**Comment:** Comments and statements like the one in the above example frequently find their way into IME reports or into accompanying cover letters. Examiners are better served by omitting this kind of polite comment that can be mischaracterized by opposing counsel to imply a sinister conspiracy.

**Defending the Report As Written:** Examiners who act defensively when faced with a comment of this nature do themselves and their reports a disservice. There is no need for the examiner to be so timid on cross-examination. In addition, the IME physician should carefully review the context of the statement to see if counsel is mischaracterizing it or twisting its meaning.

**Q.** Could you explain under oath, Doctor, what you meant by, "I hope this IME report will be useful to you"?
**A.** I was trying to be polite—something we don't see enough of. I resent the dishonest way you took the statement out of context. The entire sentence in my report reads, "I hope this IME report will be useful to you as you continue to assist the examinee."

**Example 12.55: Extraneous information in cover letter**
*Report States:*
Dear Counsel:

> At your request, I have conducted an independent forensic psychological evaluation of Mr. Subject Plaintiff 2.
>
> In compliance with *Federal Rule of Civil Procedure 26(a)(2)(b)* and with local standards of my profession regarding the preparation of expert reports, I have enclosed my report in this matter.

*Resulting Cross-examination:*
**Q.** Doctor, your IME report complies with Federal Rule of Civil Procedure 26(a)(2)(b), correct?
**A.** Yes, it does.
**Q.** What does 26(a)(2)(b) call for, Doctor?
**A.** Well, I am not a lawyer. I know that you have to list where you testified for a period of time.
**Q.** Doctor, if you don't know precisely what 26(a)(2)(b) requires, how can you testify under oath that your IME report complies with it?

**Comment:** Examiners should not put extraneous legal references into their IME reports.

**Defending the Report As Written:** Examiners who put legal references into their IME reports should be ready, willing, and able to discuss them in detail during their cross-examination.

**Q.** What does 26(a)(2)(b) call for, Doctor?
**A.** A report shall contain a complete statement of all opinions to be expressed and the basis and reasons therefore; the data or other information considered by the witness in forming the opinions; the qualifications of the witness, including a list of all publications authored by the witness within the preceding ten years; the compensation to be paid for the study and testimony; and a listing of any other cases in which the witness has testified as an expert at trial or by deposition within the preceding four years.

## 12.6 Discussions with Retaining Counsel

Referring counsel, adjusters, or brokers and the examiner sometimes discuss the case at hand before a report is issued. These conversations are perfectly legitimate. However, it is usually not good practice to document them in an IME report unless they are relevant. Opposing counsel will likely zero-in on such references and try to make it look as if the referral source improperly influenced the examiner's opinion.

**Example 12.61: Verbal report mentioned in written report**
*Report States:*

> After a verbal report, a request was made to reduce to writing the main points of that verbal report.

*Resulting Cross-examination:*
**Q.** You gave a verbal report to counsel prior to reducing it to writing?
**A.** Yes.
**Q.** Did counsel ask you to do this?
**A.** Yes.
**Q.** So, counsel could "preview" the report without actually receiving something in writing that she would have to share during discovery?
**A.** You would have to ask her about the reason.
**Q.** The verbal report you gave counsel was essentially the same as the one reduced to writing?
**A.** Yes.
**Q.** Did you memorize this seven-page, single-spaced report, or did you have notes when you discussed it with counsel?
**A.** I had notes.
**Q.** Can I see them?
**A.** I destroyed them once the report was typed up.
**Q.** As a result of your discussions with counsel, did you alter, change, modify, or revise your report when it was typed up?
**A.** Yes.
**Q.** Let's go through all the changes you made. Tell me how it was before the oral report, how it was changed, and why you made the changes, sir.

**Comment:** This examiner would have been better served by not documenting in his report the fact that a verbal report had first been made to retaining counsel.

**Defending the Report As Written:** When counsel makes a mistake during cross-examination, the examiner can pounce on the mistake and exploit it.

**Q.** So, counsel could "preview" the report without actually receiving something in writing that she would have to share during discovery?
**A.** Counsel, you know or should know that there is no discovery in workers' compensation cases in this state.

## 12.7 Additional Examples of Extraneous Language

Examiners need to self-edit their reports to remove extraneous language. This could include offers to provide treatment, piling on against a party in the case, the examiner's personal feelings, the name of any third-party broker or expert witness service, solicitation of future assignments, and snide comments directed at the examinee, opposing counsel, the examinee's providers, or anyone else. Failure to do so will result in damaging cross-examinations that are completely avoidable.

**Example 12.71: MENSA member**

*Report States:*

Member: MENSA

*Resulting Cross-examination:*

**Q.** Dr. Curran, on page 7 of your report, above your signature, you indicate that you are a member of MENSA, is that correct?
**A.** Yes.
**Q.** Why did you put that in your report?
**A.** It is part of my background that I think people would be interested in.
**Q.** MENSA is a high-IQ group only open to people with IQs over 140, correct?
**A.** No, it's 150.
**Q.** You feel you are smarter than your fellow doctors, don't you?
**A.** Well…no…not really.
**Q.** Only 3% of people have IQs over 150, correct?
**A.** Yes, but there are all kinds of intelligence. IQ is just one measurement.
**Q.** Dr. Curran, are you smarter than our judge?
**A.** I have no way of knowing that. Is that important, Counselor?
**Q.** My point exactly, Dr. Curran.

**Comment:** This IME report would have been more defensible had the examiner removed her reference to her membership in MENSA.

**Defending the Report As Written:** An experienced examiner does not permit counsel to ingratiate himself with the judge at the examiner's expense.

**Q.** Dr. Curran, are you smarter than our judge?
**A.** No, Counsel. That's why she is the judge.

**Example 12.72: Piling on: "Plaintiff bears no responsibility"**
*Report States:*

> We therefore conclude that Mr. Mack's injury was work related. He bears no responsibility for the injury he sustained.

*Resulting Cross-examination:*
**Q.** Mr. Mack fell into a five-foot-long trench at a site he was working at for two weeks, correct?
**A.** That's correct.
**Q.** You feel that the experienced laborer bears no responsibility for falling into this five-foot trench?
**A.** No legal responsibility.
**Q.** Are you testifying as a medical expert or a legal expert?
**A.** Medical expert, Counsel.
**Q.** So you are not an expert in legal responsibility in workers' compensation cases, correct?
**A.** Correct.
**Q.** So when you stated he bears no responsibility for the injury he sustained in your IME report, you were mistaken?

**Comment:** The second sentence in this excerpt is superfluous. It can be used to indicate that the examiner is biased and will say anything to help his side win. Superfluous sentences should not be included in IME reports.

**Defending the Report As Written:** Examiners need not be defensive about comments they make in their IME reports as long as they can explain them simply and directly.

**Q.** You feel that the experienced laborer bears no responsibility for falling into this five-foot trench?
**A.** No, I don't. It was covered up and anyone could have fallen into it.

**Example 12.73: Offer to provide medical care**
*Report States:*

> Given the significant relief he had with local injection, I believe it is the most appropriate form of treatment. I can certainly do them in my office.

*Resulting Cross-examination:*
**Q.** Doctor, you performed an independent medical examination and recommended yourself to provide ongoing medical care?
**A.** That's not what I said.
**Q.** You stated in your IME report, "Given the significant relief he had with local injection, I believe it is the most appropriate form of treatment. I can certainly do them in my office," correct?
**A.** That's what I said, but I was just offering to help the examinee so he didn't have to drive a long distance to get the injections.
**Q.** You would give a series of injections, not just one?
**A.** Not necessarily.
**Q.** Didn't you say in your report, "I would start with local anesthetic rather

than steroids and it will require a number of these before the problem has finally resolved"?
**A.** Yes.
**Q.** Would you profit financially from giving a series of injections to the examinee?
**A.** Any profit would be minimal.
**Q.** So, the answer is yes, you would profit?
**A.** Minimally.
**Q.** How much do you charge for each injection and how many will the examinee "need," Doctor?

**Comment:** Examiners, for several reasons, are best served by not recommending that they take over the medical treatment of the examinee.

First, this recommendation taints the impartial and independent nature of the examination. The specter of financial gain will be used to question the examiner during cross-examination.

Secondly, the referral source will most likely not be pleased with an examiner who refers himself to examinees for treatment.

Third, by offering to treat and/or treating the examinee, the examiner may be creating a physician/patient relationship with the attendant legal risk, responsibilities, and liabilities.

Dr. Christopher R. Brigham, a noted IME physician, comments on why treating examinees is not good practice:

> By definition, an independent medical examiner is not to be involved in the care of an examinee either in the past or the future. Involvement with the examinee as a treating physician may compromise the impartial nature of the assessment. Declining this involvement is best. In a very unusual situation you can speak with the client and determine if you should become involved in care. This situation would typically be limited to circumstances where no other alternatives for care exist.[1]

**Defending the Report As Written:** An IME physician who states in his report his availability to treat the examinee should be prepared to answer questions about this offer.

**Q.** Doctor, you performed an independent medical examination and recommended yourself to provide ongoing medical care?
**A.** That's not what I said, Counsel, and you know it. What I said is that the examinee is driving 60 miles one way to therapy, which I think is inappropriate. The injections can be carried out by his family physician or I can certainly do them in my office. I would ask that the fact finder take note of your picking and choosing words from my IME report. That is not a search for justice, sir.

---

[1] Brigham, et al, *The SEAK Comprehensive IME System: Essential Resources for an Efficient and Successful IME Practice* (SEAK, Inc., 1997) 199.

**Example 12.74: Examiner's personal feelings**

*Report States:*

There were some disturbing elements to this case.

*Resulting Cross-examination:*

**Q.** Were you completely objective and non-judgmental when you started working on this case?

**A.** Yes, absolutely.

**Q.** You became "disturbed" when you finished your examination and before you issued your report?

**A.** Well....it was somewhat disturbing.

**Q.** In all honesty, you were not completely objective and non-judgmental once you became disturbed?

**A.** Yes, that's fair.

**Comment:** By including his personal feelings of being disturbed, this examiner can be made to seem as no longer objective.

**Defending the Report As Written:** Examiners do not have to wait for counsel to "spring the trap" on them during their cross-examination. Examiners who can see the trap coming can avoid it by a proactive answer.

**Q.** You became "disturbed" when you finished your examination and before you issued your report?

**A.** As this was your client's seventeenth workers' compensation claim, most doctors would be disturbed as well. Don't you think so, Counsel?

**Example 12.75: Legal advice: Defendant should settle**

*Report States:*

This injury is clearly not work related. The examinee would best be advised to settle.

*Resulting Cross-examination:*

**Q.** You were hired as a medical expert in this case, correct?

**A.** Yes.

**Q.** And you rendered your expert medical opinion?

**A.** Yes.

**Q.** Then you rendered your legal opinion as well?

**A.** I did no such thing, Counselor.

**Q.** When you state in your report, "The examinee would best be advised to settle," is that a medical opinion?

**A.** No, not strictly.

**Q.** In fact, you are commenting on the relative chances of success in the legal action, correct?

**A.** Well....it was just an off-the-cuff, innocent remark.

**Q.** If the examinee followed your advice and settled this case, would you feel responsible for his actions?

**A.** Absolutely not. He would be foolish to rely on my advice. After all, I am not a lawyer.
**Q.** Precisely—just as foolish as you were in offering the advice, correct?

**Comment:** This is advice a lawyer gives, not an IME doctor. Advice regarding settlement has no place in an IME report.

**Defending the Report As Written:** Examiners, when given an opening, can expound on the meaning of what they wrote in their IME reports.

**Q.** When you state in your report, "The examinee would best be advised to settle," is that a medical opinion?
**A.** As the examinee told me, he is contemplating suicide if his four-year workers' compensation ordeal is not over soon. I would say, yes, it is a medical opinion.

**Example 12.76: Snide comment**
*Report States:*

> In the opinion of the undersigned, referring this examinee for chiropractic manipulation was an unfounded and amateurish thing to do.

*Resulting Cross-examination:*
**Q.** You felt that sending the examinee for chiropractic manipulation was a mistake, correct?
**A.** Yes.
**Q.** But that's not what you said in your report, is it?
**A.** I said it was unfounded and amateurish.
**Q.** Would you agree that those are your characterizations of what was done?
**A.** To some degree…yes.
**Q.** Those are not strictly facts, are they?
**A.** No, but I stand behind what I said.
**Q.** Other physicians would characterize this in their own way, wouldn't they?
**A.** Yes.
**Q.** Would they also be amateurish?

**Comment:** Calling a colleague an amateur makes the examiner look opinionated and pompous. This is an unnecessary statement and can be used effectively against the expert.

> In the opinion of the undersigned, referring this examinee for chiropractic manipulation was a violation of the standard of care.

**Example 12.77: Solicitation of future work**
*Report States:*

> Testimony available upon request.

*Resulting Cross-examination:*
**Q.** Doctor, how much do you charge to testify?
**A.** $1,500 for depositions and $2,500 for trial.

**Q.** How much did you charge for this IME?
**A.** $750.
**Q.** Does that include your examination, review of the records, and dictating your IME report?
**A.** Yes, it does.
**Q.** How long did all that take you in this case?
**A.** Approximately three hours.
**Q.** So, testifying after you do an IME is more lucrative than doing the IME itself?
**A.** In many cases, it is.
**Q.** Approximately how many IMEs have you done in your career, Doctor?
**A.** Approximately 2,500.
**Q.** How many times did you issue an unfavorable report for the retaining client and then get asked to testify for the client?
**A.** Not too often.
**Q.** As you sit here today, can you name two cases out of the 2,500 IMEs that you have performed in which this happened?
**A.** No.
**Q.** But when you issue a favorable report for a client, you are frequently called upon to testify, correct?
**A.** Not frequently. Maybe 10%. Most cases settle, Counsel, as you know.
**Q.** So, the only way to get the more remunerative work, testifying at deposition and trial, is by first giving the client a favorable IME report, correct?
**A.** I resent the implication of bias, Counsel.
**Q.** That is why you promote your availability to testify in your IME report, correct?
**A.** I don't promote my availability, Counsel.
**Q.** Your IME report does say, "Testimony available upon request," at the bottom of page 3, does it not?
**A.** Yes.

**Comment:** The examiner is far better served by leaving out phrases that promote or suggest his availability for additional work. As in the above example, the examiner's motives and credibility can be called into question by such self-promotion.

**Defending the Report As Written:** Examiners need not apologize for making themselves available to testify.

**Q.** That is why you promote your availability to testify in your IME report, correct?
**A.** I stated a fact that I am available to testify. It is my legal and ethical duty to make myself available. As you know, many physicians refuse to have anything to do with the legal system. If all physicians followed that practice, you would have no one to cross-examine, Counsel.

**Example 12.78: Settlement will help symptoms**

*Report States:*

Settlement of his claim or suit will result in symptomatic benefit.

*Resulting Cross-examination:*

**Q.** Doctor, you wrote in your IME report that, "Settlement of his claim or suit will result in symptomatic benefit," correct?
**A.** Yes.
**Q.** Of course, if he received a negligible amount for his settlement, he might get worse, isn't that true?
**A.** It's possible.
**Q.** How much would he have to get to have symptomatic benefit?
**A.** I couldn't say.
**Q.** Could you tell us what claims or suits of the examinee are pending?
**A.** I am not sure.
**Q.** How much did he sue for?
**A.** I don't know.
**Q.** What was his legal theory?
**A.** I don't know.
**Q.** What is the status of the suit?
**A.** I don't know.
**Q.** You don't know anything about the suit, its status, theory, amount sued for, or what would be a fair recovery, but you state that "settlement of his claim or suit will result in symptomatic benefit"?

**Comment:** Examiners are in a stronger position to defend their IME reports when they do not recommend that claims be settled or tried in a court of law. Examiners who offer opinions on how a settlement may affect the examinee or his prognosis engage in speculation, which will be difficult to defend during cross-examination.

**Defending the Report As Written:** Examiners who, for whatever reason, comment on the effect of a settlement, still have methods to fend off cross-examination.

**Q.** You don't know anything about the suit, its status, theory, amount sued for, or what would be a fair recovery, but you state that "settlement of his claim or suit will result in symptomatic benefit"?
**A.** First of all, Counsel, you left out the second half of my sentence. What I said in my report was, "Settlement of his claim or suit will result in symptomatic benefit by eliminating the stressors associated with the claim or suit." The examinee expressed considerable anxiety about his claim and expressed his desire on several occasions to put this matter behind him. In my opinion, settlement of his claim will help him reduce the litigation stressors and will result in symptomatic benefits.

# Chapter 13 Red-flag Words to Avoid

## 13.1 Executive Summary

The use of certain words in IME reports will raise red flags with the attorney whose job it is to undermine the examiner, her credibility, and her opinions. Such red-flag words should be avoided. This chapter discusses some of the most common red-flag words found in independent medical examination reports. These include the following terms.

- "Authoritative" to describe a medical text or journal. This term has special legal significance that may allow a cross-examining attorney to question the examiner about everything in the text.
- "Legal" or "legally." What is and is not legal is usually outside of the area of expertise of most examiners.
- "Draft." This term alerts counsel to the existence of draft reports that are usually extremely fertile grounds for cross-examination.
- "Work product," "confidential," or "privileged." These terms make it appear as though the examiner is trying to hide something. These are also legal terms that the examiner may have difficulty defining properly.
- "Probable" and "possible." These ambiguous words should be avoided.
- "Substantially." This is another ambiguous word to avoid.
- "Obviously" and "clearly." These terms can be used to make the expert appear patronizing or presumptuous.
- "Appears," "presumably," "supposedly," "is said," and "evidently." These terms imply uncertainty.
- "He," "she," "it," "they," and other pronouns. Pronouns are uncertain. It is best to use a proper noun.
- Royal "we." This can be used to make the expert look silly, pompous, or even dishonest.
- "It seems," "could," "apparently," "I believe," and other hedge words. It is always best to use confident language.
- "Complete," "thorough," "meticulous," "exhaustive," and other such words to describe the examiner's chart review, research, or examination. These self-serving words will hold the examiner and her report to an extremely high standard.
- "Patient." The person being examined is an "examinee" or "claimant," not a patient. There is no doctor/patient relationship.
- "Malingering." In the majority of cases, it is usually better for the examiner to merely document exaggerated pain behaviors, inconsistencies, non-organic findings, and lack of objective findings rather than making a diagnosis of malingering.

- "Alleged," "credible," and other words that directly or indirectly opine on the credibility of the examinee. The examiner is a medical expert, not a credibility expert.
- "Dictated but not read" and "electronic signature." These practices make the examiner appear to be more interested in cranking out reports and collecting fees than in precision and accuracy.

## 13.2 "Authoritative"

It is a mistake for the examiner to state in her report that a cited medical text or journal article is "authoritative." Doing so may result in allowing the cross-examiner to question the examiner about anything contained in the text in question. It is, therefore, usually best to exercise caution before stating that any reference is "authoritative."

**Example 13.21: "Authoritative" text**
*Report States:*

> This impairment evaluation was performed according to the American Medical Association's *Guides to the Evaluation of Permanent Impairment,* which is an authoritative text in the area of impairment evaluation.

*Resulting Cross-examination:*

**Q.** Doctor, your report indicates that the impairment evaluation was performed according to the AMA *Guides*, correct?
**A.** Yes.
**Q.** You, of course, recognize the AMA *Guides* as an authoritative text?
**A.** Yes.
**Q.** Which edition?
**A.** The 4th edition.
**Q.** The 5th edition is an authoritative text as well?
**A.** Yes.
**Q.** Doctor, could you read the highlighted portion of the first paragraph of page 2 of the 5th edition?
**A.** "The 5th edition includes most of the common conditions...since this edition encompasses the most current criteria and procedures for impairment assessment, it is strongly recommended that physicians use this latest edition, the 5th edition, when rating impairment."
**Q.** You accept this strong recommendation as authoritative, correct?
**A.** Yes.
**Q.** But you did not follow it when performing your impairment evaluation?

**Comment:** When an examiner states in his report that a text or journal is "authoritative," he can expect questions similar to those in this example. It is better practice to exercise caution before admitting a text is authoritative.

> This impairment evaluation was performed according to the American Medical Association's *Guides to the Evaluation of Permanent Impairment,* 4th edition.

**Defending the Report As Written:** Examiners who do not wish to be cross-examined from a text with which they are not familiar can state that they do not consider the text authoritative.

**Q.** The 5$^{th}$ edition is an authoritative text as well?
**A.** I am not familiar with the 5$^{th}$ edition.

***NOTE:*** Counsel will attempt to find alternative ways to use the text to cross-examine the examiner. For example, under the Federal Rules of Evidence, an expert can be cross-examined on the text if its authoritativeness has been established through other witnesses or judicial notice.

## 13.3 "Legal," "Illegal," "Legally," or "Illegally"

Examiners should not state in IME reports what the law is and is not. Most examiners are getting well beyond their true area of expertise when they discuss what is and is not legal in their IME reports. The examiner's role is to assist the trier of fact by drafting an expert medical report. Legalities are best left to the attorneys and judge. Please see Section 4.2 for a further explanation of how commenting on legal matters is usually beyond the examiner's true area of expertise and is likely to cause problems for the examiner.

**Example 13.31: Failure to cooperate would be "illegal"**
*Report States:*

> I advised the examinee that any false statements made to me or failure to cooperate with me would be illegal.

*Resulting Cross-examination:*
**Q.** You threatened the examinee during your IME exam, correct?
**A.** I did not.
**Q.** Did you tell her that if she failed to cooperate with you that would be illegal?
**A.** Yes.
**Q.** That's not a true statement, Doctor, is it?
**A.** Well, I am not a lawyer.
**Q.** Can you point to any law that the examinee would be breaking if she "failed to cooperate"?

**Comment:** This expert would have been better served by removing the red-flag word "illegal" from his report. A good cross-examiner will suspect that most examiners are on very thin ground when legality or illegality is the subject. This expert would have been better off staying away from trying to determine what is legal or illegal.

> I advised the examinee that I was relying on him to provide me with truthful information.

**Defending the Report As Written:** The examiner in the above example may have gone too far in explaining the need to cooperate to the examinee. This does not mean he is unable to defend his report.

**Q.** Did you tell her that if she failed to cooperate with you, that would be illegal?
**A.** Yes, I did. You are, however, taking my statement out of context. What I said was, "I advised the examinee that any false statements made to me or failure to cooperate with me would be illegal." If she makes false or misleading material misrepresentations, that could constitute insurance fraud and is certainly illegal. Failure to cooperate could result in her loss of her workers' compensation benefits on a permanent basis. In fact, she did cooperate, which is what I assume you advise your clients to do. Am I correct in that assumption, Counsel?

## 13.4 "Draft"

Opposing counsel will immediately be alerted by the use of the term "draft" in an IME report. The use of this term raises numerous questions. Were there any changes made subsequent to the issuance of the draft report? Why were these changes made? Did counsel, the adjuster, or the broker have any improper influence on any changes made? Did the examiner run his initial opinion by counsel to make sure it was helpful and what he was looking for? It is best to avoid these types of questions by not using the term "draft" in an IME report.

**Example 13.41: Draft - 8/1/2003**
*Report States:*
Draft - 8/1/2003

*Resulting Cross-examination:*
**Q.** This is your 8/1/2003 draft IME report, correct?
**A.** Yes.
**Q.** This is not the first draft of the report, correct?
**A.** Yes, that's true.
**Q.** How many prior drafts were there?
**A.** Three.
**Q.** After you did each draft you sent them to Attorney Rodgers, correct?
**A.** Yes.
**Q.** You then discussed them with her?
**A.** Yes.
**Q.** You made changes after those discussions?
**A.** Yes.
**Q.** Were any of these changes ones that Attorney Rodgers did *not* ask you to make?
**A.** No.
**Q.** Did she put her suggested changes in writing?
**A.** No.
**Q.** Ever ask why not?

**A.** No.
**Q.** Did you correct typos at her suggestions?
**A.** Yes.
**Q.** Did you add sections that were missing?
**A.** Yes.
**Q.** Did you take out sections that were not supposed to be in there?
**A.** Not that I can remember.
**Q.** Well, let's take a look at them. Could you show me drafts one, two and three? The ones that were done before Attorney Rodgers reviewed them?
**A.** They are not available.
**Q.** Where are they?
**A.** I destroyed them as a regular course of business.
**Q.** Did you discuss this with Attorney Rodgers before you destroyed them?
**A.** Yes.
**Q.** Are they still on your computer hard drive?

**Comment:** Draft reports should not be issued to an examiner's referral source. As the above example demonstrates, a draft report is an invitation for trouble.

**Defending the Report As Written:** Examiners who write draft reports can expect to be questioned as in the above example. When questioned about the changes made, examiners who are prepared can answer firmly and directly.

**Q.** You made changes after those discussions?
**A.** Yes, I did, but there were no substantive changes. Here are my three draft reports. Would you like to make them part of the record, Counsel?

## 13.5 "Work Product," "Confidential," or "Privileged"

Independent medical examiners sometimes attempt to protect the confidentiality of their reports by including a clearly written notice that the document is subject to attorney-client, work product, or doctor-patient privilege. Many times such statements are boilerplate language contained in part of a standard transmittal form. Unfortunately, such a notice is not likely to have much effect on whether the IME report will be protected from discovery. Worse, such a notice can be used against the examiner to make it appear as though the examiner has something to hide or to show that the examiner is drawing legal conclusions that he is not qualified to make.

**Example 13.51: Work product**
*Report States:*
CONFIDENTIAL: ATTORNEY WORK PRODUCT

*Resulting Cross-examination:*
**Q.** Your report is stamped, "Confidential: Attorney Work Product"?
**A.** Yes.
**Q.** You are a testifying expert in this case?
**A.** Obviously.
**Q.** This is despite the fact that the court has ordered your work produced and

discoverable?
**A.** I am not a lawyer, sir.
**Q.** But you attempted to hide your report by stamping it, "Confidential: Attorney Work Product"?
**A.** I did what I was told to by counsel.
**Q.** Did you also follow counsel's instructions when forming your independent conclusions and opinions?

**Comment:** Writing "confidential" on an IME report will give the reader the impression that one has something to hide. It will have little, if any, effect on whether the report will ultimately be discoverable. It is, therefore, best to avoid labeling expert reports as "confidential," "privileged," or "work product."

**Defending the Report As Written:** Examiners need not sit idly by when counsel is trying to paint a sinister conspiracy on cross-examination.

**Q.** But you attempted to hide your report by stamping it, "Confidential: Attorney Work Product"?
**A.** There was obviously no attempt to hide this report, which went out to multiple parties. It was stamped confidential so that my office staff would exercise caution before sending it out to persons who were not supposed to receive it.

## 13.6 "Probable" and "Possible"

The words "probable" and "possible" are ambiguous and should be avoided. The examiner would be better served by more precise language.

**Example 13.61: "Probable"**
*Report States:*

> It is probable that his current complaints were not caused by the alleged 3/6/2003 workplace injury.

*Resulting Cross-examination:*
**Q.** Your report indicates that it is "probable" that his injuries were not caused by the alleged 3/6/2003 workplace injury, correct?
**A.** Yes.
**Q.** When you say "probable," you are not 100% certain, correct?
**A.** Yes, 51% or more sure.
**Q.** So, there is a 49% chance you are wrong?

**Comment:** This report would have been more persuasive and less vulnerable to attack had the examiner used more precise language.

> It is my opinion, based upon a reasonable degree of medical certainty, that his current complaints were not caused by the alleged 3/6/2003 workplace injury.

**Defending the Report As Written:** Examiners are best served by not getting sucked into the "numbers game" on cross-examination.

**Q.** When you say "probable," you are not 100% certain, correct?
**A.** I meant more likely than not, Counsel.

**Example 13.62: "Possible"**
*Report States:*

> The purpose of our evaluation was to opine as to the extent and possible cause of the examinee's current complaints.

*Resulting Cross-examination:*
**Q.** You opined in your report about the "possible" cause of the examinee's current complaints, correct?
**A.** Yes.
**Q.** Are you aware that the term "possible" in law means less than 51% and is legally insufficient for an opinion?

**Comment:** The word "possible" should be avoided.

> The purpose of our investigation was to opine as to the extent and cause of the examinee's current complaints.

**Defending the Report As Written:** When faced with a vague phrase in a report, the examiner can, during cross-examination, explain what he really meant.

**Q.** Are you aware that the term "possible" in law means less than 51% and is legally insufficient for an opinion?
**A.** Yes, I am. That is why, although the purpose of the exam was to opine on the possible cause, once I formed my opinion, it was to a reasonable degree of medical certainty.

**Example 13.63: "Possible"**
*Report States:*

> It is possible that the examinee's carpal tunnel syndrome, left wrist, is related to her employment as an accounting clerk.

*Resulting Cross-examination:*
**Q.** You stated that it is possible that the examinee's carpal tunnel syndrome is related to her employment?
**A.** That's correct.
**Q.** You can't say that to a reasonable degree of medical certainty, correct?
**A.** That's correct.
**Q.** Thank you, Doctor.

**Comment:** IME reports that use the term "possible" on causation issues are likely to be found to be legally insufficient. The commonly accepted phrases that are legally sufficient are:

- "based upon a reasonable degree of medical certainty,"
- "based upon a reasonable degree of medical probability," and

- "more likely than not."

For more information on degree of certainty, please see Section 10.2.

**Defending the Report As Written:** Even when a report is legally insufficient as written, the examiner can still leave the door open for further evidence.

**Q.** You can't say that to a reasonable degree of medical certainty, correct?
**A.** Not at this time. However, after the proposed surgery, I will review the operative notes and the findings of the surgeon and give you a more definitive opinion, Counselor.

## 13.7 "Substantially"

"Substantially" is an ambiguous word that examiners should avoid. More precise, and therefore more persuasive, language should be used.

**Example 13.71: "Substantially"**
*Report States:*

> It is probable that his current complaints can be substantially lessened through a course of physical therapy.

*Resulting Cross-examination:*
**Q.** How would you describe "substantially lessened" in a percentage form?
**A.** I am not sure.
**Q.** "Substantially" is not a medical term?
**A.** That's correct.
**Q.** Would it be more than 1%?
**A.** Yes.
**Q.** More than 2%?
**A.** Yes.
**Q.** More than 10%?
**A.** Yes.
**Q.** More than 50%?
**A.** Probably.
**Q.** Your opinion is more like an educated guess than a scientific, precise opinion, correct?

**Comment:** This report would have been more persuasive and less vulnerable to attack had the expert used more precise language.

> It is my opinion, based upon a reasonable degree of medical certainty, that his injuries can been lessened to a degree whereby he would likely have had no permanent impairment if the examinee were to undergo a course of physical therapy.

**Defending the Report As Written:** Examiners should not let cross-examining counsel drag them into a "numbers game."

**Q.** How would you describe "substantially lessened" in a percentage form?
**A.** I would not use percentages. When the claimant regains function and can resume his activities of daily living, his complaints would be substantially lessened.

## 13.8 "Obvious" and "Clearly"

The terms "obvious" and "clearly" are red flags for attorneys. An experienced cross-examiner can use the examiner's use of these terms to make the examiner appear patronizing and presumptuous. Accordingly, these terms should be avoided.

**Example 13.81: "Obvious" what prevented return to work**
*Report States:*

> It is obvious that this patient's severe cardiac status coupled with his myocardial infarction and open-heart surgery are the major factors in prohibiting his return to work and his ongoing problems.

*Resulting Cross-examination:*
**Q.** You say it is "obvious" that the patient's severe cardiac status and his MI and open-heart surgery prohibit his return to work, correct?
**A.** Yes.
**Q.** Dr. Arthur does not think that is obvious. As a matter of fact, he disagrees with your conclusion, doesn't he?
**A.** Yes, but he is wrong.
**Q.** Just like Dr. Cooper?
**A.** Yes.
**Q.** And Dr. Ralley?
**A.** Yes.
**Q.** And Dr. Kaline?
**A.** Yes.
**Q.** And the Social Security Administration, which concluded he could return to work?
**A.** Yes.
**Q.** It appears that the only physician who examined this patient and reached the conclusion he was disabled was you, correct?
**A.** Yes.
**Q.** Yet, in the face of all of this conflicting medical opinion, you stated he was "obviously" disabled?
**A.** It was obvious to me.
**Q.** Exactly, "obvious" to you and only you, correct?

**Comment:** A better way to present this opinion avoids the use of the term "obvious."

> It is my opinion, based upon a reasonable degree of medical certainty, that this examinee's severe cardiac status coupled with his myocardial infarction and open-heart surgery are the major factors in prohibiting his return to work and his ongoing problems.

**Defending the Report As Written:** Examiners who actively listen to counsel's questions are in the best position to defend their opinions and reports during cross-examination.

**Q.** You say it is "obvious" that the patient's severe cardiac status and his MI and open-heart surgery prohibit his return to work, correct?
**A.** No, Counsel. If you look at my report, I said it was "obvious…they are the major factors in prohibiting his return to work and his ongoing problems." This is an important distinction. Would you like me to explain?

**Example 13.82: "Clearly"**
*Report States:*

…[this] clearly reveals the presence of multiple chemical sensitivity.

*Resulting Cross-examination:*
**Q.** What is the difference between "reveals" and "clearly reveals" in terms of medical certainty?
**A.** There is no difference, Counselor, it's just an expression.
**Q.** So, this is your attempt to bolster your opinion and impress the jury without the benefit of any additional scientific evidence?

**Comment:** This report would have been more effective had the expert not "piled on" with the inclusion of the word "clearly." Deleting the word "clearly" makes this report seem more objective, less biased, and more credible.

…[this] reveals the presence of multiple chemical sensitivity.

**Defending the Report As Written:** Examiners do not have to let counsel parse each of their words in an attempt to create confusion.

**Q.** So, this is your attempt to bolster your opinion and impress the jury without the benefit of any additional scientific evidence?
**A.** No, it is my attempt to write clear and simple English, something you lawyers can neither seem to accomplish nor accept.

**Example 13.83: "Obviously"**
*Report States:*

Obviously, this examinee is capable of carrying out her previous job.

*Resulting Cross-examination:*
**Q.** Your report states that "Obviously, this examinee is capable of carrying out her previous job," correct?
**A.** Yes, it does.
**Q.** When did this become obvious to you?
**A.** As soon as I reviewed the medical records.
**Q.** That was before you actually examined Mr. Grace?
**A.** Yes, but the exam confirmed it.
**Q.** You used the word "obviously" to emphasize this fact for the Judge?
**A.** In part, yes.

**Q.** Was that because you felt he would not understand the issue or because he might overlook it?

**Comment:** This examiner's use of emphasis makes his report look less objective and, therefore, less credible. This examiner would have been better served by avoiding the use of emphatic language.

**Defending the Report As Written:** Sometimes examiners use the word "obviously" because it is exactly what they mean.

**Q.** When did this become obvious to you?
**A.** When I saw that the examinee returned to her prior job without any problems.

## 13.9 "Appears"

The word "appears" implies to the reader that the writer is unsure of the facts. This uncertainty will lessen the persuasive value of the IME report. More confident language should be used.

**Example 13.91: "It appears that"**
*Report States:*

> It appears that Mr. Hall's problems, particularly with his upper and lower back, are related to a chronic weakness of the musculature coupled with what appears to be some sort of fibromyalgia syndrome.

*Resulting Cross-examination:*
**Q.** Are you sure that Mr. Hall's symptoms are coupled with fibromyalgia syndrome?
**A.** Yes.
**Q.** But when you say it "appears" that they are, you are indicating less than 100% certainty?
**A.** Yes.
**Q.** How much less?
**A.** That's hard to say.
**Q.** Here you use the term "appears" twice when stating your diagnosis.
**A.** Yes.
**Q.** That would indicate even less certainty, correct?
**A.** Yes.
**Q.** How much less certainty?
**A.** That's hard to say.
**Q.** Apparently so.

**Comment:** This examiner should have used more confident language.

> It is my opinion, based upon a reasonable degree of medical certainty, that Mr. Hall's problems, particularly with his upper and lower back, are related to a chronic weakness of the musculature coupled with fibromyalgia syndrome.

**Defending the Report As Written:** Examiners should not feel obligated to assist cross-examining counsel by agreeing to all of their characterizations and questions.

**Q.** But when you say it "appears" that they are, you are indicating less than 100% certainty?
**A.** No, that's just a figure of speech with no hidden meanings, Counsel.

## 13.10 "Presumably"

To presume is to assume. Invalid assumptions can call an examiner's opinions into question. Whenever possible, examiners should avoid making presumptions. Instead, their reports should be based upon facts.

**Example 13.101: "Presumably"**
*Report States:*

Presumably, the examinee did sustain an injury to her lumbar spine on April 14, 2002.

*Resulting Cross-examination:*
**Q.** When you say "presumably" in your IME report, you are assuming this to be correct?
**A.** Yes.
**Q.** You did base your opinion in part on this assumption?
**A.** Yes, I did.
**Q.** If this assumption was incorrect, you would want to rethink your opinion, correct?
**A.** I would consider it.
**Q.** Here is a hospital record that indicates that the examinee actually hurt her back on March 4, 2002, while lifting a lawnmower. Will you change your opinion now?

**Comment:** This report would be more persuasive if it were based upon facts and not presumptions.

**Defending the Report As Written:** When an examiner chooses an incorrect word or phrase in his IME report, he should admit his mistake, correct it, and force counsel to move on.

**Q.** When you say "presumably" in your IME report, you are assuming this to be correct?
**A.** I misspoke. The sentence in the report should read, "In my opinion, based upon a reasonable degree of medical certainty, the examinee did sustain an injury to her lumbar spine on April 14, 2002."

## 13.11 "Evidently"

"Evidently" is another commonly used term that implies uncertainty. The examiner's opinion will be more persuasive if the language in the IME report does not imply uncertainty.

**Example 13.111: "Evidently"**
*Report States:*

Evidently, x-rays of the entire spine were eventually taken and these are reported as being negative.

*Resulting Cross-examination:*
**Q.** You would agree that either the x-rays of the entire spine were taken or they were not?
**A.** Yes.
**Q.** If they were not taken, could they be negative?
**A.** No.
**Q.** So when you say "evidently" they were taken and were negative, what do you mean?
**A.** I was not there, Counselor. I am just repeating what I was told by the patient.
**Q.** The patient is not a medical doctor?
**A.** Correct.
**Q.** He may be confused or mistaken about what some x-ray technician told him three years ago?
**A.** Yes.
**Q.** You cannot testify under oath here today that the x-rays of the entire spine were taken and they were, in fact, negative, can you?
**A.** Evidently not.

**Comment:** More certain language would have been more persuasive.

X-rays of the entire spine were taken on June 6th, 2003. These x-rays were negative.

**Defending the Report As Written:** Examiners should carefully listen to each and every question counsel poses to them. Frequently, counsel will try to "sell" a question with his tone and inflection. Examiners need not fall for this tactic.

**Q.** He may be confused or mistaken about what some x-ray technician told him three years ago?
**A.** I doubt it. Your client is an intelligent professional with an excellent memory.

## 13.12 "Supposedly"

Examiners often use the term "supposedly." This is yet another term that implies uncertainty and should, therefore, be avoided.

**Example 13.121: "Supposedly"**
*Report States:*

Supposedly, the examinee received epidural steroids for her lower back.

*Resulting Cross-examination:*
**Q.** Someone told you that the examinee received epidural steroids for her lower back, correct?

**A.** That's correct.
**Q.** Are you sure about that, Doctor?
**A.** I am sure someone told me.
**Q.** Who told you that?
**A.** It's unclear in my notes—most likely, the examinee.
**Q.** But you can't be sure?
**A.** I cannot.
**Q.** If you can't be sure how you obtained this information, you certainly can't be sure whether the examinee was actually given the steroids, is that fair?
**A.** That's fair.
**Q.** All you really know for sure is that someone at some point in time mentioned that the examinee may have received steroids, correct?

**Comment:** This would have been better written and more persuasive had the examiner not used the uncertain language. Instead, the expert should have provided a source for the reported information.

> The examinee informed me that she had received epidural steroids for her lower back.

**Defending the Report As Written:** When an IME examiner has an independent recollection of a fact, he may use that recollection to bolster his IME report.

**Q.** Who told you that?
**A.** Because the only person I talked to about this case is the examinee, the examinee told me that, Counsel.

## 13.13 "Is said"

The term "is said" also implies uncertainty. The use of this term makes it appear as though the examiner obtained the crucial facts upon which he based his opinion from hearsay and rumor. This will negatively affect the persuasive value of the IME report. The term "is said" should, therefore, be avoided. Instead, the specific source of information upon which the opinion is based should be stated explicitly in the IME report.

**Example 13.131: "Is said"**
*Report States:*

> It is said that rear-end collisions do not normally result in serious back injuries.

*Resulting Cross-examination:*
**Q.** You stated in your IME report that "It is said that rear-end collisions do not normally result in serious back injuries," correct?
**A.** That's correct.
**Q.** You based your opinion on causation in part on this principle?
**A.** Yes, I did.
**Q.** Can you tell me, Doctor, who exactly said that about rear-end collisions?

**A.** It is common knowledge.
**Q.** Do you have a name you could share with us?
**A.** No, I don't.
**Q.** Can you tell us where the scientific studies were conducted?
**A.** Not off the top of my head.
**Q.** When were these studies done?
**A.** I don't know.
**Q.** So, when you said in your report, "It is said," you meant someone said something, somewhere, at some point in time?

**Comment:** "It is said" should not have been included in this report. The source of the examiner's belief should have been spelled out explicitly. The same reasoning applies to comments such as "it is thought that."

**Defending the Report As Written:** Examiners who use general phrases like "it is said," need to be able to back them up during cross-examination.

**Q.** Can you tell us, Doctor, who exactly said that about rear-end collisions?
**A.** Yes, it was Doctor Janet Savage writing in the January 2002 issue of *For the Defense*. In that article she explains that when a person is struck from the side, their sacroiliac joints are stressed considerably more than when pushed from the back. Even more importantly, the lower spine is not supported on the sides as it is in the back and therefore can move more easily when the patient is struck from the side. Conversely, in a rear-end collision, the dorsolumbar and lumbosacral spine is well supported posteriorly by the seat back and anteriorly by the seat belt and by the driver's hands on the steering wheel. Therefore, no abnormal motion occurs in the lower spine as long as the seat in which the driver is sitting does not break or the steering column collapse.

## 13.14 "He," "She," "It," "They," and Other Pronouns

The use of pronouns should be avoided. Pronouns make IME reports less explicit and can generate unnecessary confusion. It is better practice to identify all nouns explicitly.

### Example 13.141: "She"

*Report States:*

> Ms. Paulson had shortness of breath at the scene and when her supervisor, Lori, got to the scene, the situation had worsened and she had to be transported to the emergency room with a suspected myocardial infarction.

*Resulting Cross-examination:*

**Q.** Your report indicates on page 3, last paragraph, "Ms. Paulson had shortness of breath at the scene and when her supervisor, Lori, got to the scene, the situation had worsened and she had to be transported to the emergency room with a suspected myocardial infarction." Is that correct?
**A.** Yes.
**Q.** Was it Ms. Paulson that was suspected of having a myocardial infarction?
**A.** No, it was her supervisor, Lori.
**Q.** So, when you say, "she had to be transported...," you were referring to Ms.

Paulson or her supervisor?
**A.** Sorry for the ambiguity. It was Lori, her supervisor.

**Comment:** Who is "she"? Where, like here, there is more than one woman discussed in the report, it is not clear to whom "she" refers. Clarity makes an IME report more valuable and reflects positively on the examiner's credibility. The pronoun in this example should have been replaced with the actual name of the woman in question.

> Ms. Paulson had shortness of breath at the scene and when her supervisor, Lori, got to the scene, the situation had worsened and Lori had to be transported to the emergency room with a suspected myocardial infarction.

**Defending the Report As Written:** Examiners are normally best served by answering even inane and sarcastic questions simply and directly. On the other hand, examiners can, on limited occasions, give as good as they get.

**Q.** So, when you say, "she had to be transported…," you were referring to Ms. Paulson or her supervisor?
**A.** They transported Lori, Counsel, the person who was suspected of having the MI. That's not too hard to follow, is it?

**Example 13.142: "It"**
*Report States:*

> The accident occurred on August 3, 2003. There was water in the bottom of the trench. The soil was silt, sand, and clay. It was dry.

*Resulting Cross-examination:*
**Q.** Page 2 of your report states, "There was water in the bottom of the trench. The soil was silt, sand, and clay. It was dry." Am I reading that correctly?
**A.** Yes, sir.
**Q.** There was water in the bottom of the trench?
**A.** Yes.
**Q.** And "it" was dry?
**A.** Yes.
**Q.** Now please forgive me as I'm not a scientist like you, but could you please explain how soil under water is dry?
**A.** It isn't. What I was referring to was the other soil in the trench, not the soil on the bottom.
**Q.** You didn't say that though, did you? What you said was "it" was dry?
**A.** Yes, but it was implied.
**Q.** Did you intentionally not specify which soil you were referring to?
**A.** That's just the way I wrote it.
**Q.** Was it your intent to confuse people or were you just sloppy?
**A.** That's just the way I wrote it.
**Q.** Did you care whether or not anyone was confused?
**A.** I never really gave it any thought.

**Comment:** The use of the pronoun "it" in this example made the examiner's report less precise. The report would have been much better if the examiner had avoided the use of the pronoun and drafted his report with more precise language.

> The accident occurred on August 3, 2003. There was water in the bottom of the trench. The soil on the sides of the trench consisted of silt, sand, and clay. The soil on the sides of the trench was dry.

**Defending the Report As Written:** When being badgered by counsel, examiners can fight back when appropriate.

**Q.** Was it your intent to confuse people or were you just sloppy?
**A.** Confusing people is usually counsel's job and you seem particularly adept at it.

## 13.15 Royal "We"

Some examiners use the word "we" when describing an IME that only they were involved in. This is known as the royal "we" and it should be avoided. The royal "we" is not commonly used and use of it can make the examiner seem silly, pompous, or even dishonest. Unless more than one person was involved in forming the opinion, IME reports should be written in the first-person singular. For further information and examples of why IME reports should be written in the first-person singular, please see Section 11.11.

**Example 13.151: Royal "we" for a one-person firm**
*Report States:*

> After conducting our examination, we came to the conclusion that the examinee's injury was not work related.

*Resulting Cross-examination:*
**Q.** Paragraph 2 of the report you signed indicates on the final page, under the conclusion, "After conducting our examination, we came to the conclusion that the examinee's injury was not work related." Is that correct?
**A.** Yes.
**Q.** What is the name of your IME company, Dr. Evans?
**A.** Evans & Associates.
**Q.** How many associates performed this IME with you?
**A.** None.
**Q.** So, when you used the term "we," is that a misstatement or the royal "we"?
**A.** I used the term "we" because it was a firm report of Evans & Associates.
**Q.** How many associates did you consult with in forming your conclusion?
**A.** None...It was just me.
**Q.** How many full-time associates are there in your firm?
**A.** None. We have part-timers.
**Q.** How many part-time employee associates are there in your firm?
**A.** Well...see...we call them in as consultants and contractors when needed.
**Q.** Did you say "we" call them in?

**A.** I…I call them in.
**Q.** Would it be fair to say, Dr. Evans, that "Evans & Associates" is essentially a one-man show?
**A.** Yes.

**Comment:** Counsel was very effective here in making the examiner look dishonest by his use of the word "we." This report should have been written with the word "I."

> Based on a reasonable degree of medical certainty, I concluded that the examinee's injury was not work related.

**Defending the Report As Written:** Examiners should not just agree with counsel in an attempt to get the deposition over or to get the attorney to move on.

**Q.** Would it be fair to say, Dr. Evans, that "Evans & Associates" is essentially a one-man show?
**A.** No. I have a full-time staff of four. Nancy, my receptionist; Pat my nurse/assistant; Jim, my scheduling clerk; and Kathy, my administrative assistant. They are the backbone of the operation.

**Example 13.152: "It was our information"**
*Report States:*

> It was our information that Mr. Thomas was employed by ABC Builders and was working as a laborer in the construction of a home.

**Comment:** If only one person worked on this report it is far better to say:

> The information available to me indicates that Mr. Thomas was employed by ABC Builders and was working as a laborer in the construction of a home.

**Example 13.153: "We"**
*Report States:*

> We conducted a detailed physical examination.

**Comment:** Avoid the royal "we."

> I conducted a detailed physical examination.

## 13.16 "It Seems," "Could," "Apparently," "I believe," and Other Hedge Words

Please see Section 11.12 on using confident language and avoiding hedge words.

## 13.17 "Complete," "Thorough," "Meticulous," "Exhaustive," and Other Such Words

Words such as "complete," "thorough," "meticulous," and "exhaustive" when used to describe the examiner's chart review, physical examination, research, or analysis can be extremely problematic. One problem is that the examiner holds himself up to a very high standard when he uses these terms. Because these words are usually self-serving and generally do not make the report more persuasive, they should be avoided. Please see Section 11.14 on avoiding subjective characterizations of the examiner's work.

**Example 13.171: "Complete and thorough"**
*Report States:*

> The following opinion is based upon a complete and thorough examination of the medical records submitted to me for this purpose.

*Resulting Cross-examination:*
**Q.** You do two kinds of medical record reviews in connection with your IMEs, an incomplete and hasty one and a complete and thorough one, correct?
**A.** No.
**Q.** All of your medical record reviews are complete and thorough, correct?
**A.** Yes.
**Q.** You get paid by the hour?
**A.** Correct.
**Q.** So, the more complete and thorough, the more you get paid?
**A.** I get paid for the time I spend.
**Q.** The more time you spend, the more you get paid?
**A.** Yes.
**Q.** Are you certain that your medical record review was 100% complete and thorough?
**A.** Yes, I stated that already.
**Q.** Did you review the physical therapy reports from FeelBetter Rehab?
**A.** I can't recall.
**Q.** Did you review the December 21, 2002 MRI?
**A.** I reviewed the radiologist's report.
**Q.** As part of your complete and thorough review of the medical records, did you review the actual MRI film?
**A.** No.

**Comment:** Self-serving descriptions of an exam or a record review, such as "complete and thorough," add nothing to the persuasiveness of an IME report. Instead, the descriptions open up the examiner to additional cross-examination. Such words should be avoided.

> The following opinion is based upon an examination of the medical records submitted to me for this purpose.

**Defending the Report As Written:** Experienced examiners are not reluctant to occasionally give as good as they get. Examiners should *not* overdo this because it could make them appear biased.

**Q.** The more time you spend, the more you get paid?
**A.** Yes, just like you, Counsel.

## 13.18 "Patient"

An independent medical examiner is not a medical treater. There is no doctor/patient relationship in an IME. As such, the examiner should refer to the person being examined as the "examinee" or "claimant" and not the "patient."

**Example 13.181: "The patient"**
*Report States:*

> The patient asked to return to playing golf and doing push-ups. The patient was told that this would be appropriate.

*Resulting Cross-examination:*
**Q.** Doctor, when did you assume the medical care of Mr. Paul?
**A.** I didn't, Counsel. He was just seen for an independent medical examination.
**Q.** He was a patient, was he not?
**A.** No. I already told you he was just seen for an IME.
**Q.** Would you look at your IME report and count the number of times you refer to Mr. Paul as "the patient"?
**A.** Well, 13 times actually.
**Q.** Are you now saying that Mr. Paul, who you refer to as "the patient" 13 times in your report, was not a patient?
**A.** That's correct.
**Q.** He asked you for medical advice and you gave the person you refer to as "the patient" the advice, did you not?
**A.** Absolutely not.
**Q.** He asked you if he could resume playing golf and doing push-ups and you told him and I quote from page 2 of your IME report, "This would be appropriate." Correct?
**A.** Well, yes, but,...but,...I didn't see the harm in just answering the one question.
**Q.** Are you aware that he ruptured a disc in his back doing push-ups the day after you saw him?
**A.** No. He was just here for...I was just supposed to do an IME.
**Q.** Exactly.

**Comment:** Examiners performing IMEs should refer to the person examined as an "examinee" or "claimant," not as "a patient" or "the patient." Experienced examiners go to great lengths (verbal and written explanations) to make it clear to the examinee that he is *not* their patient and that no patient/physician relationship is established. Likewise, the examinee is told orally and in writing that the examiner will not provide medical advice or treatment to the examinee.

All of the explanations, releases, and other risk reduction behavior will not help the examiner who renders advice and then goes a step further and memorializes the advice in his written IME report. The examiner would have been better served by documenting the fact that he did not render medical advice.

> The examinee asked to return to playing golf and doing push-ups. He was advised by me to consult with his physician before he undertook this activity. He was reminded by me again that there is no physician/patient relationship and I will not provide medical advice or treatment. The examinee said he understood.

**Defending the Report As Written:** Using the word "patient" in an IME report need not be a devastating error if the examiner keeps his wits about him.

**Q.** Are you now saying that Mr. Paul, whom you refer to as "the patient" 13 times in your report, was not a patient?
**A.** Counsel, you are confusing the issue unintentionally or intentionally. I never refer to Mr. Paul as "my patient," just "the patient" when he saw the seven physicians for treatment. I am not saying he is not "a patient," just not "my patient."

**Example 13.182: "Patient/examinee"**
*Report States:*

> I appreciate the opportunity of seeing this patient for an independent medical examination.

*Resulting Cross-examination:*
**Q.** Doctor, was Mr. Kliner on whom you performed your IME exam, your patient?
**A.** He was examined.
**Q.** Did you intend to create a treating physician/patient relationship?
**A.** Absolutely not.
**Q.** When did you dictate your IME report?
**A.** Immediately after the examination and in front of Mr. Kliner so he could correct any mistakes in the history.
**Q.** When you dictated, "I appreciate the opportunity of seeing this patient for an independent medical examination," in front of Mr. Kliner, could that have created confusion in his mind about him being a patient and you being his doctor?
**A.** It could have.
**Q.** Was that a mistake that you would not want to repeat?
**A.** Yes.
**Q.** But you did repeat it three more times in the first page of the report you dictated in front of Mr. Kliner, correct?

**Comment:** The examiner should make it clear to the examinee (directly and in his report) that there is no physician/patient relationship.

> The independent medical examination process was explained to the examinee and he understands that no patient/treating physician relationship was established.

**Defending the Report As Written:** When the examiner makes a mistake, as in the above example, he should admit it simply and directly and force opposing counsel to move on.

**Q.** Doctor, was Mr. Kliner, on whom you performed your IME exam, your patient?
**A.** No. I mistakenly used the word "patient" when I should have properly said "examinee" throughout paragraph one of my report.

## 13.19 "Malingering"

"Malingering" is a red-flag word for opposing counsel. Examiners should take great care in its use. In the majority of cases it is usually better for the examiner to merely document exaggerated pain behaviors, inconsistencies, non-organic findings, and lack of objective findings, rather than making a diagnosis of malingering. Where the term is used, examiners need to be able to defend its use under the DSM-IV definition of malingering. For more information on documenting symptom magnification, nonorganic findings, and lack of objective findings, please see Section 10.16.

**Example 13.191: Malingering**
*Report States:*

> Mr. Bowler's behavior and presentation are consistent with malingering.

*Resulting Cross-examination:*
**Q.** Your IME report states that Mr. Bowler's presentation is consistent with malingering, correct?
**A.** Yes, that's correct.
**Q.** Why do you say he was malingering?
**A.** Well, he didn't try to return to work and it's my impression that he is just milking the system, Counselor.
**Q.** You are aware that malingering is a disorder defined in DSM-IV, correct?
**A.** Yes.
**Q.** What is that definition, Doctor?
**A.** I can't cite chapter and verse, Counselor.
**Q.** Can you tell us the essential feature of malingering?
**A.** No.
**Q.** What about the four diagnostic criteria?
**A.** Not off the top of my head.
**Q.** You are willing to swear under oath and accuse the examinee of malingering even though you can't even tell us what it is?

**Comment:** IME examiners should be very cautious in labeling an examinee as a malingerer.

> Malingering is not a clear-cut, easy to prove accusation…With the above in mind, the IME physician should not overreach the facts when drawing his or her conclusions. Statements that an examinee is malingering are very hard to prove conclusively for the reasons noted in this chapter. If an examinee displays positive Waddell's findings and other inconsistencies, it is best to note these observations without assuming the role of judge and jury. The physician can couch such observations in the IME report in several ways:
> (1) The examinee displays nonorganic findings.
> (2) Viewing this examinee superficially would lead to the impression that his or her impairment is greater than that listed above; however, nonorganic findings lead me to believe that the above noted opinions are correct.
> (3) The examinee's subjective complaints outweigh his or her objective findings; in fact, the objective findings are questionable because of their nonorganic nature.
> (4) This examinee has mostly functional, rather than structural, findings on examination.
>
> Making and defending an accusation of malingering is as difficult today as it was a century and a half ago when Alexis de Tocqueville wrote, "Nothing is so difficult to distinguish as the nuances which separate unmerited misfortune from an adversity produced vice….What profound knowledge must be presumed about the character of each man and of the circumstances in which he has lived, what knowledge, what sharp discernment, what cold inexorable reason!"[1]

Mr. Bowler's behavior and presentation are consistent with symptom magnification.

**Defending the Report As Written:** Only physicians who know and understand the term "malingering" should even consider using it in an IME report.

**Q.** Why do you say he was malingering?

**A.** Let me refer to my copy of DSM-IV, Counsel.

"The essential feature of Malingering is the intentional production of false or grossly exaggerated physical or psychological symptoms, motivated by external incentives such as avoiding military duty, avoiding work, obtaining financial compensation, evading criminal prosecution, or obtaining drugs. Under some circumstances, Malingering may represent adaptive behavior - for example, feigning illness while a captive of the enemy during wartime.

Malingering should be strongly suspected if any combination of the following is noted:

1. Medicolegal context of presentation (e.g., the person is referred by an attorney to the clinician for examination)
2. Marked discrepancy between the person's claimed stress or disability and the objective findings
3. Lack of cooperation during the diagnostic evaluation and in complying with the prescribed treatment regimen
4. The presence of Antisocial Personality Disorder."

In this case, the examinee had an absence of objective signs of neurologic impairment, no objective signs of musculoskeletal impairment, had pain behavior, and nonphysiologic findings on examination. Would you like me to explain further, Counsel?

---

[1] Thomas G. Grace, MD, ed., *Independent Medical Evaluations* (American Academy of Orthopedic Surgeons, 2001) pp. 77-78.

## 13.20 "Alleged" and "Credible"

The examiner should be careful to avoid using words that directly or indirectly opine on the credibility of the examinee. Examiners are medical experts and not credibility experts. Commenting on the credibility of the examinee is most likely outside of the examiner's true area of expertise and can be used to show the bias of the examiner. For more information on the dangers of opining on the credibility of the examinee or others, please see Section 11.17.

**Example 13.201: "Allegedly"**

*Report States:*

> The examinee allegedly was injured on March 4, 2003, in an accident at work.

*Resulting Cross-examination:*

**Q.** You stated that the examinee allegedly was injured on March 4, 2003, in an accident at work?
**A.** That's correct.
**Q.** Allegedly a seven-foot brick wall fell on the examinee?
**A.** That's the history I have.
**Q.** Allegedly he was trapped under the wall?
**A.** Yes.
**Q.** Allegedly there were two witnesses to the alleged accident?
**A.** Yes.
**Q.** Allegedly the fire and rescue teams came and helped extricate him from the rubble?
**A.** Yes.
**Q.** Allegedly he almost suffocated before he was pulled to safety?
**A.** Yes.
**Q.** Doctor, when you say "allegedly," you are not questioning the accident in this case, are you?

**Comment:** An examiner who uses the words "allegedly" or "claimed" indiscriminately can be made to look foolish or even biased. These terms imply that the examiner doesn't believe the examinee. The examiner could instead say:

> The examinee, according to history, was injured when a seven-foot brick wall fell on him on March 4, 2003, in an accident at work.

**Defending the Report As Written:** IME examiners are almost never at an accident scene. Thus, many examiners use terms like "allegedly" or "claimed" to cover the rare instance of staged accidents or fraud.

**Q.** You stated that the examinee allegedly was injured on March 4, 2003, in an accident at work?
**A.** That's correct. I use the term "allegedly" because I was not personally present to see the accident.

**Example 13.202: "Not credible"**
*Report States:*

The examinee's claim of constant, unbearable pain is not credible.

*Resulting Cross-examination:*
**Q.** You find that the examinee's claim of constant, unbearable pain is not credible?
**A.** That's correct.
**Q.** Who is in the best position to know how much pain the examinee is in?
**A.** The examinee.
**Q.** Do you actually believe you are a lie detector and can tell when people are not telling the truth about pain?

**Comment:** The issue of credibility of the claimant is best addressed by objective evidence. Letting the record speak for itself permits the fact finder to draw her own conclusions about the credibility of the examinee. This avoids making the examiner appear biased.

> The examinee's claim of constant, unbearable pain is not consistent with the medical records, surveillance material, and the history provided by the examinee.

**Defending the Report As Written:** A significant part of the examiner's job is to give an unbiased opinion on issues such as pain, disability, and impairment. Being prepared to defend the opinion is crucial for success.

**Q.** Do you actually believe that you are a lie detector and can tell when people are not telling the truth about their pain?
**A.** My opinion is based on my education, training, experience, review of the records, and physical examination. Here the musculoskeletal and neurological examinations were negative. There was no atrophy and no wasting of the muscles. The MMPI-2 is consistent with faked-bad. The surveillance videos show the examinee performing tasks that he said he was unable to do because of the constant unbearable pain. All of the diagnostic tests were negative. Based on this, I concluded to a reasonable degree of medical certainty that the examinee's complaints of pain were not credible.

## 13.21 "Dictated But Not Read" and "Electronic Signature"

Examiners should personally read, review, and sign all of their IME reports. If this is not done, the impression is that the examiner is not overly concerned about the quality of the report but just wants to get his fee as quickly and easily as possible. For examples of the types of cross-examination these practices can generate, please see Section 14.4.

# Chapter 14 Preparation of IME Reports and the Influence of the Referral Source

## 14.1 Executive Summary

An examiner's credibility can be severely damaged if opposing counsel can show that the examiner's client improperly influenced the examiner and his report. The authors recommend the following.

- Do not circulate draft reports to the referral source. If a draft report is circulated, opposing counsel will attempt to show that the final report's contents were improperly influenced by the referral source.
- Do not discard circulated draft reports or cover letters from the referral source. Destroying these may be illegal and will certainly have a negative influence on the examiner's credibility.
- Do not agree to change the substance of the report at the request of the referral source. If a mistake was made, issue a supplemental report and explicitly correct the previous mistake. If additional information is requested, write an addendum and label it as such.
- If the referral source presses for improper changes in a report, ask the referral source to make its request in writing.
- Review and sign all reports personally.
- Do not work for referral sources who "improve" and "finalize" the report and then attach the examiner's on-file electronic signature.

## 14.2 Draft Reports

Draft reports should not be provided to the referral source. If a draft report is provided, opposing counsel will attempt to show that the referral source influenced the contents of the later report. This can devastate the examiner's credibility. For more information on the dangers of circulating a draft report to the referral source, please see Section 13.4.

**Example 14.21: Draft report had been provided to retaining counsel**

*Report States*:

Final Draft

*Resulting Cross-examination:*

**Q.** Your IME report indicates that this is your final draft, correct?
**A.** Yes, it does.
**Q.** Before you issued a report in this case, you called retaining counsel and gave him an oral report?
**A.** Well, we discussed the case.

**Q.** And your preliminary findings?
**A.** Yes.
**Q.** Retaining counsel then instructed you to write a report?
**A.** He asked me to write a report.
**Q.** Which you did?
**A.** Yes.
**Q.** That was your preliminary draft report, correct?
**A.** Yes, it was.
**Q.** When was that dated?
**A.** April 16, 2002.
**Q.** You sent counsel a copy of the preliminary draft report?
**A.** Yes.
**Q.** You then discussed the report in detail, correct?
**A.** I don't know if I would say it was in detail.
**Q.** Approximately how long did the conversation take?
**A.** About 45 minutes.
**Q.** I don't see a copy of the preliminary draft report in your file which we subpoenaed. Where is it, Doctor?
**A.** I destroyed it.
**Q.** After you talked to counsel?
**A.** Yes.
**Q.** You then made some changes to the preliminary draft report?
**A.** Yes.
**Q.** Can you tell me what you changed, altered, modified, added, and/or deleted from the first report?
**A.** That would be difficult to do without the report in front of me.
**Q.** That's why you destroyed the report. So nobody could compare it to later ones?
**A.** No, that's not why I destroyed it.
**Q.** Did counsel ask you to correct, modify, change, alter, add, or delete from your original report?
**A.** Yes, but it was not anything significant.
**Q.** Did you refuse to make any of counsel's requested changes to the report?
**A.** Not that I recall.
**Q.** So whatever changes he asked for you made?
**A.** It sounds sinister when you put it that way.
**Q.** Maybe it sounds sinister because it is sinister. How many drafts did you and counsel have to do to arrive at this final draft?
**A.** Three total.
**Q.** Why don't you go to the board and tell us the insignificant changes from report 1 to report 2 to report 3?

**Comment:** Examiners who send draft reports to retaining counsel and later finalize their reports run the risk of this type of cross-examination. It is not hard for counsel to paint a conspiracy of silence between the examiner and retaining counsel. Many experienced examiners do not circulate draft reports to retaining counsel and put a catchall phrase at the end of their report, such as:

> The above report is based upon the available information at this time. If more information becomes available at a later date, the information may or may not affect the opinions rendered above.

**Defending the Report As Written:** Examiners who destroy or delete preliminary or draft reports may place themselves in legal jeopardy and must, at a minimum, be able to explain their actions.

**Q.** I don't see a copy of the preliminary draft report in your file which we subpoenaed. Where is it?
**A.** I discarded the draft report once the report was finalized. I do this in all cases as my regular course of business. Keeping copies of all of these old draft reports just takes up too much room.

## 14.3 Requests for "Corrections," "Clarifications," and "Improvements"

IME physicians may encounter requests to modify, alter, add to, or correct their IME reports. IME brokers, scheduling companies, or clients may have quality control employees review reports before they are "finalized." How should IME physicians deal with these requests?

The issue in many of these cases is where to draw the line. Unfortunately, many of the requests fall into a "gray area" with few, if any, hard and fast rules or guidelines. An IME physician should remember that her reputation and credibility are worth more than any one client. The "gut test" may help to guide the IME physician. If the request feels wrong, it is recommended that the examiner ask the referral source to put its request for changes in writing. It is very unlikely that an examiner will ever receive such a document.

Dr. Stephen F. Freifeld, MD, explains how he deals with requests for modifications, alterations, or corrections to an IME report.

1. Modifications: The opinion is what has been written and the report is unchangeable once it is rendered with one exception. If you made a mistake during the course of either the examination or the record review, a supplemental report should be sent stating a mistake was made. It may be a typographical error, or an incorrect statement, or the overlooking of material that was sent and mistakenly construed during the first evaluation.

   Other than the incidence in which you have made a mistake, or your staff has made a typographical or incorrect statement, the report is not subject to modification.

2. Alterations: Alterations are also unacceptable except insofar as the English language has been crucified. In that case a supplemental statement to clarify a previous statement will be rendered. The original report remains as it was but the supplemental report will clarify it.

3. Corrections: Corrections come under the same heading as modifications, or alterations. They are generally not acceptable except

in the incidence in which a mistake has been made.

The other circumstance is receipt of a further record, or piece of material or evidence, which was not considered initially and which would cause a change in the opinion. Such materials should be treated as a separate report starting where the change in opinion has occurred and why it has occurred.

4. Pressure from the Referral Source to slant your opinion in their favor: Don't.[1]

**Example 14.31: Addendum**

*Report States:*

At your request, I am writing an addendum to my report of 2/17/1999.

*Resulting Cross-examination:*

**Q.** You were requested by the insurer to write an addendum to your IME report of 2/17/1999, is that correct?
**A.** Yes, that's correct.
**Q.** Do you know why the insurer waited for 6 months before requesting an addendum?
**A.** No. You would have to ask them.
**Q.** Between the time you wrote your 2/17/1999 report, and the addendum dated 8/20/1999, what new medical records, reports, or test results did you review?
**A.** None.
**Q.** Did you re-examine the examinee during that 6-month period?
**A.** No.
**Q.** So when you wrote the addendum, you had no new or additional information available to you, correct?
**A.** That's true.
**Q.** In your 2/17/1999 report, you found the shoulder injury causally related to the auto accident, correct?
**A.** Yes.
**Q.** So the insurer was then on the hook for the medical care and continuing disability?
**A.** I suppose. I am not a lawyer.
**Q.** Having performed over 400 IMEs, you are familiar with the medical-legal aspects of IME reports and their implications?
**A.** Yes, but I repeat, I am not a lawyer.
**Q.** Keeping in mind that you are not a lawyer, was it your idea to comment on the pre-existing shoulder injury being the major contributing cause of the examinee's ongoing impairment?
**A.** The insurer may have requested my opinion on that issue.
**Q.** May have or did, Doctor?
**A.** I believe they did.
**Q.** In your 2/17/1999 report, you never mentioned the pre-existing injury being the major contributing cause of the examinee's impairment, you reviewed no new medical information, and didn't re-examine the claimant, and all of a

[1] *SEAK IME Summit Handbook,* 11/3/2001-11/4/2001, Dallas, TX, p. 195.

sudden, six months later, you decide it's the pre-existing impairment that's causing his ongoing impairment?
**A.** I wasn't asked previously to comment on that issue.
**Q.** You changed your opinion and accommodated one of the insurers that sends you tons of business with an addendum to help them move to discontinue the examinee's weekly benefits, isn't that the truth of the matter, Doctor?

**Comment:** Opposing lawyers and judges will normally take a long, hard look at addenda to IME reports. The suspicion is that the insurer was not provided with what it needed and then asked for "clarification." This healthy suspicion is exacerbated when the IME physician is provided with no new or additional information and is asked in essence to re-write or expound on the prior report.

To reduce these suspicions, examiners should consider meeting them head-on with full disclosure.

> On 8/1/1999, I was requested by the Umbrella Insurance Company to comment on "whether the pre-existing shoulder injury is responsible for any portion of the examinee's shoulder impairment." A copy of the insurer's request is appended to my report and marked "A."

**Defending the Report As Written:** Examiners, when faced with defending an "addendum," should consider attempting to short-circuit the questioning of their motives.

**Q.** You were requested by the insurer to write an addendum to your IME report of 2/17/1999, is that correct?
**A.** On 8/1/1999, I was requested by the insurer to comment on what effect, if any, the pre-existing shoulder injury was playing in his impairment. I have a copy of the request, Counsel. Should we make it part of the record?

**Example 14.32: Improper contact with examiner**
*Duhon v. Snelling Personnel Services,* 97-347 (La.App. 3 Cir. 10/8/97), 702 So.2d 922 (1997)
Some statutes have specific prohibitions against contacting/interfering with IME physicians. For example, Louisiana Statute La.R.S. 23:1317.1(E)(2) provides that direct contact with the IME physician is prohibited. The provision reads:

> (2) Except to schedule the deposition or further discovery as described above, the office of the independent medical examiner shall not be contacted regarding the claimant by any party, attorney, or agent.

In the case *Duhon v. Snelling Personnel Services,* the court found contact by the adjuster with the IME physician was improper but was not sufficient to exclude the report. The court stated:

> The claims adjuster, in this case, corresponded with Dr. Bernauer on more than one occasion. However, the hearing officer concluded the improper contacts occurred *after* Dr. Bernauer formulated his medical opinion. Our review of the record convinces us the hearing officer was correct in this regard. Therefore, we do not find it appropriate to exclude Dr. Bernauer's report as plaintiff suggests.

> We caution, however, had the improper contact occurred before Dr. Bernauer formulated his conclusions, sanctions would have been appropriate. Improper contact with an independent medical examiner is expressly prohibited by statute, and we will not hesitate to exclude such reports when circumstances indicate even the slightest possibility that the physician's opinion or neutrality may have been compromised. At 926.

See also *Heimann v. Roadway Express, Inc.,* 2002 WL 31268195 (N.D. Ill.) (2002), in which the court refused to exclude an IME report finding that the employee failed to show that the examiner had an unauthorized ex parte communication with the employer's workers' compensation insurer.

**Example 14.33: Tainting of IME: Surveillance video**

*Fabre v. ICF Kaiser International,* WL 31664773 (La.App.1 Cir. 2002)
When an IME physician is contacted by an adjuster, attorney, or other representative in an attempt to influence his opinion, this ex parte contact may be improper and taint the IME process.

In the case *Fabre v. ICF Kaiser International,* an adjuster sent the physician who conducted the IME a surveillance videotape of the claimant. This tape influenced the IME report and the physician's opinion on the need for back surgery. The court found the adjuster's action tainted the IME. The court stated:

> Surveillance tapes were recorded of Fabre's activities on May $8^{th}$, $9^{th}$, and June 5, 2000, and sent to all of his treating physicians, including the IME physician prior to his report, without the consent of Fabre's attorney. ICF alleges that it was an error for the WCJ to disregard the IME report even if "tainted" by the tapes.
>
> The WCJ found that the adjuster's action made the IME report of no value because it had been tainted by consideration of the tapes, since an IME is supposed to be unbiased. The WCJ held that a proper way of handling the tapes would have been to bring them to the WCJ's attention and then set up a deposition so that claimant and claimant's attorney could be present while the doctor viewed the video; thereby ensuring the doctor's evaluation was "an even playing field."
>
> We agree with the WCJ who stated that for the adjuster to take it upon herself to send the IME doctor a surveillance video and then ask him to look at the tape to see if it changes his mind "is beyond the parameters of what they are able to do. They are not to have any contact with an independent medical examiner." After Dr. Ioppolo viewed the tapes he sent a letter stating that Fabre had unrestricted movement, and that the tapes demonstrating him bending, lifting and pushing a cart, unloading and loading a car, and walking. He felt that this activity was not indicative of someone having a great deal of pain and, thus, Fabre would not be a surgical candidate. The WCJ ruled that this tainted report would not considered in her decision. The WCJ found that, in her opinion, there was nothing in the tapes to dispute his injury. The WCJ found that after three days of video, the only significant activity filmed was Fabre pushing a grocery cart, which any three year old can do and loading the bags into the back of the truck one at a time. The WCJ noted that Fabre sat on the tailgate to arrange the groceries instead of stretching across the rear of the truck. He also picked up an empty aquarium, and later leaned over to connect a trailer hitch to his pickup. The WCJ commented that hitch seemed to be a ball type attachment and the video did not show that he had to pull or strain to hitch the trailer. At 6.

IME physicians need to have a full and complete understanding of who may contact them and in what fashion they may be contacted during the IME process. The rules will vary from jurisdiction to jurisdiction and from forum to forum.

## 14.4 Review and Finalization by the Referral Source

Some referral sources transcribe and/or finalize the IME report for the examiner. This is not overly problematic as long as the report is not in any way changed and the examiner reviews and signs the report himself.

Some referral sources may have signature stamps or electronic signatures of the examiner so that they can sign the report once it is transcribed. They may also perform "quality control" reviews in which the examiner's report is reviewed and possibly modified after transcriptions. Such practices are extremely problematic. The authors recommend that examiners not perform examinations for referral sources that use such practices.

**Example 14.41: "Dictated but not read"**
*Report States:*
Dictated but not read.

*Resulting Cross-examination:*
**Q.** Doctor, you performed this IME exam for Quality IMEs, Inc., correct?
**A.** Yes, I did.
**Q.** You dictated the report and Quality IMEs, Inc., typed it for you?
**A.** Yes.
**Q.** They correct minor mistakes you might inadvertently make?
**A.** Such as?
**Q.** Substituting "he" for "she," tenses, dates?
**A.** They may.
**Q.** Of course, they have you sign off on the report after they make the corrections, correct?
**A.** Yes.
**Q.** Could you then explain, Doctor, why your report states, "dictated but not read"?

**Comment:** "Dictated but not read" is a serious mistake for IME physicians. It indicates that the examiner is too busy to check his work. This problem is even more severe when the examiner is working for an IME company. The impression is that the examiner is not overly concerned about the quality of the report but just wants to get his fee as quickly and easily as possible.

**Defending the Report As Written:** Examiners who use "dictated but not read" are hard pressed to defend this action.

**Q.** Could you then explain, Doctor, why your report states, "dictated but not read"?
**A.** That's because I carefully dictated the report to a medical transcriptionist who has 23 years of experience. She is excellent and I have every confidence in

her ability. If there are any questions, she calls me and I clarify the point on the phone.

**Example 14.42: Electronic signature**

*Report States:*

Electronic signature. Original on file.

*Resulting Cross-examination:*

**Q.** You did this IME examination and report for Impartial IME, Inc., correct?
**A.** Yes, that's correct.
**Q.** You dictated the report into a special 800-line they provide?
**A.** Yes.
**Q.** After the dictation, Impartial IME, Inc., types up your report?
**A.** Yes, they transcribe it.
**Q.** It then is sent to their quality control nurse, correct?
**A.** Yes.
**Q.** She corrects mistakes?
**A.** Yes, she does.
**Q.** Does she correct these mistakes without consulting you?
**A.** No.
**Q.** So when she corrects a typographical error, she calls you and says, "Dr. Dennis, the word 'two,' 't-w-o,' was spelled 'too,' 't-o-o,' on page three. Is it OK to correct that?"
**A.** No, not exactly.
**Q.** The simple mistakes she corrects without calling you?
**A.** Yes.
**Q.** The routine mistakes as well?
**A.** Yes.
**Q.** If she doesn't call you, you don't even know how she is changing your report, correct?
**A.** Well, they wouldn't make any major changes without my OK.
**Q.** Could you define what a major change is, Doctor?
**A.** That would be hard to say.
**Q.** Then they just put your electronic signature on the report without you seeing and reading the report?
**A.** They use my signature.
**Q.** And then you swear under the pains and penalties of perjury that the report that the IME company "corrected" and that went through "quality control" is accurate?

**Comment:** Examiners should personally review and sign off on all their IME reports.

**Defending the Report As Written:** Examiners who provide an electronic signature should have tight control of what their name is attached to.

**Q.** The simple mistakes she corrects without calling you?
**A.** All changes are faxed to me so I can sign off on them.

## 14.5 Cover Letter from Referral Source

Opposing counsel will want to review the cover letter from the referral source that accompanied the medical records or the separate correspondence that requested the report and certain opinions from the examiner. Counsel is looking to show through these documents that the referral source in some way improperly influenced the examiner's opinion and report. Such correspondence should not be removed or purged from an examiner's file.

**Example 14.51: Missing cover letter**

*Report States:*

> To specifically address the eight questions raised in your letter, the patient's history and medical treatment are contained in my current note.

*Resulting Cross-examination:*

**Q.** Doctor, you received a subpoena duces tecum in this case, correct?
**A.** Yes.
**Q.** Number 1 in the subpoena was for you to have with you "any and all documents/letters and/or tangible materials which have been provided to you regarding the examinee."
Number 2 is the subpoena for you to have with you "your entire file, including but not limited to any and all reports and notes you have made regarding your opinions and conclusions in this case."
Is that correct?
**A.** Yes.
**Q.** Did you tender these materials to me?
**A.** Yes. I gave you my complete file, Counsel, and I want it back when this deposition is over.
**Q.** Where is the cover letter from the insurer, Doctor?
**A.** If there is no cover letter in the file, there is none.
**Q.** Doctor, you said in your IME report, page 7, paragraph #2, "To specifically address the eight questions raised in your letter, the patient's history and medical treatment are contained in my current note." Isn't that what you wrote?
**A.** Yes.
**Q.** Where is the missing cover letter with the eight questions, Doctor, and why is it not contained in the "complete" file you tendered to me?

**Comment***:* Examiners should be prepared to produce their files when subpoenaed. When she receives a subpoena duces tecum, an examiner should go through a brief checklist before responding:

- ✓ What were you requested to produce?
- ✓ Is the material in your file?
- ✓ Have you produced all of the material subpoenaed?
- ✓ Have you removed anything from the file?

An examiner should produce her entire file and should *not* "clean out" the file before turning it over to opposing counsel. Examiners should expect to be asked about missing cover letters, billing records, etc. When these are referenced in the IME report and not produced, the examiner can expect to be asked about them, about what they contained, and why she chose not to produce them. Opposing counsel often prefers that the missing records are not found because he can then paint a sinister conspiracy picture. As in the Enron/Arthur Andersen case and Watergate, the cover-up is almost always worse than the crime.

**Defending the Report As Written:** When faced with a mistake, the examiner should admit the error and not permit counsel to blow the mistake into a bigger issue than it actually was.

**Q.** Where is the missing cover letter with the eight questions and why is it not contained in your "complete file" you tendered to me?
**A.** Sorry. Here it is. I asked my assistant to make a copy of it so I could refer to it during my deposition and I forgot to put it back into the file.

**Example 14.52: Instructions from insurer**
*Lindsey v. Metropolitan Life Insurance Company,* 909 F.Supp. 1408 (1995)
IME physicians who claim that they received from the insurer no cover letter or letter of instruction with the file can expect to be closely questioned on this issue.

In the case *Lindsey v. Metropolitan Life Insurance Company,* a physician explained how he proceeded without a letter of instruction. His forced explanation strained credulity.

> **Q.** Do you recall receiving any insurance instruction at all about what you were to do or not to do in the Lindsey case?
> * * * [objection omitted]
> **A.** Right. We never received instructions. I remember we did receive information at some stage, it may have been at the first review or later reviews, where the examiner had a very specific question about the ability to drive a car for some hours at a time, and we took special care to look into that question and try and address it in the report.
> **Q.** Okay. Well--
> **A.** I know there was other information provided.
> **Q.** Did you make any finding at all in any form that Sam Lindsey was either disabled or not disabled under the Met Life policy?
> **A.** We didn't make any--arrive at any conclusions nor state any conclusions in that regard.
> **Q.** Did you even attempt to do so?
> **A.** No.
> **Q.** And why is that?
> **A.** Because our basic previous agreement was we would provide a medical review of a medical question and we didn't consider--I didn't consider the presence or absence of some legally defined disability to be a medical question.
> **Q.** How did you even know when you got the Lindsey file that the file was being sent to you as a disability claim or did you know that?
> **A.** We knew it had something to do with disability because prior discussions with Vocational Resources were that the unit of Met Life sending the cases did not handle life insurance or health insurance problems, and, therefore, didn't need to know about causes of death. In addition, obviously, Mr. Lindsey was still alive, and they also didn't need to know about present necessity or necessity of

treatment or paying the bill.

**Q.** Is that the only way you in [sic] knew it was a disability claim?

**A.** Yeah. At 1425.

# Chapter 15 Catching Mistakes Before They Catch You

## 15.1 Executive Summary

Examiners need to proof their IME reports for mistakes. Every mistake made in an IME report will lessen the report's persuasive value and the credibility of the examiner who wrote it. Opposing counsel will argue that if the examiner could make one mistake in his report, he may have made other mistakes and his entire report may be suspect. Opposing counsel will also use the mistakes to show that the examiner was sloppy or even ill-informed. Common mistakes that need to be corrected in the proofreading process include:

- substantive mistakes,
- bad grammar,
- typographical or transcription errors, and
- misspelled words.

Mistakes can and should be avoided. They are best avoided by careful proofing before the report is finalized and sent to the client.

When an examiner is confronted with an apparent mistake, he should either gracefully admit the mistake or explain to counsel why no mistake was made. Just because counsel accuses an examiner of being mistaken does not mean that the examiner is, in fact, mistaken.

## 15.2 Substantive Mistakes

An examiner's substantive mistakes in a report may not only result in the report and testimony being excluded, but they may also be a permanent albatross hung on the examiner's professional career. They may even result in a lawsuit against the examiner for negligence or in actions against the examiner's license. Examiners should carefully draft and proof their reports so that substantive mistakes are avoided.

**Example 15.21: AMA *Guides* 5$^{th}$ edition**

*Report States:*

> In determining his impairment rating for the lumbosacral region, *The Guides to the Evaluation of Permanent Impairment,* 5$^{th}$ edition, was utilized. I used the DRE method and found that Mr. Sidell would likely fall into the DRE lumbar Category III.

*Resulting Cross-examination:*

**Q.** You used the DRE method under the AMA *Guides,* 5$^{th}$ edition, instead of the Range of Motion Method to rate the permanent impairment in this examinee, correct?

**A.** Yes, I did.
**Q.** Table 15-3 on page 384 sets out three criteria to satisfy using the DRE method for Lumbar Category III, does it not?
**A.** Let me get my copy of the *Guides*. Yes, it does.
**Q.** Did this examinee have the significant signs of radiculopathy set forth in Table 15-3?
**A.** He had signs of radiculopathy.
**Q.** Were the signs significant?
**A.** Possibly.
**Q.** He didn't have a fracture, correct?
**A.** That's correct.
**Q.** He did not undergo surgery for radiculopathy with the result that he is asymptomatic.
**A.** He did not.
**Q.** These are the three criteria set forth in DRE category 3, are they not?
**A.** Yes, they are.
**Q.** As you incorrectly chose to discuss the DRE method to rate the impairment instead of the correct ROM method, your rating of the impairment is mistaken, is it not, Doctor?

**Comment:** IME examiners who use the AMA *Guides* to rate impairment in their reports should have a full and complete understanding of all aspects of the *Guides*. The examiner who makes a mistake as in the above example runs the risk of destroying her credibility as a trusted IME examiner.

**Defending the Report As Written:** When an examiner makes a technical mistake in her IME report, she should admit it and force counsel to move on. However, just because a different table or category was used does not necessarily mean the rating is wrong. The *Guides* leaves a fair amount of discretion in the hands of the examiner.

**Q.** As you incorrectly chose to discuss the DRE method to rate the impairment instead of the correct ROM method, your rating of the impairment is mistaken, is it not, Doctor?
**A.** No. I used the DRE method because Section 15.2, page 379, says "The DRE method is the principal methodology used to evaluate an individual who has had a distinct injury. When the cause of the impairment is not easily determined and if the impairment can be well characterized by the DRE method, the evaluator should use the DRE method." There are five examples when the ROM method is preferred. Of course, that is a judgment call. If one felt the radicular signs were not "significant," then the ROM method could have been used. Would you like me to calculate the impairment based on the ROM method, Counselor?
**Q.** Yes, I would, since you used the wrong method.
**A.** I have completed my calculations using the ranges of motion that were recorded in the medical record and find the ROM method provides for 12% impairment of the whole person, which is similar to the DRE category III recommendation of 11% to 13% whole person. Do you have any other questions, Counselor?

***Note:*** The AMA *Guides* DRE method can cause some confusion because terms such as "specific injury," "significant signs," or "loss of muscle strength" allow for interpretation. Therefore, the examiner must be able to support her decision to use a specific approach. In this example, if the examiner decided that the radicular signs were not significant or that the recurrent radiculopathy was not due to a recurrent disc herniation in the same spinal region, then the ROM method should have been used because none of the three criteria for using DRE in Table 15-3 would have been met. It was fortunate for the examiner that the impairments were similar for the DRE and ROM methods in this case.

**Example 15.22: Bladder dysfunction**

*Report States:*

> The bladder dysfunction in the examinee is caused by the lesion at the L5-S1 level.

*Resulting Cross-examination:*

**Q.** You stated in your IME report that the examinee's bladder dysfunction is caused by the lesion at the L5-S1 level, correct?

**A.** Yes, I did.

**Q.** Isn't it true, Doctor, based on our anatomy, the corticospinal tract is nowhere near to be found at the L5-S1 level, particularly that which would affect bladder dysfunction? The spinal cord ends at the lower first or upper second lumbar vertebrae. Thus, a central nervous system lesion would have to occur above this level for corticospinal tract damage. By the time one arrives at the L5-S1 level, we are dealing with nerve roots and not the spinal cord and it is therefore anatomically impossible to have corticospinal damage at this level?

**Comment:** Examiners who make technical mistakes on the medicine will have short careers as IME physicians.

**Defending the Report As Written:** When faced with a direct attack on their medical knowledge and expertise, examiners must be able to explain that they are not mistaken when that is the truth.

**Q.** Isn't it true, Doctor, based on our anatomy, the corticospinal tract is nowhere near to be found at the L5-S1 level particularly that which would affect bladder dysfunction? The spinal cord ends at the lower first or upper second lumbar vertebrae. Thus, a central nervous system lesion would have to occur above this level for corticospinal tract damage. By the time one arrives at the L5-S1 level, we are dealing with nerve roots and not the spinal cord and it is therefore anatomically impossible to have corticospinal damage at this level?

**A.** The examinee in this case had a cauda equina syndrome where the lesion compressed the entire cauda equina and not the spinal cord. Both spinal cord damage (corticospinal tract damage) and cauda equina syndrome (nerve root compression) interrupt the brain's ability to communicate with the bladder and give similar neurologic deficits. This led to his neurogenic bladder and incontinence.

***Note:*** The AMA *Guides* has a confusing discussion of corticospinal tract involvement and cauda equina syndrome. In the 4th edition, the AMA *Guides* uses the term "cauda equina syndrome" appropriately for lumbosacral DRE categories VI and VII, but it also uses the term inappropriately for cervicothoracic and thoracolumbar categories VI and VII ("corticospinal tract involvement" should have been the term used).

In the 5th edition's DRE system discussion, section 15.7 is entitled "Rating Corticospinal Tract Damage." The section actually applies to cervical and thoracic injuries with spinal cord involvement and also to lumbar injuries with cauda equina involvement. The text does not make this distinction, but Example 15-18 of the L2 burst fracture properly labels the injury as cauda equina syndrome.

The "loose" use of the terms "cauda equina syndrome" and "corticospinal tract damage" in the *Guides* has caused many doctors to use the terms as if they are synonyms, leading to embarrassing deposition events as in this example.

**Example 15.23: Misconduct charge resulting from mistakes in IME reports**
*Kirschner v. Mills,* 274 A.D.2d 786, 711 N.Y.S.2d 65 (2000)
Physicians conducting IMEs can be subject to professional disciplinary action for:

1. the opinions they express in their IME reports and
2. their actions during the exam.

In the case *Kirschner v. Mills,* the court found the dentist guilty of misconduct for failure to wear gloves during an IME exam.

> Petitioner was found guilty of that portion of the second specification charging him with failing to wear protective gloves while performing an IME on patient S.L. This was supported by testimony from S.L., whom the panel found to be "direct, forthright, and credible," that petitioner did not wear gloves during the IME. The violation of accepted practice was supported by the testimony of petitioner's own expert, John Dodes, a dentist, who opined that it was necessary to wear gloves "anytime you put your hands on a patient." Accordingly, we find the requisite evidence to sustain this charge. At 768.

The court then dealt with three IME reports authored by the dentist regarding TMJ.

> The charges found to constitute gross incompetence and incompetence on more than one occasion are premised on statements made by petitioner in IME reports pertaining to examinations of F.M., S.L., and G.G., and involved six statements of his opinion related to the etiology and existence, or lack thereof, of TMJ-related complaints by these examinees. Those statements of opinion read as follows:
>
> (1) that if pain is present in the absence of jaw movement then it is wrong to attribute the primary source of this pain to the temporomandibular joint or function thereof (Third specification, par I[a]);
> (2) that a panoramic x-ray is of no diagnostic benefit in the study of the temporomandibular joint (Third Specification, par I[c]);
> (3) that trauma to the joint does not constitute a valid basis for dysfunction of the temporomandibular joint (Third Specification, par II[a]);
> (4) that bilateral pain in the absence of bilateral trauma thereto is always pain that is referred from a primary source that is common to both the right and left

> sides of the jaw (Third Specification, par II[b]);
> (5) that an inferior and anterior positioning of the condyle is one which lends itself to hypermobility (Third Specification, par III[b]); and
> (6) that orthodontic treatment in childhood resulted in condylar misarticulation (Third Specification, par III[c]). At 789, 790.

The court found the expert testimony insufficient to support the charges of gross incompetence for the opinions expressed in the IME reports on TMJ.

## 15.3 Grammatical Mistakes

Examiners should check the grammar in their IME reports. Bad grammar in an IME report can be used by opposing counsel during cross-examination to lessen an examiner's credibility. Opposing counsel will try to show that the bad grammar is a result of rushing, sloppiness, ignorance, or worse. Bad grammar in a report will also damage the examiner's standing with and value to retaining counsel, the adjuster, or other referral sources. To avoid grammatical errors, examiners should have their reports proofed for grammar by both their computer word processor and a third person, such as a competent assistant.

**Example 15.31: Sloppiness**
*Report States:*

> EMTs arrived at the accident 4:47 P.M. to include Carol Stephenson, paramedic and Charlie Hess, intermediate.

**Comment:** This is sloppy work and damages the expert's credibility. The damage to credibility is avoided with a little grammatical proofing.

> The EMTs arrived at 4:47 P.M. The EMTs consisted of Carol Stephenson, paramedic, and Charlie Hess, intermediate.

**Example 15.32: Improper tense**
*Report States:*

1. Care by paramedics and intermediate EMS staff was appropriate.
2. All care provided by the Midland Medical Center staff including John Johnson is appropriate.

*Resulting Cross-examination:*
**Q.** Can you please describe for the jury the treatment the plaintiff is currently receiving at the Midland Medical Center?
**A.** I'm not aware that he is continuing to receive any treatment at Midland.
**Q.** Doctor, I refer you to page 7 of your report, third paragraph, number 1: "Care by paramedics and intermediate EMS staff was appropriate. All care provided by the Midland Medical Center staff including John Johnson *is* appropriate."
**A.** I apologize, that's just a little mistake. What I meant to say is that the treatment provided *was* appropriate.
**Q.** You consider it a little mistake when you write in your report that the claimant is continuing treatment at a medical center that he hasn't been to in

over three years?
**A.** It was a typo.

**Comment:** There is no getting away from the fact that the examiner made a mistake. The mistake in his report will be used to show that the examiner may have made other mistakes. The result is a needless loss of credibility. This could have been avoided with careful proofing.

**Defending the Report As Written:** When examiners carefully prepare for their testimony, they will catch many of their typographical errors. Examiners are best served by correcting them quickly.

**Q.** Can you please describe for the jury the treatment the plaintiff is currently receiving at the Midland Medical Center?
**A.** There is a typographical error in my report. It should have read "the treatment provided was appropriate." He is not currently receiving treatment. I apologize for the mistake.

**Example 15.33: Missing apostrophe**
*Report States:*
Patients repeated serial examinations were unremarkable.

*Resulting Cross-examination:*
**Q.** What is the relevance of the other patients in this case?
**A.** Other patients?
**Q.** Doctor, I refer you to page 4 of your report, fourth paragraph, "Patients repeated serial examinations were unremarkable." Am I reading that correctly?
**A.** Yes, that should be "patient's" with an apostrophe. I am only talking about one patient.
**Q.** That's not what you wrote in your report, however. You refer to "patients," plural, in your report.
**A.** That appears to be incorrect. I'm sorry for the confusion.
**Q.** That's not the only reason I'm baffled by your report. On page 6....

**Comment:** Here the examiner is forced to apologize for confusing counsel. This is not a high point in his cross-examination testimony.

**Defending the Report As Written:** When confronted with an obvious mistake in an IME report, the examiner has two choices.

1. Apologize and move on.
2. Fight back.

The apology is the preferred method of dealing with an obvious mistake. Some examiners, however, have great difficulty in admitting *they* made a mistake. Blaming others for the mistake is looked at as a weak response.

**Q.** That's not what you wrote in your report, however. You refer to "patients," plural, in your report.
**A.** That's what I dictated. There was an apparent transcription error.

**Example 15.34: Bad grammar**
*Report States:*

> This examiner's examination of Mrs. Elderly was timely and complete in the privacy of her own home.

**Comment:** This sentence is unacceptable.

**Example 15.35: "Who names he does not recall"**
*Report States:*

> He then went to Dr. Colman who treated him with medicines who names he does not recall.

*Resulting Cross-examination:*
**Q.** Doctor, did you dictate your April 17, 2002, IME report?
**A.** Yes, I did.
**Q.** Did you read it before you signed it?
**A.** Yes, that is my practice.
**Q.** Did you exercise the same degree of precision and professionalism in your proofreading as you did in your examination, evaluation, diagnosis, and forming your opinion?
**A.** I said that I read it, Counsel, not proofread it.
**Q.** The difference being, Doctor?
**A.** Proofreading implies that I read it closely and carefully.
**Q.** You didn't do that because of how busy you are, Doctor?
**A.** Yes, I am very busy.
**Q.** You made a mistake when you dictated, "He then went to Dr. Colman who treated him with medicines who names he does not recall."
**A.** That doesn't sound correct, but it could have been a simple transcription mistake.
**Q.** You didn't mean to say he went to Dr. Colman whose name he does not recall?
**A.** No, that doesn't make any sense.
**Q.** What did you say, Doctor?
**A.** "He then went to Dr. Colman who treated him with medicines <u>whose names</u> he does not recall." No, wait. That should be "<u>which names</u> he does not recall."
**Q.** Is that your final answer, Doctor?

**Comment:** Examiners who dictate IME reports should have a precise, detail-oriented person proofread their reports before the reports are mailed. While a single mistake like the one in the above example does not seem too important, what if the examiner had 4, 5, or 8 typographical or grammatical errors in a 3-page report? The fact finder will quickly lose faith in the examiner, his work product, and most importantly, his opinion.

**Defending the Report As Written:** Prior to being deposed or testifying at a hearing or trial, the examiner should carefully re-read his report so he is prepared for questions about mistakes.

**Q.** Did you dictate your April 17, 2002, IME report?
**A.** Yes, I did.
**Q.** Did you read it before you signed it?
**A.** I would like to correct a mistake. It should read, page 1, line 17, "the names of which he does not recall." I did proofread it, but missed the error. It is my mistake.

## 15.4 Typographical or Transcription Errors

Examiners should proof their reports carefully for typographical errors. Then they should have someone else proof their reports. Typographical errors in an IME report may indicate to the reader that the examiner was rushed, sloppy, or did not take her assignment seriously. Consider the following examples.

**Example 15.41: 12 packs of cigarettes per day**
*Report States:*
The examinee smoked 12 packs of cigarettes per day for past 20 years.

*Resulting Cross-examination:*
**Q.** You took a careful history in this case, correct?
**A.** Yes.
**Q.** Did you take it yourself?
**A.** Yes.
**Q.** Did you carefully review the IME report after it was typed up?
**A.** Yes.
**Q.** Do you stand behind the accuracy of this report?
**A.** Yes.
**Q.** Your report says the examinee smoked 12 packs of cigarettes a day, correct?
**A.** No, that's a mistake.
**Q.** It may be a mistake, but that is what it says, correct?
**A.** Yes. It should read 1-2 packs of cigarettes a day.
**Q.** Can you tell us how many other mistakes there are in this report?

**Comment:** Typographical errors are 100 percent avoidable and absolutely must be eliminated from an IME report.

**Defending the Report As Written:** An examiner who signed off on a mistake in his IME report should be able to explain how the mistake happened.

**Q.** Your report says the examinee smoked 12 packs of cigarettes a day, correct?
**A.** No, that's a mistake. That is why I stopped using the voice recognition software. It just wasn't accurate.

**Example 15.42: Incorrect date**
*Report States:*

On 6/1/697 the neck mass was noted to be much smaller with no tenderness and the patient was instructed not to return in 2-3 months.

*Resulting Cross-examination:*

**Q.** Your report is replete with sloppy typographical errors, is it not?
**A.** No. That's just not true.
**Q.** When it reads, "on 6/1/697 the neck mass was…," that's a typo, correct?
**A.** Yes.
**Q.** On the next line when it says, "the patient was instructed not to return in 2-3 months," that's a typo, correct?
**A.** Yes. I had a new transcriptionist and she was not used to my style.
**Q.** Your report is in fact replete with typographical errors, correct?

**Comment:** Careful proofreading would have eliminated this embarrassing and damaging line of questioning.

On 6/1/97, the neck mass was noted to be much smaller with no tenderness and the patient was instructed to return in 2-3 months.

**Defending the Report As Written:** When faced with a series of typographical errors, the examiner's apology may have to be more extensive and self-effacing.

**Q.** Your report is, in fact, replete with typographical errors, correct?
**A.** Yes, it is. There is no excuse for these mistakes. It is an embarrassment and I will make sure it doesn't happen again.

**Example 15.43: Dictation or voice recognition software error**
*Report States:*

These are all soft tissue injuries and shoulder resolve on their own.

*Resulting Cross-examination:*

**Q.** Doctor, on page 5 of your IME report, you state, "These are all soft tissue injuries and shoulder resolve on their own." Is that correct?
**A.** That's what it says.
**Q.** That's an error?
**A.** It's just a dictation/proofreading error.
**Q.** How many more errors are there in your IME report, Doctor?
**A.** Honestly, I don't know.

**Comment:** Examiners and their staffs should take great pains to read and proofread each report carefully. Dictation and transcription errors make the examiner look sloppy and unprofessional.

**Defending the Report As Written:** When faced with an obvious mistake they have made, examiners should admit it and correct the mistake simply and directly. Any attempt to minimize the mistake or blame others is a losing proposition.

**Q.** Doctor, on page 5 of your IME report, you state, "These are all soft tissue injuries and shoulder resolve on their own." Is that correct?
**A.** That's my error. I should have caught that in proofing the report. The report should read, "....injuries and should resolve on their own."

**Example 15.44: "Medical treatment has been appropriated"**
*Report States:*

> The current medical treatment that the claimant has had so far has been appropriated.

*Resulting Cross-examination:*
**Q.** Doctor, you dictated your IME report but didn't bother to read it before you signed it, correct?
**A.** No. I read it—each and every word—before I signed it.
**Q.** Did you read the sentence contained on page 7, of your report that reads, "The current medical treatment that the claimant has had so far has been appropriated"?
**A.** I read the report and didn't notice the typo. It's no big deal, Counsel.
**Q.** Did you read the sentence on the same page, page 7 of your report that reads, "occasional message therapy is indicated"?
**A.** Again, Counsel, I read the report and didn't notice the typo.
**Q.** No big deal again?
**A.** Well, it's a typo.
**Q.** Would you take a moment and look at page 7 of your report again where I have highlighted eight other sentences? Do you agree that each one of the sentences has at least one error in it?
**A.** Yes.
**Q.** So, by your own admission, page 7 of your report contains ten mistakes?
**A.** Ten typographical errors.
**Q.** Do you know how many mistakes are contained on the other eight pages of your IME report?
**A.** No, I don't know.
**Q.** Doctor, do you still maintain under oath that you read each and every word of the report before you signed it?

**Comment:** Examiners should proofread their IME reports before signing and submitting them. When time does not permit the physician to proofread the report, an experienced medical proofreader who is detail-oriented should proofread the report.

**Defending the Report As Written:** When examiners prepare to testify at deposition, hearing, or trial, they should carefully review their IME reports. If the physician in the above example had done so, he could have avoided the embarrassing cross-examination. Examiners should scrupulously tell the truth when testifying. This will also help avoid the loss of credibility of the physician who is caught in a "little lie"—not proofreading his report.

**Q.** Doctor, you dictated your IME report but didn't bother to read it before you signed it, correct?

**A.** Unfortunately, that is correct. I changed my policy after I noticed reports like this one with many typographical errors.

**Example 15.45: "Tie anxiety"**
*Report States:*

> In review of the records and tie anxiety and depressants agents were recommended.

*Resulting Cross-examination:*
**Q.** Doctor, when on page 1 of your IME report you state, "In review of the records and tie anxiety and depressants agents were recommended," those are mistakes, correct?
**A.** Yes, they are transcription errors.
**Q.** How many more transcription errors are there in your report?

**Comment:** Examiners should carefully proofread and have a second party proofread their reports.

**Defending the Report As Written:** The examiner in the above example was correct to admit the errors simply and directly. When faced with the follow-up question, the physician should take his time before replying. This serves two purposes:

1. it permits him to give an accurate answer (as opposed to an educated guess) and
2. it slows down the rhythm and momentum of opposing counsel.

**Q.** How many more transcription errors are there in your report?
**A.** I will need 20-30 minutes to proofread the report carefully. Would you like me to start now, Counsel?

**Example 15.46: "Marshall arts"**
*Report States:*

> He states that due to the accident of 12/18/99 he is not able to cook or to participate in sports (baseball, Marshall arts, and run).

**Comment:** Transcription errors can be minimized if the examiner personally reviews the report prior to signing.

> He states that due to the accident of 12/18/99 he is not able to cook or to participate in sports (baseball, martial arts, and run).

## 15.5 Spelling

Spelling mistakes in an IME report are inexcusable. Because it is often difficult to proof one's own work, two persons, including the examiner herself, should personally proof each report before it is signed. Any spelling error that is not caught will make the examiner look sloppy or inattentive and will needlessly damage the examiner's credibility. Consider the following example.

**Example 15.51: Misspelling**
*Report States:*

This is exactly the seneiro in this examinee.

*Resulting Cross-examination:*

**Q.** Doctor, did you conduct a careful investigation before forming your opinions and issuing your reports?
**A.** Yes.
**Q.** Did you feel that you were rushed in any way?
**A.** No.
**Q.** Did you carefully review your report for errors before it was submitted?
**A.** Yes, of course.
**Q.** Page 3 of your report, second line, states, "this is exactly the seneiro, s-e-n-e-i-r-o, in this patient." Am I reading that correctly?
**A.** Yes.
**Q.** What's a seneiro, Doctor? I couldn't find the word in my dictionary.
**A.** That's just a typo, it is supposed to say "scenario."
**Q.** So what you're saying is that that's a mistake in your report, is that correct?
**A.** Yes.
**Q.** The report that you just testified was carefully reviewed by you?
**A.** Yes.
**Q.** Are there any other mistakes in your report?
**A.** I don't know.

**Comment:** The expert should have proofed the report and corrected the spelling error prior to signing the report.

This is exactly the scenario in this examinee.

**Example 15.52: He/she**
*Report States:*

The examinee is a 53-year-old obese female adult who was seen in my office… At times he fell asleep while the history from his mother was taking place.

*Resulting Cross-examination:*

**Q.** You examined a 53-year-old obese female adult for this IME, correct?
**A.** Yes, I did.
**Q.** So when you say on page 7 of the report, "He fell asleep," that is a mistake?
**A.** That's a typographical error. Just left off the "s." It should have read "she," not "he."
**Q.** This was a female you examined, correct?
**A.** Yes, it was.
**Q.** If "he" for "she" was truly a typographical error, Doctor, how do you explain the "his" instead of "her"?

**Comment:** Errors such as the above happen fairly frequently and are truly embarrassing for the IME examiner. Computer spell checks will not find mistakes of this nature. Careful review for context and internal inconsistencies is required.

## 15.6 Run-on Sentences

Run-on sentences make an IME report difficult to read and may result in a needless loss of credibility. Please consider the following example.

**Example 15.61: Run-on sentence**

*Report States:*

> It is therefore my orthopedic opinion, to a reasonable degree of medical probability, that any portion of her low back pain that is related to trauma would certainly be related to the accident of January 1999 and not to either of the subsequent accidents, however, it must be stated that her apparent pelvic obliquity and thoracolumbar scoliosis is a very frequent initiator of low back pain and also the most probable cause of continuation of that pain, any continued low back pain should be apportioned to her idiopathic scoliosis as well as to the January 1999 motor vehicle accident, I do not feel that any of the low back pain should be apportioned to either the 10/31/99 or 2/2/00 motor vehicle accidents.

*Resulting Cross-examination:*

**Q.** Your opinion consists of a ten-line, 123-word sentence, Doctor?

**A.** Ten lines is correct. I haven't counted the words.

**Q.** Did you intentionally write your opinion in this fashion to confuse the fact finder or was it a mistake, Doctor?

**A.** It could have been written more clearly.

**Q.** Could you go to the board with the blow-up of your 123-word sentence and put in the proper punctuation so we could try to understand what you were trying to say?

**Comment:** This type of embarrassing cross-examination could have been avoided had the examiner taken the time to proofread his IME report and eliminate this run-on sentence.

> *Corrected Opinion:*
>
> It is therefore my orthopedic opinion, to a reasonable degree of medical probability, that any portion of her low back pain that is related to trauma would certainly be related to the accident of January 1999 and not to either of the subsequent accidents. It must be stated that her apparent pelvic obliquity and thoracolumbar scoliosis are very frequent initiators of low back pain and also the most probable causes of continuation of that pain. Therefore, any continued low back pain should be apportioned to her idiopathic scoliosis as well as to the January 1999 motor vehicle accident. I do not feel that any of the low back pain should be apportioned to either the 10/31/99 or 2/2/00 motor vehicle accidents.

**Defending the Report As Written:** Counsel generally asks the questions and the IME examiner answers them. When humiliating or unreasonable requests are made, the examiner can refuse them.

**Q.** Could you go to the board with the blow-up of your 123-word sentence and put in the proper punctuation so we could try to understand what you were trying to say?
**A.** No, I will not. I am a physician, not an English teacher, and I find your request unreasonable and humiliating. If you continue in this fashion, Counsel, I will be forced to terminate this deposition.

# Chapter 16 Defeating Counsel's Tactics

## 16.1 Executive Summary

Examiners can expect that opposing counsel will use any and all tactics, fair and unfair, to attempt to discredit them. These include the following.

- Painting the examiner as an "insurance doctor" who always testifies for the defense and always testifies the same way.
- Accusing the examiner of trying to trick the examinee when the examiner administered tests for symptom magnification, such as axial loading.
- Emphasizing exaggerations in the report and using them to imply the dishonesty of the examiner.
- Pouncing on superfluous pronouncements in the report and using these to prove the bias of the examiner.
- Attempting to show that the examiner's conclusions were foregone and designed merely to assist the referral source.
- Accusing the examiner of interfering with the examinee's legal representation.
- Alleging that the examiner hurt the examinee during the examination.
- Bringing out prior bad acts of the examiner, so-called skeletons in the closet.
- Taking cheap shots at the examiner with marginally relevant or irrelevant personal attacks or attempts to belittle the examiner.
- Investigating the legal authority of the examiner to conduct the examination.
- Following the money. Close questioning regarding the money earned from IMEs.
- Impeaching the examiner with prior inconsistent statements.
- Highlighting multiple "textbook normal" measurements in the report to imply that the examiner was exaggerating—or worse.
- Raising the specter of misconduct by pointing out that the examination was performed "in secret" without any other witnesses being present.
- Pointing out that the examiner did not know what medications the examinee was on on the day in question and how the medications could affect the accuracy of the examiner's findings.
- Showing that the examiner could not have performed a thorough examination because he spent too little time with the examinee and performed too many IMEs in one day.
- Reviewing other potential causes for the injury that the examiner did not explicitly rule out.

- Closely questioning the examiner on how he scored the pain drawing and trying to show that this is an arbitrary test.
- Proving that the examiner did not have a detailed job description before he opined on causation and work capacity.
- Contrasting the examiner's opinions with those of several other doctors to show that the examiner is out alone in left field.
- Attempting to get the examiner to buy into the notion that his opinion is merely guesswork with some sort of a numerical margin of error.
- Zeroing-in on any computer-generated language or templates used to show that the report is not a result of a careful, individualized examination, but is rather a computer-generated "form" document.
- Questioning the validity of the factual assumptions upon which the examiner based his opinions.
- Getting the examiner to agree on as many points as possible before attacking the examiner and his report.

The above tactics are defended by the following.

- Being truthful and consistent and calling cases as one sees them.
- Avoid giving opposing counsel ammunition for cross-examination.
- Remaining calm and collected during cross-examination.
- Making concessions when appropriate.
- Forming a well-reasoned opinion.
- Being prepared to defend one's examination, methodology, findings, and conclusions.

## 16.2 Tactics and Defenses

### *Tactic 1: Insurance doctor*

Counsel will try to show that the examiner is biased because she always (or almost always) examines and testifies for an insurance company or for the defense. This tactic is defensed by accepting referrals from both plaintiffs and insurance companies and opining in all cases honestly and objectively.

**Example 16.21: Insurance doctor**

*Report States:*

It is my medical opinion that the examinee suffers from no psychiatric condition due to her alleged job-related injury.

*Resulting Cross-examination:*

**Q.** Doctor, you found no causal relationship in your IME report, correct?
**A.** Yes.
**Q.** You consider yourself an impartial medical evaluator?

**A.** Yes, I do.
**Q.** You are an insurance doctor, correct?
**A.** I don't accept that mischaracterization.
**Q.** You no longer see private patients?
**A.** Correct.
**Q.** You stated in your deposition that 95% of your work is done for insurance companies, correct?
**A.** I don't have exact figures but that's my best approximation.
**Q.** You don't examine for employees?
**A.** I usually am not asked to do so.
**Q.** Doctor, when I called last week and spoke to your assistant, Mary Ellen, she told me your policy is that you don't examine for plaintiffs. That is your policy, is it not?

**Comment:** Counsel wants to make it clear to the fact finder that, in fact, the examiner is an "insurance doctor." The more the doctor tries to fight off this label, the less credibility he has. In fact, the fact finder probably already knows who the insurance doctors and plaintiff's doctors are and makes allowances for the biases of each. The IME examiner who sees both plaintiffs and defendants and calls them as he sees them retains the most credibility and will have the longest and most successful career.

> The first requirement is that the IME physician must be independent. Attorneys categorize physicians in one of three ways:
> (1) plaintiff's physicians;
> (2) insurance company physicians; and
> (3) all the rest.
> Physicians in the first two categories earn their reputations by receiving numerous referrals from, and consistently generating reports favorable to, one side or the other. No matter how qualified the physician or detailed the examination and report, the opinions of an IME physician who has a reputation of being a "plaintiff" or "insurance company" physician simply will not be accepted by the other side. Above all else, the IME physician's reputation for impartiality must be beyond reproach.[1]

**Defending the Report As Written:** IME exams are almost always done for insurance companies and defense attorneys. When the "defense doctor" tactic is used, experienced examiners may strike back.

**Q.** You are an insurance doctor, correct?
**A.** No more than Dr. Kulkin, who you hired, is a "plaintiff's doctor."

**Example 16.22: Number of IMEs and payment for IMEs**
*Douponce v. Drake,* 183 F.R.D. 565 (1998)
IME physicians can expect that they will be questioned about the number of IMEs they performed for insurance companies and how much they were paid for them. If the examiner gets a reputation as an "insurance doctor," the plaintiff's attorney may push hard to prove bias.

---

[1] Grace, *Independent Medical Evaluations* (American Academy of Orthopedic Surgeons, 2001) p. 6.

In the case *Douponce v. Drake*, the U.S. District Court (Colorado) dealt with an IME physician who had performed at least 164 IME exams in three years for defense counsel and insurance companies. Counsel subpoenaed the IME physician's records. The court ruled that:

> Much of the information plaintiff seeks in the subpoena is the subject of Rule 26(a)(2) disclosures. The remainder of the information sought is largely irrelevant. Plaintiff, however, is entitled to know how many independent medical examinations Dr. Larson performed within the last three years and what he was paid for those examinations. Plaintiff may also have copies of the independent medical examination reports as long as the patients' names are redacted to protect their privacy. At 567.

Interestingly, the court then went on to order:

> State Farm is to produce records of payments to Front Range Orthopedic as set forth in paragraph one of plaintiff's subpoena, but only in the format maintained by State Farm. State Farm is also to identify the number of independent medical examinations Dr. Larson has performed at the request of State Farm in 1995, 1996, 1997 and 1998, within **twenty (20) days** of the within order. At 568.

**Example 16.23: Going after the insurer**
*Leeson v. State Farm Mutual Automobile Insurance Company,* 190 Ill.App.3d 359, 546 N.E.2d 782, 137 Ill.Dec. 837 (1989)
Just how far will opposing counsel go to "get the goods" on an insurer or examiner ordering or using IMEs?

In the case *Leeson v. State Farm Mutual Automobile Insurance Company,* the Illinois Court dealt with a bad faith case in which the plaintiffs alleged the insurer was using IMEs to delay settling claims. The plaintiffs filed a very broad set of interrogatories.

> Specifically, these interrogatories requested:
> (a) the total number of claims for medical payments processed through the Des Plaines office
> (b) the number of claims processed through the Des Plaines office where an independent medical examination was conducted
> (c)-(e) the number of claims in which an independent medical examination was conducted and the full amount of the claim or the available benefits were paid, no benefits were paid, or partial benefits were paid
> (f) of the claims where an independent examination was conducted, the number of lawsuits filed against the defendant for recovery of medical benefits
> (g) the name, address and telephone number of all doctors used by the Des Plaines office to conduct the independent medical examinations
> (l) the minimum education, training and experience required of those conducting the independent medical examinations
> (m)-(n) whether independent medical examinations are routinely conducted on all claims for medical expenses and, if so, at what time after the claim was submitted was the examination undertaken
> (o) if independent medical examinations are not routinely conducted, the name, address, telephone number, employer, department, occupation and job title of those responsible for determining which claims require an independent medical examination
> (p) if it is determined that an independent medical examination is required, how

long after the claim is submitted is the exam conducted
(q) the minimum dollar value of a claim that will have an independent medical examination conducted
(r) the maximum dollar value of a claim for benefits that will not have an independent medical examination conducted. At 785.

### *Tactic 2: Attempt to trick examinee*

Counsel here will try to show the fact finder that the examiner used a series of "tricks" during his examination in an attempt to trap the unwary and unsophisticated examinee. This tactic is defensed by explaining the common acceptance of medical testing for symptom magnification, by explaining the necessity of such testing, and by resisting counsel's characterization that the examiner was somehow a dishonest person out to trick the examinee. For more on defending the use of distraction and other tests, please see Section 10.16.

**Example 16.24: Attempt to trick examinee**

*Report States:*

The examinee was tested for non-organic physical findings with a series of distraction and other tests.

*Resulting Cross-examination:*

**Q.** Doctor, you tried a series of tests to trick the examinee, didn't you?
**A.** I did not.
**Q.** You pressed down on the examinee's head and then asked her to tell you if that increased her back pain, didn't you?
**A.** Yes, I did.
**Q.** Before you did this test you knew that this should not increase her back pain, correct?
**A.** Yes.
**Q.** She didn't fall for this trick, did she, Doctor?
**A.** If you mean did she complain of more pain, she did not.
**Q.** You then tried straight leg raising with her sitting up and lying down in an attempt to trick her into some discrepancy, correct?
**A.** I performed the straight leg raising tests.
**Q.** She didn't fall for that trick, either, did she?
**A.** There were no discrepancies.
**Q.** You then tried to trick her by having her twist her torso at the hips with the shoulder and pelvis in the same plane and asked her if this increased her back pain?
**A.** I performed this test.
**Q.** Even though you knew it should not increase her back pain?
**A.** Yes.
**Q.** She didn't fall for this trick, either, correct?
**A.** She reported no additional complaints of back pain.
**Q.** By the way, she did complain of leg pain, didn't she?
**A.** Yes.
**Q.** What does that indicate, Doctor?
**A.** It can indicate legitimate nerve root irritation.

**Q.** Did you state that in your IME report, Doctor?
**A.** No.
**Q.** You then stuck her left leg with a needle to see if she could move the leg more than she told you, correct?
**A.** I performed a pain test.
**Q.** Did she move the leg more than she previously told you she could?
**A.** No.
**Q.** She didn't fall for that trick either?
**A.** She didn't move the leg more than she previously said she could.
**Q.** Doctor, the significance of the fact that you tried to trick the examinee, who has a seventh-grade education, with all of these sophisticated medical tests, and she passed all the tests, is that she is an honest, straightforward woman who is in the pain she complains of, isn't it?

**Comment:** Counsel here is attempting to get the fact finder a little upset about the tricks and tests the impartial examiner used during his examination. If the fact finder finds even one of the tests to be improper, he may discount the IME exam and report.

**Defending the Report As Written:** The examiner needs to set the record straight when faced with this type of tactic by counsel.

**Q.** Doctor, you tried a series of tests to trick the examinee, didn't you?
**A.** An important part of my job as an independent medical examiner is not to accept at face-value all of the complaints of the examinee. These tests are used to objectively document, in a standardized way, examinees who have symptoms without objective findings. The Waddell Tests are used extensively by IME physicians to note exaggeration. In this case, Counsel, the tests showed that the examinee was not exaggerating her symptoms.

### *Tactic 3: Exaggeration of examiner*

Counsel, with the use of this tactic, will try to demonstrate for the fact finder that the examiner exaggerated key aspects of his IME report. If counsel can make this assertion stick, the entire IME report will become suspect. To defense this tactic, examiners should take care to avoid exaggerations. For more information on the potential difficulties that can be caused by the use of absolute words, which are themselves often exaggerations, please see Section 11.6.

**Example 16.25: "Totally" disabled**

*Report States:*

> As a result of this injury, this examinee went from a normal, healthy mother to a totally disabled human being.

*Resulting Cross-examination:*

**Q.** Doctor, your IME report indicates that the examinee is a "totally disabled human being," correct?
**A.** Yes, it does.

**Q.** That is an exaggeration on your part, correct?
**A.** Not in my opinion.
**Q.** Did you utilize the *Barthel Index* to measure what activities of daily living she could perform?
**A.** No.
**Q.** What about the *Index of Independence in Activities of Daily Living* or *The Functional Status Rating System* or the *OARS Multidimensional Functional Assessment Questionnaire?* Did you use any of these to come up with your "totally disabled human being" opinion?
**A.** No, I did not.
**Q.** Is the examinee able to take care of her own self-care, teeth, and personal hygiene without assistance?
**A.** Yes.
**Q.** So she is not totally disabled in that regard?
**A.** Correct, as far as that goes.
**Q.** What about communication? Is she able to see, hear, speak, and write?
**A.** For the most part, yes.
**Q.** Not a totally disabled human being in that regard?
**A.** No.
**Q.** She also has complete sensory function?
**A.** Yes.
**Q.** She is a single parent and able to care for her seven-year-old daughter, Karen, is she not?
**A.** For the most part, yes.
**Q.** Doctor, I ask you again. When you said this examinee was a "totally disabled human being," you were exaggerating, were you not?

**Comment:** Counsel here selected a poor choice of words by the examiner to show that the examiner was, in fact, exaggerating, imprecise with medical-legal terminology, and less than candid when pressed to explain.

**Defending the Report As Written:** When faced with the above tactic, the examiner needs to talk about the medicine and not agree to play "word games" with opposing counsel.

**Q.** That's an exaggeration on your part, correct?
**A.** This examinee has the following diagnosis:

1. Paresthesias down the right arm.
2. Severe cervical sprain with possible disc bulging, though no MRIs were done.
3. Lumbar sprain, for the most part improved, and not treatable at this time.
4. Impingement syndrome of the right shoulder.
5. Fracture of the right wrist, healed.
6. Impingement of the left shoulder (resolved).
7. Severe, persistent, and permanent sympathetic dystrophy of the right lower extremity with extreme tenderness and extreme impairment.
8. Fixed ankle contracture.
9. Fixed knee contracture.

10. Complete atrophy of the right lower extremity.
11. Hypersensitivity of the skin.
12. Tremors, probably secondary to anxiety and depression.
13. Torn lateral meniscus.
14. Internal derangement of the knee.
15. Probable fracture of the patella or "separation" of the patella.

Unfortunately, Counsel, there is no exaggeration. In my opinion, the examinee is a totally disabled human being.

### *Tactic 4: Pounce on superfluous pronouncements*

An examiner who makes a pronouncement in his IME report should expect counsel to pounce on this during cross-examination. Counsel will try to show that this pronouncement is the examiner's personal belief, which has interfered with his medical analysis, opinions, and conclusions.

Pronouncements are usually extraneous and should not be placed in IME reports. If the pronouncement is already in the report, the examiner needs to be prepared to defend the truth of the pronouncement. For more information on the dangers of including speeches and other extraneous information in an IME report, please see Chapter 12.

**Example 16.26: Pronouncement in report**

*Report States:*

> The examinee has a history and findings of fibromyalgia. In fact, like many of the other five million women complaining of fibromyalgia, she has a pre-occupation with pain in the absence of significant physical findings.

*Resulting Cross-examination:*

**Q.** Doctor, do you believe that fibromyalgia exists?

**A.** Well, I believe that millions of mostly women are complaining about it and seeking benefits for it.

**Q.** Do you believe the examinee has fibromyalgia?

**A.** No, I do not.

**Q.** So when the American College of Rheumatology published their criteria for the classification of fibromyalgia, they were wrong?

**A.** They needed a condition to bill for because fibromyalgia is the second most common disorder women go to rheumatologists for. So they created one.

**Q.** Do you still maintain, Doctor, that your IME report on the examinee's history and findings of fibromyalgia is impartial and unbiased?

**Comment:** The examiner in the above example has clearly evidenced that he has an axe to grind with women who file fibromyalgia claims. His credibility will be impacted.

> The examinee was diagnosed with fibromyalgia by Dr. Jones. For the reasons stated below, I disagree with this diagnosis.

**Defending the Report As Written:** When faced with this type of confrontational cross-examination, the examiner is best served by remaining calm and letting the medicine and science speak for themselves.

**Q.** Do you believe the examinee has fibromyalgia?
**A.** No, I do not because she does not have chronic widespread pain involving all four quadrants of the body as called for in the American College of Rheumatology 1990 criteria for the classification of fibromyalgia.

### *Tactic 5: Examiner is an advocate*

Counsel will try to show that the examiner's sole purpose was to "build a case" that the examinee is not disabled and that, even if she is, it is not causally related to her injury. Counsel will show that the methods chosen to evaluate the medical records, perform the exam, and write the report were done in a biased fashion to reach a specific result. The more that counsel can show the examiner is an advocate, the less credibility the examiner and his report will have. This tactic is defensed by presenting honest, well-grounded opinions and by being prepared to defend these opinions during cross-examination.

**Example 16.27: Examiner accused of working backwards to justify pre-ordained opinion**
*Report States:*

**Factitious Disorder and Malingering should be diagnosed.** Data supporting this conclusion include, but are not limited to, the following:

1. Ongoing litigation.
2. Personality disorder.
3. History of substance abuse or dependence.
4. History of antisocial behaviors.
5. Broad and vague, ever-expanding complaints.
6. Exaggerated and dramatic presentation.
7. Withholding important past history.
8. Manipulation of information.
9. Pain frequently noticed to be out of proportion to physical findings.
10. Functional overlay.
11. Symptom magnification.
12. No objective disease process that could possibly result in presentation and degree of dysfunction.
13. Presentation of discrepant information.
14. Discrepancies in her history of physical and psychiatric conditions.
15. Lack of validity.
16. Bizarre symptom complex.
17. Pain complaints without objective findings.
18. Avoids giving an accurate history.
19. Leaves out and changes details.
20. Evidence of manipulation of benefits. Ongoing litigation.

*Resulting Cross-examination:*
**Q.** Doctor, you concluded in your IME report that the examinee was a malingerer, correct?
**A.** Yes, I did.
**Q.** You listed 20 reasons for that conclusion on page 23 of your report?
**A.** Yes.
**Q.** But those 20 reasons weren't enough, so you stated "Data supporting this conclusion include, but are <u>not limited to,</u> the following…"?
**A.** That's what I said. The "are not limited to" just means that there may be more reasons in the records that I didn't find.
**Q.** You did make a diligent search for this type of information, didn't you?
**A.** I don't understand, Counsel.
**Q.** When you reviewed her medical records, you stated in your report "brackets refer to comments of this examiner; bold refers to emphasis placed by this examiner; bullets added for clarity," correct?
**A.** Yes, that's what I said.
**Q.** Each and every one of the materials you bracketed or bolded was information you felt could be used to bolster your ultimate conclusion?
**A.** That's not fair.
**Q.** You stated, "She denies visual disturbance [though later in the record she said her vision was blurring]," correct?
**A.** Yes, that's what she said.
**Q.** On page 21, you bolded, **"Self-diagnosed fibromyalgia,"** did you not?
**A.** I did.
**Q.** You even stretched and twisted the facts and statements to make the examinee look bad, did you not?
**A.** I resent that statement, Counsel.
**Q.** On page 24 you quoted the examinee as saying, "Her last migraine was several years ago"?
**A.** Yes, I did.
**Q.** But you then bolded your own comment directly after that, **"There are documented headaches just prior to the accident,"** correct?
**A.** Yes.
**Q.** You knew when you did this that there is a big difference between a headache and a migraine?
**A.** Sometimes.
**Q.** You bolded information about her cocaine use 22 years previously?
**A.** Yes, I did.
**Q.** Doctor, your 32-page IME report is full of your use of innuendos, half-truths, and biased comments made to help you reach your pre-determined opinion that there is nothing wrong with the examinee and she doesn't deserve any benefits, correct?

**Comment:** Counsel here is trying to show the fact finder that the examiner worked backwards—first finding no disability and then culling and manipulating the records and test results to reach that opinion. If the fact finder finds the examiner acted as an advocate, his IME report will be discounted.

**Defending the Report As Written:** When faced with this type of frontal assault, the examiner may choose to fight fire with fire.

**Q.** You did make a diligent search for this type of information, didn't you?
**A.** Counsel, the examinee has been a manipulative, cunning liar her entire adult life. There are probably hundreds of lies and inconsistencies in her records and statements. Due to space limitations, I only put in the highlights. Would you like me to go through all of them?

### *Tactic 6: Interference with legal representation*

Counsel here will use this tactic to try to show the fact finder that the examiner intentionally interfered with the legal advice and instructions given to her by counsel. To defense this tactic, examiners need to be prepared to explain why the information they requested from the examinee was necessary.

**Example 16.28: Interference with legal representation**

*Report States:*

The examinee signed the informed consent and medical release forms, filled out the detailed questionnaire, and my IME satisfaction survey.

*Resulting Cross-examination:*

**Q.** You had the examinee sign four forms and fill out a detailed questionnaire and a satisfaction survey, correct?
**A.** Yes, we…
**Q.** This was after the examinee told you her lawyer specifically advised her not to sign anything or fill out any forms?
**A.** It was her choice, Counsel.
**Q.** I take that as a yes?
**A.** Take it any way you want.
**Q.** As a matter of fact, you threatened the examinee in order to get her to fill out these forms against the advice of counsel, didn't you, Doctor?
**A.** I did no such thing. You're pushing it, Counsel.
**Q.** Didn't you tell the examinee that if she didn't sign and fill out the forms you would not proceed with the exam and you would send a letter to the insurer saying she was uncooperative?
**A.** That's my policy.
**Q.** You also told her that when the insurer got the letter, they would stop her weekly workers' compensation checks, didn't you, Doctor?

**Comment:** Counsel here is trying to point out the adversarial nature of the exam process to the fact finder. If the fact finder feels that the examiner "browbeat" the claimant into doing things against the advice of counsel and against her self-interest, she may not give too much weight to the IME report itself.

**Defending the Report As Written:** Examiners need to be prepared to explain the legitimate reasons why they need the cooperation of the examinee.

**Q.** This was after the examinee told you her lawyer advised her not to sign anything or fill out any forms?
**A.** I cannot complete the examination without the cooperation of the examinee. That's what I told her. Your client was free to either follow your advice and withhold information or cooperate and tell the truth.

### *Tactic 7: Hurt the examinee*

Counsel here will try to show that the examiner hurt the claimant during the IME exam. Being "too rough," even if it didn't cause any permanent damage, may not sit too well with the fact finder. This tactic is defensed by being prepared to explain the various safeguards the examiner employs to ensure that the examinee is not injured during the examination.

**Example 16.29: Hurt the examinee**
*Report States:*
The examinee tolerated the 45-minute IME examination well.

*Resulting Cross-examination:*
**Q.** Doctor, are you concerned about the fact that you hurt the claimant during your IME examination?
**A.** I am not, as it is not true.
**Q.** Here is a report by her treating doctor who she saw three hours after your exam. In the report he recounts her injury at your office and restricts her to bed rest. Do you still maintain, Doctor, that you didn't hurt her?

**Comment:** Counsel here is making a serious allegation against the examiner. If the fact finder believes the examinee, the factfinder is likely to be upset with the examiner and discount his entire exam and report. The examiner may also face potential civil liability for malpractice.

**Defending the Report As Written:** When faced with this type of spurious allegation, the examiner needs to do more than just deny it. In a "she said, he said" situation, there is no telling who the judge will believe.

**Q.** Doctor, are you concerned about the fact that you hurt the claimant during your IME examination?
**A.** Counsel, I would be concerned for the welfare of the claimant if your statement was true. However, the examinee was told orally not to do anything during the exam that would result in harm and to stop the examination at any time she had a concern. This was witnessed by my nurse and documented in my report. She was also told to notify us immediately of any difficulties during the examination. She at no time during or after the examination did this. At the end of the examination, she read and signed the satisfaction survey. In the form she answered the following three questions:

1. Were you pleased with the manner in which this evaluation was performed? (She checked "yes" she was.)
2. Were you treated with dignity and respect by the staff? (She checked "yes" she was.)
3. Did you experience any difficulties during the examination?

(She checked "no" she did not.)
She then signed and dated the form. Counsel, would you like to make this form part of the record?

### *Tactic 8: Skeletons in the closet*

IME physicians, in addition to defending their IME reports, may, in some cases, have to defend themselves. Physicians who have had serious criminal, professional, financial, personal, and even health problems may have to reply to questions on these difficult issues. Examiners with serious skeletons in the closet should strongly consider another line of work. The defense to this tactic is to ask retaining counsel to get a ruling through a motion in limine that the information regarding the examiner's prior bad act is inadmissible or, failing that, the examiner should be prepared to make the prior bad act seem less damning by pointing out that the event in question occurred a long, long time ago.

**Example 16.210: Skeletons in the closet**
*Cross-examination:*
**Q.** Doctor, did you ride over here with defense counsel?
**A.** Yes, we rode in the same car.
**Q.** You had testified earlier that there was a series of questions that you were going to refuse to answer, what questions were those?
**A.** There are certain questions about my personal life which my attorney has advised me not to answer.
**Q.** Such as what?
**A.** I can only give you a general response to your question. It is a matter of public record that I was arrested in September of 2001. Anything having to do with that arrest, beyond that which is public record, I'm probably not going to answer on the advice of my own attorney.
**Q.** All right. The arrest we're referencing is an arrest that took place September 17$^{th}$, which would have been 12 days after the deposition in this case; is that correct?
**A.** Yes.
**Q.** Okay. And the arrest, as reflected by the newspaper, which you indicated was public record, September 18$^{th}$ states, "University physician was arrested Monday afternoon after officials said they found drugs on him during a security checkpoint, and was charged with possession of cocaine and methadone." The police report is public record, isn't it, Doctor?
**A.** I guess so.
**Q.** Have you read the police report, or are you aware of its contents?
**A.** I don't believe I am aware of its contents.
**Q.** Has anyone advised that you were quoted by the officer as saying quote, I fucked up, end quote?
**A.** No, I'm not aware that the officer wrote that.
**Q.** Did you tell the officer that?
**A.** I don't have a recollection of telling the officer that, so I don't know.
**Q.** Have you been formally charged for that crime?
**A.** I don't know how to answer that.

**Q.** Why not?
**A.** Well, I thought when I was arrested that is being formally charged.
**Q.** Is that currently an open case, is that currently ongoing?
**A.** Yes.
**Q.** Where were you going on that particular day? It was at the airport and you were about to board a plane, what was your destination?
**A.** My instruction from my attorney, again, was to not discuss in deposition anything having to do with the events of that day. So I'm kind of at a loss. I don't know whether that's pertinent or relevant or not.
**Q.** So if I were to ask you questions such as where were you going, how long were you going to stay, why did you have the items on you, where did you obtain the items, those would all be questions that you would not answer upon advice of counsel?
**A.** Correct.
**Q.** Also the question: That would be six days after the 9-11 terrorist attack, when security at airports was at its absolute height in the history of the United States; is that correct, the date of the event for which you were arrested?
**Q.** Go ahead. Or is that one of the topics that you're not going to answer upon advice of counsel?
**A.** It's not that it's a topic that I wouldn't answer on the advice of counsel, obviously, what occurred on 9-11-2001 is very well-known, but I'm not in a position to tell you whether some six days later, security precautions at the Southland airport or other airports were at their height as compared to now.
**Q.** Wouldn't you agree that security was greater after September 11th and definitely on September 17th, 2001, in airports across the country, secondary to the terrorist attack; would you agree with that statement?
**A.** I'll just try to answer as best I can. It is my belief that on September 17th, 2001, security at airports around the country, including Southland, was greater than it was on September 10th, 2001.
**Q.** After your arrest you were an inpatient at Long Grove Clinic, a drug rehabilitation facility; is that correct?
**A.** I decline to answer, again, on advice of counsel.
**Q.** And were you under treatment for addiction to narcotics?
**A.** Again, I must decline to answer on the advice of counsel.
**Q.** Have you ever been addicted to either cocaine, methadone, or any other narcotic?
**A.** Once again, I must decline to answer on the advice of counsel.
**Q.** How long would you have been, if the answer to that question is yes, addicted to cocaine, methadone, or any other narcotic or mind-altering drug?
**A.** I can't answer, again, based on the advice of my own attorney.
**Q.** Were you treated by the medical director at the Long Grove Clinic?
**A.** Can't answer on the advice of my attorney.
**Q.** Did you have a diagnosis that was given to you?
**A.** Can't answer on the advice of my attorney.
**Q.** Doctor, would you agree that both cocaine and methadone are mind-altering drugs?
**A.** They can be, yes.
**Q.** How—if cocaine is to be, let's say, taken in through the nose, snorted, you would agree that that is a mind-altering drug, or not, maybe not?

**A.** Oh, no, I'm sorry, maybe I misinterpreted your question. The drugs themselves are known to have at least properties which can alter cerebral function.
**Q.** Meaning concentration, memory, and focus?
**A.** Those drugs can affect concentration, memory and focus, attention.
**Q.** Methadone is a scheduled narcotic, Class 2, correct?
**A.** Yes, I believe so.
**Q.** Now, when your deposition was taken, you were employed with the University; is that correct?
**A.** Yes.
**Q.** And in what capacity?
**A.** As a psychiatrist.
**Q.** And you are no longer so employed; is that correct?
**A.** I retired from the University as of December 31/January 1st of this last year.
**Q.** And at whose request—or what prompted you to retire?
**A.** What prompted me to retire?
**Q.** Did they suggest that you leave?
**A.** As you may recall, I was a tenured professor at the University, so I had certain rights, privileges, job security, whatever you want to call them, so the decision to retire was my decision. And there were a number of factors which went into that decision.
**Q.** Are you employed currently?
**A.** I have been engaged in private practice for the last number of months, and as of today found out that I'm being offered a job by the state, which I plan, at least at this point, to accept.
**Q.** Doing what?
**A.** Practicing psychiatry, treating.
**Q.** For whom?
**A.** Patients.
**Q.** Where?
**A.** It's with the Department of Corrections.
**Q.** Will you be maintaining a private practice in addition to your employment with the Department of Corrections?
**A.** Yes. It's my understanding that the employment with the Department of Corrections does not preclude me from engaging in private practice as well.
**Q.** Are you still licensed by the Board of Medicine to practice psychiatry?
**A.** Yes.
**Q.** Prior to September 17th, in your deposition you indicated that you had a salary and additional income from testimony that approximated $250,000 a year. Currently, what is your monthly income generated from your forensic practice, the 6 to 12 cases?
**A.** Well, it fluctuates, as you might imagine. There have been a couple of months where I've made twenty grand, there have been a couple months where I made $3,000 or $4,000.
**Q.** So as I understand it, you're refusing to answer the question with regard to what you did with your patients regarding narcotics that they may have brought back and given to you; is that correct?
**A.** On the advice of my counsel, yes, I have to decline to answer questions about how I treated my patients with regard to their bringing back narcotics.

**Q.** During the year 2001 up to and including April 5th, 2001, September 5th, 2001, and today's date, did you use narcotics taken from your patients for personal use, yourself, without a prescription?
**A.** I can't answer that question based on the advice of counsel. I can only tell you that at no time that I treated patients or performed an evaluation on this particular lady, was I impaired with any mind-altering substance.
**Q.** But you were impaired at other times?
**A.** I can't answer that question.
**Q.** Did you keep a calendar on when you were impaired?
**A.** Can't answer that question. Any time I say I can't answer, it's based on the advice of counsel. I just want to make that known.

**Comment:** IME physicians who have serious "skeletons in the closet" may have to look for other work because few attorneys are likely to retain them once they become aware of their problems.

### *Tactic 9: Cheap shots*

In this tactic, counsel will take whatever type of a cheap shot he can come up with in an effort to demean and undermine the credibility of the expert. This tactic is defensed by taking the high road. When confronted by a cheap shot, examiners should attempt to make opposing counsel sound like a jerk for unfairly belittling the examiner.

**Example 16.211: Examiner is strange**

*Report States:*

> In addition to my training as a forensic psychiatrist, I specialize in spontaneous past-life regressions.

*Resulting Cross-examination:*

**Q.** Doctor, one of your specialties, besides doing IME exams is spontaneous past-life regressions?
**A.** Yes.
**Q.** What exactly is that, Doctor?
**A.** With this technique I hypnotize my patients and take them back to a past life they have had. In one case I took a phobic patient back to his past life as a soldier in the Civil War. Once we explored his past traumatic death, we could deal with his phobias.
**Q.** Do you light candles and hold hands too?

**Comment:** Counsel using this tactic attempts to portray the doctor as strange, unusual, or possibly having his own problems or issues. Would a fact finder find the doctor in the above example credible?

**Defending the Report As Written:** When faced with this tactic, the examiner is best served by short answers and by downplaying the significance of the specialty.

**Q.** Do you light candles and hold hands too?
**A.** I don't think your belittling, adolescent tone is appropriate and professional.

However, I will answer your question. I use hypnosis to help patients deal with their fears. It works and I've helped a lot of people with it. That's the bottom line. As you well know, hypnosis wasn't used in this case. Anytime you'd like to get back to discussing the case, I'm sure the hearing officer would appreciate it.

### *Tactic 10: Licensure*

Counsel here will try to shake up the examiner by questioning his legal right to perform the examination. The fact finder may also wonder why the insurance company had to bring in an "out-of-stater" to do an IME. The tactic is defensed by obtaining licensure in any and all states where IMEs are performed or, if applicable, by pointing out why a license was not required. If the examiner does not maintain a license at the time of trial, that can also be problematic.

**Example 16.212: Licensed to practice in-state**

*Report States:*

> I, Carol Duff, MD, being a physician duly licensed to practice in the state of New York, hereby affirm under the penalties of perjury that the statements contained herein are true and accurate.

*Resulting Cross-examination:*

**Q.** Doctor, you are licensed to practice in the State of New York according to your CV, correct?
**A.** Yes.
**Q.** But you performed the examination in the State of Maine, correct?
**A.** True.
**Q.** You are not licensed to practice in Maine?
**A.** True.
**Q.** Are you familiar with the restrictive rules and regulations about when physicians can perform IMEs in Maine?
**A.** No, I am not.
**Q.** So you don't know which laws, rules, and regulations you may have violated, Doctor?

**Comment:** While IME physicians are not generally considered to be "practicing medicine," they are subject to state laws, rules, and regulations concerning IME exams. Christopher R. Brigham, MD, gives sound advice when he states:

> Physicians performing IMEs should obtain copies of their jurisdiction's statutes, regulations, and IME cases and seek legal advice concerning these laws. It is only by obtaining these documents and studying them that a physician can comply with the laws of his or her jurisdiction and reduce the risk of legal difficulties.[2]

---

[2] Brigham, et al, *The Comprehensive IME System* (SEAK, Inc., 1997) p. 134.

**Defending the Report As Written:** When faced with this type of ambiguous tactic, the examiner should make his point directly to the fact finders.

**Q.** You are not licensed to practice in Maine?
**A.** I am not licensed to treat patients in Maine. This was an IME. There was no doctor/patient relationship and no treatment was provided. This was all communicated to the examinee and is well documented in my report.

**Example 16.213: Lack of medical license**
*Rogers v. Professional Erectors,* 945 P.2d 1045 (1997)
When an IME examiner is not qualified as a physician at the time of trial, his report may not be admissible. In the case *Rogers v. Professional Erectors,* the Oklahoma Court stated:

> The court appointed Dr. M as an independent medical examiner (IME) with instructions to determine, among other things, whether "Claimant's liver condition has been aggravated by his job." Dr. M examined Claimant and issued his report, concluding the injury did not cause any damage to Claimant's liver. Prior to trial, Dr. M lost his license to practice medicine. At trial, Employer offered Dr. M's report into evidence, and Claimant objected on the grounds of competency and probative value. At 1046, 1047.

The court held it was an error to admit the IME report of a witness who was not a licensed physician at the time of trial.

### *Tactic 11: Forensic income: Alleged improper retention of income*

IME examiners can anticipate that opposing counsel will ask the standard questions about IME income, i.e.:

1. the charge per IME,
2. the percentage of work one's forensic practice comprises, and
3. the amount of forensic income per year.

This tactic is defensed by being prepared to give forthright, accurate responses. This will force counsel to move on. Examiners should not plead ignorance when asked about fees or billing as this will not be believable. Evasiveness to these questions should also be avoided as it will only make matters worse.

**Example 16.214: Forensic income: alleged improper retaining of income**
*Cross-examination:*
**Q.** Doctor, are you currently employed?
**A.** I work for myself in private practice and have recently agreed to go to work in Daytona Beach, Florida.
**Q.** In what capacity?
**A.** As a psychiatrist.
**Q.** Are you currently treating patients?
**A.** No.
**Q.** And have you treated patients since January 1$^{st}$ of this year?

**A.** No.
**Q.** When you say you work for yourself, what do you mean, you're doing evaluations?
**A.** Medical-legal type work.
**Q.** Doctor, pursuant to a Freedom of Information Act request, we received a document which is Claimant's Composite Exhibit 3, actually I'm referencing the first worksheet of dc 153, which I would like marked as Plaintiff's Exhibit 1, and I would like to give that to you and ask you to take a look at it.
**A.** I see it.
**Q.** Have you seen that document before?
**A.** Yes.
**Q.** And when did you see it? When was the last time or the first time?
**A.** Probably several months ago, something like that.
**Q.** Meaning when roughly?
**A.** This year.
**Q.** March, April?
**A.** I can't give you a specific recollection of when I first saw it.
**Q.** Why did you first see it? How were you given that document?
**A.** The University did an investigation regarding my outside activities and made a request or communication for monies to be returned to them based on my outside activities and generated that list to give me some numbers.
**Q.** This list was created by your secretary, at your request, wasn't it?
**A.** No.
**Q.** Was the information input into the computer at your suggestion and request?
**A.** No.
**Q.** Where did this information come from?
**A.** I believe it came from her computer.
**Q.** You did not ask her to track the money that you received from outside activity; she just chose to do it on her own?
**A.** I have no recollection and do not believe I asked her to track the monies that I made on outside activities. I was tracking it, at least at that time.
**Q.** How were you tracking it?
**A.** I had a—back when I was do doing that I would keep a file of, like if I had a case, whether that person had paid or not.
**Q.** So that you could bill them if they hadn't paid?
**A.** Right.
**Q.** What did you do with that information?
**A.** Once the case was gone, the file would be disposed of.
**Q.** How would you know what to report to the IRS as your income if you kept no records?
**A.** The 1099s that were supplied to me at the end of the year.
**Q.** Did you ever receive any of this money in cash?
**A.** I don't think I ever received money in cash.
**Q.** This totals $1.3 million. That $1.3 million was requested by the University that you pay back; correct?
**A.** Yes.
**Q.** Have you responded to that request?
**A.** I have an attorney that represents me and I'm not going to be able to give

you much more information than that. But my attorney is certainly—
**Q.** Why not?
**A.** I believe I have certain Fifth Amendment rights and—
**Q.** You mean regarding this list and what occurred?
**A.** Yes. And again, I can't vouch for the accuracy of that list or the completeness of that list or basically anything about that list.
**Q.** Let's talk about your calendars. You have calendars which reflect when you worked for the University in 1998 and 1999, 2000, and 2001 and through the end of 2001, which indicate on the calendars if you did a deposition or a trial or an evaluation, don't you?
**A.** No, but I had calendars—
**Q.** What happened to them?
**A.** —which would keep my schedule. When those years were over with, I would again dispose of those calendars.
**Q.** So you threw the calendars away?
**A.** Both the calendars, and when the files were over with, I threw the files away.
**Q.** When did you throw the calendar away for the year 2001?
**A.** I can't give you an exact—
**Q.** Do you have it?
**A.** I don't believe I have it, no.
**Q.** So when we took your deposition in September of last year, the 2001 calendar which listed depositions or hearings—or depositions or trial testimony, that 2001 calendar still existed, didn't it?
**A.** In September of 2001?
**Q.** Yes?
**A.** Probably, yes.
**Q.** And now it doesn't?
**A.** Probably not.
**Q.** Who was the first person that contacted you or advised you that this list existed and that the money was expected to be paid back?
**A.** I think I got a letter first that did not include the list that said an audit had been done of some form and that they wanted me to pay back that $1.28 million, or whatever figure is they're using.
**Q.** In fact you've been sent three bills, haven't you?
**A.** I don't know that, either.
**Q.** Do you plan to pay the money back?
**A.** That's a subject between my attorney and me, and again, I'm not going to be able to discuss it with you. I'm going to assert my Fifth Amendment rights.
**Q.** You're aware that University regulations require that you file reports listing your outside activities; correct?
**A.** Yes.
**Q.** Did you in fact report all your outside activities as required by the University rules?
**A.** I'm not going to be able to answer that question.
**Q.** Why not?
**A.** Fifth Amendment rights.
**Q.** Just to cut to the chase, because we're tired, if I were to ask you any questions with regard to whether in fact you diverted $1.3 million from the

university, whether in fact you filled out the proper paperwork as required by the University rules and State statutes, any questions along those lines, would I be correct in assuming that you would assert the Fifth Amendment and not respond?
**A.** Two things. One, I'm not going to talk about my income anymore. I talked about that as much as I'm going to in the previous deposition about my income.
Secondly, yes, I would like to assert my Fifth Amendment rights regarding any and all outside activities that I may or may not have conducted while employed at the University.
**Q.** Doctor, during the time in which you were in treatment for drug addiction in a private facility in the northeast, you still continued to practice medicine, didn't you?
**OBJECTION**
**Q.** Doctor, did you or did you not practice medicine by testifying in two forensic cases while you were an inpatient in the northeast the latter part of 2001, specifically from September to the end of the year? Let me be specific. When were you an inpatient?
**OBJECTION**
**Q.** Doctor, did you in fact testify in two separate cases while you were an inpatient receiving treatment up in the northeast in the hospital the latter part of 2001?
**A.** Once again I'm going to have to assert my Fifth Amendment rights regarding whether or not I was in treatment. So as I mentioned to you in a previous deposition, anything having to do with that time frame in my life I'm not going to be able to answer.

**Comment:** As you can see by the above example, the resourcefulness and doggedness of opposing counsel should not be underestimated. While few IME examinations and reports result in this type of cross-examination, some do.

***Tactic 12: Impeachment with inconsistent prior written statement***
IME examiners should expect that opposing counsel will search for all of their prior writings to uncover anything that is inconsistent with the examiner's IME report. When uncovered, this prior writing will be used to impeach or discredit the examiner. *Impeachment* is a very effective cross-examination technique. If done well, the cross-examiner will show that the examiner was either lying before or is lying now. Either way, the examiner is a liar. This tactic is defensed by:

1. always being consistent,
2. being prepared to explain a legitimate reason for the inconsistency, and
3. being prepared to show that counsel is taking a statement out of context.

**Example 16.215: Impeachment from prior writing**

*Report States:*

> The claimant may have experienced a mild cervical strain in the low-impact collision. No damage to a vertebra could have been done in this low-impact collision.

*Resulting Cross-examination:*

**Q.** Now, let me ask you these questions. Tell me if you agree with this statement, Doctor. "Diagnosis is almost always uncertain." Do you agree with that or disagree?

**A.** I disagree with that.

**Q.** You disagree?

**A.** Yes.

**Q.** Really? Let me ask you this. Do you agree with this? You can damage a vertebral structure in a low impact collision. Do you agree with that or disagree?

**A.** The statement is too general. In general, you can get damage from almost anything, but the probability is something else.

**Q.** Let me ask you this: However you define low impact, whatever you mean, whatever you mean by low impact, would you agree that under your definition you can damage a structure in the disc as a result of what you call a low impact?

**A.** That would be highly unlikely.

**Q.** You don't agree with that statement then either, do you? You disagree with that statement; is that right?

**A.** I think we probably were close to that, yes.

**Q.** Now, do you agree with this statement, "Compression, nerve compression is what causes the symptoms"? Do you agree with that?

**A.** That causes what symptoms?

**Q.** Well, let's use these problems, pain in the right neck area, the numbness in the finger, that it's compression?

**A.** In this particular situation, that is the pain pattern and distribution. It does not fit a nerve pattern. There's no indication whatsoever of a nerve root injury.

**Q.** Let me ask you this, it's not the disc bulging or herniation by itself that causes this problem, is it? That's not what happened?

**A.** No.

**Q.** That is, you can have—I could be standing here with a herniated disc the way you define it, the pulposus coming through the ligament, and be pain-free?

**A.** That's correct.

**Q.** All right. And the reason that's correct is because it's the compression on the nerve root in the neck that causes the pain and the symptoms we're talking about; is that right?

**A.** The compression of the structure that can give the rest of the spinal cord pain, nerve, whatever, yes.

**Q.** Okay. And would you agree with this, that it's the objective findings that mean there's a structural injury, meaning to the disc, the objective finding, that's how you determine it?

**A.** No, it's the totality of the findings when you look at how they fit together with a single source.

**Q.** Okay. Now, let me suggest this, Doctor. The statements that I just gave

you that you disagreed with, I've taken from a book, an article that you've written. What do you think about that?
**A.** I think you may have taken it partially out of context, but I know which one you're talking about.
**Q.** Oh, okay. And now do you disagree with the statements that I just gave you that you wrote?
**A.** No, you still have to have the context of it.
**Q.** Let's go through this then.
**Q.** Now, this would be an article you wrote: Disc related injury or not, question mark. That's you, Jeff Packard, MD, neurologist?
**A.** Yes, I believe it was a talk I gave to the Bar Association.
**Q.** Okay. So this is the written version of the talk?
**A.** I made a handout.
**Q.** And when did you do this?
**A.** It was '97.
**Q.** Okay. Sounds right to me.
**A.** Can't remember.
**Q.** It's very recently, correct?
**A.** Fairly recently.
**Q.** And on page one it says, and I quote, "a medical diagnosis can therefore best be described as a conclusion based upon probability. This means that there will always be a degree of uncertainty in any diagnosis." Do you agree with that now?
**A.** Yes. The important word here is "probability."
**Q.** All right. The sentence means there will always be a degree of uncertainty in any diagnosis. Now, by any diagnosis, I assume that means your diagnosis, Dr. Ruth's diagnosis, Dr. Hallac's diagnosis, or anybody's; is that correct?
**A.** Yes, but it can be anywhere from zero to one.
**Q.** And zero is if you have a broken arm, that's zero?
**A.** Yes.
**Q.** And something like this, which you wrote and gave this talk on, is at the other end where there are differences and uncertainty in this type of diagnosis and that's what this whole paper is about, isn't it, the uncertainty of diagnosis?
**A.** Yes.
**Q.** In a cervical injury, a disc injury, that's what you wrote the whole paper about?
**A.** I wrote it to give an idea of how we treated it.
**Q.** You wrote it to give the scenario that we're involved with here almost identically, right?
**A.** I hate to say so, it's almost.
**Q.** What we're talking about here, except this is a back and here we're dealing with a neck?
**A.** That's right.
**Q.** Okay. Now, on page two it says there are situations where actual structural damage occurs even at fairly low impact, correct?
**A.** Yes.
**Q.** And that's what you wrote? I didn't write that, you wrote it?
**A.** You used the term low, I said fairly low.
**Q.** Now, on page six you say: "In the case of a structural injury to one or more

nerves there will be objective findings referable to the structure being injured"?
**A.** Yes.
**Q.** Okay. And you agree with that, obviously, because you wrote that?
**A.** Yes.
**Q.** Now, in this paper, this article anticipates the scenario where you have two doctors, one doctor looking at all the films and you talk about all we've talked about here, x-rays, MRIs, myelograms. One doctor looks at it and says it's a strain, correct?
**A.** Uh-huh.
**Q.** And in this scenario, this eleven-page paper, the other doctor looks at everything and says it's a herniated disc?
**MR. FRIED:** Right? Isn't that what you wrote in '97, that scenario?
**A.** I cannot remember how I put it out, but I put it up as a bit of a discussion to show why people do write things that sometimes mean the same thing.
**Q.** Right. And you end it where the scenario where there's one doctor that has concluded based on all the same evidence that he's looked at, that there are degenerative changes and that there was a strain from the accident, and the other doctor disagrees, is surgically inclined and feels it's a degenerated disc?
**MR. FRIED:** That's what this is all about, correct?
**A.** That's part of what it's about, sure.
**Q.** And that's exactly what we're talking about here?

**Comment:** IME physicians who write or lecture should anticipate that their articles, lectures, and course outlines will at some point be used by opposing counsel to cross-examine them. For this reason, many IME physicians are cautious about where they speak and what they say and write. IME physicians who write one thing and testify to another are subject to impeachment, as in the above example. A less global statement in the IME report would have been more difficult to attack successfully.

> The claimant may have experienced a mild cervical strain in the low-impact collision. In my opinion, no damage to the vertebral structure was done in this low-impact collision.

**Defending the Report As Written:** When faced during cross-examination with statements that they have previously written, experienced IME physicians distinguish them, when appropriate, from the case at hand.

**Q.** Do you agree with this? You can damage a vertebral structure in a low impact collision? Do you agree with that or disagree?
**A.** Counsel, if you are referring to the article I wrote in 1997, you are comparing apples to oranges. First, there's no vertebral structure in this case. Secondly, the article was about back injuries and we are dealing with a neck injury.

### *Tactic 13: All normal findings*

Counsel will try to show that the results of the examiner's findings are too perfect. The implication is that the examiner is exaggerating or, even worse, that exact measurements were not even taken. This tactic is defensed by taking and documenting all measurements and findings accurately. Once this is done, any suggestions by counsel that the examiner made up numbers should be actively resisted.

**Example 16.216: All normal findings**
*Report States:*

The range of motion for the wrist, elbow, and hip were all within normal limits.

*Resulting Cross-examination:*
**Q.** Doctor, your IME report indicates that the examinee's range of motion in his hips, wrist, and elbow were all within normal limits, correct?
**A.** Yes.
**Q.** As a matter of fact, not only were your findings within normal limits, they were exactly as set forth in the AMA *Guides* and precisely symmetrical.
**A.** I am not sure I follow.
**Q.** Your wrist/elbow examination results were as follows:

**WRIST/ELBOW EXAMINATION:**

Range of motion [degrees]:

| | Left | Right |
|---|---|---|
| Elbow Flexion | 150 | 150 |
| Elbow Extension | 0 | 0 |
| Elbow Supination | 85 | 85 |
| Elbow Pronation | 85 | 85 |
| Wrist Extension (Dorsiflexion) | 65 | 65 |
| Wrist Flexion (Volar/Palmar Flexion) | 70 | 70 |
| Wrist Ulnar Deviation | 35 | 35 |
| Wrist Radial Deviation | 20 | 20 |

Correct?
**A.** Yes.
**Q.** These are precisely symmetrical and precisely perfectly normal.
**A.** They speak for themselves.
**Q.** Your hip examination results were as follows.

**HIP EXAMINATION:**
Hip flexion
L: 110
R: 110
External rotation
L: 50
R: 50
Internal rotation
L: 35

R: 35
Hip Abduction
L: 50
R: 50
Hip Adduction
L: 30
R: 30

Again, precisely symmetrical and precisely perfectly normal?
**A.** They speak for themselves.
**Q.** Doctor, is it your testimony today that the examinee's ranges of motion of her wrist, elbow, and hips were precisely the same from side to side and precisely what the textbooks define as normal?

**Comment:** Counsel here is attacking the veracity and findings of the examiner. The fact finder might start to be concerned about all of these "textbook" findings.

**Defending the Report As Written:** When faced with a frontal assault on his veracity, the examiner should respond in an equally strong manner.

**Q.** Doctor, is it your testimony today that the examinee's range of motion in her hips, wrist, and elbow were all within normal limits?
**A.** Counsel, I signed this report and I am testifying under oath here today that the measurements recorded were the measurements observed at the time of the examination. In this case, they were equal, symmetrical, and similar to the normal range as reported in the AMA *Guides*. Are you suggesting that I should have inappropriately reported the measures?

### *Tactic 14: No third party present*

Counsel here will try to imply that the examiner "did something wrong" in not having an office staff member or nurse present during the exam. Depending on the nature of the examination, this can get the attention of the fact finder and the examiner. This tactic is defensed by always having a staff member present during the physical examination. When this is not done, the examiner should be prepared to state the legitimate reasons why it was not done.

**Example 16.217: No third party present**
*Report States:*

> I spent 20 minutes examining the claimant's genitalia. No one else was present during the examination.

*Resulting Cross-examination:*
**Q.** Doctor, you do sometimes have a staff member or nurse present when you do IME exams?
**A.** Yes, I do.

**Q.** This is both for your protection and the protection of the examinee?
**A.** Yes, it is.
**Q.** But for this 20-minute examination of the claimant's genitalia, you chose to have no one else present for the examination?

**Comment:** Counsel here is raising the specter of improper action by the examiner. This is a risky tactic that is just as likely to backfire as it is to affect the credibility of the examiner and his report.

**Defending the Report As Written:** When faced with this type of implicit smear tactic, the examiner can and should meet it head on.

**Q.** But for this 20-minute examination of the claimant's genitalia, you chose to have no one else present for the examination?
**A.** Counsel, I asked the claimant if he would like my nurse to be present in the exam room and he said no, that he would be embarrassed. I protected his privacy and resent the implication of your question. As a gentleman, I am sure you agree with my effort to respect your client's privacy.

### *Tactic 15: Effect of medication*

Counsel here will try to show that the examinee's true condition was masked by the medication she had taken prior to the examination. This tactic is defensed by precisely documenting the medications that the examinee was taking on the date of the examination and by being prepared to explain the possible significance of these medications in terms of the findings made during the examination.

**Example 16.218: Effect of medication**
*Report States:*
Medications: Oxycontin, Vioxx, and Flexeric.

*Resulting Cross-examination:*
**Q.** Doctor, you noted in your 27-page IME report the medications the examinee was taking?
**A.** Yes, I did: Oxycontin, Vioxx, and Flexeric.
**Q.** These are powerful opioid analgesics?
**A.** Some are.
**Q.** The opioid analgesics can have the effect of masking pain symptoms and enhancing the ability to perform certain movements?
**A.** Yes, depending on how much medication the examinee took prior to the examination.
**Q.** Did you, during your extensive interview and examination, ask the examinee which medications and what dosage she took before you examined her?
**A.** I did not.
**Q.** So you can't really say if the movement, range of motion, and absence of pain you described in your IME report were, in fact, the results of the medication she took prior to the examination?

**Comment:** Counsel here is trying to point out to the fact finder that the examinee was probably heavily medicated when she was examined, so the examiner's findings may be suspect. The report would have been clearer if the examiner had been more specific.

> Medications: Oxycontin, Vioxx, and Flexeric. Examinee states that on advice of her lawyer she has not taken any of these medications today.

**Defending the Report As Written:** Experienced examiners specifically ask claimants the medications they are taking and the medications they took prior to the examination.

**Q.** Did you, during your extensive interview and examination, ask the examinee which medications and what dosage she took before you examined her?
**A.** Yes, I did. She told me she took no medications on the date of the examination on the advice of her lawyer.

### *Tactic 16: Number of examinees*

Here counsel tries to point out to the fact finder that the IME examinees are given "short shrift" by the doctor who is cranking out IMEs in assembly-line fashion. The more the process is perceived to be like an assembly line, the less professional the evaluation will appear. The other implications from this are that the examiner is just trying to make as much money as quickly as possible and that the examiner is biased because a large part of his practice is IME-related. This tactic is defensed by spending adequate time on the evaluation, documenting the examination times, and being prepared to justify why the time spent with the examinee was adequate.

**Example 16.219: Number of examinees per day**

*Report States:*

> I spent approximately ten minutes interviewing the examinee and approximately ten minutes examining him.

*Resulting Cross-examination:*

**Q.** Doctor, according to your IME report, you spent twenty minutes with the examinee?
**A.** Approximately twenty minutes.
**Q.** If I told you the examinee's wife was in the waiting room and timed how long her spouse was with you and that she has sworn in an affidavit it was no more than fifteen minutes, would you say she is mistaken?
**A.** No. Fifteen to twenty minutes, I said, approximately.
**Q.** You do IMEs one day a week, correct?
**A.** That is correct.
**Q.** How many do you schedule for your IME day?
**A.** Well, my IME administrator, Susan, handles that.
**Q.** That's Susan Ames?
**A.** Yes.

**Q.** She says she schedules fifteen to seventeen IMEs for your IME day?
**A.** That sounds about right.
**Q.** When you see new patients, how many do you see a day?
**A.** Approximately five to eight.
**Q.** Could you explain how you see twice as many IME examinees as you do private patients? Is your IME evaluation less thorough than the one you do for private patients?

**Comment:** Counsel has used this tactic to show that the examinee was in and out quickly, the examiner was dishonest about the amount of time he spent, and that the doctor's private patients were treated more thoroughly.

**Defending the Report As Written:** When faced with the time-spent tactic, the examiner should remind the fact finder that his role as an IME examiner is a limited one.

**Q.** Could you explain how you see twice as many IME examinees as you do private patients? Is your IME evaluation less thorough than the one you do for private patients?
**A.** In the IME setting, I am not a treating physician and do not have to concern myself with a treatment plan, prescribing medication, and follow-up visits. I answer the questions I am asked to comment on. This process simply takes less time than treating patients, especially when dealing with clients like yours with an injury to just one part of the body, in her case, her finger.

**Example 16.220: Amount of IME work**
*Azarian v. Witte,* 140 Md.App. 70, 779 A.2d 1043 (2001)
Examiners should expect to be closely questioned about the amount of IME work they do and have done.

In the case *Azarian v. Witte,* the issue revolved around whether the physician devoted more than 20% of his time to testifying in personal injury cases. Dr. Honick testified as follows:

> **Q.** And can we agree, sir, that you have testified in court between 300 and 400 times?
> **A.** Over a 30 year period, between 300 and 400.
> **Q.** Can we also agree that you had your deposition taken, like many of these transcripts here in this box, again more than 300 to 400 times, during your career?
> **A.** Probably. That's what orthopedists do as far as their profession.
> **Q.** Can we agree that probably in the neighborhood of 60 to 70 percent of your patients are referred to you by attorneys?
> **A.** I think it is probably more in the likelihood of 50 to 60. Again, I don't—
> **Q.** I am not going to quibble over that.
> **A.** But it's i[n] that ball park.
> **Q.** Okay. And that of your practice that are referred by attorneys, they are referred for purposes of evaluations and what are called independent medical examinations?
> **A.** I would say that half of the ones that are referred to me by attorneys are probably evaluations only, and where no treatment is required or requested. At 1053, 1054.

***

**Q.** Can we agree that as of July 29th, 1997 that approximately 30 to 40 percent of your practice would be doing independent medical examinations and evaluations?
**A.** In 1997?
**Q.** Yes, sir.
**A.** Probably.
**Q.** And can we agree, sir, that for 1997, 1998, and 1999, that that figure has been consistent; that approximately 30 to 40 percent are patients that you see for independent medical evaluations and examinations?
**A.** I guess so. Again, I don't keep statistics. I am just giving you a guesstimate.
**Q.** And when you gave those guesstimates under oath in other cases, and in giving a guesstimate here, you were trying to be as accurate as possible; is that correct?
**A.** Yes.
**Q.** Now, when we talk about doing independent medical examination and evaluations, we are talking about a patient coming into you, whether it is from an attorney, or a workers' compensation insurance carrier, or another insurance company, and they usually come with paperwork, with records, from other physicians who have seen the patient, right?
**A.** Paperwork usually arrives well ahead of time.
**Q.** So you have to sit down and go over that paperwork, and review it, in order to prepare to effectively and competently examine the patient when they come into the office, correct?
**A.** The paperwork allows me to effectively take a good history, or get a good history of what has happened since the injury occurred.
**Q.** But it makes it easier for you to know what is going on?
**A.** It gives me background information.
**Q.** And that after you complete that examination, you have to prepare a report either to the attorney or to the workmen's compensation carrier, or whoever sent the patient, correct?
**A.** That's correct.
**Q.** And that would then summarize your findings, and opinions, right?
**A.** Correct.
**Q.** And then as needed you have to then provide additional assistance in the litigation process to either the insurance carrier or to the attorney to discuss your report over the phone, or perhaps in a face-to-face conference, in order to educate them and apprise them as to what that report means?
**A.** Seldom does it get that far. Usually my reports are pretty straightforward, but occasionally I have to speak to an attorney or adjustor, or whatever.

***

**Q.** Now, in addition to doing independent medical examinations and evaluations, you have your own patients that are referred to you by these attorneys and by others for treatment; is that right?
**A.** That's correct.
**Q.** That there is this section, which is the independent evaluation section, and then there is the section of patients from attorneys for treatment.
**A.** Nowadays, I guess it would be five percent or so.
**Q.** Okay. How about in '96, '97, and '98? At 1054, 1055.

The court ruled that the statutory phrase "directly involve testimony," as pertaining to the 20% limitation on professional activities of attesting experts in personal injury claims, did not include all activities that could lead to testimony. Thus, the witness was not disqualified as an attesting expert.

### *Tactic 17: Other potential causes*

An effective tactic of counsel is to try to get the examiner to talk about other potential medical conditions. The more potential causes counsel can elicit from the examiner, the more difficult it may be for the fact finder to accept the examiner's opinion on causation. This tactic is defensed by forming well-grounded opinions and by being prepared to defend these opinions during cross-examination.

**Example 16.221: Other potential causes**

*Report States:*

> It is my opinion expressed to a reasonable degree of medical certainty that the examinee's carpal tunnel syndrome is causally related to her employment at the ACME Building Company and her work as a carpenter.

*Resulting Cross-examination:*

**Q.** Doctor, did you consider alternative causes for the examinee's carpal tunnel syndrome?

**A.** Well, I concluded it was probably from the use of carpentry tools.

**Q.** Doctor, are you familiar with the other systemic and anatomic causes of carpal tunnel syndrome?

**A.** Yes, I am.

**Q.** What are some of the other potential causes?

**A.** Actually there are quite a few including tendinitis, osteoarthritis, rheumatoid disease, diabetes, small wrist dimension, collagen-vascular, neoplasms, thyroid disease, tubercular granuloma, gout, radial head fracture, renal disease, hematoma, gynecological disorders, pregnancy, obesity, alcoholism, Dupuytren's disease, and medications.

**Q.** Thank you, Doctor. Would you go through each one of these potential causes and tell us if you considered them and how and why you ruled them out in this case?

**Comment:** The examiner in the above example is, in effect, cross-examining himself.

**Defending the Report As Written:** Counsel is using the doctor's knowledge of the subject area to call into question his opinion on causation. There is no reason to assist counsel in this fashion.

**Q.** Doctor, did you consider alternative causes for the examinee's carpal tunnel syndrome?

**A.** Yes. I considered three broad categories:

1. systemic causes, which I ruled out,
2. anatomic causes, which I ruled out, and
3. ergonomic causes.

After taking the history from the examinee, including the forceful repetition, awkward postures, and vibration she had at work, I confirmed my opinion that her carpal tunnel syndrome was work-related.

### *Tactic 18: Pain drawing*

Counsel here will try to show the fact finder that the use of a pain drawing is at best an imprecise way to test for symptom magnification. This tactic is defensed by being able to defend the use of the pain drawing and by being prepared to point out the other reasons upon which the examiner's symptom magnification opinion was based.

**Example 16.222: Pain drawing/symptom magnification**

*Report States:*

> The examinee completed a pain drawing using symbols to describe sensations. The examinee's drawing demonstrated symptom magnification.

*Resulting Cross-examination:*

**Q.** Doctor, you had the examinee fill out a pain drawing, correct?
**A.** Yes, I did.
**Q.** Because of the manner in which the examinee filled in the marks for her pain drawing, you concluded she displayed symptom magnification?
**A.** Yes, I did.
**Q.** By putting too many Xs, she demonstrated "unreal drawings"?
**A.** Yes.
**Q.** By not coloring within the lines, she demonstrated "expansion" and "magnification"?
**A.** Yes.
**Q.** By circling a painful area, she demonstrated "I particularly hurt here" indicators?
**A.** Yes, she did.
**Q.** When you scored the exam using the Ransford Method, she demonstrated symptom magnification?
**A.** Exactly.
**Q.** By the way, did you actually score the pain drawing?
**A.** No. But it clearly indicated evidence of a behavioral overlay.
**Q.** Do you know how to score the pain drawing, Doctor?
**A.** Not exactly.
**Q.** By the way, are you aware that the method you described for evaluating the pain drawing was originally done in 1976?
**A.** No, I was not aware of that.
**Q.** Are you aware that since 1976, three new methods have been developed to score pain drawings?
**A.** No.
**Q.** You are not familiar with the Modified Ransford Method, the Pain Sites Method, and the Body Map System?
**A.** No, I am not.
**Q.** Are you familiar with the medical literature done since 1976 about the validity of pain drawings?
**A.** No, I am not, but I feel I might be enlightened.
**Q.** An article was done in *Spine*, Volume 20, #2, pages 236-243 (1995) by Parker entitled, "The Use of the Pain Drawing As a Screening Measure to Predict Psychological Distress in Chronic Low Back Pain." Have you had a chance to look at that seminal article, Doctor?

**A.** No, I have not.
**Q.** Too busy doing IMEs?
**A.** No, treating patients.
**Q.** Do you agree with the article's conclusion, Doctor, that:
"No one score for the Pain Drawing was able to accurately identify normal patients and those at risk or distressed. This both indicates that none of the six new measures is valid for use as a method of predicting psychological distress in patients with chronic low back pain. Therefore, we conclude that the Pain Drawing has major limitations when used as a screening measure for psychological distress or to differentiate between organic and nonorganic patterns of pain. In our experience, the Pain Drawing has high face validity for patients and can act as an introduction to further psychometric assessment. In addition, it can confirm a presented clinical picture, but we argue that further investigation is needed to establish what the Pain Drawing actually measures?" At 241.

**Comment:** Examiners who use tests to draw conclusions for their IME reports should be familiar with the tests, their scoring, and their efficacy. Examiners can get themselves into serious trouble when, as in the above example, opposing counsel seems to know more about scoring the pain drawing than the examiner.

**Defending the Report As Written:** An examiner should deal with this type of tactic directly by defending his interpretation of the pain drawing and pointing out the other reasons supporting the examiner's opinions on symptom magnification.

**Q.** Because of the manner in which the examinee filled in the marks for her pain drawing, you concluded she displayed symptom magnification?
**A.** Counsel, this was one of eight separate tests that I did for symptom magnification. I used:

- the pain drawing,
- the Pain Disability Index,
- the McGill Pain Questionnaire,
- the Multidimensional Pain Inventory,
- the Minnesota Multiphasic Personality Inventory,
- the Center for Epidemiologic Studies - Depressed Mood Scale,
- the Dartmouth Pain Questionnaire, and
- the Vanderbilt Pain Management Inventory.

And they all came out positive for symptom magnification.

### *Tactic 19: Lack of information about job*

Counsel will try to show that because the examiner is not familiar with the claimant's job duties, his opinion on causation and/or disability is suspect. This tactic is defensed by only giving opinions dependent on an accurate job description when the examiner actually has such a description. Where it is not necessary to have an accurate job description, the examiner needs to be prepared to explain why this is the case.

**Example 16.223: Lack of information about job**

*Report States:*

The development of carpal tunnel syndrome in this examinee is unrelated to his employment at the Pilot Construction Company.

*Resulting Cross-examination:*

**Q.** You found no causal relationship between the examinee's employment and his development of carpal tunnel syndrome, correct?
**A.** That's correct.
**Q.** What was the examinee's position at Pilot Construction?
**A.** He was some kind of a builder.
**Q.** Do you know if he used a screw gun?
**A.** I do not.
**Q.** Are you aware that he consistently used hand tools that vibrated?
**A.** He didn't tell me that.
**Q.** Did you ask him about the kind of tools he used?
**A.** No, I did not.
**Q.** Do you know how much his wrist was flexed or extended at work?
**A.** I do not know.
**Q.** How much forceful repetition was he involved with?
**A.** I don't know.
**Q.** Can you tell us what exactly he did do at this job?
**A.** I am not really sure.
**Q.** Despite knowing next to nothing about the examinee's job duties, you found no causal relationship between his work and his development of carpal tunnel syndrome?

**Comment:** The more specific information the examiner has concerning the claimant's job duties, the better position he is in to opine and defend his opinion on causation.

**Defending the Report As Written:** The examiner may be able to defend his report even when he is not furnished with crucial information about the examinee's job duties.

**Q.** Despite knowing next to nothing about the examinee's job duties, you found no causal relationship between his work and his development of carpal tunnel syndrome?
**A.** I considered the time-relatedness here to be determinative. As the clinical presentation did not manifest itself until 1½ years after he left this job, it was too remote to be related. That is why I was not overly concerned about what his precise duties were at Pilot Construction.

### *Tactic 20: Contrast with opinion of other doctors*

Counsel here will try to show that the opinion expressed by the examiner stands in stark contrast to the great weight of the other medical opinions expressed in the claim. Counsel will want to make this point for the benefit of the fact finder and also to see if she can browbeat the examiner into changing or modifying his opinion. This tactic is defensed by the examiner maintaining confidence in his opinions and being prepared to explain why he believes that his opinion is correct.

**Example 16.224: Contrast with opinion of other doctors**

*Report States:*

The stress that the examinee experienced between 6/17/2002 and 9/20/2002 did not cause his myocardial infarction.

*Resulting Cross-examination:*

**Q.** You found no causal relationship between the stress that the examinee experienced and his myocardial infarction of 9/20/2002, correct?
**A.** Yes, that's correct.
**Q.** Dr. Byrne found that the myocardial infarction was causally related to the examinee's stress and that the stress significantly accelerated and aggravated the examinee's underlying coronary atherosclerosis. You don't agree?
**A.** I do not.
**Q.** Dr. Mathews found that acute psychosocial stress results in high levels of catecholamines which lead to rupture of a cholesterol plaque and clot formation producing myocardial infarction. You don't agree?
**A.** I do not.
**Q.** Dr. Barker, examining for the Social Security Administration, found causal relationship. You don't agree?
**A.** I do not.
**Q.** You also don't agree with Drs. Eckman, Kramer, Doner, and Dudley?
**A.** I do not.
**Q.** Isn't it fair to say that of the eight physicians who examined the claimant, you are the only physician who found no causal relationship between the stress and the myocardial infarction?

**Comment:** Counsel here is trying to show the fact finder that the examiner's opinion is inconsistent with those of other physicians who examined the claimant. This argument becomes more powerful when the other physicians examined the claimant for disinterested parties who had nothing to gain from their opinions.

**Defending the Report As Written:** When faced with this tactic, the examiner can point out that just because "more doctors" say something does not make it correct or true.

**Q.** Isn't it fair to say that of the eight physicians who examined the claimant, you are the only physician who found no causal relationship between the stress and the myocardial infarction?
**A.** Counsel, when workers' compensation first started in Germany, 2,000 books and papers were published on "traumatic cancer." That didn't make those doctors right. My opinion in this case is based on my training, experience, review of the records, and examination.

***Tactic 21: Margin of error***

Counsel here will try to point out to the fact finder that medicine is not an exact science. The examiner is then forced to deal with "margin of error" questions. This tactic is defensed by not acknowledging a margin of error where none exists and by not accepting counsel's invitation to play numbers games.

**Example 16.225: Margin of error**

*Report States:*

The examinee has a 4% permanent impairment under the AMA *Guides* (5th edition) for his joint instability of the PIP joint of the right middle finger.

*Resulting Cross-examination:*

**Q.** Doctor, you would agree that medicine is not an exact science?
**A.** Yes.
**Q.** You rated this examinee at 4% permanent impairment, did you not?
**A.** Yes, I did.
**Q.** As medicine is not an exact science, what is your margin of error?
**A.** It would be minimal.
**Q.** Could you be off by 1%?
**A.** Yes.
**Q.** Could you be off by 2%?
**A.** Yes.
**Q.** What about 3%?
**A.** Yes.
**Q.** What about 10%?
**A.** No, that's too much.
**Q.** So you could be off as much as 3% to 9% on this rating?
**A.** I do not feel comfortable with those numbers.
**Q.** By the way, on your margin of error, let's say 5%, that would be plus or minus. So the rating could be -1% to 9%?

**Comment:** Counsel here is combining two tactics. First, the use of the "margin of error," and second, the "numbers game."

**Defending the Report As Written:** Examiners should avoid playing these games with counsel when at all possible. The examiner's opinion is what it is.

**Q.** As medicine is not an exact science, what is your margin of error?
**A.** I used the best objective guide to rating permanent impairment, the AMA *Guides*. Under Section 16.4e, Finger Motion Impairment, and Section 16.7a, Bone and Joint Deformities, the rating is 4%. Would you like me to explain how the 4% is calculated?

***Tactic 22: Attacking use of computer-generated standard language and templates***

Counsel may inquire if the examiner used a form, checklist, or template to prepare the IME report. He may then ask to see the template and compare it with the final report. Sophisticated counsel may ask to see not only the general template, but also the specialized paragraphs—statements that the examiner has on the computer for common conditions (e.g., carpal tunnel syndrome, fibromyalgia, chronic fatigue syndrome, low-impact collision, etc.). The more counsel can get the examiner to talk about forms, checklists, and templates, the less originality and credibility the IME report will retain. This is an effective tactic. Just because a computer was used doesn't mean that there is anything wrong with the report. Problems will arise when the computer generates inaccurate or inconsistent language. This tactic is defensed by admitting the use of the computer to assist in the preparation of the report while at the same time defending the accuracy of the report. For more information on the potential dangers of using computer-generated language, templates, and boilerplate language, please see Sections 11.20 and 17.2.

**Example 16.226: Template**

*Report States:*

> The cause(s) for the development of carpal tunnel syndrome still remains a controversial subject. There are a number of speculations, theories, and hypoytheses for the development of carpal tunnel syndrome. The matter is debated in scientific meetings devoted to this subject. However, to this date, not a single well-run scientific research study has proven a direct relationship between the development of this illness and a particular job or vocation.
>
> In my own experience, covering more than 30 years of treating this problem, I have noticed that the majority of my patients have been housewives or retired individuals with no particular job or vocation.

*Resulting Cross-examination:*

**Q.** The two paragraphs in your IME report about the cause(s) of carpal tunnel syndrome are standard parts of your IME reports, correct?
**A.** I use them in carpal tunnel syndrome cases.
**Q.** These are part of the template you use to create these reports?
**A.** If you mean checklist, yes.
**Q.** This is more than a checklist, isn't it, Doctor?
**A.** Not really.
**Q.** The examinee here is not a housewife or retired individual with no job or vocation. He is a 38-year-old builder, correct?
**A.** Yes.
**Q.** So, the part about retired housewives doesn't really apply?
**A.** I guess not.
**Q.** It's in there because it's part of the template?
**A.** Again with the template.
**Q.** As a matter of fact, you even have the word "hypoytheses" misspelled in all of these reports?
**A.** So what?
**Q.** That shows that you are just using the same paragraphs over and over again

even with the same misspellings?
**A.** If you say so.
**Q.** Let's go over the other standard paragraphs you have in your IME template.

**Comment:** Counsel in the above example has cast serious doubt about the process and procedure used by the examiner in writing his IME report. The examiner's denials are disingenuous and damage his credibility.

**Defending the Report As Written:** When faced with an attack as in the above example, the examiner is best served by telling the truth, making a small concession, and forcing counsel to move on.

**Q.** The two paragraphs in your IME report about the cause(s) of carpal tunnel syndrome are standard parts of your IME reports, correct?
**A.** Yes, they are, but that doesn't mean they are not true.

### *Tactic 23: Attacking assumptions*

Counsel may try to attack one or more of the factual assumptions that the examiner relied on to formulate his opinion. This is a simple, direct, and effective tactic to attack the examiner, his opinions, and conclusions. This tactic is defensed by admitting the obvious; that is, if the factual assumptions upon which the examiner based his opinions are incorrect, the examiner *may* have to alter his opinions.

**Example 16.227: Attacking assumptions**

*Report States:*

> The degenerative disc disease of the lumbar spine and cervical spine are pre-existing and associated with the degenerative process and are consistent with the examinee's age of 57 years.

*Resulting Cross-examination:*
**Q.** You indicated that the degenerative disc disease of the lumbar spine and cervical spine are pre-existing and associated with the degenerative process and are consistent with the examinee's age of 57, correct?
**A.** Yes, I did.
**Q.** Are you aware, Doctor, that the examinee is in fact 37, not 57? Here is a copy of her birth certificate. Will you now change your opinion on causation?

**Comment:** Examiners need to pay particular attention to these kinds of facts. While medicine may not be an exact science or art, the age of the examinee is a precise fact. If discrepancies exist in the records, the examiner should attempt to clarify them with the examinee.

**Defending the Report As Written:** Examiners may be faced with new facts that render prior assumptions incorrect. When faced with these "new facts," the examiner need not necessarily change his opinion.

**Q.** Are you aware, Doctor, that the examinee is in fact 37, not 57? Here is a copy of her birth certificate. Will you now change your opinion on causation?

**A.** I will consider the new information and will add it to the results of my examination, review of the records, and diagnostic testing.

### *Tactic 24: Getting the examiner to agree on issues*

Counsel, when starting his cross-examination, may first try to get the examiner to agree on as many issues as possible before attacking the examiner. This tactic narrows the dispute and highlights for the fact finder the true issue in dispute. It is defensed by breaking counsel's rhythm, qualifying responses, and not agreeing with a simple "yes" unless the examiner is 100% in agreement with opposing counsel's questions.

**Example 16.228: Getting the examiner to agree on issues**
*Report States:*

> The fall of 7/24/2002 caused the biomalleolar fracture of the right ankle. The surgical treatment was complicated by the examinee's severe osteomyelitis. The right BK amputation was necessitated to control and manage the osteomyelitis.

*Resulting Cross-examination:*
**Q.** Doctor, do you agree that there is a very good correlation between the objective findings and the examinee's symptoms?
**A.** Yes, I do.
**Q.** The fall of 7/24/2002 caused the biomalleolar fracture of the right ankle?
**A.** Yes.
**Q.** Surgical treatment for the fracture was both reasonable and necessary?
**A.** Yes.
**Q.** The surgical treatment was complicated by the examinee's osteomyelitis?
**A.** Yes.
**Q.** The examinee's diabetes was a contributing factor to the osteomyelitis?
**A.** Yes, it was.
**Q.** The foot and ankle were stable and showed no evidence of neuropathic changes prior to the injury?
**A.** Yes.
**Q.** Would you agree, Doctor, that the fracture of the ankle set up a chain of events that ultimately necessitated the below-knee amputation and that if it were not for the injury of 7/24/2002, she would still have an intact functional right lower extremity?

**Comment:** Counsel in the above example first obtained six crucial admissions from the examiner before he got to the true issue in dispute. Counsel also built up momentum during this cross-examination and attempted to make it difficult for the examiner to deny causation.

**Defending the Report As Written:** When faced with this tactic, the examiner should attempt to break the momentum of the cross-examiner. This will slow down the examination and make the answer to the final question seem less than inevitable.

**Q.** The foot and ankle were stable and showed no evidence of neuropathic changes prior to the injury?
**A.** That's not really accurate. The ankle showed instability and the foot had clear neuropathic changes including avascular necrosis and resorption of most of the talus. Would you like me to explain what I mean?

### *Tactic 25: Violation of ethics*

Counsel here will try to show that the examiner knew about unethical activity by another examiner but did not report it to the proper authorities.

**Example 16.229: Examiner accused of not properly reporting unethical activity**

*Report States:*

> The psychological tests administered were the WAIS-R and the WRAT-R, which are out-of-date and have been replaced. The ethical guidelines of the American Psychological Association (APA) state that only the latest psychological testing instruments should be employed.

*Resulting Cross-examination:*
**Q.** Doctor, you concluded in your IME report that Dr. Lewis improperly administered out-of-date psychological tests to the examinee, correct?
**A.** Yes, I did.
**Q.** Did you report the ethical violations of Dr. Lewis under Section 1.05 of the APA Ethical Standards?
**A.** No, I did not.
**Q.** Was that because there was no ethical violation or did you yourself commit one by your failure to report it?

**Comment:** Examiners should be very careful when they accuse other doctors of unethical activities in their IME reports. If there are truly unethical activities, the IME examiner may be forced to report the activities to the proper authorities. The failure to do so can result in a cross-examination such as in the above example.

**Defending the Report As Written:** When faced with an accusation of a failure to report unethical activity, the examiner can use all the standards in question.

**Q.** Did you report the ethical violations of Dr. Lewis under Section 1.05 of the APA Ethical Standards?
**A.** I followed 1.04 and called Dr. Lewis and engaged in the appropriate informal resolution of ethical violations process.

# Chapter 17 Trick and Difficult Cross-Examination Questions for Independent Medical Examiners

## 17.1 Executive Summary

Examiners should be well-prepared for cross-examination. Questions on cross-examination should be answered truthfully and artfully. Part of proper preparation requires becoming familiar with some of the most difficult questions examiners are likely to be asked on cross-examination. These include the following.

- Questions about any missing IME credentials, such as ABIME certification.
- A request for an admission that the examinee's treating physician is in a much better position to offer an opinion in this case than an examiner who only saw the examinee once, for a brief period of time.
- Highlighting any medical terms that may seem inapplicable to a lay person serving as a fact finder. For instance, describing a seriously injured person as being in "no acute distress."
- Asking the examiner to guarantee future outcomes.
- Following the money. Questions about how much money the examiner is making from IMEs.
- Asking the examiner to define all medical-legal and other terms used in the report.
- Questions regarding impairment guidelines that show the guidelines are unreliable because different editions will yield different ratings for the same condition.
- Close questioning on any observations made of the examinee arriving at and leaving the exam. Such observations may leave the impression that the examiner spied on the examinee.
- Inquiries that show that the examiner has no independent memory of the examinee beyond the report.
- A line of questioning that shows that the examiner is not an expert in "the truth."
- Questions which show that the examiner no longer treats patients and is merely an "insurance doctor."
- Requests for the examiner to cite supporting literature.
- Asking the examiner how many IMEs are done in a day to show that the examiner is trying to maximize income, is rushing, and cannot possibly produce informed opinions.
- Questions highlighting how the examiner treats patients and

examinees differently.
- Inquiries concerning the expert's forensic history that show that the examiner always testifies for one side and always testifies the same way.
- Conspiracy theory. Questions highlighting all contacts with the referral source may attempt to show that the referral source improperly influenced the contents of the report.
- Questions outside of the examiner's true area of expertise.
- Asking to what extent the examinee's pain inhibits concentration.
- Accusations of HIPAA non-compliance.
- Cheap shots, such as how often an examiner is sexually aroused by an examinee.
- A line of questioning that fleshes out the examiner's biases. For example, bias toward early return to work.
- Questions about past complaints against the examiner arising out of IMEs.

## 17.2 Responses to 27 Trick and Difficult Cross-Examination Questions for Independent Medical Examiners

***Question 1: Lack of ABIME certification***
**Question:** Are you a Certified Independent Medical Examiner, Doctor?

**Reply 1 (Novice):** What's a Certified Independent Medical Examiner?
**Reply 2 (Aggressive):** I am a board certified orthopedic surgeon. That should be more than enough certification to do an IME, don't you think?
**Reply 3 (Artful):** I have 32 years experience as a neurosurgeon, am a clinical professor at Harvard, and have conducted over 1,000 independent medical examinations. I have not applied for certification in IMEs. That didn't exist when I started doing these exams in the 1970s.

**Lesson:** Counsel here is trying to question the credentials of the examiner. He will go through the fact that over 2,300 physicians have passed a rigorous written certification examination administered by the American Board of Independent Medical Examiners. Counsel may also point out that because the examiner is not ABIME certified, he is also not bound to abide by the ABIME guidelines of conduct. This question is also designed to plant a seed of doubt in the mind of the fact finder and, if possible, to put the examiner on the defensive.

- The *novice* reply evidences that the examiner is not even aware of the existence of certification for IME examiners. Ignorance does not add to credibility.

- The *aggressive* reply sounds arrogant and may put off the fact finder.
- The *artful* reply is not defensive and uses the question as an opportunity to restate the examiner's impressive credentials and offer a legitimate reason why the examiner is not certified.

***Question 2: Treating physician vs. IME examiner***
**Question:** Since you only saw the examinee once, for 30 minutes, and her treating doctor saw her numerous times over a three-year period, isn't the treating physician in the best position to opine on the examinee's disability, impairment, and work capacity?

**Reply 1 (Novice):** Yes, she is.
**Reply 2 (Defensive):** Just because she is the treating physician doesn't mean she knows more than I do.
**Reply 3 (Artful):** The treating physician did not enjoy the advantage of having all of the medical records available to her before developing her opinion. Furthermore, I was asked to answer specific questions. It is possible that her treating physician may not have my extensive training and experience in the areas of disability, work capacity, and impairment or have specific training in rating and evaluating disability impairment and work capacity. Therefore, in this case, the answer to your question is no, the treating physician is not in a better position than I am to opine on the examinee's disability, impairment, and work capacity.

**Lesson:** Here counsel is trying to allege, imply, or infer that because the treating physician has had more contact with the examinee, she is in a better position to opine on the issues raised by the IME process. In fact, many IME examiners have had extensive training and experience in dealing with evaluating and rating impairment and disability. They have no allegiance to the examinee and have no patient-physician relationship. Examiners also have the benefit of hindsight, which the treating physician often does not have.

- The *novice* reply is a major concession that could dramatically influence the outcome of the case.
- The *defensive* reply is a weak denial without any reasons or specifics to back it up. It is not persuasive.
- The *artful* reply is a strong answer because it provides specific reasons and information to back it up. Notice as well how the examiner gave his explanation first and then provided his "no" answer. This helps to ensure that the examiner's explanation is not cut off.

*Question 3: No acute distress*
**Question:** You found the examinee, who has had four back operations and has chronic, unremitting pain, in "no acute distress"?

**Reply 1 (Volunteering Novice):** Yes, I did. I think he is a malingerer.
**Reply 2 (Aggressive):** I am the one who examined him, Counsel, not you. He seemed fine to me.
**Reply 3 (Artful):** Yes, I did. Would you like me to explain?

**Lesson:** Counsel here is trying to contrast the objective medical facts (e.g., four back operations and chronic pain) with the apparently incongruous finding by the examiner of "no acute distress." While "no acute distress" in a medical sense means no urgent care or immediate surgery is needed, most laypersons, lawyers, and fact finders may be unaware of this fine distinction.

- The *volunteering novice* reply opens the examiner up to an entirely new line of questioning about the definition and diagnosis of malingering as it applies to the examinee.
- The *aggressive* reply sounds arrogant and condescending. It opens up the hostile examiner to a cross-examination about how an examinee who has had four back operations and suffers from chronic pain syndrome could be "fine." Saying the examinee looked "fine" was probably not accurate and is an example of what can happen when an examiner loses his cool and does not carefully consider his response to a cross-examination question.
- The *artful* reply is simple, direct, and places opposing counsel in an awkward position. Counsel could ask the very dangerous question why or he could ignore the baiting and run the risk that the fact finder will assume counsel was trying to hide something. When the examiner has a valid explanation ready, "Would you like me to explain?" can be a very effective way to turn the tables on opposing counsel.

*Question 4: No guarantee patient will not be re-injured*
**Question:** You released the examinee to return to full-time employment. Can you guarantee that he will not be re-injured when he returns to work?

**Reply 1 (Evasive):** Do you mean re-injured right away or at some time in the future?
**Reply 2 (Aggressive):** Medicine is an art and a science. If you want guarantees, you should go to Walmart.
**Reply 3 (Artful):** It is my opinion that he is medically fit to return to work at this time. However, as I stated in my report, page 7, there is no guarantee that he will not be re-injured once he returns to work. The consensus of the medical literature now recommends that patients with low back problems

return to work as quickly as possible, even when they have some ongoing symptoms. Would you like me to explain the studies?

**Lesson:** Counsel here is trying to show several things to the fact finder. First, that the examiner will not swear under oath that the examinee will not be re-injured. Second, that the examiner is so concerned about the risk of re-injury he has put a disclaimer in his IME report. While most fact finders are sophisticated enough to know that physicians do not guarantee anything, this question raises the specter of re-injury. The more the examiner is forced to backpedal on the safety of return to work, the less attractive the option becomes for the fact finder preparing a written decision.

- The *evasive* reply invites extended cross-examination on both areas suggested by the examiner—"right away" and "some time in the future."
- The *aggressive* reply is offensive and is the type of response cross-examination counsel hopes for.
- The *artful* reply answers the question, cites the statement in the IME report, and offers to provide a scientific basis for the return-to-work opinion. Counsel will be very reluctant to ask for the studies.

***Question 5: Income from IMEs***
**Question:** What was your income in the last 12 months from performing IMEs?

**Reply 1 (Evasive):** Do you mean net or gross?
**Reply 2 (Evasive):** I don't really know. My spouse handles the billing and collections.
**Reply 3 (Artful):** Approximately $40,000, gross.

**Lesson:** Counsel here is usually not overly concerned with the actual amount earned doing IMEs. She is, in fact, trying to rattle the examiner and force him into a mistake or into a defensive posture.

- The first *evasive* answer will lead to at least two additional questions about net and gross, and perhaps an explanation of the difference. The more counsel can get the examiner to talk about money and the high cost of doing business, e.g., overhead, the more the examiner may reveal himself to be highly motivated by money, new business, and repeat business.
- The second *evasive* reply is exactly the reply counsel is trying to elicit. With this reply, counsel can inquire into why this examiner is the only person who doesn't know how much he is earning. While the reply may be truthful, it is not believable and

will be met with suspicion by the fact finder, who knows exactly how much his gross salary is, the deductions taken, and how many years, months, days, and hours he has left until he is eligible for retirement.

- This simple and direct *artful* reply is truthful, informed, and will force counsel to move on. Examiners should be prepared to answer this question in a direct fashion. That is, they need to know how much money they are making from their IME practices.

***Question 6: Definitions of causation and apportionment terms***

**Question:** When you opined on causation and apportionment in your report, you used the terms "precipitation," "acceleration," "aggravation," "recurrence," and "exacerbation." Could you define these terms?

**Reply 1 (Novice):** Well, the term "aggravation" means a worsening of a condition and so does "exacerbation." What were the other terms you mentioned?
**Reply 2 (Aggressive):** Is this an open-book exam, Counselor, or are you the only one who can read the answers off a piece of paper?
**Reply 3 (Artful):** Yes. When I use the term "precipitation," I mean an injury or exposure causes a "latent" or potential disease to become manifest. "Acceleration" is an injury or exposure which hastens clinical appearance of an underlying disease process. "Aggravation" is a permanent worsening of a prior condition by a particular event or exposure. "Exacerbation" is a temporary worsening of a prior condition by exposure or injury, and "recurrences" are signs of symptoms attributable to a prior illness or injury that occur in the absence of a new provocative event.

**Lesson:** Counsel here is trying to trip up the examiner by asking him to define medical-legal terms that the examiner used in his report. Examiners need to be able to define every term they use in their reports in a simple and direct fashion. Using terms that one cannot define and distinguish is a prescription for disaster. Note that the definitions of these terms may vary from text to text and from jurisdiction to jurisdiction. The above definitions are from *Disability Evaluation,* second edition, Demeter, Mosby 2003 (p. 99). Contrast these definitions with those found in the AMA *Guides,* fifth edition, and other texts.

- The *novice* reply indicates that the examiner is not familiar with these terms. He can expect counsel to question him until he either makes a crucial mistake or admits he cannot define the terms he used in the report.
- The *aggressive* reply is non-responsive and will lead to additional questioning. For instance, "Does that mean you don't

know the answer or that you know it but don't want to tell us what it is?"

- The *artful* reply indicates that the examiner is familiar with the terms he used in his report and is prepared to discuss them if pushed by counsel.

***Question 7: Different editions of* Guides, *different impairment ratings***
**Question:** Using the fourth edition of the AMA *Guides,* you rated lumbar radiculopathy at 10% of the whole person, using the fifth edition of the AMA *Guides,* you rated the same condition at 5% impairment of the whole person. If the sixth edition says it's 1%, is that how you will rate lumbar radiculopathy in the future?

**Reply 1 (Novice):** Yes, I guess I will.
**Reply 2 (Evasive):** I will face that problem if and when the *Guides* changes in the sixth edition.
**Reply 3 (Artful):** In this case, the examinee's radiculopathy resolved with conservative non-surgical treatment. In the fifth edition, using the DRE method, the rating is done when the examinee reached maximum medical improvement. This accounts for the difference between the 10% in the fourth edition and the 5% in the fifth edition. Since the sixth edition is not available, I can't answer that question.

**Lesson:** Counsel here is trying to show that the examiner blindly "follows the book" when doing impairment ratings using the AMA *Guides*. The line of questioning leads to asking the examiner if there is any number that the AMA *Guides* would use that the examiner would not follow. For more information on questioning on impairment rating evaluations, please see Section 10.13.

- The *novice* reply falls directly into the trap set by counsel. The examiner will have to eventually admit he "follows the book" using little or no discretion. More importantly, he may also have to admit that the ratings in the book may bear no relationship to reality.
- The *evasive* reply will lead to additional questioning. Note how the examiner did not say that he would not follow the 1% rating.
- The *artful* reply gives a reasoned explanation to the real question asked—why 10% under the fourth edition and 5% under the fifth edition? Refusing to answer a hypothetical question posed as a factual question is legitimate. *NOTE:* The analysis for the artful reply is derived from *The Guides Casebook*, second edition, Brigham, AMA Press 2002, Case 15-6, (pp. 153-157).

***Question 8: Secret observation of examinee entering and leaving examiner's office***

**Question:** You based your opinion on your observation of the examinee entering and leaving your office?

**Reply 1 (Novice):** I couldn't help seeing what I saw.
**Reply 2 (Aggressive):** If your client didn't want to be caught, he should have either told the truth or been more careful.
**Reply 3 (Artful):** It was one of the factors I considered. I also considered my review of the records, the history, my examination, and the diagnostic test results before I formed my opinion.

**Lesson:** Counsel here is trying to imply that the examiner was lying in wait to try to "catch" the examinee in a discrepancy between what he stated during his examination and his true state. A classic example would be an examinee who alleged severe knee or leg problems during the examination and, once it was over, ran down the office steps two at a time. If counsel can get the examiner to act defensively, the fact finder may start to question whether the personal observation was "fair play" or a "trap" set by the examiner, who is a bought-and-paid-for agent of the insurance company. In fact, many experts consider personal observation of the examinee a legitimate and important function of the examination.

> The IME physician and the office staff, if possible, should observe the patient entering and leaving the examination room or the clinic to assess whether the patient's symptoms or reaction to his or her physical condition changes or is inconsistent with the presentation during the physical examination. For example, an observation that a patient who limps only in the examination room but not on the way in or out of the clinic should be included in the IME report under the physical observation section.[1]

For more information on the potential pitfalls resulting from "spying" on an examinee, please see Example 8.53.

- The *novice* reply is defensive and invites questioning about whether the physician accidentally observes all of the examinees.
- The *aggressive* reply makes the examiner sound like a bought-and-paid-for agent of the insurance company (like a surveillance company) involved in a cat and mouse game with the examinee.
- The *artful* reply is simple and direct and not defensive. In addition, it reinforces the numerous other legitimate reasons that reinforce the examiner's opinions.

---

[1] Grace, *Independent Medical Evaluations* (American Academy of Orthopedic Surgeons, 2001) p. 9.

***Question 9:* Dictionary of Occupational Titles *and other definitions***
**Question:** Your IME report indicates that the examinee can return to medium work. How much can he lift and how often can he do this in an eight-hour day?

**Reply 1 (Novice):** Not too much—as tolerated.
**Reply 2 (Aggressive):** The examinee is a finish carpenter. If you ever had one of these guys working on your house, you would know, Counsel, the heaviest thing they lift is their paycheck.
**Reply 3 (Artful):** The examinee can lift up to 50 lbs. occasionally (defined as less than 1/3 of the workday or sometimes described as 1 to 100 lifts), up to 20 lbs. frequently (defined as 1/3 to 2/3 of the workday or sometimes described as 101 to 500 lifts), and constantly up to 10 lbs. (defined as 100% of the workday or sometimes described as more than 500 lifts). The total number of lifts also depends on the shape and location of the object being lifted and the environment in which the lifting occurs.

**Lesson:** IME examiners who use medical-legal terms of art or "magic words" should be familiar with their meanings and be able to explain them. Although the U.S. Department of Labor *Dictionary of Occupational Titles,* fourth edition (1986), is somewhat out of date, it is still used by IME examiners to evaluate lifting and carrying at work. Examiners should be prepared to be questioned on the meanings of the terms "sedentary," "light," "medium," "heavy," and "very heavy work" if used in their reports. As always, an examiner should not use any term in her report that she cannot simply, directly, and readily explain during cross-examination. For more information on work capacity opinions and the *Dictionary of Occupational Titles*, please see Section 10.14.

- The *novice* reply evidences that the examiner is not familiar with the technical meaning of these terms.
- The *aggressive* reply is offensive and is unlikely to win over the fact finder unless he himself is undertaking remodeling work.
- The *artful* reply indicates that the examiner is very familiar with the technical meaning of the term and reinforces the examiner's skills, experience, and expertise.

***Question 10: Independent memory of the examinee***
**Question:** In your examination, you don't list the height or weight of the examinee. Do you have an independent recollection of the examinee?

**Reply 1 (Novice):** I see so many examinees for IMEs, it's hard to place this one.
**Reply 2 (Evasive):** What's the difference how tall she was and how much she weighed? She had a hand injury.

**Reply 3 (Artful):** Yes, I do. We requested permission to photocopy her driver's license to identify the examinee. Here is a copy of the picture—5'4", 117 pounds.

**Lesson:** Counsel here is trying to point out to the fact finder that the examiner sees so many IME claimants that she can't even remember who she is testifying about. The effect of this admission is that the examiner who has no independent recollection of the examinee has to rely exclusively on her report when testifying. Any facts not in the report will be difficult, if not impossible, to assert. Some examiners take a digital photo of the examinee and incorporate this into the report. This is of benefit to the client and can also help refresh the memory of the examiner prior to testifying.

- The *novice* reply falls directly into the trap of opposing counsel.
- The *evasive* reply is argumentative and invites additional questioning: "I take that as a no. You don't have an independent recollection of the examinee?"
- The *artful* reply makes use of the examinee's photo to refresh the recollection of the examiner. Supplying the height and weight lessens the impact of having omitted it from the IME report.

***Question 11: Expert in determining the truth?***
**Question:** Do you believe the examinee's complaints of severe pain?

**Reply 1 (Direct):** I have no way of really knowing.
**Reply 2 (Aggressive):** Isn't it curious how almost all disability claimants say they are in severe pain?
**Reply 3 (Artful):** I do believe that the examinee has some residual pain, but the pain complaints were disproportional to the objective clinical findings.

**Lesson:** Counsel here is trying to either gain an admission from the examiner that the claimant has severe pain or that the examiner does not believe the claimant is telling the truth. Many experts advise examiners not to be dragged into the truth vs. lying controversy. Examiners have specific and extensive medical training, but they are not human lie detectors.

> The IME physician should not judge whether the examinee is telling the truth or lying about his or her complaints. Some people are consummate liars, others are terrible truth-tellers, and there are a whole lot of people in between. The IME physician does not have enough time during the evaluation to make these distinctions or any judgments about honesty with any degree of accuracy.[2]

---

[2] Ibid., p. 7.

For more information on the dangers of becoming an expert in "the truth," please see Section 11.17.

- The *direct* reply is honest and straightforward. It opens up the examiner to a line of questioning that, "If the examinee is telling the truth, he is disabled, correct?"
- The *aggressive* reply is offensive and evidences a clear defense bias on behalf of the examiner.
- The *artful* reply is honest and avoids getting dragged into the truth-telling business. The examiner states the factors upon which his opinion is based and does not try to figure out if the examinee is telling the truth.

***Question 12: Last time treated a patient***
**Question:** When was the last time you actually treated a patient, Doctor?

**Reply 1 (Novice):** I don't treat patients. I perform insurance exams on examinees.
**Reply 2 (Defensive):** I volunteer once a year at the medical tent for our local marathon. Can I count that?
**Reply 3 (Artful):** Approximately two years ago, when I retired after 37 years of orthopedic surgery. I couldn't do surgery anymore because of arthritis in my hand.

**Lesson:** Counsel here is trying to show the fact finder that the examiner is "not really a doctor" in the traditional sense of the word. Physicians who continue to see patients regularly generally have more credibility than so-called "IME doctors" who only do forensic work.

**Q.** When was the last time you actually treated a patient?
**A.** About 45 minutes ago.

Physicians who are full-time IME examiners may be nonplussed by the question and get defensive. This is exactly what counsel is trying to achieve. The more defensive the examiner gets, the more suspicious the fact finder becomes.

- The *novice* reply is exactly the point counsel is trying to make for the fact finder.
- The *defensive* reply is damaging because when the examiner has to search his memory for the name of a person he could say he treated, he is tacitly admitting two things. First, that he really doesn't treat patients anymore, and, second (and even more damaging), that this is a really bad thing to admit.
- The *artful* reply is simple, direct, and explains to the fact finder

that the examiner probably treated thousands of patients over 37 years and was forced to stop practicing because of a physical disability.

***Question 13: Do you keep up with the literature?***
**Question:** Do you keep up with the medical literature on fibromyalgia?

**Reply 1 (Novice):** Not really.
**Reply 2 (Novice):** Nothing of significance has been published since the 1990 criteria from the *American College of Rheumatology.*
**Reply 3 (Artful):** I continue to read about this disorder as well as others.

**Lesson:** Here counsel is trying to either get the examiner to admit that she is not current and thus her opinion on the medical condition is suspect, or, alternatively, that she keeps current. If the examiner is not current, counsel can pound away at her on cross-examination about all the new articles and literature she is unaware of and how they may impact her opinion on causation and disability. Alternatively, if the examiner states that she is current, she may then be faced with a computer-generated list of 100 articles on the topic and be asked which ones she has read.

- The first *novice* reply is a significant and potentially devastating admission by an examiner who is supposed to be a medical expert.
- The second *novice* reply shows the examiner has some familiarity with the literature, but it invites cross-examination regarding each and every article and book written since 1990.
- The *artful* reply indicates that the examiner reads some of the literature and gently reminds the fact finder that medicine is a very large topic on which to keep current. If pressed further, the examiner can state that thousands of medical journals are published each year and it is not practical to read them all.

***Question 14: Result of unfavorable opinions on future referrals***
**Question:** How many unfavorable IMEs would it take before this insurance company stopped using you?

**Reply 1 (Novice):** I am not sure, maybe one or two.
**Reply 2 (Aggressive):** How would I know that? Why don't you ask the insurance company?
**Reply 3 (Artful):** I call these IMEs as I see them. I don't concern myself with what you characterize as favorable or unfavorable IMEs.

**Lesson:** Here counsel is trying to plant a seed of doubt with the fact finder. He would like the fact finder to say to herself, "If he issued 'too many' unfavorable reports, the insurance company would definitely drop him." If counsel can make that connection with the fact finder, the questions become "How many is too many?" and "Is this one of them?"

- The *novice* reply makes the case counsel is trying to drive home.
- The *aggressive* reply feels good to say, but it concedes by omission that there is a number not to be exceeded. If such a number exists and the examiner doesn't even know what it is, he would err on the side of caution and not take a chance with unfavorable reports.
- The *artful* reply refuses to play the numbers game with counsel and makes two important points for the fact finder. First, that the examiner is honest and calls them as he sees them. Second, that the characterization of favorable or unfavorable may be simplistic or simply unfair.

***Question 15: Number of IMEs in a day***
**Question:** When you do IMEs at Efficient IME, Inc., how many do you do a day?

**Reply 1 (Direct):** Anywhere from five to fifteen a day.
**Reply 2 (Aggressive):** As many as they can schedule that day.
**Reply 3 (Artful):** I limit them to scheduling five per day.

**Lesson:** Counsel here is trying to portray the process of doing IMEs at an IME company as a cold, efficient, and sometimes sordid business. The object is to try to show that the business and the physician are trying to make as much money as possible, as quickly as possible, with as little work as possible. Counsel will have the physician describe the set-up where the exams took place, the fact that he is given only a few minutes to review the records, perform the exam, and dictate his report. If counsel can convey this "IME factory"-type of atmosphere, the credibility of the examiner and the weight given to his report will be severely limited.

- The *direct* reply is honest and opens up the examiner to the line of attack listed in the above lesson. Can an IME examiner be accurate, complete, and unbiased doing five to fifteen IMEs a day for an IME company? Of course, depending on the complexities at issue, the answer could very well be "yes."
- The *aggressive* reply helps make the case that money is the name of the game and all else is secondary.
- The *artful* reply evidences that the examiner has set up professional requirements and limits and is at least attempting to set boundaries with the IME company. This will serve him well when he is cross-examined about his relationship with the IME

company. If he can honestly say that the IME company would like to set up ten a day, but he limits them to five, this will help to re-establish his credibility and independence.

***Question 16: Scientific and medical studies supporting opinion***

**Question:** What scientific or medical studies support the opinion you expressed in your IME report?

**Reply 1 (Novice):** None that I know of.
**Reply 2 (Aggressive):** This is a simple cervical disc disease case. What additional support do I need?
**Reply 3 (Artful):** Two studies come to mind:

1. Simeone, "Surgical Management of Cervical Disc Disease," *Seminars Spine Surgery* (1989), and
2. Burden, "Conservative Treatment of Cervical Disc Disease," *Seminars Spine Surgery* (1989).

**Lesson:** Here counsel is trying to point out to the fact finder that there is rarely a scientific or medical study that supports the opinion expressed by the examiner.

> The lack of scientific certainty in regard to causation decisions in musculoskeletal impairment and disability cases explains why in the same case (same facts), well-qualified physicians testify that work definitely caused an employee's problem, while other equally well-qualified physicians testify that there is no scientific way to say that the employee's job caused the problem in question. This obviously contradictory testimony by two seemingly well-qualified IME physicians causes the non-physicians involved to conclude that either one or both of the physicians are ignorant of the science of epidemiology and causation, or that one or both are biased.[3]

For more information on citing authority to support findings and conclusions in an IME report, please see Chapter 9.

- The *novice* makes the exact point that counsel is trying to drive home.
- The *aggressive* reply is potentially offensive for calling it a simple matter and for referring to it as a "case." Either or both of these phrases could adversely affect the fact finder.
- The *artful* reply makes the point that the examiner is familiar with the supportive medical literature. This may make the difference in a close "case."

[3] Ibid., pp. 67–68.

***Question 17: Treating patients and examinees differently***
**Question:** Do you treat examinees present for IMEs the same way you treat your own patients?

**Reply 1 (Novice):** Yes, I do.
**Reply 2 (Aggressive):** I probably treat the examinees better.
**Reply 3 (Artful):** I treat both with dignity and respect. The goal for patients is treatment, which is different for examinees who I don't treat, but evaluate.

**Lesson:** Counsel here is trying to get the fact finder to think how she would like to be treated if she were an examinee or patient of the examiner. Contrasting the manner of treatment can be effective despite the fact that patients are seen to be treated and examinees are seen to be evaluated. Forcing the examiner to make artificial distinctions and excuses for different levels of service can also be an effective cross-examination technique.

- The *novice* reply opens the examiner up to extensive questioning by counsel. Inquiries will include if the examiner observes his patients coming and going from his office, performs distraction tests to question veracity, searches for and documents all inconsistencies, deals with issues of causation, malingering, etc. It also overlooks the deliberate mischaracterization of "treating examinees."
- The *aggressive* reply is too clever and flippant to be effective. The fact finder is probably thinking "I'd hate to see how he treats his patients if this is the way he treats examinees." The examiner may be forced to either explain the reply or to admit it was just an exaggeration.
- The *artful* reply makes it clear that both patients and examinees are treated with dignity and respect. It also makes the important distinction between treatment and evaluation.

***Question 18: Past testimony favorable to "other" side***
**Question:** When was the last time you found that an examinee was permanently or totally disabled due to a work-related injury?

**Reply 1 (Novice):** I think I did the last time I did an exam for a plaintiff seven years ago.
**Reply 2 (Aggressive):** I can't testify that they are permanently and totally disabled if they aren't, Counsel.
**Reply 3 (Artful):** Approximately three years ago in the *Leahy* claim.

**Lesson:** Counsel here is trying to drive home two points. First, the examiner rarely, if ever, finds the examinee permanently and totally disabled due to a compensable injury. Second, even if he did so find, the insurance company would never have him testify to this opinion.

Counsel is trying to get the fact finder to think to himself, "This doctor has been before me dozens of times and never testified to anything even close to that."

- The *novice* reply helps drive home the point that when testifying for insurers, examiners rarely find the claimant permanently and totally disabled. On the other hand, when testifying for plaintiffs, this kind of testimony is not at all unusual. The implication is clear: "He who pays, gets the opinion."
- The *aggressive* reply is too strident to be effective. The use of the word "they" will be offensive to many fact finders. This examiner will be open to questions about why in 2,500 IMEs he has never found one permanently and totally disabled client. The implication is powerful. Lying and saying he did so will seal the examiner's fate when he is asked to name the claimant or to produce the file.
- The *artful* reply concedes it has been some time, but it does include a specific reference. If asked why it has been three years, the examiner could explain he is reluctant to "sentence" people to lifetime disability and would prefer to try to help get them back to work.

***Question 19: Contact with insurer***

**Question:** Could you tell us all the contacts you or your staff have had with the insurance company concerning this claim?

**Reply 1 (Novice):** It was just the initial phone call, the letter sending along the records, a couple of calls for the adjuster, and the date she dropped off the surveillance videos. I also gave them an oral report.
**Reply 2 (Jail):** None that I know of.
**Reply 3 (Artful):** All contact has been in writing. The letter with the records, the questions to be answered, and my report back to them. These have all been produced to you already.

**Lesson:** Counsel here is trying to show that the examiner has met and talked to the insurer on many occasions and is in fact part of the "litigation team." Counsel is trying to plant the seed with the fact finder that either the contact was improper or that it has influenced the IME report. Please see Chapter 14 on the dangers of close contact with the referral source.

- The *novice* reply helps connect the dots for the fact finder so that the picture of close cooperation is clearly painted.
- The *jail* reply is an outright lie and will be exposed as such. It would be an extremely rare case in which there was no contact

(e.g., letters, faxes, e-mails, or calls).

- The *artful* reply makes the point that there is no sinister conspiracy and that, in fact, everything is in writing and open to discovery and inspection.

***Question 20: Computer-generated standard language***

**Question:** What portions of your 24-page IME report are computer-generated standard language that you use over and over again?

**Reply 1 (Novice):** Not too much.
**Reply 2 (Evasive):** Each claim is different and I dictate a new report each time.
**Reply 3 (Artful):** The introduction, my qualifications, and the disclosure statement at the end are standard language that I use in most reports as applicable.

**Lesson:** Counsel here is trying to paint the picture of a cookie-cutter operation in which computer-generated paragraphs and pages are used over and over again by the examiner in a rush to the same or similar conclusions. While there is nothing inherently wrong with some standard language, the question becomes how much is too much? If the fact finder and the examiner are talking about standard language, counsel has achieved his goal. For more information regarding the dangers of computer-generated standard language and templates, please see Section 11.20.

- The *novice* reply will invite a line-by-line, paragraph-by-paragraph, page-by-page review of the report. The examiner will be forced to admit that he was mistaken and large portions of the report are standard.
- The *evasive* reply is not accurate and will be proven so by counsel. How will the examiner explain the 1½ pages of general information on fibromyalgia in the report? Can he maintain that he dictates a new 1½-page report for each fibromyalgia claim? Is this claim credible? What happens when he is confronted with numerous past reports containing the same exact language?
- The *artful* reply is simple and direct and makes a small concession about some standard language. The examiner is not evasive and is more credible, not less, after this reply.

***Question 21: Causation for mental disorder***

**Question:** Is the examinee's depression that you mention in your IME report causally related to his workers' compensation injury?

**Reply 1 (Novice):** Yes, it is.
**Reply 2 (Evasive):** It might be.
**Reply 3 (Artful):** As I am not a psychiatrist, this is outside my area of expertise.

**Lesson:** Counsel here is trying to use the IME examiner's passing comment, "the examinee evidences depression," to help make a significant part of his case. If the examiner helps tie in the depression, the insurer could be liable for all of the reasonable and necessary medical treatment for the depression and also weekly workers' compensation benefits if the depression worsens. This one passing comment and the reply to this question could have a major impact on the value and course of the claim.

- The *novice* reply is a very significant admission that could cost the insurer thousands or hundreds of thousands of dollars.
- The *evasive* reply opens up the examiner to an extensive line of questioning. Counsel will try to extract an admission that the examiner is not sure if it is or is not related. This type of admission may be enough to "tip the scales" in favor of the claimant on this issue.
- The *artful* reply keeps the examiner from being drawn into an area where:

    - he is not an expert,
    - he has not formed an opinion, and
    - he does not want to express an opinion.

Counsel is likely to try to draw the examiner into this area again, but the experienced examiner will be vigilant in his refusal. The examiner understands that answering just one question on this topic will ensnare him into this controversy.

***Question 22: Pain and concentration***
**Question:** How much will the examinee's pain affect his ability to concentrate at work?

**Reply 1 (Novice):** Not too much.
**Reply 2 (Aggressive):** Let's get him back to work and see.
**Reply 3 (Artful):** The examinee said he was in pain when I examined him and when I administered a battery of tests for 1½ hours. His concentration was excellent. I do not feel his pain will affect his ability to concentrate.

**Lesson:** Counsel here is trying to tell the fact finder that a person in chronic pain may have great difficulty in concentrating on the job. The significance of this fact is greatly enhanced if concentration is necessary for the job to be done well and safely. This is the kind of point fact finders use to justify the examinee's inability to return to former employment.

- The *novice* reply opens the floodgates to the numbers game (e.g., 10%, 20%, 50%, etc.). Once the examiner admits that concentration will be impacted, the damage is done. The only question then becomes how severe is the damage?
- The *aggressive* reply is direct and has some logic to it. It does not dispute the fact that concentration may be affected. This is a major unintentional concession.
- The *artful* reply does not buy into the characterization of the question by counsel (e.g., not "if it will impact," but "how much it will impact"). This is crucial for an effective response. The reply is direct and is tied into the performance the examiner personally observed. This reply is difficult to overcome with generalities.

***Question 23: HIPAA and reports***

**Question:** Why didn't you follow the HIPAA law and regulations and take care to limit the PHI used?

**Reply 1 (Novice):** Does HIPAA apply to IME reports? If I did something wrong, I am sorry.
**Reply 2 (Aggressive):** What the hell is PHI?
**Reply 3 (Artful):** I did follow HIPAA and put the Protected Health Information, or PHI, both the social history and family history, in a separate appendix to my report.

**Lesson:** As with any new sweeping legislation, there are ambiguities and contradictions present with HIPAA. Clarification of these will be an evolving process that will occur over years through legal and regulatory decisions.

The HIPAA privacy rule does impact workers' compensation. Although workers' compensation insurers, workers' compensation administrative agencies, or employers are exempted from the privacy rule, a physician can be held liable as a covered entity for the improper disclosure of health information to insurers and other entities in the workers' compensation system.

However, covered entities (physicians) are permitted to disclose protected health information for such purposes as authorized by, and to the extent necessary to comply with, workers' compensation law under 45 CFR 164.512(l). In addition, the Privacy Rule generally permits covered entities to disclose protected health information in the course of any judicial or administrative proceeding in response to a court order, subpoena, or other lawful process under 45 CFR 164.512(e).

Furthermore, there are provisions under 45 CFR 164.530 for safeguards. These provide that the covered entity must reasonably safeguard health information to limit incidental uses or disclosures made pursuant to otherwise permitted or required uses for disclosure, and must mitigate, to the extent possible, any harmful effect that is known to the covered entity of a use or disclosure of protected health information. As such, if the provider has reason to expect that health information disclosed might be provided to and utilized by others (e.g., an employer) these safeguards may be applicable.

- The *novice* reply admits unfamiliarity with HIPAA, is defensive, and does not inspire confidence.
- The *aggressive* reply is offensive and may not sit well with the fact finder.
- The *artful* reply evidences some knowledge of HIPAA and an attempt to comply.

***Question 24: Sexual arousal***
**Question:** How often have you been sexually aroused by an examinee?

**Reply 1 (Novice):** Not too often. Have you seen what most of these people look like?
**Reply 2 (Sarcastic):** Not often enough.
**Reply 3 (Artful):** Never. I'm a medical professional, and the examinee is just that to me, a person to be examined. 80% of the examinees I see are men.

**Lesson:** This is a real cheap shot. Counsel here is trying to get the examiner flustered, upset, or otherwise distracted by asking an off-the-wall question. This would almost always occur at a deposition where no judge would be present. While the question bears no relationship to the issues, it usually does have its desired effect, especially if it is the first question asked in the deposition.

- The *novice* reply is an admission that may offend the sensibilities of some fact finders.
- The *sarcastic* reply is funny, but it makes the examiner seem less professional and dignified.
- The *artful* reply is a strong response that reinforces the professionalism of the examiner.

***Question 25: Biased toward getting employees back to work***
**Question:** You like to get employees back to work as soon as possible, correct?

**Reply 1 (Novice):** Yes, I do.
**Reply 2 (Aggressive):** Most employees need the encouragement, especially if they have a lawyer.
**Reply 3 (Artful):** I like to help get people back to work when they can return to work and do the job, yes.

**Lesson:** Counsel here is trying to paint the picture of a hard-nosed examiner who tries to push employees back to work before they are ready. If counsel can show the fact finder that this is the examiner's propensity, it will damage the credibility of the examiner.

- The *novice* reply falls into the "as soon as possible" trap of counsel.
- The *aggressive* reply demonstrates a clear bias by the examiner.
- The *artful* reply ties the return to work to the ability to work. If pressed further, the examiner can cite the Canadian Medical Association's policy statement: "Prolonged absence from one's normal roles, including absence from the workplace, is detrimental to a person's mental, physical, and social well-being…."[4]

***Question 26: Complaints against examiner***
**Question:** How many complaints have been filed against you as an independent medical examiner?

**Reply 1 (Novice):** Which ones do you mean? Complaints from examinees, insurers, judges, or the workers' compensation division?
**Reply 2 (Evasive):** What do you mean by complaints?
**Reply 3 (Artful):** Two in the last 20 years.

**Lesson:** Counsel here is trying to accomplish three things with this question.

1. Shake up the examiner.
2. Get the examiner talking about complaints filed against him.
3. Divert attention away from the IME report.

- The *novice* reply provides additional information with which to cross-examine the examiner. Counsel will likely say, "Let's take them one at a time."
- The *evasive* reply is just postponing the inevitable. Trying to say he doesn't know what a "complaint" is may not sit well with the fact finder.

---

[4] "The Physician's Role in Helping Patients Return to Work After Illness or Injury," *Canadian Medical Association Journal,* 156:680 A-F (1997).

- The *artful* reply is simple and direct and will force counsel to either move on or run the risk of further inquiry. Further questioning could elicit a response such as this: "Both were by disgruntled examinees and were summarily dismissed."

***Question 27: Malpractice insurance***
**Question:** Do you carry malpractice insurance for your IME business?

**Reply 1 (Novice):** I didn't know it was available. Could I talk to you about that later?
**Reply 2 (Aggressive):** I have no reason to. I did not do anything wrong.
**Reply 3 (Artful):** I have an errors and omissions policy for independent medical evaluations that I do. I don't have an "IME business."

**Lesson:** Counsel is trying to raise doubts in the mind of the examiner and, more importantly, in the mind of the fact finder. Questions that may arise are: "Should he carry this insurance?," "Does he have a separate IME business?," and "Why does he need insurance?"

- The *novice* reply evidences a lack of knowledge, experience, and sophistication.
- The *aggressive* reply is arrogant and offensive.
- The *artful* reply acknowledges his coverage and corrects the mischaracterization of the "IME business."

# Chapter 18 Model Reports[1]

**Report #1: Personal Injury—Upper Extremity Injuries**

This report is most notable for the following.

- A well-drafted first page with easy-to-read identifying information, a summary of the diagnoses, and page references to other sections of the report.
- Superb formatting makes the report easy to read.
- Good use of headnotes. It's easy to find the information the reader is looking for.
- Digital images of the examinee's injured finger and diagnostic studies incorporated into the report. A picture says a thousand words. The digital images add greatly to the report.
- It is a well-written report using measured, objective language. The examining physician does not exaggerate or take pot shots at the examinee. The issues of symptom magnification and inconsistencies in the history provided are dealt with professionally and in a non-judgmental manner.
- Easy-to-read, detailed, well-formatted review of the available medical records.

While this is an excellent report, all reports can be improved. Areas of possible improvement follow.

- This examiner should be careful with the boilerplate language in the report. See especially the "Disclosure Statement" at the end of the report. This language may not be appropriate in every case, thus the examiner should review this language in each report prior to signing the report.
- Some of the conclusions would be stronger if they were buttressed with reasoning. For example, the examiner's opinion that the prognosis was "fair" would have been stronger if the examiner explicitly stated why the prognosis was "fair" and not "poor" or "good."
- The times stated in the report are all expressed in five-minute intervals. This is probably not accurate. It would be better to clearly state that the times are "approximate" or to precisely state the times to the exact minute. This will make the examiner appear more precise and his opinions will appear more believable.

---

[1] The names and other information in the following reports have been changed.

## Independent Medical Examination

| | |
|---|---|
| Examinee: | Martha Jane Formaggio |
| Identification Number: | 123456789 |
| Date of Birth: | 01/24/40 |
| Date of Examination: | 04/25/01 |
| Examining Physician: | Thomas S. Eagan, M.D., P.C. |
| Examination Location: | 215 County Highway 128, Gloversville, NY 12078 |
| Date of Injury: | 11/26/99 |
| Client Organization: | Buntz Claims Services, Ltd. |
| Referral Source: | Judy Buntz |
| Date Exam Requested: | 04/06/01 |

### Summary

Diagnosis

1. Dislocation Right Shoulder.
2. Lower Brachial Plexus Injury Right Shoulder.
3. Chip Fracture Nasal Bone.
4. Diabetes.
5. Hypertension.
6. Morbid Obesity.
7. Degenerative Arthritis Right Shoulder (pre-existing).
8. Rotator Cuff Tear Right Shoulder.
9. Fracture Left Clavicle.
10. Cervical Spondylosis.
11. Carpal Tunnel Syndrome Right.



### Introduction

This 61-year-old, right-handed woman was referred for an independent medical evaluation (IME) by the above client. The independent medical examination process was explained to the examinee, and she understands that no patient/treating physician relationship was established. Ms. Formaggio was advised that the information provided will not be confidential and a report will be sent to the requesting client. Informed consent was obtained with signed permission. This consent included the obtaining of photographs during the examination.

Ms. Formaggio arrived at 3:15 PM, the interview commenced at 4:10 PM, followed by the physical examination, which started at 4:45 PM and was completed by 5:10 PM. Ms. Formaggio was cooperative. History was provided by the examinee, who was a fair historian. The information she provided was not always consistent with the medical records provided.

Accompanying Ms. Formaggio was Jayne, her daughter, who remained in the examining room the entire time. A questionnaire and pain inventories were partially completed by the examinee.

A staff member, Deborah, was present throughout the physical examination. Ms. Formaggio reported no difficulties occurring during the examination.

The client provided the following clinical records: Everett Hospital, Joseph Arsenault, MD, John Flogger, MD, Robert Lancaster, MD, Acton Medical Center Hospital, Rosa Sanders, MD, Frederick Evers, MD, Edward Laramy, MD, Charles Davies, MD, Marc Smith, MD, Dr. John Casazza, Dr. Everett Forester, Eric Zigler, MD, Mark Browning, MD, Andrea Beachum, MD, SmithKline Beecham, Pedro Berchowitzc, MD, Donald Winer, MD, Gerald Williamson, MD, Philip Benson, MD, Montclaire Psychiatric Associates, Jennifer Levon, MD, Elizabeth Sanders, MD, Michele Daniels, MSN, Kathleen Vickers, MD, and Medical Acupuncture Clinic.

These records were carefully reviewed. No medical records subsequent to 03/09/01 were available for review.

## Medical Record Review

Type of Encounter: C=Consult, H=Hospital, I=IME/Impairment Assessment, M=Medical Visit, O=Operation, R=Report/Letter, P=PT/OT Visit, S=Diagnostic Study, X=X-ray (Imaging) Study, *=Other

| Date | Provider | Type | Summary |
|---|---|---|---|
| 11/26/99 | Prehospital Care Report | * | Pt states she tripped and fell landing on R shoulder....she can't feel her hand. |
| 11/26/99 | Everett Hospital | H | ...R shoulder pain... |
| 11/26/99 | Everett Hospital | H | ...diagnosis...R shoulder dislocation axillary nerve injury. |
| 11/26/99 | Arsenault, MD | X | Right Shoulder–Routine, Right Clavicle and Right |

| | | | |
|---|---|---|---|
| | | | Humerus…anterior dislocation…no…fracture… |
| 11/26/99 | Flogger, MD | X | Right Shoulder Routine. Normal position post reduction right humerus. Nasal Bones Routine. Chip fracture anterior aspect nasal bones. |
| 11/26/99 | Arsenault, MD | X | Right Ankle Routine.… no…fracture…no significant soft tissue swelling… |
| 11/26/99 | Arsenault, MD | X | Right Tibia/Fib Uni. Right Lower Leg.…no…fracture… |
| 11/27/99 | Everett Hospital | H | …R arm feeling "dead." |
| 11/27/99 | Everett Hospital | H | …no movement in RUE. Brachial Plexus injury. |
| 11/29/99 | Lancaster, MD | M | She had immediate numbness in the arm and it felt dead. …brachial plexus palsy secondary to a dislocation ...probably contused. |
| 11/29/99 | Lancaster, MD | M | …R breast tumor (benign). |
| 11/30/99 | Lancaster, MD | M | She has US Healthcare which we don't participate… She had gone to Acton Med Emergency…they are going to schedule her for an MRI.…she had almost complete brachial plexus neuropraxia. |
| 11/30/99 | Sanders, MD | X | Shoulder, Right-Routine. Degenerative changes of the AC joint.…irregularity about the greater tuberosity most likely from a previous trauma. |
| 11/30/99 | Sanders, MD | X | Spine Cervical 4-5 Views .…chronic disc disease at C5-C6… …fracture of the mid-shaft of the left clavicle. |
| 12/02/99 | Laramy, MD | S | MRI Shoulder-Right.…tear… supraspinatus tendon… …inferior labral…injury/tear .…tear…long head biceps… |
| 12/02/99 | Davies, MD | S | MRI Spine-Cervical. Spondylosis…biforaminal |

| | | | |
|---|---|---|---|
| | | | encroachment at C5-6… |
| 12/06/99 | Smith, MD | M | She…fell…had immediate pain as well as noticing that strength in the arm and sensation were just not there....lot of discomfort in the shoulder…can't move her hand… …can't lift her arm …no evidence of vascular injury…She does not volitionally move at all at the elbow or shoulder….no volitional movement of the hand….no sensation in the C6, C7, C8 or T1 distributions. I cannot elicit any deep tendon reflexes… MRI of the cervical spine… spondylotic changes… …brachial plexus injury… active Tinel's…suggests that there is at least some continuity of fibers in the brachial plexus. …wait and see how much of this returns. …plan…EMG's…five or six for this to be a valid test…I am hopeful that this is an injury that will improve on its own without any need for surgery. |
| 12/06/99 | Casazza, MD | M | …injury to the brachial plexus. |
| 12/08/99 | Casazza, MD | M | …MRI…tears of the rotator cuff… |
| 12/21/99 | Zigler, MD | M | …immediate severe pain in the right shoulder…severe electric shock-like pain down the right upper extremity…. pain and hyperesthesia in the forearm and hand…. MRI…full thickness tear of the supraspinatus tendon and…infraspinatus tendon. MRI…cervical spondylosis… |

| | | | |
|---|---|---|---|
| | | | borderline canal stenosis… …arthroscopic knee… bilateral carpal tunnel release. …history of an irregular heartbeat…chronic heartburn, hiatal hernia…good range of motion of the cervical spine… …patchy sensory loss in the right upper extremity, most dense in the ulnar distribution of the hand.…infraclavicular stretch/contusion injury of the brachial plexus…effects multiple cords and nerves ….arrange for evaluation in our anesthesia pain clinic for treatment of her severe neuropathic pain.…she will improve significantly in the proximal upper extremity, but the lower cord function may be most seriously impaired on a long term basis. |
| 12/21/99 | Browning, MD | * | Severe diffuse right brachial plexus injury, especially… lower trunk.…NCS and EMG findings indicate that the radial, musculocutaneous, median and ulnar nerves are in partial continuity. This has favorable prognosis implications. |
| 01/04/00 | Berchowitzc, MD | M | Brachial plexus injury especially of the lower cords including the ulnar nerve distribution, some involvement of the median nerve distribution. The radial nerve appears to be spared at least partially. Rotator cuff tear.…Gerald Williamson… …recommended rotator cuff repair surgery…recommend …rotator cuff repaired… |

| | | | |
|---|---|---|---|
| 01/04/00 | Winer, MD | X | Shoulder…Right….mild degenerative changes of the glenohumeral joint and of the acromioclavicular joint. Clavicle left. No clavicular fracture is seen. |
| 01/04/00 | Williamson, MD | M | …most of her ability to not raise her arm has to do with her rotator cuff and not her brachial plexus….her weakness in her shoulder is primarily the responsibility of her rotator cuff. |
| 01/12/00 | Benson, MD | S | MRI Right Shoulder. Rotator cuff tear which involves the supraspinatus tendon and a part of the infraspinatus tendon. |
| 01/21/00 | Berchowitzc, MD | M | …improved…biceps is 4/5…wrist extension is also about 3+-4/5….EDS and EDP function at the fingers which is improved….3/5 pronator strength, 3/5 supinator strength as well….hand is still somewhat numb to light touch throughout the median and ulnar nerve distributions…. MRI… Some of the brachial plexus nerves…appear to be normal in size…infraspinatus …torn…put her in touch with our hand therapists… |
| 02/02/00 | Williamson, MD | O | The biceps tendon was completely absent. We then identified the rotator cuff tear….two traction sutures…and mobilized…by bluntly lysing adhesions on the superficial surface. We then incised the rotator interval all the way to the base of the coracoid…also released the undersurface of the tendon |

| | | | |
|---|---|---|---|
| | | | and muscle belly by releasing the capsule just distal to the labrum…placed a longitudinal incision between supra and infraspinatus at the area of retraction… |
| 02/24/00 | Daniels, MSN/ Vickers, MD | M | …MRI performed on January 12, 2000, of the brachioplexus, revealed no gross abnormality of the right brachioplexus. …bilateral carpal release in the 1990's, irregular heartbeat… hypertension, chronic heartburn, hiatal hernia, diabetes…appendectomy…. chronic pain as the result of…right brachial plexus injury and status post rotator cuff tear. |
| 03/02/00 | Zigler, MD | M | …underwent operative repair of her right rotator cuff… progressive improvement in function of the right upper extremity.…recovered quite strong biceps and triceps strength, good supination and pronation, reasonably good wrist extension and wrist flexion…moderate improvement in median nerve function in the hand.…FCU now has 3+ function.… chronic pain in the ulnar aspect of the forearm and hand.…making excellent progress in terms of spontaneous recovery of her brachial plexus injury. |
| 03/06/00 | Williamson, MD | M | …passive range of motion is excellent. |
| 03/24/00 | Chisolm, MD | M | Right rotator cuff tear status post-repair. Right brachial plexopathy with main involvement of the lower |

| | | | |
|---|---|---|---|
| | | | trunk by exam and early EMG. |
| 03/31/00 | Sanders, MD | O | Colonoscopy; Upper Endoscopy…Duodenitis. |
| 04/07/00 | Browning, MD | * | EMG. Strength in the right was deltoid 3, extensor digitorum communis 5, ulnar hand muscles 3- and median hand muscles 2.…diminished pinprick perception over the inner 2/3 of the right hand and forearm. Right median motor studies were normal… prolonged median distal motor latency.…mild chronic denervation…axillary…musc ulocutaneous…radial … median…very severe denervation in ulnar muscles. Generalized brachial plexopathy…lower trunk most affected. …modest but defined improvement in ulnar nerve function… |
| 04/12/00 | Berchowitzc, MD | M | …weakness in extension and finger flexion is improved. …pain in her right hand.…3/5 strength in finger adduction. …positive Froment's sign. Two point discrimination is intact to approximately 5-6 mm spacing in a median and ulnar nerve distribution in the hand.…improvement with regard to her electrodiagnostic findings. This is quite reassuring…in terms of the regaining of strength, as well as for prognostic reasons. |
| 04/17/00 | Williamson, MD | M | …no lag sign with her arm at 90…fairly reasonable external rotation strength… |
| 06/19/00 | Williamson, MD | M | …active flexion to 90 degrees.…strength is actually a good 4/5. |

| | | | |
|---|---|---|---|
| 08/25/00 | Beachum, MD | M | ...complains of edema.... probably at this point due to her obesity... |
| 10/06/00 | Bird, MD | * | EMG. Right median motor ...prolonged distal motor latency. Right brachial plexopathy....only minimal abnormalities at the upper and middle trunk level....chronic denervation in muscles innervated by lower trunk ....collateral sprouting from remaining motor axons. Moderate right median neuropathy at the wrist (carpal tunnel syndrome). |
| 10/11/00 | Berchowitzc, MD | M | ...numbness and tingling in the ulnar aspect of her hand...medial aspect of her forearm....she appears to be quite symptomatic, even though her function is not significantly impaired. |
| 12/18/00 | Williamson, MD | M | ...really don't know what the cause of her pain is....she has virtually complete overhead function... |
| 01/09/01 | Zigler, MD | M | ...fairly dense sensory loss in the ulnar aspect of the right hand...weakness of selected ulnar innervated intrinsic hand muscles. Her thumb functions quite well...Dr. David Kline...New Orleans ...he recommended...possible proximal ulnar nerve neurolysis and transposition of the ulnar nerve at the elbow. |
| 03/09/01 | Sanders, MD | O | Mild gastritis. |

## History (per Examinee)

### Pre-Existing Status

She denies any previous problems or injuries, including any other work- or liability-related injuries. Ms. Formaggio also denies having any difficulties similar to those she is now experiencing until the injury.

### Injury

She reports that on 11/26/99 she came in contact with a cart at WalMart located at the Lancaster Farms Shopping Center. She was inside the store. It was very crowded. All she can remember is making contact with something hitting her right shin and she flew through the air. She came down landing flat on her nose with her right arm stretched over her head.

She could not move. There was no loss of consciousness. She had excruciating pain in her right shoulder and the right shin and ankle. Her left shoulder was also painful. Her nose was bleeding. Her arm was paralyzed. She couldn't move her right arm.

Following the injury, she was taken by ambulance to Everett Hospital.

### Clinical Chronology

She was in a great deal of pain at Everett ER. She was x-rayed and told her right shoulder was dislocated. It was reduced. Dr. Lancaster, Schenectady orthopedic surgeon came in. Pain medication was given. A sling was given. She was sent home. She was told she had a fracture of the nose.

She continued to experience pain and electroshocks radiating up her entire arm. Because of this she returned to Everett Hospital Emergency Room. She was met by Dr. Lancaster. He gave her stronger medication and told her to follow up in his office.

The pain was still so bad that she went to Acton Medical Center Hospital. Her arm "wouldn't do anything." She went to AMCH within the next couple of days.

She was seen by Dr. Smith, neurosurgeon at Acton Medical Center Hospital. She was sent for an MRI and x-rays. She followed up with Dr. Smith in his office. She was set up for EMG's. She was also referred to Dr. Casazza, Acton orthopedic surgeon. Dr. Casazza told her that she would never be able to move the arm again and might need an arthrodesis procedure of the right arm.

She previously lived in the Acton area, several of her children continued to live in the Acton area. She was visiting them from her new home in Nottingham, PA.

She had a lump on the right anterior leg, which got larger. There was throbbing. She returned to Pennsylvania. This was evaluated and she was told that it was not a blood clot. Her home in Pennsylvania is 260 miles from Acton.

She went to the University of Pennsylvania in Philadelphia and saw Dr. Zigler, neurosurgeon. He had EMG's performed. He said that she also needed orthopedic care because a rotator cuff tear was noted on the MRI. She saw a hand surgeon and also Dr. Williamson, a shoulder surgeon.

Dr. Williamson said that there was a very bad rotator cuff injury. He said that he couldn't promise what kind of result she would have but that she should have surgery.

On February 2, 2000, she had surgery performed on her right shoulder.

She was in physical therapy prior to and after this surgery. Her leg continued to bother her. She had a test for a blood clot but this was okay.

She was depressed because of the loss of use of her hand. She was seen by a psychiatrist. She was treated with pills. Her stomach became irritated from this medicine. She subsequently had gastroscopy. She had to cut back on these medications.

Her psychiatrist is now deceased. She sees a psychotherapist every two weeks. "I am a very depressed person. It's like living with a tourniquet around my arm, like someone is pulling on it. It's like sleeping on your arm and not being able to wake it up."

She has tried acupuncture on two occasions, physiatry, and pain management. She had a second opinion with a neurosurgeon in New Orleans. He offered to "cut the nerves in her neck."

She saw Dr. David Kline, a specialist in New Orleans. He performed testing and evaluation. He told her that success from a surgical procedure would be low. He discouraged surgery.

She returned to Dr. Zigler, neurosurgeon in Philadelphia. He placed her back in therapy. Eventually physical therapy told her that it made no sense for her to come anymore, because she was not improving.

She asked Dr. Zigler to amputate her hand. He told her that this would not work because she would still get phantom pain in her hand.

She now sees Dr. Fried in Nottingham. Dr. Williamson said to come back if her arm is hurting.

The physical therapy ended a week ago.

She is also seeing a Dr. Niescien for a dietary program.

## Current Status

The examinee's chief complaint is pain and numbness in the right arm and hand. She reports difficulties with pain that is primarily located in the right shoulder, right arm, and right hand. The pain is described as pulling and throbbing. The pain is not worsened by anything, it is pretty much the same all the time. It is improved by ice packs. The pain is reported as constant.

On a scale from 0 (no pain) to 10 (excruciating pain), the examinee reports the pain now is a 10. During the past month the pain averaged 10, with a high of 10 and a low of 8.

The examinee also reports difficulties with the left shoulder and with pain. She also reports difficulties with breathing because her nose feels blocked. Her right hand turns blue when she holds it in a dependent position. She has other problems with hypertension, diabetes, and irritation of her stomach.

## Functional Status

She reports greatest difficulties with the following tasks: buttoning her bra, tweezing her eyebrows, tying her shoes, and taking care of herself with personal hygiene. She can't get in and out of the bathtub easily. She has difficulty doing her hair and makeup. She used to cook, decorate cakes, garden, and bowl, which she can no longer do.

## Occupational History

At the time of the injury she was not employed. She had previously worked eight years ago as a bank teller. She worked there for less than one year. Prior to that she worked in her father's store for fifteen to twenty years. She has previously sold real estate. She and her husband also have real estate properties, which she states she takes care of. She then corrected herself and stated that she used to take care of these. She has a high-school-graduate education. In terms of current work status, she is not working.

She reports no work restrictions placed upon her.

**Social History**

The examinee lives in Nottingham, Pennsylvania with her husband. The activities of a typical day include getting up, watching television, going to doctor visits, and going for rides in the car once in a while. She denies performing any other work activities or vigorous recreational pursuits. The examinee does not smoke. She denies any problems with alcohol or illicit drug usage.

**Past Medical History**

| | |
|---|---|
| Medical: | Hypertension. (Controlled)<br>Diabetes.<br>Hiatal hernia.<br>Chronic heartburn.<br>History of irregular heartbeat. |
| Surgery: | Cholecystectomy.<br>Complete hysterectomy age 48.<br>Appendectomy.<br>Bilateral carpal tunnel releases.<br>Bilateral Arthroscopic knee surgery. |
| Medications (other): | Catapress.<br>Prevacid.<br>Lipitor.<br>Aceybutolol. |
| Allergies: | None known. |

**Review of Systems**

Noncontributory.

**Family History**

Mother alive at age 82 with Diabetes Mellitus. Father deceased age 64 with cancer of the urethra.

## Physical Examination

### Observations

The examinee is a well-developed well-nourished overweight female. She appears healthy. Examination of the hands reveals no callus. No assistive devices were used. Weight was reported as 296 pounds and height was reported as 5 feet 3 inches.

### Behavioral Observations

The examinee was pleasant, cooperative, and attentive. Affect was normal. During the visit she appeared comfortable. She sat continuously for up to 45 minutes during the interview. There was no significant pain behavior. Nonphysiologic findings were present, as noted below.

### Structural Examination

In the standing neutral position cervical, thoracic, and lumbar curves were well maintained. Extremities appeared grossly normal. The shoulders were symmetric and pelvis was level. Gait was normal, with no antalgia.

Examination focused on the right upper extremity.

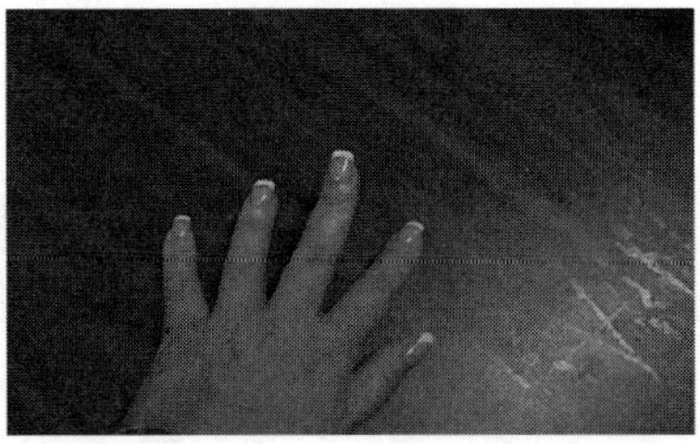

### Regional Examination

### Observations

There was no gross deformity or obvious abnormality. The examinee was morbidly obese.

The examinee tends to position her right upper extremity in front of her. The long finger remains in full extension. The remainder of the hand is in a position of function. The right hand shows slight increased redness and coolness.

There was a 13 cm surgical incision along the lateral aspect of the acromion of the right shoulder.

**Range of Motion**

Range of motion was restricted.

The following measurements were obtained:

| **RANGE OF MOTION (Right Shoulder Region)** | | |
|---|---|---|
| | **Normal Active ROM**<br>**ROM-0-ROM** | **Examination** |
| Sagittal | Extension-0-flexion<br>(40)-0-(150) | (35)-0-(85) |
| Frontal | Abduction-0-adduction<br>(150)-0-(30) | (45)-0-(10) |
| Rotation | External-0-internal<br>Rotation rotation<br>(90)-0-(80) | (10)-0-(90) |

| **RANGE OF MOTION (Left Shoulder Region)** | | |
|---|---|---|
| | **Normal Active ROM**<br>**ROM-0-ROM** | **Examination** |
| Sagittal | Extension-0-flexion<br>(40)-0-(150) | (70)-0-(170) |
| Frontal | Abduction-0-adduction<br>(150)-0-(30) | (170)-0-(30) |
| Rotation | External-0-internal<br>Rotation rotation<br>(90)-0-(80) | (45)-0-(90) |

| **RANGE OF MOTION (Right Elbow Region)** | | |
|---|---|---|
| | **Normal Active ROM**<br>**ROM-0-ROM** | **Examination** |
| Sagittal | Extension-0-flexion<br>(0)-0-(150) | (0)-0-(40-80) |

| **RANGE OF MOTION (Right Forearm Region)** | | |
|---|---|---|
| | **Normal Active ROM**<br>**ROM-0-ROM** | **Examination** |
| Rotation | Supination-0-pronation<br>(80)-0-(80) | (70)-0-(90) |

| RANGE OF MOTION (Wrist Region) | | |
|---|---|---|
| | **Normal Active ROM ROM-0-ROM** | **Examination** |
| Sagittal | Dorsal-0-palmar<br>Extension flexion<br>(60)-0-(60) | (10)-0-(25) |
| Frontal | Radial-0-ulnar<br>Deviation deviation<br>(20)-0-(30) | (10)-0-(12) |

*Palpation*

Mild tenderness is reported on palpation diffusely of the right anterior shoulder and diffusely of the right arm, wrist, and hand.

**Objective Findings**

Positive physical findings included: atrophy of the muscles of the 1st web space between the thumb and index finger. Surgical scar of the right shoulder. Surgical scar of the right palm.

**Neurological Examination**

There is atrophy of the 1st web space. There is a well healed vertical surgical incision in the palm measuring 3 cm. (Previous carpal tunnel release.) There is normal sensation of the entire thumb with 5 mm 2 point discrimination. The examinee is able to hold her fingers in extension. She volunteers the fact that there is no abduction or adduction of her fingers. There is fair pinch strength between her thumb and index finger.

The long finger remains in extension. The index, ring, and little fingers come 3 cm from the palm. There is normal sensation of the right shoulder and upper arm. There are diffuse paresthesias of the entire forearm. Sensation of the radial aspect of the index finger is intact. There is fair sensation of the remaining portion of the hand and the median nerve distribution. There is decreased sensation of the ulnar supplied aspect of the hand. Radial pulse is intact. Right biceps reflex intact, right brachioradialis reflex intact, right triceps reflex is not obtainable. Left biceps, triceps and brachioradialis reflexes are intact.

Knee and ankle jerk reflexes are intact. Measurements of the upper extremities: right upper arm 42 cm, left upper arm 42 cm, right forearm 29 cm, left forearm 30 cm. There are no visible abnormalities of the right lower leg in the region of the previous contusion.

### Nonphysiological Examination

Nonphysiological findings were present in the form of posturing of the right upper extremity.

## Diagnostic Studies

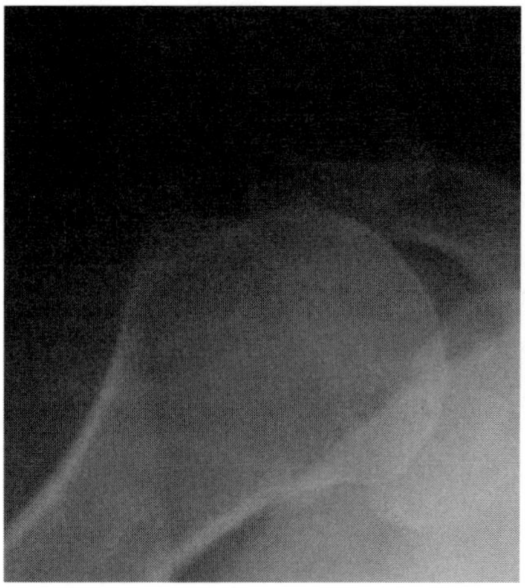

X-ray Right Shoulder

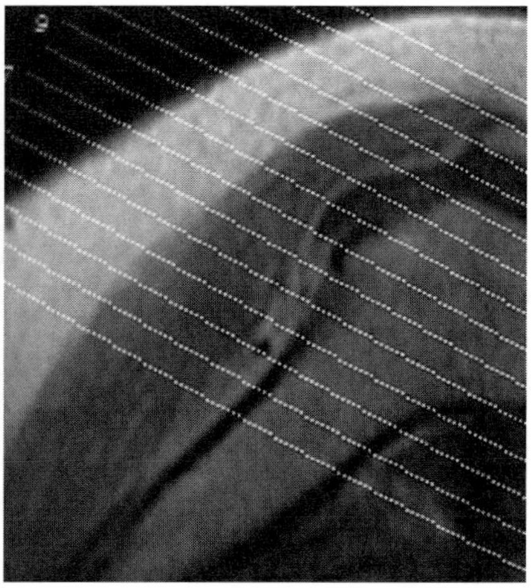

MRI Right Shoulder

## Pain Status Inventories

### Pain Drawing

The examinee completed a pain drawing (attached), using symbols to describe sensations. This drawing did reveal findings suggestive of symptom magnification.

### Pain Disability Index

The Pain Disability Index uses rating scales to measure the extent of perceived disability in seven areas of life. The results are as follows:

| Area | Perceived Disability |
|---|---|
| Family/home responsibilities | 100% |
| Recreation | 100% |
| Social activity | 80% |
| Occupation | 100% |

| | |
|---|---|
| Sexual activity | 100% |
| Self-care | 80% |
| Life-support activities | 50% |

The total score is 61 out of a possible 70, for a total index of 87%. This indicated a high level of perceived disability.

**Oswestry Function Test**

The score on the Oswestry Function Test was 20 out of a possible 30, giving 67%, indicating a perception of severely disabled.

**Short-Form McGill Pain Questionnaire**

The McGill Pain Questionnaire specifies fifteen potential pain descriptors. The examinee rates the intensity of each descriptor on a scale of 0 to 3. The total of all descriptors was 22, the total of the eleven somatic descriptors was 19, averaging 90%, and the total of the four affective descriptors was 3, averaging 100%.

This is consistent with a behavioral component to her distress.

**CES-D**

The Center for Epidemiologic Studies Depressed Mood Scale was administered. The examinee scored 46, which is consistent with a depressed mood.

## Conclusions

**Diagnoses**

1. Dislocation Right Shoulder.
2. Lower Brachial Plexus Injury Right Shoulder.
3. Chip Fracture Nasal Bone.
4. Diabetes.
5. Hypertension.
6. Morbid Obesity.
7. Degenerative Arthritis Right Shoulder (pre-existing).
8. Rotator Cuff Tear Right Shoulder.
9. Fracture Left Clavicle.
10. Cervical Spondylosis.
11. Carpal Tunnel Syndrome Right.

The subjective complaints are not entirely consistent with the objective findings. Symptom magnification was evident. The examinee's lack of use of her right upper extremity are out of proportion to her physical examination and EMG findings. Her function is not significantly impaired.

This is a case of a morbidly obese diabetic woman who fell sustaining an anterior dislocation of the right shoulder. There was stretching of the brachial plexus with initial complete neurapraxia. A soft tissue injury of the shoulder occurred.

The examinee had significant pre-existing problems with the right upper extremity prior to these injuries. These included degenerative arthritis of the right shoulder with attrition of the rotator cuff and biceps tendon, and median nerve compression of the wrist. The carpal tunnel syndrome is more commonly seen in diabetics.

The rotator cuff tear was massive. This may occur with a shoulder dislocation, but sometimes this may be pre-existing and aggravate the shoulder dislocation. Without a rotator cuff in place the shoulder dislocation is more likely to occur because there is not a competent rotator cuff to help hold the shoulder in place. In my opinion, it is more likely than not that this massive rotator cuff tear was to a large extent already present in her right shoulder.

A massive retracted tear was found. A great deal of surgical dissection had to be performed to mobilize this tear for repair. The x-rays at the time showed pre-existing arthritis of the AC joint and a spur of the greater tuberosity, this indicates that there was already degenerative process going on in the shoulder that caused a chronic tear.

A fresh massive tear is straightforward to repair and does not take extensive surgical dissection and mobilization to bring the rotator cuff to a position that it can be repaired. A great deal of releasing and surgical dissection had to be performed to repair the supraspinatus and infraspinatus tendons. This indicates that the tear had been there for a long time. The presence of atrophy of the supraspinatus tendon indicates pre-existing disease. Atrophy takes a long time to occur. The absence of a biceps tendon also indicates that it was gone from previous attrition due to degenerative disease of the shoulder. If there was a fresh tear of the biceps tendon which is adjacent to the rotator cuff, the tendon would have been visible at surgery. A biceps tendon that had already worn out over a long period of time would not have been visible. Many rotator cuff tears are asymptomatic. In this sedentary morbidly obese woman it would not be unusual to find an asymptomatic tear. This soft tissue fall did irritate the right shoulder joint and caused an aggravation of the pre-existing tear. The examinee has had an excellent result of surgical repair of the rotator cuff of the right shoulder. The examinee's shoulder is now in better condition than it was prior to her fall. The shoulder function is not significantly impaired. There is good strength and range of motion.

In regards to the brachial plexus injury, the nerves of the brachial plexus were stretched. There was excellent recovery of the upper and middle portions of the brachial plexus. The lower portion in the distribution of the ulnar nerve was permanently damaged. However, the examinee already had significant nerve damage in her upper extremity from a previous carpal tunnel syndrome. She did not provide information regarding the fact that she had previous bilateral carpal tunnel releases. When I pointed out to her that she had a surgical scar on her palm she then recalled that she had carpal tunnel surgery. Carpal tunnel syndrome with median nerve compression in a diabetic leaves the patient with some loss of sensation and strength of the hand. This indicates that there were significant pre-existing problems with the examinee's right hand prior to these injuries.

The examinee does have an impairment of her right hand in the form of ulnar nerve distribution damage. This does add to the weakness of the hand and loss of sensation in the ulnar aspect of the hand and forearm. However, this leads only to a mild functional disability of the right upper extremity.

The examinee's pain inventories, including the pain diagram, and posturing of the right upper extremity indicate symptom magnification. The diagnosis of symptom magnification syndrome is not intended to discredit the subjective complaint of pain, its possible basis in organic pathology, or the existence of a certain degree of objective disability. This individual reports symptoms that are essentially nonnegotiable, that serve to control the environment, and that result in significant amplification of perceived and expressed functional limitations. This should not be interpreted to suggest an intentional misrepresentation of pain and disability, but more likely represents a learned pattern of illness behavior.

In regards to the examinee's reports of chronic pain of her extremity, pain is an entirely subjective complaint which cannot be verified. In most cases the pain of this type of injury gradually subsides to a very low level. The pain status inventories indicate a magnification of symptoms. There may be some pain present, but in my opinion this condition would not cause a great deal of pain at this time.

The examinee had an injury to the brachial plexus. The brachial plexus refers to a group of nerves as they exit the neck and enter the upper arm in the region of the shoulder. They consist of five nerve roots: C5, C6, C7, C8, and T1. They supply the sensation and motor power of the upper extremity.

Plexus refers to the fact that there is crisscrossing of these nerve roots as they form the individually named nerves that supply the upper extremity. Low energy injuries, such as a fall onto the shoulder, typically cause mostly reversible injuries such as neuropraxia or stretching of the nerves. Various degrees of axonotmesis may be caused. This refers to tearing of the nerves within their substance. Because of its anatomy, the lower structures of the brachial plexus suffer more significant injuries than do the proximal located roots, trunks, and cords.

Most of the nerve injury in this case was reversible. The initial flail extremity recovered so that the examinee has good control of the upper portion of the arm and is essentially left with an ulnar nerve deficiency. This causes numbness along the ring and little fingers of the hand and inner aspect of the forearm and weakness of grip of the hand.

Good neurological function remains of the right upper extremity. There is minimal functional limitation of the right upper extremity on the basis of neurological injury. I base my opinion on the fact that in clinical practice I have seen many patients with ulnar nerve deficient arms who are able to work and function. This includes people who work in factories and farmers who work at full capacity with heavy manual labor.

The upper extremity of this examinee had many problems prior to this injury. This included carpal tunnel syndrome, which required surgery on both hands. This is performed to relieve compression at the wrist on a major nerve of the hand. It is inconsistent that the examinee did not mention this until the scar was pointed out to her on her hand.

The x-rays show that there were degenerative changes of the right upper extremity that took many years to form including degenerative arthritis of the AC joint and of the shoulder joint itself. These degenerative changes contribute to the wearing out of the rotator cuff. A high percentage of people in the regular adult population with these findings have torn rotator cuffs. In a sedentary individual such as this (as documented by her obesity) the examinee didn't know that she had a torn rotator cuff. Further evidence that this torn rotator cuff was pre-existing is the fact that there was atrophy of the supraspinatus muscle and by the fact that the surgeon had to perform a good deal of mobilization of the cuff at the time of the repair. These changes take years rather than a few months to form.

In regards to the outcome of her rotator cuff injuries, the examinee has had a good repair and has no functional limitations of her shoulder because of the successful repair.

## Causation

Based upon the available information, to a reasonable degree of medical certainty, there is causal relationship between the examinee's current complaints and the reported injury, to the extent that there is an ulnar nerve distribution injury.

## Prognosis

The overall prognosis is fair.

## Maximum Medical Improvement

The examinee has achieved maximum medical improvement. MMI is defined as the date after which further recovery and restoration of function can no longer be anticipated, based upon a reasonable degree of medical probability.

## Work Capacity

This examinee has at least a sedentary work capacity as defined in the *Dictionary of Occupational Titles*, U.S. Department of Labor.

The following work restrictions are suggested: no repetitive usage of the right hand and no repetitive lifting with the right hand.

## Appropriateness of Care

The client has asked that I specifically address the issue of appropriateness of medical care. Based on the specifics of this care, it is my professional opinion that care has been consistent with the usual standards of care for this problem.

## Recommendations

### Diagnostic/Consultation

No further diagnostic testing or consultation is indicated.

### Therapeutic

No further treatment is required.

## Qualifications

My comments are based upon the specifics of this case and my knowledge, skills and abilities in this domain. I am a practicing orthopaedic surgeon. During the past twenty years I have analyzed and performed five hundred Independent Medical Examinations and Impairment Evaluations. I am frequently called to testify for both plaintiffs and defendants in civil and workman's compensation matters.

I am certified by the American Board of Orthopaedic Surgery and by the American Board of Independent Medical Examiners. I am a fellow of the American Academy of Orthopaedic Surgeons. My curriculum vitae is attached.

## Disclosure Statements

The above analysis is based upon the available information at this time, including the history given by the examinee, the medical records and tests provided, the results of pain status inventories, and the physical findings. It is assumed that the information provided to me is correct. If more information becomes available at a later date, an additional report may be requested. Such information may or may not change the opinions rendered in this evaluation.

My opinions are based upon reasonable medical certainty. Medicine is both an art and a science, and although an individual may appear to be fit for work activity, there is no guarantee that the person will not be reinjured or suffer additional injury. If applicable, employers should follow the processes established in the Americans with Disabilities Act, Title I. The opinions on work capacity are to facilitate job placement and do not necessarily reflect an in-depth direct threat analysis. Comments on appropriateness of care are professional opinions based upon the specifics of the case and should not be generalized, nor necessarily be considered supportive or critical of, the involved providers or disciplines.

Any medical recommendations offered are provided as guidance and not as medical orders. The opinions expressed do not constitute a recommendation that specific claims or administrative action be made or enforced.

I declare under penalty of perjury that the information contained in this report and its attachments is true and correct, to the best of my knowledge and belief, except as to information that I have received from others. As to that information, I declare under penalty of perjury that the information accurately describes the information provided to me, and except as noted in this report, that I believe to be true. I further declare under penalty of perjury that to the best of my knowledge and belief, the contents of this report and bill are true and correct. The foregoing was signed in the County of Fulton,

State of New York on the date of this letter.

Thank you for asking me to see this examinee in consultation. If you have any further questions, please do not hesitate to contact me.

Sincerely,

Thomas S. Eagan, M.D., P.C.

Enclosures: Pain drawing
Multidimensional Pain Inventory results

## Report #2: Racial Discrimination—Emotional Distress

This report is most notable for the following.

- It is concise.
- Exact quotes of the examinee are thoroughly documented.
- Clear explanations of the significance of the numerous psychological tests and their results.
- The examiner's conclusions are supported by specific references to literature.
- The examiner's opinion of probable malingering is objectively supported by the numerous standardized tests administered to the examinee.
- Good list of documents reviewed. Each document is specifically identified.
- Technical terms are explained. For example, "soto voce" is defined as a soft voice. This makes the report easier to understand by the lay reader for whom it is written.
- Inconsistencies found are specifically documented. For example, the six symptoms reported in the testing (looking around room while speaking, losing train of thought, etc.) were documented as not being consistent with what was observed during the interview.
- Headnotes break up the report.

Areas of possible improvement include the following.

- Avoid legal references, such as "Work Product," "Federal Rules of Civil Procedure 26 (a)(2)(b)," and "F.S. 490." Unless the examiner is an attorney, legal references are usually outside of the examiner's true area of expertise.
- More precise language could have been used in some areas to make the report more powerful and persuasive. For example, instead of basing the report on an "extended" clinical interview with the examinee, it could have been based on a "214-minute" interview.
- The transmittal letter for this work could have been shorter with less extraneous information (for example, the reference to "local standards of my profession regarding to the preparation of expert reports"). When it comes to transmittal letters, anything more than one sentence is probably too long.
- Possible overstating of the examiner's conclusions. These are stated "with psychological certainty." A more defensible opinion might be stated "to a reasonable degree of psychological

certainty."

- Avoid colloquial language (for example, "he is a moody, anxious, irritable fellow"). Colloquial language is inappropriate in an IME report and may diminish the credibility of the examiner and his report.
- The final conclusion could have been more clearly written. As it is currently written ("In summary, it is my professional judgment that as a psychological certainty there is <u>not</u> a definitive connection between Mr. Plaintiff 2's alleged symptoms and events alleged to have occurred in the workplace. A more reliable explanation is his character logical interpersonal mistrust combined with the presence of malingering."), the final conclusion is not completely clear.
- The use of bold in the headnotes may make the report more visually pleasing and easier to read.

---

January 14, 2004

Mr. Oliver Wendell Holmes, Esq.
Dewey, Cheatem & Howe, LLP
2003 Lawyers' Tower
1001 Elm Street
Miami, Florida 12345

In re: Plaintiff 1, Plaintiff 2 & Plaintiff 3 v Defendant
Case Number: 00-0000 CIV Rhenquist

REFERENCE: SUBJECT PLAINTIFF 2

***WORK PRODUCT***

Dear Counsel:

At your request I have conducted an independent forensic psychological evaluation of the plaintiff Mr. Subject Plaintiff 2.

In compliance with *Federal Rule of Civil Procedure 26 (a) (2) (b)* and with local standards of my profession regarding the preparation of expert reports, I have attached the following:

1. My narrative report, prepared and signed by me, of my evaluation of Mr. Plaintiff 2, which includes references to and a delineation of:

- meeting times,
- collateral sources of information (documents),
- tests administered, and
- my conclusions and the basis therefore.

2. A copy of my qualifications as an expert reflected in my current *c.v.*

3. A listing of other federal cases in which I have been accepted as an expert witness, to be found following the text of my c.v.

Respectfully,

Jerome H. Poliacoff, Ph.D., P.A.
*Florida Licensed Psychologist 123456*

*CONFIDENTIAL REPORT*

In re: Plaintiff 1, Plaintiff 2 & Plaintiff 3 v. Defendant
Case Number: 00-0000 CIV Rhenquist

REFERENCE: SUBJECT PLAINTIFF 2

Statement of Purpose:

Mr. Subject Plaintiff 2 [hereinafter also: *'Plaintiff'*] has filed a complaint against Defendant (hereinafter also *'DEFENDANT'*).

Mr. Plaintiff 2 is alleging that [1] he was denied a promotion, or that promotions were delayed because of his race [African American], [2] he was denied a promotion in retaliation for filing a Charge of Discrimination, and [3] he was subject to a racially hostile environment during his employment with DEFENDANT.

As a consequence of these alleged actions by DEFENDANT, Mr. Plaintiff 2 claims that he *"has in the past, present and future will suffer emotional pain and suffering, inconvenience, mental anguish,* [and] *loss of enjoyment of life...."*[2]

In order to evaluate the degree to which, if any, Mr. Plaintiff 2 is suffering any psychological effects owing to DEFENDANT's alleged actions, I conducted an independent psychological evaluation of Mr. Plaintiff 2.

Psychological Findings:

Based upon:

- my extended clinical interview with Mr. Plaintiff 2, and
- my review of psychological test data generated by his responses to test questions completed by Mr. Plaintiff 2, and
- my review of collateral material and interviews with collateral informants,

I can state with psychological certainty that:

Mr. Plaintiff 2 is not suffering from any psychological symptoms that are consistent with, or attributable to, alleged discriminatory actions in his former place of employment.

Mr. Plaintiff 2 is grossly overstating, if not making up, the presence of any symptoms consistent with his claims of psychological distress for the purpose of gaining compensation in this litigation.

---

[2] From: Second Amended Complaint, ¶ 100 [page 123]; ¶ 101 [page 124]; and ¶ 102 [page 125].

His cognitive style and personality organization is characteristically tense, accompanied by an undercurrent of sadness and anger. He is a moody, anxious, irritable fellow who feels unappreciated and misunderstood and who takes a pessimistic outlook on life. While he may wish to blame his state of unhappiness on his perception of his lack of vocational advancement any true psychological problems and symptoms that can be teased out of his litigation presentation are more readily attributable to a childhood in which he was the casualty of both parental violence and sexual victimization.

<u>*Sources of Information:*</u>

*Interviews and Testing*:

Mr. Plaintiff 2 appeared for testing on December 25th and was interviewed on December 26th, 2002.

At the first meeting Mr. Plaintiff 2 was given the following objective test instruments to complete:

- *The Minnesota Multiphasic Personality Inventory - 2 (MMPI-2)*
- *The Millon Clinical Multiaxial Inventory (MCMI-III)*
- *The Millon Behavioral Health Inventory (MBHI)*
- *The Trauma Symptom Inventory (TSI)*
- *The Malingering Probability Scale (MPS)*
- *The Validity Indicator Profile (VIP).*

Because of the invalid scoring profiles on the MMPI-2 and the MPS and because he had endorsed so many improbable symptoms or symptom combinations which yielded an invalid MMPI-2 profile, an additional test, to rule out the presence of malingering, the Structured Interview of Reported Symptoms (SIRS), was administered at the end of the formal interview process.

*Documents reviewed:*

The following documents were provided by defense counsel and reviewed:

Amended Complaint [Home County]
Amended Complaint [Federal]
Defendant's Answer to Plaintiffs' Amended Complaint
Plaintiff Plaintiff 2's Response to Defendant's First Set of Interrogatories
Plaintiffs' Second Amended Complaint
Second Amended Complaint [Federal]

Defendant's Answer to Plaintiffs' Second Amended Complaint
**Memorandum of Law in Support of Motion for Summary Judgment & Appendix of Evidence**
Defendant's Answer to Plaintiff's Second Amended Complaint
Defendant's Motion for Summary Judgment
Expert's [Dr. Skinner, Ph.D.] report, c.v. & deposition [June 20, 2003]
Collateral empirical research review, including:
    Articles referenced by Plaintiffs' expert
    APA Psych Info Search
Materials related to "APT Test", including:
    Document: "*Validation of the APT Management Trainee-Executive Profile,*" and sub-test components
Deposition transcripts of:
        Lyle Lovett
        Barry Gibbs
        Nicholas Claus
        Walt Disney
        Larry the "Plaintiff" #1
        Eddie the "Plaintiff" #3
Personnel Records of three [3] plaintiffs: Plaintiff 1, Plaintiff 2, & Plaintiff #3
Defendant's Motion to Compel Rule 35 Mental Examination of Plaintiff 1, Plaintiff 2 and Plaintiff 3 and
Brief in Support of Plaintiff's Memorandum of Law in Opposition to Motion to Compel Rule 35 Mental Examination of Plaintiffs
Defendant's Reply to Plaintiff's Memorandum of Law in Opposition to Motion to Compel Rule 35 Mental Examination of Plaintiffs
Plaintiff's Appeal of and Objection to Magistrate Judge O'Connor's Order of October 24, 2003
Defendant's Memorandum in Response to Plaintiff's Appeal of and Objections to Magistrate Judge O'Connor's Order of October 24, 2003

*Behavioral Observations, Pertinent Record Information, Test Results*

*Behavioral Observations & Interview:*

*Informed Consent:* At the first visit for the purpose of completing the various questionnaires Mr. Plaintiff 2 was informed as to the limits of confidentiality, i.e., that this was not a therapeutic relationship and that as his mental status was placed at issue as part of his claim, he was not entitled to the protections of privilege as might otherwise be afforded by *F.S. 490.*

Mr. Plaintiff 2 was given a written statement[3] concerning these limitations and was advised to review them with his attorney.

*Appearance:* Mr. Plaintiff 2 is a well-groomed, muscular, and handsome but grim looking African American male, who is forty-two years of age.

He arrived early for his testing and interview sessions and at each appeared initially put out or impatient that he was here at all. Throughout, he spoke in a *soto voce* [soft voice] that was at times difficult to hear at first listening. His responses to questions were given with just sufficient information to be acceptable but nothing of his personal history or feelings were forthcoming without continued or repeated inquiry.

He was easily engaged despite his continued emotional distance and guardedness. He apparently felt comfortable enough to take and make a business call initiated during a brief break and continued even though signals were given that it was time to resume.

*History:* Mr. Plaintiff 2 is currently employed by XYZ Corp. in Hialeah, a company not dissimilar to Defendant where he had worked previously. Prior to his work in the XYZ manufacturing industry he did "*nothing steady*" having worked for ACME, Inc. and for his father's nightclub business "*collecting tickets at the door.*"

Mr. Plaintiff 2 was born in the Caribbean and raised in France, coming to live in Florida as a late teen.

He reports that his parents are not divorced, but separated since 1985, his father living in Caribbean where he owns a retail business, having formerly been a policeman; and, his mother lives in South Florida with him [Mr. Plaintiff 2]. She is not working as she is disabled having suffered a stroke in 1983.

He has three older sisters. The oldest ran away from home at age sixteen and hasn't been seen in years; the middle sister, age 47, lives in France; and, the youngest [but older than Mr. Plaintiff 2] is a nurse, living in Florida.

Mr. Plaintiff 2 reports having completed his A.A. degree at the Institution of Middle Learning, in Tampa, Florida.

---

[3] A copy of that written statement may be found in APPENDIX 1, following the main body of this report

Early in the interview I asked Mr. Plaintiff 2 where or how he had developed such a soft voice. He replied, initially, that he had learned to talk softly so as not to be perceived as *"talking back to my father."* His father was *"strict,"* prone to *"yelling and hitting."*

Mr. Plaintiff 2 reports not having very many close friends because *"I don't trust a lot of people," "I see what people do."* Mr. Plaintiff 2 is not married, *"Everybody has problems."* During the inquiry about significant relationships, family, and marriage, Mr. Plaintiff 2 did not initially disclose that he had two children [out of wedlock from a previous relationship] aged eleven and eight who he only spoke about later in the interview when he was being asked about perceived changes in his affective life.

Much like his delayed disclosure of having children, he delayed reporting any history of sexual victimization. When asked about any psychiatric history in his family, he briefly reported that he *"had a cousin in France that liked to mess with kids."* Only on further inquiry did Mr. Plaintiff 2 reveal that he had been sexually victimized by his cousin.

*Pertinent Record Information:*

*Criminal History and Reporting:* In a similar non-disclosing fashion Mr. Plaintiff 2 reported, only when asked, that he had been arrested for *"some tickets"* and had his license suspended; and for *"domestic violence, a girlfriend didn't like getting dumped."*

In fact the police report reflects that he was the intruder to his ex-friend's residence, and that when there committed battery on the ex-girlfriend and her male friend. The police report also reveals that when arrested for the *"domestic violence,"* Mr. Plaintiff 2 had in his possession thirteen twenty dollar bills all with the same serial number [i.e., counterfeit], which led to his being reported to the Secret Service.

Problematic for Mr. Plaintiff 2, and reflected in his personnel records, but certainly not reported by Mr. Plaintiff 2, was that he served at least twelve days in jail and as a consequence missed work and was terminated from employment by DEFENDANT (although apparently rehired upon reapplication for employment).

*Workplace Complaint:* Mr. Plaintiff 2 reports that he filed this lawsuit because he started *"thinking about not getting promoted, my sales numbers were in the 1%-2% and other people were getting promoted."* His perception was that "*Caucasians were getting promoted*" and he wasn't. His conversation with Larry the "Plaintiff" #1 [another plaintiff in this suit] led him to believe that *"he was feeling the same way."*

His report to this examiner about racial discrimination allegations was vague. Equally vague are his allegations contained in his deposition of September 11th, 2002.

In that deposition when asked if he had heard [or been the object of] any racially derogatory terms,[4] he replied, *"Not personally, no,"* but that he had heard from Mr. Plaintiff 1 that racially derogatory terms were used by other employees in DEFENDANT[5].

When asked about a racially hostile work environment Mr. Plaintiff 2 replied *"I haven't been appreciated by them [DEFENDANT] that's pretty hostile,"* [6] *and "knowing I'm working that hard and not getting promoted, of course that's hostile to me."*[7]

When asked about any emotional impact of alleged racially discriminatory actions in the workplace, Mr. Plaintiff 2 reported his disappointment about not having achieved more vocationally, *"My family members kept telling me something is wrong* [i.e., not being promoted], *all those years I could've been but I wasn't" now "Anything I do, anywhere I go I don't trust people."* Not unlike his co-plaintiff Mr. Plaintiff 1, Mr. Plaintiff 2 reports continued thoughts and worries around the theme of *"If I was promoted like I should have been,"* and not about any racially discriminatory behaviors by others to him.

When asked about the causes of any emotional distress or effects to his personality Mr. Plaintiff 2 readily acknowledged that any distress had *"more to do with my father, you had to speak softly to my father, he would yell....I got beaten...I got the most, any time I was in trouble."*

*Test Results:*

Some individuals, particularly in the context of litigation, may over-report or misrepresent trauma histories or trauma-related symptomatology.[8] For this reason one of the first issues to evaluate is for the possibility of malingering.

---

[4] Deposition of Plaintiff #1, Pages 102 line 25, & 103 lines 1-3.
[5] Op. cit., Page 136, lines 16-25.
[6] Op. cit., Page 105, lines 1-2.
[7] Op. cit., Page 136, lines 2-3.
[8] See: Fairbank, S.A., McCaffrey, R.J., & Keane, T.M. (1985). Psychometric detection of fabricated symptoms of post-traumatic stress disorder in Vietnam veterans. *Journal of Clinical Psychology, 43*, 44-55. Hyer, L.A., Fallon, J.H., Harrison, W.R., & Boudewyns, P.A, (1987). MMPI over-reporting by Vietnam combat veterans. *Journal of Clinical Psychology, 43*, 79-83.

*VIP:* In this evaluation, as measured by the *Validity Indicator Profile* (VIP),[9] which is used as a general assessment of response style designed to identify valid from invalid responding efforts, Mr. Plaintiff 2 appeared to have exhibited good, consistent effort throughout the Verbal portion of test.

However the results of the Non-Verbal subtest may not be an accurate reflection of his abstract reasoning abilities, or his perceptual accuracy or attention to detail. His performance on this test is indicative of careless responding which may have been due to any number of possible factors [distracting internal stimuli, fatigue, or an insufficient investment in the test process].

*MPS:* His responses to the *Malingering Probability Scales* (MPS)[10]

---

[9] Richard Frederick (1997). *VIP Validity Indicator Profile Tutorial.* National Computer Systems, Minneapolis, MN.

The *VIP* was originally designed as a measure of malingering to be used in the detection of intentionally feigned or grossly exaggerated neuropsychological symptoms.

Scoring rules for the *VIP* were developed using a sample of more than 1,000 clinical and non-clinical subjects. Results were then cross-validated using an independent sample of 312 cases comprised of five (5) criterion groups: traumatic brain-injured patients, suspected malingerers, normal subjects, a 'faking bad' group, and a group of random responders.

The use of the *VIP* has now been expanded to a general assessment of response style. Using six (6) primary scale indicators, an individual's performance is classified into either valid or invalid.

Using statistical modeling, the characteristics of the individual's performance curve are further classified to discriminate invalid responding into one of three (3) categories: *Careless Responding*, *Irrelevant Responding*, and *Malingering.*

The *VIP* is comprised of two subtests, a 78-item Verbal test and a 100-item Nonverbal test. All items have two response options and are randomly ordered with respect to difficulty. These subtests, called the *VIP Nonverbal (VIPNV)* and the *VIP Verbal (VIPV),* are validity measures that can be used when assessing cognitive abilities.

It is designed to provide a broad spectrum of information about a person's performance and effort in achieving that performance during an assessment battery in order to indicate whether the testing should be considered representative of the individual's true overall abilities.

[10] Leigh Silverton and Chris Gruber (1998). *Malingering Probability Scale (MPS) Manual.* Western Psychological Services, Los Angeles, CA.

The *MPS* is a 139-item objective inventory that is designed to assess whether an individual is attempting to produce false evidence of psychological distress.

The norms for this instrument were derived from a population of more than 1,000 adults, nationally representative in terms of gender, age, educational level, and region. In addition, numerous validation studies were conducted on a sample of more than 600 individuals including prison inmates, normals, outpatients, inpatients,

provide a clearer explanation of his careless responding to that portion of the testing [non-verbal] that did not appear to be related to anything emotional or psychological.

Specifically, he responded in a fashion that indicates a high [88%] likelihood that he attempted to use his responses to the MPS statements to exaggerate or fabricate symptomatic complaints.

Scores as high as Mr. Plaintiff 2 achieved reflect the endorsement of many "*pseudo symptoms.*" Pseudo symptoms are complaints that often sound like legitimate signs of distress, but are not connected with the mental disorders tested by the MPS as they have been documented by psychologists and psychiatrists.

People who are truly suffering from a mental disorder may at times say "*Yes*" to one or two of these pseudo symptoms, but seldom endorse them at the rate that Mr. Plaintiff 2 has. In situations such as the present litigation where there is an incentive to malinger, the likelihood of exaggerated responding is 97% over the base rate assumption of 76%.

*MMPI-2:* His responses to the MMPI-2, scored both by the NCS and Caldwell scoring systems, are such that the test is invalid for clinical or evaluative [of personality or symptom problems] purposes.

Mr. Plaintiff 2 was clearly able to read and comprehend the individual test items, he was attentive in considering his responses, and he consistently matched the item numbers in the test booklet to the corresponding numbers on the answer sheet and therefore his elevated scores on scales F and F-Back [the two rare answer scales] cannot be attributed to his inability to understand the content or to respond to the format of the inventory.

According to the Caldwell interpretation, the absence of substantial elevation on the VRIN together with his very high fake bad score reflect that a major part of the elevation on scale F derived from a purposeful, consistent effort to exaggerate his disturbance.

His profile, a T score of higher than 95 on the F scale [his is greater

---

and worker compensation claimants. The scale has been validated against multiple measures and criteria.

The *MPS* approaches the assessment of malingering by evaluating a person's tendencies to answer questions in an inconsistent fashion and to endorse statements that describe spurious yet seemingly authentic symptoms.

The domains or areas of distress that are measured include depression and anxiety, dissociative disorders, post-traumatic stress disorder, and schizophrenia.

than 109] accompanied by highest scales of 8 and 6 with lesser but substantial elevations [i.e., typically T scores in the 80 to 90 range] on 7, 1, 4, and 9 are consistent with empirical findings[11] that such profiles are associated with extremely disturbed individuals who manifest hallucinations, delusions, and general confusion, particularly so when dealing with an inpatient psychiatric population, and in an outpatient setting with individuals who are malingering.

*SIRS:* Results of the MMPI-2 would indicate, if not malingering, the presence of such severe psychopathology as to require immediate psychiatric hospitalization. To further rule out the presence of malingering [and rule in the presence of such severe psychopathology as to require hospitalization] a third test, the Structured Interview of Reported Symptoms[12] (SIRS) was administered as part of the clinical interview.

Mr. Plaintiff 2 did not endorse or respond to items reflecting the presence of rare symptoms, rare or improbable symptom combinations, or improbable symptoms. He did, however, report blatant symptoms [difficulties fighting evil forces, others talking behind his back, various signs of depression], a wide range of symptoms, and inconsistent symptoms [reporting that he (1) always looked around the room when speaking, (2) loses his train of thought when speaking, (3) always gestures or moves his hands when speaking, (4) stutters and stumbles on words, (5) sighs when he talks, and (6) moves his feet a lot], none of which were observed either during the testing or interview portions of the evaluation.

The overall scoring puts him in the "probable" range of malingering as measured by the SIRS.

---

[11] Ganellan, R., Wasliw, G., Haywood, T. & Grossman, L., (1993). *Can psychosis be malingered on the Rorschach?* (Paper presented at the 101st Annual Convention of the American Psychological Association, Toronto, Ontario, Canada).
Graham, J., Watts, D. & Timbrook, R., (1991). Detecting fake-good and fake-bad MMPI-2 profiles. *Journal of Personality Assessment.* Vol. 57, 264-277.
Meyer, Robert G.; Deitsch, Sarah M., (1995). The assessment of malingering in psychodiagnostic evaluations: Research-based concepts and methods for consultants. *Consulting Psychology Journal: Practice & Research*. Vol. 47(4), 234-245.

[12] The Structured Interview of Reported Symptoms [Rogers, Richard; Bagby, R. Michael; and Dickens, Susan E. (1992). Psychological Assessment Resources. Odessa, Florida] is designed to evaluate malingering and other forms of dissimulation. The SIRS provides valuable data on feigning (malingering and factitious disorders with psychological symptoms) and honest responding.

*Integration of Results and Findings:*

Specific stressor types aside (e.g., alleged discrimination), the extant trauma literature suggests that the amount of post stressor symptomatology an individual may experience is a function of at least four broad variables:

- characteristics of the stressor,
- variables specific to the victim,
- subjective responses to the stressor, and
- the response of others to the victim.

*Characteristics of the alleged stressor:* While Mr. Plaintiff 2's complaint before the Court is that he was subject to a racially hostile environment, his expressed complaint appears to be less about having overheard reports by others about persons using racially derogatory terms [which were not directed at him] than he is about not having been promoted when he thought he should have been. One is hard pressed to determine from his interview, deposition, or other materials what exactly the basis for his complaint is in that he reports no direct action taken against him.

*Variables specific to the victim:* Clearly Mr. Plaintiff 2 brings to the situation personality characteristics that allow him to distort his reality to fit his wishes. The results of the MCMI-III [a test which addresses personality organization, or AXIS II diagnoses on the DSM-IV] describe a man who has had a checkered history of disappointments in his personal and family life; who has deficits in social attainments, as well as a tendency to precipitate self-defeating vicious circles. His interpersonal mistrust is self-professed in the interview and further documented in his responses on the MCMI-III. These are characteristics developed over time, and are not symptoms of reactions to transient stressors.

A good example of Mr. Plaintiff 2's feeling of being misunderstood and unappreciated by others, yet blaming them nevertheless for his own limitations, are his complaints that the testing for managerial responsibilities was a *"test that must have been written by a white guy because it has nothing to do with things that African Americans know about,"*[13] *"I know the way it was written, a white person prepared it. It was only meant for white people to pass it so they could be managers and not the Blacks."*[14]

The test he complains about is comprised, in part, of the MMPI-2, on which there have been more studies[15] of ethnic differences using the MMPI

[13] Deposition of Plaintiff #3, Page 192, lines 17-20.
[14] Op. cit., Page 196, lines 21-24.
[15] Hall, Gordon C., Bansal, A., Lopez, Irene R. (1999). *Ethnicity and*

and the MMPI-2 than any other measure. Unlike the original MMPI, in the 1989-91 revision of the MMPI, ethnic minority persons were included in the standardization sample of the MMPI-2.[16]

*Subjective responses to the alleged stressor:* Mr. Plaintiff 2's alleged emotional problems were certainly not of sufficient intensity or distress for him to want to seek medical or psychiatric care at the time of the deposition in 2002, and by the time of this interview, over a year later, he had still not, despite assertions that he would,[17] sought intervention amelioration for his self-proclaimed problems.

*The Response of Others to the Victim:* By Mr. Plaintiff 2's account, he does not have close relationships with others because *"I don't trust a lot of people"* and one infers that the Subject Plaintiff 2's significant others has not changed very much over time.

<u>Conclusions:</u>

Having reviewed the available collateral sources of information; having administered and reviewed the results of various psychological tests; and having interviewed the plaintiff, Mr. Plaintiff 2, I offer the following conclusion:

[1] Mr. Plaintiff 2's alleged complaints cannot reliably be understood to have arisen solely, if at all, as a result of the actions which he alleges occurred in his workplace [i.e., Mr. Plaintiff 2's current emotional state is <u>not</u> consistent with the possibility that the alleged workplace events produced the current claimed intense symptom pattern].

[2] There is abundant empirical evidence of Mr. Plaintiff 2's direct, intentional effort to malinger.

While it is ultimately up to the jury, or trier of fact, to decide whether or not the claims made by Mr. Plaintiff 2 constitute, under the law, a racially hostile environment, or that he was the object of racial discrimination, the fact remains that Mr. Plaintiff 2 has a hard time telling a complete narrative – he reports that he was subject to racial hostility because he heard from others that other employees acted that way, and that as a consequence of these alleged conditions he is suffering emotional damages [for which he has yet to

---

*psychopathology: A meta-analytic review of 31 years of comparative MMPI/MMPI-2 research.* Psychological Assessment, June 1999 Vol. 11, No. 2, 186-197.

[16] Butcher, J. N., Dahlstrom, W. G., Graham, J. R., Tellegen, A. & Kaemmer, B. (1989). *MMPI-2: Manual for administration and scoring.* Minneapolis: University of Minnesota Press.

[17] Deposition of Plaintiff #3, Page 139, lines 12-13.

seek any intervention for] that by testing are evidently fabricated.

In summary, it is my professional judgment that as a psychological certainty there is not a definitive connection between Mr. Plaintiff 2's alleged symptoms and events alleged to have occurred in the workplace. A more reliable explanation is his character logical interpersonal mistrust combined with the presence of malingering.

Respectfully submitted,

Jerome H. Poliacoff, Ph.D., P.A.
Florida Licensed Psychologist # PY11111

## Report #3: Workers' Compensation—Personal Injury

This report is most notable for the following.

- A good statement at the beginning of the report documents the non-treating purpose of the exam to the examinee and states that the examinee was advised not to do anything that might injure her.
- The report is well-organized with headnotes.
- Easy-to-read font.
- Several quotes from the examinee are included. These quotes help support the report.
- Thorough review of the medical records. Each record obtained by the examiner is summarized in detail.
- This report, apparently drafted for an insurance adjuster, found a causal relationship between the workplace injury and the examinee's difficulties. This proves the objectivity and honesty of the evaluator.

While this is an excellent report, all reports can be improved. Areas of possible improvement include the following.

- Use more precise language. Avoid words such as "approximately," "includes," and "appears."
- The report reads as though it has been dictated. It doesn't read as well as a report that was written.
- The examiner failed to weigh and measure examinee. It would have been more precise to measure these without simply taking the examinee's word for them.
- Range of motion measurements provided are all in round numbers. Exact numbers would be more precise.
- The examiner expressed no confidence that he had reviewed all relevant medical records. For examp!e, he only reviewed the x-rays the examinee brought with her.

---

January 6, 2003

Dear Ms. Susan Pepersmith,

At your request, Ms. Connie Johnson was evaluated by me for independent medical examination and possible permanent partial impairment rating on January 6, 2003. The history was obtained from Ms. Connie Johnson and by reviewing the medical records sent to me.

Some readers of this report may wish to proceed directly to the Summary section that begins on page 14 of the Impression section, which begins on page 16. The data contained in the earlier sections of this report provide the basis for the opinions rendered.

The patient was advised that the purpose of the evaluation was to provide medical information so that appropriate assistance could be provided and administrative decisions could be made, and not to provide treatment. This evaluation does not constitute or replace a general medical exam. The patient was advised not to engage in any physical maneuvers beyond her tolerance or that she thought might injure herself.

HISTORY OF PRESENT ILLNESS

This 36-year-old, right-handed individual is partially college-educated, single, and childless. She complains of pain in the region of the right shoulder. Ms. Connie Johnson attributes her symptoms to the effects of an injury which occurred on the job on 9/6/01. At the time of that injury, Ms. Connie Johnson said, "It started when I was lifting boxes of books from the floor to the shelf." Ms. Connie Johnson states she lifted approximately 40 boxes of books, weighing about 30 pounds each. She notes she had "no problems at the time. Four or five hours later, when I went home, I felt the pain (in my right shoulder). I couldn't move my (right) arm or anything."

Later that day, Ms. Connie Johnson sought treatment at the immediate care center. She was seen by Dr. Jones. She reports he prescribed medication. She rested at home for three days, and then returned to work.

Ms. Connie Johnson said her shoulder symptoms "didn't go away." She returned to the clinic in 4/02. She was referred to Dr. Allen, an orthopedic surgeon. He sent her for treatment with physical therapy, which "helped, but (______)? said to stop it." The therapy was discontinued because "I'm a diabetic, and my eyes tend to bleed with pressure."

Ms. Connie Johnson reports Dr. Allen attempted to treat hear with a "cortisone shot," which "didn't help."

Ms. Connie Johnson was last seen by Dr. Allen on approximately 10/02 or 11/02. She has completed formal treatment for her right shoulder condition.

Ms. Connie Johnson denies having seen any other health care providers or undergoing any additional investigations regarding the diagnosis or treatment of her condition.

PRESENT COMPLAINTS

Ms. Connie Johnson complains of right shoulder pain. The pain occurs "when I do any kind stuff. It just hurts." Most of the pain is in the right lateral arm. Occasionally, it radiated to the elbow. The pain occurs several times a day. It may be precipitated by activities, such as washing her hair, or holding up a newspaper to read.

Ms. Connie Johnson states she can sleep on her right side for "only a little while, then it (my right shoulder) hurts. So, I gotta move."

Regarding strength about the right shoulder, she said, "It's not as good as before because I got the pain."

Ms. Connie Johnson denies any problems with sensation in the right upper extremity.

Ms. Connie Johnson denies having had any symptoms affecting the right shoulder prior to the 9/6/01 injury.

When asked how her shoulder is now compared to how it was a few months ago, Ms. Connie Johnson said, "It's worse. It didn't hurt as much when I do stuff."

Ms. Connie Johnson currently treats her right shoulder symptoms by "moving it around to get it going."

She takes medications for this.

Ms. Connie Johnson functional inquiry is otherwise negative or noncontributory. In particular, she denies any motor or sensory symptoms referable to either upper extremity. She denies any symptoms specifically affecting the left shoulder. She denies problems with neck pain, talking, or swallowing. She reports problems with vision, which she attributes to complications of diabetes mellitus and laser surgery.

Ms. Connie Johnson denies any motor or sensory symptoms referable to the lower extremities, or problems with low back pain.

Regarding her bowel and bladder, Ms. Connie Johnson said, "I've always had bowel problems . . . many years (diarrhea)."

HISTORY OF PAST HEALTH

Ms. Connie Johnson has been diagnosed with diabetes mellitus since age 26. Adverse effects of diabetes have mainly affected her eyes.

In the early 1990's, Ms. Connie Johnson underwent bowel and bladder surgery.

Ms. Connie Johnson denies having had any other serious medical illnesses, operations, accidents or injuries.

Current medications include Glucovance 2.5/500 mg one bid, Glucophage XR 500 mg one qhs, Actos 30 mg one qam, Protonix 40 mg one qam, and captopril 25 mg two qam and one qhs.

Ms. Connie Johnson has no known allergies.

PERSONAL AND SOCIAL HISTORY

Ms. Connie Johnson smokes four cigarettes a day. She drinks no alcohol.

When asked what she does for fun, Ms. Connie Johnson said, "I used to go bowling, but I cannot, because I cannot use my (right) arm." She last bowled prior to the 9/6/01 injury.

Ms. Connie Johnson enjoys shopping and going to movies.

FAMILY HISTORY

Ms. Connie Johnson is the fourth of four children. She has a brother and two sisters. She has no children. Her siblings and parents are in good health, except for her mother having diabetes mellitus.

WORK HISTORY

Ms. Connie Johnson has worked as a clerk for a department store chain for about eight years. For the past 5 ¾ years she has been a regular employee. Prior to that, she was an emergency hire. At the time of that 9/6/01 injury, she was working full-time. She last worked on 6/5/02. At that time, she was placed on off-duty status because "Dr. Allen said I can do light-duty, but there's no light-duty for me." Light-duty includes no lifting more than 15 pounds with the right upper extremity because of her shoulder condition.

When asked about plans for return to work, Ms. Connie Johnson initially said, "I just hope my arm will get better so I can go back to my same job."

When I reminded her that Dr. Allen's work restriction was permanent, Ms. Connie Johnson acknowledged that she has been "talking about looking for another job," but has not yet done so.

Prior to working for the book warehouse, Ms. Connie Johnson did "all different kinds of jobs," including working as a cashier and doing office work.

WORK ATTITUTES

Ms. Connie Johnson said about her job in the warehouse, "I liked it. I've been doing it for about eight years."

PHYSICAL EXAMINATION

On examination, Ms. Connie Johnson was a well-developed, overweight woman in no acute distress. She was alert, cooperative, and fully oriented. Her spontaneous speech was fluent and well articulated. She was neatly dressed and well-groomed. She wore a t-shirt, shorts, and sandals. She moved easily during the examination and on and off the examining table.

The general physical exam showed Ms. Connie Johnson's heart sounds were normal. There were no murmurs. Her chest was clear to auscultation. Her blood pressure was 130/85 mmHg in the right arm sitting. By her own report, she is 5'1" tall, and weighs 170 pounds. Ms. Connie Johnson has a marked central pattern of fat distribution.

On neurologic exam, Ms. Connie Johnson was normocephalic. Her neck was supple. There were no cervical bruits.

The cranial nerve exam showed the pupils to be 3.0 mm in diameter and reactive to light. Visual fields were full to confrontation. The funduscopic exam was noteworthy for changes consistent with diabetic retinopathy and laser surgery. The changes appear more extensive on the left than the right. There was a full range of extraocular movement and no nystagmus. Facial sensation and movement were intact. The ear canals and drums were normal. The palate elevated in the midline. The tongue protruded in the midline.

Motor exam showed normal power, tone, and bulk throughout. There were no abnormal involuntary movements.

A focused examination was performed about the right shoulder. There was no swelling, deformity, or discoloration. There was no focal tenderness. The range of motion was measured about both shoulders.

**SHOULDER RANGE OF MOTION**

| | Right | Left |
|---|---|---|
| Flexion | 150 | 180 |
| Extension | 45 | 50 |
| Abduction | 120 | 180 |
| Adduction | 30 | 40 |
| External Rotation | 70 | 90 |
| Internal Rotation | 30 | 80 |

There was a slightly greater passive range of motion than active range of motion about the right shoulder.

Hawkins sign was positive on the right.

Deep tendon reflexes were 1+ and symmetrical throughout. Plantar responses were down going bilaterally.

Sensation was intact to touch and pinprick in all dermatomes of both upper and both lower extremities. However, sensation to pinprick was decreased distally in the upper and lower extremities (stocking-glove distribution).

Stance and gait were normal.

PAIN STATUS INVENTORY

On a pain diagram completed by Ms. Connie Johnson she notes the presence of pain over the anterior aspect of the right shoulder and arm.

Ms. Connie Johnson completed a short-form McGill pain questionnaire rating 15 pain descriptors on a scale from 0 (none) to 3 (severe). Some descriptors were selected more than once. The minimum sum of 11 sensory descriptors was 9, for an average of 0.82. The maximum sum of 11 sensory descriptors was 10, for an average of 0.9. The sum of four affective descriptors was 6, for an average of 1.5. Sensory descriptors selected by Ms. Connie Johnson included: shooting, sharp, aching, heavy, and throbbing. Affective descriptors included: sickening, fearful, tiring/exhausting, and punishing/cruel.

On a present pain intensity index, rating overall pain from 0 (no pain) to 5 (excruciating), Ms. Connie Johnson rated her overall pain level at 3 (distressing).

On a visual analog scale, Ms. Connie Johnson placed a mark at a point corresponding to a pain level of 7.4 on a 10-point scale, with 10 being the worst possible pain.

Ms. Connie Johnson completed an AMA impairment impact inventory (pain questionnaire). The pain severity score was 12/20. The activities limitation score was 7/30. The emotional distress score was 5/10.

X-RAY EXAMINATION

I reviewed the imaging studies Ms. Connie Johnson brought with her.

On 6/14/95 plain x-rays of both hands and both wrists were performed on Ms. Connie Johnson. No significant abnormality is apparent.

On 4/11/02 plain x-rays of the right shoulder were performed on Ms. Connie Johnson. No significant abnormality is apparent.

REVIEW OF MEDICAL RECORDS

I reviewed the medical records sent to me regarding Ms. Connie Johnson These records are comprised of approximately 45 pages.

On approximately 11/2/01 (the date is not clear) a WC-1 report was submitted regarding an injury which occurred and which was reported on 9/6/01. The report indicates, "lifting boxes. Lifting and carrying boxes from floor to shelf." Ms. Connie Johnson was noted to have sustained a right shoulder strain. She sought treatment from Dr. Jones. She had been employed for 4.8 years as a stocker by the Thomas Book Warehouse at the time of this injury.

There is a copy of a position description for the position of stocker. It is primarily a qualitative description.

On 9/17/01 a reopen initial WC-2 report was submitted by Dr. Allen, of the Urgent Care Clinic, regarding treatment rendered to Ms. Connie Johnson beginning on 9/6/01 for the injury of that date. The report indicates, "In the warehouse, I was lifting boxes onto shelf and felt pain in my right shoulder." Reference was made to attached notes.

On 9/6/01 Ms. Johnson was seen by Dr. Allen in the Urgent Care Clinic. She reported injuring her right shoulder after lifting boxes onto shelves at work.

The boxes were filled with books. She did it for about half an hour. She began to experience pain about three hours after the activity. The pain was mostly with abduction of the shoulder. She was examined. Findings included tenderness near the right AC joint. There was a decreased range of motion secondary to pain. She was diagnosed with sprain and tendonitis of the right shoulder. Naprosyn was prescribed.

There are copies of interim WC-2 reports from the office of Dr. Allen regarding ongoing treatment rendered to Ms. Connie Johnson related to the 9/6/01 injury.

On 9/14/01, Ms. Connie Johnson was seen in follow-up by Dr. Allen. The pain in her right shoulder had previously been rated at 10/10. It was now approximately 5/10. (The copy is not clear.) She was examined. Findings included limited internal rotation. The assessment was right shoulder tendonitis. Naprosyn was prescribed. Follow-up in one week was planned.

On 9/21/01 Ms. Connie Johnson was seen in follow-up by Dr. Allen. Right shoulder symptoms persisted. The pain was on the top of the shoulder. She was examined. Findings included mildly decreased range of internal rotation. Her range of motion appeared otherwise normal. There was mild tenderness over the AC joint. The assessment was right shoulder pain – improving. Ms. Connie Johnson was released to return to work as of 9/24/01.

On 3/28/02 Ms. Connie Johnson returned to Dr. Allen. Only the first page of this two-page report is included among these records. Ms. Connie Johnson complained of right shoulder pain rated 6-7/10. The pain was at the top of the shoulder. She said her symptoms never went away.

On 4/25/02 a report was submitted by Dr. George Davis, an orthopedic surgeon, regarding evaluation of Ms. Johnson on 4/11/02 at the request of Dr. Allen. Ms. Connie Johnson was 35 years old. She complained of right shoulder pain, which she attributed to the effect of an injury which occurred on the job on 9/6/01 after lifting boxes at work. She reported experiencing sharp pain of the right shoulder radiating to the upper arm, which had not resolved since the accident. She reported occasional cracking and popping sounds in the right shoulder, and difficulty with sleep, as well as activities of daily living. She denied neck pain or arm numbness. She felt the symptoms were no better, despite the passage of time. Her history of past health was noteworthy for diabetes, irregular heartbeat, hypertension, and a sensitive stomach. Ms. Connie Johnson was examined. Findings included restricted right shoulder range of motion with elevation to 140 degrees. Internal rotation was performed to the lumbar spine. Impingement tests were positive on the right. Passive range of motion about the right arm was good, without signs of capsular adhesions. Plain x-rays of the right shoulder were reviewed and noted to be negative. The impression was right shoulder bursitis/tendonitis from industrial occurrence on 9/6/02. Treatment with physical therapy and possible treatment with an injection were recommended, along with light-duty work. Follow-up as-needed was planned. Dr. Davis stated if Dr.Allen wanted to transfer Ms. Johnson's care, he would accept her.

On 4/11/02 plain x-rays of the right shoulder were performed on Ms. Connie Johnson at the request of Dr. Davis. The films were read by Dr. Davis as negative right shoulder.

There are copies of notes regarding ongoing follow-up of Ms. Connie Johnson by Dr. Davis. They are handwritten and marginally legible.

On 5/13/02 Ms. Connie Johnson was seen in follow-up by Dr. Davis. Persistent intermittent right shoulder symptoms were noted. Treatment with physical therapy was planned. If symptoms persisted, an injection would be administered.

On 5/23/02 Dr. Davis submitted a disability certificate for Ms. Connie Johnson covering the period between 4/11-5/24/02, indicating she could return to light-duty work with no heavy lifting or carrying, and no climbing until further notice.

On 6/20/02 Ms. Connie Johnson was seen in follow-up by Dr. Davis. Right shoulder symptoms persisted. She had not attended physical therapy. She had been off work, as there was no light-duty. She was otherwise OK, except for her eyes and diabetic problems. She was examined. Findings included right shoulder range of motion to 120 degrees (flexion? Abduction?). Internal rotation was performed to the hip. Impingement signs were positive. The assessment was right shoulder bursitis/tendonitis. Ms. Connie Johnson was referred for treatment with physical therapy.

On 6/20/02 Dr. Davis extended the period of light-duty work.

There are copies of notes regarding physical therapy treatment provided to Ms. Connie Johnson at the Coray Rehabilitation Center. Treatment appeared to begin on 7/8/02.

On 8/15/02 a physical therapy progress report was submitted by Brad Stoner. He noted Ms. Connie Johnson had been attending outpatient physical therapy. She received a total of eight treatments thus far. She reported her overall condition improved by about 20%. Symptoms otherwise persisted. More treatment would be provided, if requested, by Dr. Davis.

On 8/19/02 Dr. Davis submitted a request for additional treatment with physical therapy, with eight treatments between 9/9-10/11/02.

On 8/29/02 you wrote to Dr. Davis after their meeting on that date, clarifying medical issues regarding Ms. Connie Johnson and her shoulder condition alleged to the 9/6/01 injury. The diagnosis was noted to be right shoulder tendonitis and bursitis, with subsequent adhesive capsulitis. She had been unable to participate fully in the rehab of her right shoulder due to a pre-existing medical condition involving unstable diabetes mellitus with retinal hemorrhaging, requiring ongoing laser surgeries. It was noted the slightest increase in pressure caused her to bleed again. Thus, she had been unable to do the work hardening program. She was also unable to use the Thera-band in rehab. Manipulation under anesthesia to assist in recovery of adhesive capsulitis was also said to be not viable related to her diabetic condition. When seen in follow up on 9/17/02, the plan was to administer a cortisone injection to the right shoulder. Unfortunately, even if the steroid injection and physical therapy had been completed, Ms. Connie Johnson was noted to be not capable of performing her regular job secondary to diabetes. Ms. Connie Johnson indicated she would be contacting Dr. Willem Holz, who was handling her diabetic eye surgeries, to obtain permanent restrictions regarding that issue. Dr. Davis noted, in conclusion, the injuries Ms. Johnson sustained to the right shoulder on 9/6/01 would most likely have healed by now, and she would have been able to return to her job as a stocker if it were not for the unfortunate pre-existing issues of her diabetes. On 9/2/02, Dr. Davis signed his name to a letter and crossed out the portion indicating that, by now, the right shoulder condition would likely have healed by now were it not for the diabetes. Dr. Davis stated that the date by which Ms. Connie Johnson's shoulder condition would heal was unknown.

On 9/6/02 a functional capacity assessment form was completed by Dr. Willem Holz, an ophthalmologist, regarding Ms. Connie Johnson, noting she could lift and carry up to ten pounds maximum, on an occasional basis. She was to do minimal bending or stooping. These restrictions were said to be permanent.

On 9/17/02 Ms. Connie Johnson wrote to Dr. Holz thanking him for seeing her in a follow-up visit. Ms. Connie Johnson's right shoulder adhesive capsulitis was reportedly resolved. The physical therapist felt she would benefit from continued therapy for strengthening. Dr. Holz reportedly felt Ms. Connie Johnson made good progress in therapy, but discontinued this due to the overlapping diagnosis of a diabetic eye disorder. She had a recent laser surgery to the eyes due to retinal hemorrhages from such movements as bending forward to the pick up a soda, and pulling weeds. A cortisone injection was administered to the right shoulder area. Ms. Connie Johnson was instructed to monitor her blood glucose more frequently and stay in contact with her diabetic educator. Dr. Holz signed a copy of this letter, indicating agreement with its contents, on 10/16/02.

On 10/3/02 a report was submitted by Dr. Rabe, an orthopedic surgeon, following his review of records sent to him regarding Ms. Connie Johnson. Included was a report of a functional capacity evaluation in which it was felt Ms. Connie Johnson occasionally could do a variety of activities, and lift up to ten pounds. This was exclusively for her right shoulder. Dr. Rabe then addressed several questions, and noted that Ms. Connie Johnson's unstable diabetic condition prevented her from completing the recommended treatment for her shoulder. He thought it was likely she was medically stable. She was not doing active rehab. There was no active treatment. She was more than one year post-injury. He thought it was unlikely her condition would change in the indefinite future. He reviewed the records and noted range of motion measurements were documented in the physical therapy report of 8/15/02. Findings included limitation of shoulder flexion to 160 degrees. There was also limitation of internal rotation. He stated that limitation of flexion to 160 degrees represented 1% impairment of the upper extremity. Assuming there was a similar impairment in abduction, that would also represent 1%. He estimated Ms. Connie Johnson would have 1-2% impairment of the upper extremity for limitation of internal rotation, and possibly another percent impairment in one of the other ranges of motion. Therefore, an estimated permanent impairment would be on the order of 4-5% of the upper extremity. He emphasized this was not a formal rating, but an estimate of what he thought her rating would be if it were done formally. He noted the majority of patients in their 30's, such as Ms. Connie Johnson, with a diagnosis of shoulder tendonitis would be able to resume their previous occupations. Therefore, he said it was medically probable, but by no means certain, that if she were able to participate fully in physical therapy and exercise programs as recommended, she would be able to resume her previous occupation.

On 10/14/02 Dr. Davis completed a functional capacity assessment form, indicating Ms. Connie Johnson could lift and carry up to ten pounds maximum, on a frequent basis. Dr. Davis stated this limitation was based exclusively on Ms. Connie Johnson's right shoulder condition, and did not include restrictions due to her eye condition.

On 10/14/02 you wrote to Dr. Davis following your visit of this date. Ms. Connie Johnson's right shoulder had a good range of motion. She continued to complain of pain, which ranged from 0 to 5-6/10. She reported no help from the recent cortisone injection. Dr. Davis felt she had attained maximum medical improvement, and had permanent partial disability with work restrictions. On 10/23/02 Dr. Davis signed a copy of this letter, indicating agreement with its content.

Thank you for your letter regarding this case. You noted Ms. Connie Johnson is a 36-year-old stocker for the Book Warehouse. On 9/6/01 she injured her right shoulder after lifting and carrying heavy boxes. You summarized Ms. Connie Johnson's subsequent clinical course, and note that she had been unable to participate fully in rehabilitation of her shoulder due to a pre-existing medical condition, specifically diabetes mellitus with retinal hemorrhaging, requiring ongoing laser surgeries. The slightest increase in pressure caused her eyes to bleed. You note Dr. Davis deemed Ms. Connie Johnson at maximum medical improvement with permanent partial impairment, and outlined permanent work restrictions for her shoulder. Following my examination of Ms. Connie Johnson and review of the records sent to me, you have asked me to address several questions.

SUMMARY

Ms. Connie Johnson is a 36-year-old woman who complains of right shoulder pain. She attributes her symptoms to the effects of an injury which occurred on the job on 9/6/01. At the time of that injury, Ms. Connie Johnson reportedly lifted approximately 40 boxes, weighing about 30 pounds each, from floor to shelf. Following the onset of symptoms, Ms. Connie Johnson sought treatment at the Urgent Care Clinic. She was seen by Dr. Jones in the clinic on the injury date. Dr. Jones diagnosed sprain and tendonitis of the right shoulder, and prescribed Naprosyn.

On 9/14 and 9/21/01 Ms. Connie Johnson was seen in follow-up by Dr. Allen. Shoulder symptoms had improved. Ms. Connie Johnson was off work between approximately 9/6-9/24/01.

On 3/28/02 Ms. Connie Johnson returned to Dr. Allen for persistent right shoulder symptoms. She was referred to Dr. Davis, an orthopedic surgeon.

On 4/11/02 Ms. Connie Johnson was evaluated by Dr. Davis. Findings included a decreased range of motion about the right shoulder, and positive impingement signs. She was diagnosed with right shoulder bursitis/tendonitis from industrial occurrence on 9/6/02. Treatment with physical therapy was recommended.

On 4/11/02 plain x-rays of the right shoulder were performed on Ms. Connie Johnson and found to be normal.

Ms. Connie Johnson was seen in follow-up by Dr. Davis on dates including 5/13 and 6/20/02. Continued treatment with physical therapy was recommended.

On 5/23/02 Dr. Davis indicated Ms. Connie Johnson should be on light-duty work as of 4/11/02. Subsequent notes continued to extend the period of light-duty.

On 9/6/02 a functional capacity assessment form was completed by Dr. Holz, an ophthalmologist, who noted Ms. Connie Johnson could lift and carry up to ten pounds maximum on an occasional basis. She was to do minimal bending or stooping. This work restriction was permanent (and was related to complications of diabetic retinopathy).

On approximately 9/17/02 Dr. Noyes administered a steroid injection to Ms. Connie Johnson's right shoulder. Ms. Connie Johnson denies any significant improvement as a result of this.

Ms. Connie Johnson was apparently unable to participate in physical therapy treatment related to problems with diabetic retinopathy.

On 10/3/02 a report was submitted by Dr. Rabe, an orthopedic surgeon, following his review of Ms. Connie Johnson's medical records. Dr. Rabe estimated Ms. Connie Johnson would have a permanent impairment on the order of 4-5% of the right upper extremity for her shoulder condition. He emphasized this was not a formal rating, but only an estimate. He noted the majority of patients in their 30's, such as Ms. Connie Johnson, with a diagnosis of shoulder tendonitis would be able to resume their previous occupations. Therefore, he said it was medically probable that if she were able to participate fully in physical therapy, she would be able to resume her previous occupation.

On 10/14/02 Dr. Rabe completed a functional capacity assessment form, indicating Ms. Connie Johnson could lift and carry up to ten pounds maximum on a frequent basis. Dr. Rabe stated this limitation was based exclusively on Ms. Connie Johnson's right shoulder condition, and did not include restrictions due to her eye condition.

On 10/30/02 Dr. Davis signed a note indicating he agreed with Dr. Rabe's opinions.

Ms. Connie Johnson's examination is noteworthy for a decreased range of motion about the right shoulder due to complaints of pain, centralized fat distribution, decreased sensation to pinprick in a glove and stocking distribution, and retinal changes consistent with diabetic retinopathy and laser surgery.

IMPRESSION

Ms. Connie Johnson's history, physical examination, and results of ancillary studies are most consistent with the diagnosis of chronic right shoulder tendonitis/subacromial bursitis.

Other diagnoses which apply in Ms. Connie Johnson's case include diabetes mellitus and complications of diabetes mellitus, including diabetic retinopathy and probable small fiber peripheral neuropathy.

RECOMMENDATIONS FOR FURTHER EVALUATION

No additional specific investigations are indicated in Ms. Connie Johnson's case at this time related to the effects of the 9/6/01 injury.

TREATMENT RECOMMENDATIONS

In general, Ms. Connie Johnson should be encouraged to remain active and continue to participate in an appropriate home exercise program daily, aimed at maintaining strength and flexibility about the right shoulder, within the limits imposed by Dr. Davis, regarding lifting with the right upper extremity. Ms. Connie Johnson indicates she is doing stretching exercises regularly to maintain her range of motion.

In view of Ms. Connie Johnson's general medical conditions, I agree with Dr. Davis that additional specific formal treatment directed toward the right shoulder condition is either not indicated, or contraindicated.

CAUSATION

Based on the history provided by Ms. Connie Johnson, and the information contained in the medical records, there is a probable causal relationship between her right shoulder condition and the occupational injury of 9/6/01.

Although diabetes mellitus may be regarded as a risk factor for the development of some shoulder conditions, including adhesive capsulitis, this does not appear to apply in Ms. Connie Johnson's case.

PROGNOSIS

Ms. Connie Johnson is approximately one year four months post-injury. She experiences some persistent right shoulder symptoms, which are predominantly activity-related. Overall, her condition has not changed significantly in some months (particularly based on the information contained in the medical records), and medical conditions unrelated to the 9/6/01 injury preclude more aggressive treatment of her right shoulder condition. Considering this data, the current pattern of symptoms will likely continue.

ANSWERS TO SPECIFIC QUESTIONS

I have attempted to address the questions which you have raised in your consultation request in the body of this report including questions concerning Ms. Connie Johnson's history, findings on examination, diagnosis, recommendations for further evaluation, treatment recommendations, causation, and prognosis.

In addition, you ask what is Ms. Connie Johnson's current diagnosis and prognosis.

I have attempted to address these questions in the Impression and Prognosis sections above. In addition, in the Prognosis section, I note Ms. Connie Johnson's condition has not changed significantly in several months. Although Ms. Connie Johnson's right shoulder has somewhat more limited range of motion now than that documented in the physical therapy report of 8/15/02, in that report, reference was made to "maximum assisted right shoulder flexion." This is not the same as active range of motion. In view of this, it is unlikely there has been any significant change in Ms. Connie Johnson's actual condition.

You ask my opinion as to whether or not Ms. Connie Johnson's current symptoms and alleged disability status continues to be the result of the industrial injury of 9/6/01, or whether or not it may be the result of some other cause, such as diabetes.

Ms. Connie Johnson's disability is related to a combination of factors, including the 9/6/01 injury, and diabetic retinopathy. Were it not for diabetic retinopathy, Ms. Connie Johnson would be able to participate in a more aggressive physical therapy program, and improve range of motion and function about the right shoulder. Her current right shoulder condition contributes to her present disability status.

The lifting and carrying limit of ten pounds occasionally to frequently in general, primarily related to the problem of diabetic retinopathy. Were that not the case, Ms. Connie Johnson would be able to lift and carry more than ten pounds at least with the left upper extremity. With respect to the 9/6/01 injury, per se, work restrictions may include no lifting and carrying of more than 10-15 pounds with the right upper extremity on more than an occasional basis, and no lifting above shoulder height.

Although the work restrictions for both the condition of diabetic retinopathy and her shoulder injury are similar, they are not entirely the same as reflected in the discussion above. Unfortunately, the problem of diabetic retinopathy appears to preclude more aggressive treatment of her work-related shoulder condition.

You ask if Ms. Connie Johnson's current medical treatment for her industrial injury to her shoulder appropriate. If not, you ask me to explain.

Ms. Connie Johnson is presently not receiving any formal treatment. However, she states she is participating in a stretching program regularly. This is appropriate. Unfortunately, problems with diabetic retinopathy appear to preclude more aggressive treatment of her right shoulder.

You ask if I have any recommendations for further treatment.

Attempts to treat Ms. Connie Johnson have included oral non-sterioidal anti-inflammatories, a steroid injection, and a limited course of treatment with physical therapy. Treatment with active physical therapy generally represents the corner stone of management of conditions such as Ms. Connie Johnson's. Unfortunately, problems with diabetic retinopathy would appear to preclude this. Surgical treatment would not be indicated, particularly because she would be unable to participate in post-operative physical therapy. Considering this situation, I have no additional recommendations regarding further formal treatment.

In my opinion, you ask if Ms. Connie Johnson's condition would deteriorate if treatments for her industrial injury were discontinued.

Ms. Connie Johnson has discontinued treatment for her shoulder condition due to the presence of a non-work-related condition (diabetic retinopathy). Although Ms. Connie Johnson feels that her symptoms are subjectively worse now than they were several months ago, the information contained in the medical records does not tend to support a significant change in her condition during this time. The physical therapy progress report of 8/15/02 indicates Ms. Connie Johnson complained of pain about the right shoulder with active elevation above 90 degrees. (That is presently true-- Ms. Connie Johnson limits shoulder elevation to 150 degrees.) The maximum assisted right shoulder flexion noted in the 8/15/02 report was 160 degrees. This is consistent with the current findings of a slightly greater passive range of motion than that demonstrated actively.

In summary, Ms. Connie Johnson's condition has not deteriorated in the absence of further formal treatment.

Ms. Connie Johnson should be encouraged to continue her home stretching program. Aside from this, Ms. Connie Johnson is not a candidate for additional specific treatment directed toward her right shoulder.

You ask my opinion as to whether Ms. Connie Johnson has achieved stationary and stable status/maximum medical improvement for her shoulder injury.

Based on the history provided by Ms. Connie Johnson and the information contained in the medical records, including the report of 10/23/02, Ms. Connie Johnson has obtained maximum medical improvement for her shoulder injury.

Ms. Connie Johnson is stationary and stable, you ask my opinion as to the extent of any permanent impairment sustained by her, in accordance with the AMA Guides to the Evaluation of Permanent Impairment, Fifth Edition. In the event that I find there are pre-existing factors involved in her impairment, you ask me to apportion their degree of contribution.

Ms. Connie Johnson is stable for rating purposes. She will be rated using the Guides to the Evaluation of Permanent Impairment, Fifth Edition. In the event that I find there are pre-existing factors involved in her impairment, you ask to apportion their degree of contribution.

Ms. Connie Johnson is stable for rating purposes. She will be rated using the Guides to the Evaluation of Permanent Impairment, Fifth Edition, published by the American Medical Association.

Referring to Figure 16-40, on page 476, limitation of right shoulder flexion to 150 degrees represents 2% impairment of the upper extremity. Limitation of extension to 45 degrees represents 1% impairment of the upper extremity (with rounding).

Referring to Figure 16-43, on page 477, limitation of abduction to 120 degrees represents 3% impairment of the upper extremity. Limitation of adduction to 30 degrees represents 1% impairment of the upper extremity.

Referring to Figure 16-46, on page 479, limitation of internal rotation to 30 degrees represents 2% impairment of the upper extremity.

These impairment values are additive, for a total of 8% impairment of the upper extremity.

Based on the history provided by Ms. Connie Johnson, and the information contained in the medical records, the issue of apportionment does not apply to this impairment rating.

This impairment rating is somewhat higher than that estimated by Dr. Rabe in his report of 10/3/02 following his review of Ms. Connie Johnson's medical records. Dr. Rabe based his estimate on range of motion measurements referenced in the physical therapy report of 8/15/02. However, the limited measurements documented were based on "maximum assisted" movement. Whereas, the measurements used for impairment rating purposes are active and unassisted.

In my professional opinion, you ask if Ms. Connie Johnson has, or will have, any permanent restrictions from returning to her normal and customary duties as a stocker resulting from the industrial injury of 9/6/01.

Permanent restrictions would apply in Ms. Connie Johnson's case related to the persistence of her right shoulder condition. In the absence of her ocular condition (diabetic retinopathy), solely related to the effects of her right shoulder condition, it is likely Ms. Connie Johnson would be able to return to work with a lifting and carrying limit of up to 15 pounds occasionally to frequently, and no lifting above shoulder height. With respect to the right upper extremity, there would be no lifting limit related solely to the use of the left upper extremity.

ADDITIONAL COMMENTS

The above analysis is based upon the history provided by Ms. Connie Johnson findings on examination and the information contained in the medical records sent to me. It is assumed that the material provided is correct. If more information becomes available at a later date, an additional report may be requested. Such information may or may not change the opinions rendered in this evaluation

The opinions I have expressed are based upon reasonable medical probability and are totally independent of the requesting agent.

Please do not hesitate to contact me if you have any questions regarding this report.

Thank you for asking me to see Ms. Connie Johnson.

Kevin Keefe, MD
Certified Independent Medical Examiner

**Report #4: Workers' Compensation—Hearing Loss**

This report is most notable for the following.

- It is concise and well written.
- There is no superfluous or extraneous information.
- The report is nicely formatted.

While this is an excellent report, all reports can be improved. Areas of possible improvement include the following points.

- The medical records reviewed were not itemized.
- The report would be better if it explicitly explained how the disability percentage was calculated.

---

September 1, 2003

Ms. Sylvia Obendorf
Obendorf, Siefert, & Kresge
1212 President Street
Apple Valley, New Jersey 10023

Re: Case 12-34578

Thank you very much for referring this individual. He is a 52 year old man who comes for evaluation regarding loss of hearing in his right ear.

EMPLOYMENT HISTORY: He has worked for the City of East Courtland for 21 years as a firefighter. He last worked 1-28-03.

PAST MEDICAL HISTORY: He has hypertension previously treated with Norvasc. (His antihypertensive medication has recently been changed and he does not recall its name.) He has a history of hepatitis C. He denies history of ear, nose, or general nose or throat problems, "no." He has no known allergies. He smoked for about five years until 1979. He does not use tobacco products at this time. Family History: He has no known family history of hearing loss. He has had prior audiograms. The audiogram of 6-2-99 was included with the medical records; I will comment on it later in this report.

PRESENT COMPLAINTS: He notes hearing loss mostly on the right side which he first noted in approximately 1999. He currently has "constant ringing right ear only." He notes the incident to be described occurred on 8-21-01.

HISTORY OF INCIDENT: "I was filling some air tanks. When air bleeds from the tanks, it makes a loud, hissing noise. I noticed the ringing in my right ear; it started immediately." This operation entails taking air from smaller tanks ("bleeding the air out") before refilling them from a larger tank.

At that time of the incident he went to the company doctor, "I believe the next day, did all kinds of tests; did not give a definite answer as to what was wrong."

Initially he stated to me that he had no ringing in his ears before the incident, "no." Later he stated that while he did have some ringing before the incident, "it didn't linger; now it is constant and hearing loss is worse."

PHYSICAL EXAMINATION: The ear canals are clear, the tympanic membranes intact and normal in appearance. The nose showed a good airway without obstruction. The septum is not obstructing. The mucous membranes and turbinates are clear. The pharynx and nasopharynx are clear without discharge. He heard normal conversation well.

MEDICAL RECORDS: The medical records include a handwritten note from Edward Haynes, D.O., et al, ear, nose and throat, dated 5-27-99 and an audiogram of 6-2-99. It gives a history of "ringing right ear for about a few years, varies (illegible word that may be "more" or "worse"), hearing varies on right."

Following the audiogram, which revealed normal hearing in the left ear and a mild hearing loss in the right ear with bilaterally normal speech discrimination ability, he underwent an MRI of the brain, open MRI of internal auditory canals. The report of 6-22-99 states the MRI was normal.

The incident in which he was filling the tanks occurred on 8-21-01. The report indicates "I noticed my right ear was ringing due to the noise from bleeding residual air from the tank system; the noise referred to above is loud and piercing."

There is also indication in the record of a diagnosis of hepatitis C in 1998.

AUDIOGRAM: The audiogram shows left normal hearing from 250-8000 Hz at all frequencies tested. Speech discrimination testing in the left ear is normal.

The right ear shows sensorineural hearing loss from 250-8000 Hz with a moderately severe decrease in speech discrimination ability.

The audiogram was conducted by a certified audiologist under my supervision using an audiometer calibrated to ANSI standards, in an enclosure meeting ANSI background noise requirements. The reliability was good.

DIAGNOSIS: Right sensorineural hearing loss. Left normal hearing.

OPINION: This individual has normal hearing in the left ear. He had no specific complaints about his left ear.

In the right ear he has sensorineural hearing loss with accompanying tinnitus. The hearing loss in his right ear is unrelated to the incident of 8-21-01. It is not due to either acute or chronic noise exposure. Hearing loss of this type does not occur from such exposure.

It is noted that in 1999 he had a variable hearing loss in the right ear. The medical probability is that he has a condition known as fluctuating hearing loss or cochlear hydrops in which the hearing level may drop to a greater level with each succeeding episode of hydrops. Following an episode, hearing may or may not recover to its original level.

Although the MRI in 1999 was negative, he should be counseled to have an MRI with gadolinium contrast to be sure that he is not harboring a cerebropontine angle or internal auditory canal lesion.

Fluctuating hearing loss may occur from such a lesion although it is unusual. Ordinarily the hearing loss is due to obstruction of the outflow system in the inner ear and can be treated with a combination of medication and/or surgical treatment.

CONCLUSION:

1) Right-sided hearing loss and tinnitus unrelated to his occupation. It has nothing to do with the sound that occurred from bleeding air from tanks.
2) He should have further work-up as noted above through his own physicians.
3) He has not suffered any permanent hearing loss related to his occupation.

Using the NJ 1980 workers' compensation guidelines to assess hearing loss disability, he has 22.5% right, 0% left and 0% binaural.

The opinions expressed in this report are within a reasonable degree of medical probability.

If you have any questions, please feel free to contact me.

Sincerely,

Richard Gilnett, MD

RG/mkh
enc.

**Report #5: Workers' Compensation (Claimant)—Chiropractic**

This report is most notable for the following.

- Superbly drafted identifying information.
- Superb formatting makes it easy to read.
- Very good use of headnotes. It is easy to find the information the reader is looking for.
- Digital images of the examinee are incorporated into the report. A picture says a thousand words. The digital images add greatly to the report.
- Charts and graphs make the report stand out and help communicate the basis of the expert's opinions.
- The documentation of the tests demonstrates the thoroughness of the examination that was performed.
- Conclusions are supported by citations to texts and articles.

While this is an excellent report, all reports can be improved. Areas of possible improvement follow.

- The times of arrival and departure are exactly on the hour. This is not believable. More precise times are more believable (e.g., 4:57 P.M. instead of 5:00 P.M.).
- The issues covered in the report and the opinions expressed are somewhat difficult to find and read.
- Boilerplate language concerning the appropriate use of the AMA *Guides* might be better left out.

---

**Steven Babitsky, 12/30/02**

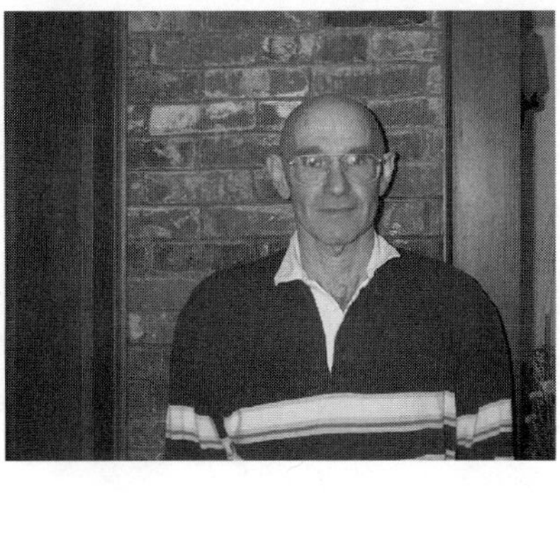

## INDEPENDENT MEDICAL EXAMINATION

| | |
|---|---|
| EXAMINEE: | Steven Babitsky |
| EXAMINEE'S DATE OF BIRTH: | 08/25/62 |
| DATE OF EXAMINATION: | 12/30/02 |
| DATE OF INJURY: | 11/01/99 |
| REFERRING INDIVIDUAL: | Mr. James J. Mangraviti, Jr. |
| REFERRING ORGANIZATION: | SEAK, Inc.<br>Legal & Medical Information Systems |
| REFERRING ORGANIZATION'S ADDRESS: | Post Office Box 729<br>Falmouth, MA 02541 |
| REFERENCE NO.: | 10100 |
| EXAMINING PHYSICIAN: | Preston B. Fitzgerald, Sr., D.C., CDE I, CICE, CIFCME |
| LOCATION OF EXAMINATION: | Manning, South Carolina 29102 |
| TYPE OF EXAMINATION: | Workers' Compensation |

## INTRODUCTION AND BACKGROUND

Mr. Babitsky is a 40-year-old male who was referred for the purposes of an independent medical examination (IME) by the above client. The independent medical examination process was explained to Mr. Babitsky. He understands that no patient/treating physician relationship was established. Mr. Babitsky was advised that the information he provided will not be held in confidence and that a written report will be sent to the requesting client.

Mr. Babitsky arrived at our offices at 2:00 p.m. where he was interviewed and examined. Mr. Babitsky left our offices at 5:00 p.m. Mr. Babitsky was cooperative. He was a good historian in relating his history. The information as provided by Mr. Babitsky was consistent with the medical records in my possession and reviewed at the time of or prior to the examination.

Mr. Babitsky was driven to the examination by himself.

A questionnaire and pain inventories were completed by the examinee. To ensure accuracy, the clinical history was dictated in his presence. Throughout the physical examination a staff member, Sonja Torez, was present. Mr. Babitsky reported no difficulties occurring during the examination. This examination was performed at the request of the above referring client.

## PREEXISTING STATUS

Mr. Babitsky had a disc herniation in 1995 at L4-5. He denies any prior work or liability-related injuries. He denies any significant prior injuries.

Mr. Babitsky stated that at the time of his injury on 11/01/99 his was not under any self-imposed restrictions in his activities to avoid re-injury to his lower back and right leg.

## HISTORY

The following history is as elicited from Mr. Babitsky.

### History of Injury:

Mr. Babitsky reported that he was at a football practice on November 1, 1999, on his job as a coach at LMA, when he threw a football approximately

15 yards. He felt a "pop" in his lower back. He had an immediate "sharp" pain in his low back and down his right leg. He had to go home and go to bed and took over-the-counter medications. The following day he came here for treatment, where he was x-rayed, examined, given physical therapy, and returned the next day for physical therapy and manipulations. Pain increased, so he returned to Carolina Spine, Dr. Don Johnson, and had surgery on November 23, 1999. On January 1, 2000, he was lifting his right knee to put on pants when he felt a "pop" in his lower back. He then again had surgery on January 6, 2000. He has had frequent pain and discomfort in his lower back and both legs. Ibuprofen only gives temporary relief.

**Past Medical History**

| | |
|---|---|
| Medical: | None |
| Surgical: | 1st back surgery - August 1995, low back problems.<br>2nd surgery - November 23, 1999, due to injury from work on November 1, 1999.<br>3rd surgery - January 6, 2000, due to injury on November 1, 2000, when pulling on pants. |
| Allergies: | None |
| Medications: | Ibuprofen – over-the-counter. Takes five days per week. |

## REVIEW AND SUMMARY OF MEDICAL RECORDS

Mr. Babitsky's records that were sent by the above client arrived at our office on December 30, 2002. These records were reviewed carefully. The records that were available for review fell between the dates of November 2, 1999 and April 11, 2001. No other records were available for review.

I had the opportunity to review the following records:

1. Records from Corrine Daley, D.C., of Daley Rehab Clinic, 4009 N. Doyle Ave., Dixon, Iowa, dated 11/02/99 through 12/15/99.

2. Records from Karl Petersen, Sr., M.D., of Midwestern Health, 1515 W. Shawnee Rd., Morristown, Iowa, dated 11/05/99 through 04/11/01.

3. MRI reports from Maria Lorenz, M.D., Ph.D., and Holly Folgam, M.D., of MRI Specialists, 4028 Doyle Ave., Dixon, Iowa, dated 11/08/99 and 01/04/00.

4. History and Physical from St. Elizabeth's Hospital, 1001 W. Lincoln Ave., Dixon, Iowa, dated 01/06/00.

5. Report of Operation from St. Elizabeth's Hospital, 1001 W. Lincoln Ave., Dixon, Iowa, dated 11/23/99 through 01/09/00.

6. Discharge Summary from St. Elizabeth's Hospital, 1001 W. Lincoln Ave., Dixon, Iowa, dated 01/09/00.

**Summary of Diagnostic Studies:**

| Date | Study | Findings |
|---|---|---|
| 11/08/ 99 | MRI Lumbar Spine, W/O and W/ Contrast Disc Imaging Referred by: Donald Johnson, M.D. | OVERVIEW: Overview of the lumbar spine shows there is normal bony alignment and normal marrow signal with no evidence of a congenital anomaly of the spine. The visualized paraspinal soft tissues are unremarkable. Images of the hips, sacroiliac joints, piriformis muscles, and proximal sciatic nerves reveal no abnormality.<br><br>THORACIC SPINE: Views of the distal thoracic spine show a normal spinal cord and conus medullaris, normal vertebra, and no evidence of abnormal discs.<br><br>LUMBAR SPINE OVERVIEW: There are changes of laminectomy and discectomy at L4-5. There is loss of height and signal in the discs at L1-2, L4-5 and L5-S1, the remaining discs showing loss of signal.<br><br>L1-2. Images at this level show mild concentric bulging of the disc. No compression of neural structures is noted.<br><br>L2-3, L3-4. There is normal disc space height and signal without disc bulge or herniation of disc material beyond its |

| | | |
|---|---|---|
| | | normal confines. There is no evidence of entrapment of the nerve roots in the exit foramen, lateral recess or in the central canal.<br><br>L4-5. Images demonstrate changes of laminectomy and discectomy. There is a board-based recurrent disc herniation which is located centrally. Furthermore, there is a migrated free fragment of disc located approximately half way up the dorsal aspect of the L4 vertebral body on the right. There is peripheral enhancement surrounding this free fragment. It compresses the thecal sac markedly on the right side.<br><br>L5-S1. Images show mild disc bulging, slightly more prominent on the left than right without evidence for focal disc herniation.<br><br>OPINION: MRI of the lumbar spine demonstrates post operative changes at L4-5 with a recurrent central disc herniation, as well as a right parasagittal free fragment above the disc level, compressing the thecal sac and nerve roots on the right. |
| 11/23/99 | PORTABLE LUMBAR SPINE 1 VIEW/797039 East Cooper Regional Medical Center | A portable lateral view of the lumbar spine was obtained at 4:10 pm on 11/23/99. No previous lumbar spine exams are available at this institution for comparison - the usual numbering of five lumbar spine segments will be assumed. Surgical retractors are present posterior to the lower lumbar region with the tip of a surgical probe projecting posterior to the spinal canal at the level of the L4-5 disc space. The L4-5 disc space appears narrowed and there also appears to be slights retrolisthesis at this level. |

| | | |
|---|---|---|
| 01/04/00 | MRI Lumbar Spine, W/O and W/ Contrast Disc Imaging Referred by: Donald Johnson, M.D. | OVERVIEW: Overview of the lumbar spine shows there is normal bony alignment and normal marrow signal with no evidence of a congenital anomaly of the spine. The visualized paraspinal soft tissues are unremarkable. Images of the hips, sacroiliac joints, piriformis muscles, and proximal sciatic nerves reveal no abnormality.<br><br>THORACIC SPINE: Views of the distal thoracic spine show a normal spinal cord and conus medullaris, normal vertebra, and no evidence of abnormal discs.<br><br>L1-2, L2-3, L3-4. There is normal disc space height and signal without disc bulge or herniation of disc material beyond its normal confines. There is no evidence of entrapment of the nerve roots in the exit foramen, lateral recess or in the central canal.<br><br>L4-5. There has been surgical intervention at this level. It appears to have occurred in the interval between this examination and the examination of 11/8/99. Fluid collection can be seen in subcutaneous tissue immediately behind the spine, as well as evidence of edema in the paraspinal muscles adjacent to the spinous process of L5 with evidence of enhancing tissue extending along the lateral aspect of the thecal sac into the lateral recess and ventral to the thecal sac itself. On the previous examination, there was clear evidence of a large free fragment in this region. On this examination, there is evidence of a somewhat mixed low signal and enhancing tissue mass in the same location, as well as enhancing mass ventral to the thecal sac on the left side at this level. I believe that the |

| | | |
|---|---|---|
| | | findings are post- operative and predominantly inflammatory with possibly a collection of blood and/or granulation tissue as an explanation for these changes. They are materially different from the previous examination and different in location and do not show the typical pattern of a recurrent disc herniation. |
| 01/04/00 | MRI Lumbar Spine, W/O and W/ Contrast Disc Imaging Referred by: Donald Johnson, M.D. | L5-S1. There is evidence of annular tearing and a bulging disc at this level, but no evidence of compression.<br><br>OPINION: MRI of the lumbar spine demonstrates surgical changes at the level of L4-5 with accumulation of soft tissue in the lateral recess on both sides, particularly on the right ventral to the thecal sac. The abnormality appears to be largely due to post operative change and is probably not due to residual disc herniation. Follow up examination is recommended if there is change in clinical symptoms in that changes in the early post operative period are difficult to interpret, even with the use of gadolinium. |

**Summary of Therapeutic Interventions**

| Date | Therapy/Procedure | Result of Therapy |
|---|---|---|
| 11/23/99 | Microscopic hemilaminotomy with discectomy and removal of large free fragment L4-5, right. | Preoperative DX:<br>1. HNP L4-L5 right<br>2. Status post laminectomy/discectomy, L4-L5, left<br><br>INTERPRETATION: Complications: None. EBL:20cc. |

| | | |
|---|---|---|
| 01/06/00 | A redo laminectomy discectomy at 4-5 with interbody fusion. East Cooper Regional Medical Center Donald Johnson, M.D. | INTERPRETATION:<br>DISCHARGE DX:<br>1. Status post fusion L4-L5.<br>2. Status post laminectomy discectomy x 2.<br><br>HOSPITAL COURSE: The patient was taken to the OR on 01/07 where he underwent a redo laminectomy discectomy at 4-5 with interbody fusion. Postoperatively, he did very well. He progressed through physical therapy without difficulty. He was finally discharged on the second postoperative day doing well. He is to follow up in 1 week. He was given Lortab prn pain and Cipro. He was doing well at the time of discharge. |

## CURRENT STATUS

### Current Complaints

1. The examinee's chief complaint is low back pain 2-3 days a week. This pain began November 1, 1999. He reports that the pain is located in the low back. The pain is an intermittent "dull/ache" pain. It is aggravated by lifting, bending, twisting, prolonged standing and relieved by over-the-counter Ibuprofen and rest. On an eleven-point scale with 0 representing no pain and 10 representing excruciating pain he rates the pain a 5.

2. The examinee also complains of pain in both legs and hips. This pain began November 1, 1999. The pain is a constant dull ache. It is aggravated by lifting, stooping, kneeling, and prolonged standing and temporary relieved by rest and over-the-counter Ibuprofen. On an eleven-points scale with 0 representing no pain and 10 representing excruciating pain he rates the pain a 7.

**Functional Status**

Mr. Babitsky reports having the greatest difficulties with engaging in coaching activities that require him to bend and rotate at the waist, prolonged walking and standing on the right leg. He also has profound difficulty with doing lifting that requires him to bend at the waist.

**Physical Examination**

**Vital Signs**

Temperature - 97.4
Pulse - 70
Blood Pressure - 130/74

**Observations**

Mr. Babitsky is a well-developed male who was in obvious pain and distress.

**Behavioral Observations**

Mr. Babitsky was pleasant and cooperative during the examination. He demonstrated a normal affect. During the visit he appeared comfortable and demonstrated pain behaviors that were appropriate and confirm clinical findings of the lower back and right leg. The pain behavior that was observed was mild limping right leg.

He scored a +1 in pain behavior assessment. This indicates that the pain behaviors are appropriate and tend to confirm the clinical findings of the lumbar spine and lower extremities (legs).

**Structural Examination:**

His observed gait was mild limp right leg. There was no antalgic posture noted. There was significant loss of lumbar lordosis and deconditioning of the lumbosacral muscles. There was a surgical scar of 10 cm.

## Range of Motion

Range of motion was tested using dual inclinometers and the results of the maximal ROM in each plane follows. The ROMs indicated below in Table 1 meet the validity criteria as delineated in the AMA's *Guide to the Evaluation of Permanent Impairment, 5th Edition* in all ranges.

| Lumbar ROM | | |
|---|---|---|
| Flexion | 20 | 33% of Normal (60°) |
| Extension | 12 | 50% of Normal (25°) |
| Left Lateral Flexion | 8 | 33% of Normal (25°) |
| Right Lateral Flexion | 8 | 33% of Normal (25°) |

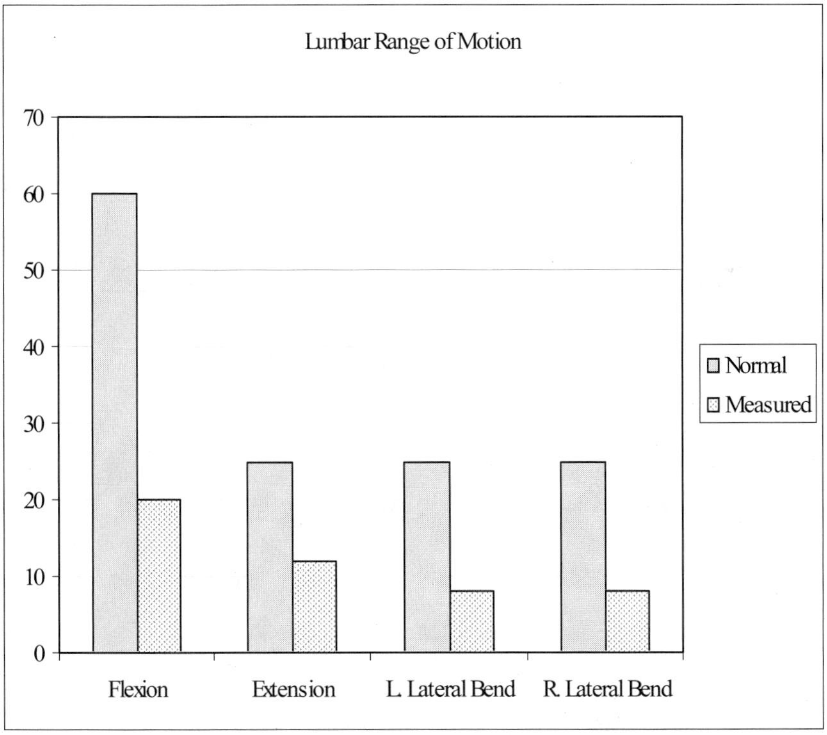


| | Flexion | Extension | L. Lateral Bend | R. Lateral Bend |
|---|---|---|---|---|
| Normal | 60 | 25 | 25 | 25 |
| Measured | 20 | 12 | 8 | 8 |

## ORTHOPEDIC EXAMINATION:

### Lumbar Spine:

**Lumbar palpation examination:**

Muscle spasms and tenderness detected to palpation in the lumbar paraspinal musculature on range of motion with pain.

Muscle spasms and tenderness detected in the gluteus musculature on range of motion with pain.

Tenderness to palpation detected in the lumbar spinous processes of L2, L3, L4, and L5.

Tenderness detected in the lumbar facets of L2, L3, L4, and L5 bilaterally.

Lumbar joint pain and tenderness, joint asymmetry, range of motion joint abnormality, connective tissue tone, texture, and temperature abnormality were detected.

Deconditioning to the lumbar spine, loss of lumbar lordosis and loss of muscle tone.

SI joint pain and tenderness, joint asymmetry, range of motion joint abnormality, connective tissue tone, texture, and temperature abnormality were detected bilaterally.

Limited mobility of the SI joint with pain noted bilaterally.

### Lower Extremity Right Lower Thigh and Calf:

The patient exhibited a mild limp on toe off and heel off.

Circumferential mensuration was as follows:

| | | Left | Right |
|---|---|---|---|
| leg: | 10 cm above superior pole of patella: | 51 cm | 47 cm |
| | 10 cm below inferior pole of patella: | 44½ cm | 42 cm |

There are 4 cm of atrophy noted in the right thigh.

There are 2½ cm of atrophy noted in the right lower calf.

There is a 60% 3/5 right muscle strength deficit and sensory loss.

| | |
|---|---|
| Supraspinatus tendonitis test | NEGATIVE |
| Codman arm drop | NEGATIVE |
| Apprehension test | NEGATIVE |
| Yergason's test | NEGATIVE |
| Apley's test | NEGATIVE |
| Drawer test | NEGATIVE |
| McMurray's test | NEGATIVE |

**RELIABILITY TESTS:**

| | |
|---|---|
| Libman's | NEGATIVE |
| Mannkopf's | NEGATIVE |
| Burn's Bench | NEGATIVE |
| Waddel's | NEGATIVE |

**NEUROLOGICAL TESTING:**

Neurological testing consisted of 1) muscle testing, 2) reflex testing and 3) sensation testing.

**SENSORY DERMATOME LEVELS:**

A hypoesthesia was noted along the L5 right nerve distribution.

Upper extremities along the sensory dermatome distribution, sensory dermatome level testing was within normal diagnostic perimeters for upper appendages.

**DEEP TENDON REFLEXES:**

The Deep Tendon Reflexes tested as follows:

| | |
|---|---|
| Patellar Reflexes 1+/3 right | 2+/3 left |
| Achilles Reflexes 0+/3 right | 2+/3 left |

**MUSCLE TESTING**:

C5, C6, C7, C8 and T1 upper extremity strengths of the muscles involved were tested and found to be symmetrical and equal.

L4, L5, S1 lower extremities strengths of the muscles involved were tested and found to be weaker on the right leg and unequal compared to the left leg.

**ORTHOPEDIC TESTING:**

Valsalva's test was positive L2, L3, L4, and L5.
Kemp's was positive L2, L3, L4, and L5.
Straight leg raise was painful at greater than 60 degrees, positive on the right.
Confirmatory straight leg raise test was positive on the right.
Soto-Hall's test was positive in the lumbar spine.

**VASCULAR TESTING:**

The following tests were done to determine any abnormalities of the lower extremities:

There were no abnormal clinical signs of the arteries of the lower extremities.

**Jamar Dynamometer**

Mr. Babitsky was tested for grip strength using the Jamar Dynamometer. Mr. Babitsky is right-hand dominant. His best performance was obtained at position 4 and the data are presented in Table 1.

**Table 1**
**Grip Strengths of Right and Left Upper Extremities**

| | Left Hand | Mean Value Left Hand | Right Hand (Dominant) | Mean Value Right Hand |
|---|---|---|---|---|
| **1** | 54 lbs | | 60 lbs | |
| **2** | 56 lbs | 58 lbs | 60 lbs | 60 lbs |
| **3** | 58 lbs | | 60 lbs | |
| **4** | 60 lbs | | 60 lbs | |
| **5** | 60 lbs | | 60 lbs | |

Mr. Babitsky made a concentrated and maximal effort to comply with this test protocol. This is evidenced by the minimal variance between trials for each hand. His grip strength fell well within the average ranges for males in his age group.

Mr. Babitsky's performance on the five-position Jamar Dynamometry tests produced curves that demonstrate symmetry between the efforts of the right and left hands, Figure 1. These curves represent the expected research trends and indicate a maximal attempt at the task and the ability to use repeated grip mechanics. I concluded that Mr. Babitsky gave maximum effort to provide grip strength data.

**Figure 1**

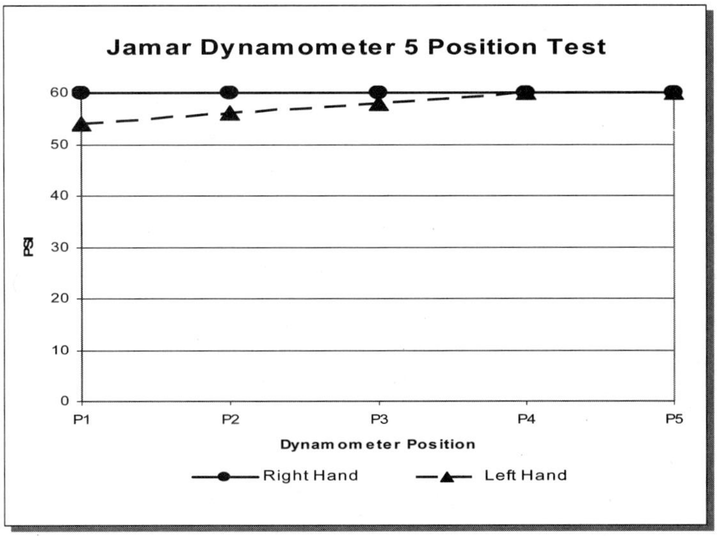


**Pain Status Inventories**

Mr. Babitsky completed the following self-report questionnaires:

**Pain Drawing** [18]

Mr. Babitsky completed a Pain Drawing. Using the scoring mechanisms for this diagram, he scored a 2, which suggests good psychometrics. Scores of less than 2 are considered indicative of normal psychometrics.

**CES-D** [19]

The CES-D is a psychometric instrument designed to screen for depression and an affective overlay that may result in symptom magnification. Scores of greater than "16" suggests depression and may suggest a need for

[18] Ransford A, Cairns D, Mooney V. *The Pain Drawing as an Aid to the Psychologic Evaluation of Patients With Low-Back Pain.* Spine 1(2):1976: 127-134
[19] Radloff L. *The CES-D Scale: a self report depression scale for research in the general population.* 1977 Appl Psychol Measurement. 1997 1:385-401

additional investigation. The examinee scored a 22.

**Conclusions**

**Diagnostic Impressions:**

1. **The examinee had a non-occupational acquired disc herniation at L4-5 in 1995 that required surgical intervention and stabilization.**

2. **The examinee sustained on 11/01/99 an occupationally acquired broad-based disc re-herniation at L4-L5 that has migrated a free fragment of disc material located above the disc space on the right side requiring a microscopic hemilaminotomy with discectomy and removal of large free fragment L4-5, right on 11/23/99.**

3. **The examinee experienced a change of condition to his lower back and right leg for the worse (deterioration) in January 2000 resulting in a L4-L5 disc re-herniation requiring a third surgery with a redo laminectomy discectomy at L4-5 with interbody fusion on 01/06/00.**

4. **Occupationally acquired persistent recurrent low back and right leg pain with some clinical response to surgical repair (Post-laminectomy syndrome), which occurred on 11/01/99 and deteriorated (worsened) in January 2000.**

5. **Occupationally acquired on lumbar and right leg deconditioning which occurred on 11/01/99 and deteriorated (worsened) in January 2000.**

6. **Occupationally acquired sensory and motor deficits(weakness of the right leg) of the right L5 nerve of the right leg with atrophy (loss of size of upper thigh by 4 cm and 2 ½ cm in the calf) and gait impairment (mild limp of the right leg) which occurred on 11/01/99 and deteriorated (worsened) in January 2000.**

**The examinee's subjective complaints were consistent with the objective findings.**

**The Work Loss Data Institute's Official Disability Guidelines™ Seventh Edition,** 2003, ODG covers all diagnostic codes in ICD-9-CM and integrates actual experience data from the US Federal Government including OSHA and the CDC National Health Interview Survey - over 3 million cases in all. Additionally, the pathways for each condition are identified that provide the different treatment options with their resultant duration of disability, including consideration for severity and type of job.

**722.1 Displacement of thoracic or lumbar intervertebral disc without myelopathy**
*ICD-10 Code(s): M51.1, M51.2*
**Description:** Displacement of a disc in the upper or lower back which may put pressure on the adjacent spinal nerve causing pain and sometimes sensory loss.
Other names: Herniated disc, Herniated nucleus pulposus (HNP), Disc bulge, Disc rupture, Disc protrusion.

The Work Loss Data Institute's Official Disability Guidelines™ Seventh Edition, 2003, ISBN 1-880891-45-X states that the average medical cost for this type of injury is:
**Medical Costs:** $10,106 (average of 214,494 cases).

**Causation**

Based upon the available information, to a reasonable degree of chiropractic orthopedic probability, there is a probable causal relationship between the current complaints and the injury to the low back, hips, and legs on November 1, 1999.

**Maximal Medical Improvement**

Maximum Medical Improvement (MMI) is defined as the date after which further recovery and restoration of function can no longer be anticipated, based upon reasonable chiropractic orthopaedic probability.

It is my clinical and professional opinion that maximum medical improvement has been achieved as of December 30, 2002.

**Permanent Impairment Evaluation**

The impairment, meaning any anatomical, physiological, or psychological abnormality that impairs the ability to work, is hereby described:

> This impairment rating was determined by consulting the American Medical Association, *Guides to the Evaluation of Permanent Impairments*, 5th Edition, as well as my past experience, and my extensive training in impairment rating.

There is not any specific category or table in the AMA *Guides* that outline Mr. Babitsky's particular pathologies to the lower back, right thigh and right calf. I have used my professional judgment to determine the permanent impairments assigned. I used Table 15-7 on page 404 and the DRE Method from the AMA *Guides* to determine the lumbar impairment:

| **Table 15-7 Criteria for Rating Whole Person Impairment Percent Due to Specific Spine Disorders to Be Used as Part of the ROM Method** | |
|---|---|
| | **% Impairment of the Whole Person** |
| **Disorder** | **Lumbar** |
| **Intervertebral disc or other soft-tissue lesion. Multiple operations with residual signs or symptoms. Third or subsequent operation.** | **I have utilized up to 5-8% for multiple surgeries.** |

**Diagnostic Related Estimate Lumbar Spine, Category V on page 387 of the *Fifth Edition Guides to the Evaluation of Permanent Impairment.***

| **Diagnostic Related Estimate Lumbar Category V** | **Impairment Rating** |
|---|---|
| **DRE Category V** | **I have utilized up to 31% based on my professional judgment and the clinical findings.** |

| **Table 17-6** Impairment Due to Unilateral Leg Muscle Atrophy | | |
|---|---|---|
| **Difference in Circumference (cm)** | **Impairment Degree** | **Whole Person (Lower Extremity) Impairment (%)** |
| **a. Thigh:** The circumference is measured 10 cm above the patella with the knee fully extended and the muscles relaxed. | | |
| 3+ | **Severe** | 13% leg impairment to the right thigh which is a **5% whole person impairment** |

**b. Calf:** The maximum circumference on the normal side is compared with the circumference at the same level on the affected side.

| | | |
|---|---|---|
| **2-2.9** | **Moderate** | 13% impairment to the right calf which is a **4% whole person impairment** |

## IMPAIRMENT RATING SUMMARY

**38% whole person impairment of the lumbar spine converting to a regional impairment of 51%.**

**13% lower extremity (right thigh) impairment, which equals a 5% whole person impairment.**

**13% lower extremity (right calf) impairment, which equals a 4% whole person impairment.**

**Impairment percentages derived from the *Guides* criteria should not be used as direct estimates of disability. Impairment percentages estimate the extent of the impairment on whole person functioning and account for basic activities of daily living, not including work. The complexity of work activities requires individual analyses. Impairment assessment is a necessary *first step* for determining disability.**

## QUALIFICATIONS:

My comments are based on my knowledge, skills and abilities in this domain. I serve as a postgraduate faculty lecturer for National University of Health Sciences in Independent Medical Examination, Chiropractic Forensics, Disability Examination and Current Concepts in Vertebrobasilar Complications following Spinal Manipulation. I have trained hundreds of medical, chiropractic, osteopathic and physical therapists, and occupational therapists on how to use the AMA *Guides to the Evaluation of Permanent Impairment*. I have published and spoken extensively in this field, and am featured in a video tape production and related topics - Medical School for Lawyers - Chiropractic Evaluation and Treatment. I am the author of a 120-hour program in the field of Chiropractic Forensics - Impairment Rating, Disability Rating, & Forensic Rating for the Doctor of Chiropractic. During the past fifteen years I have analyzed and performed several thousand impairment evaluations using the AMA *Guides to the Evaluation of Permanent Impairment*, using the Third, Fourth, and Fifth Editions. I have performed hundreds of functional capacity evaluations using the National

Association's Disability Evaluation Professionals' protocols. I have served as the Chiropractic Commissioner for the Commission on Disability Examiner Certification since 1994.

I was on the Editorial Advisory Board of the Work Loss Data Institute for the Official Disability Guidelines (ODG), Seventh Edition, 2002, ISBN 1-880891-38-7, and Eighth Edition, 2003, ISBN 1-880891-45-X on establishing disability guidelines and Chiropractic "Best Practice" Guidelines to identify treatments and services that are reasonable and medically necessary to effectively treat a particular injury. These chiropractic guidelines in ODG are based primarily on input from the 80 members of the interdisciplinary ODG Editorial Advisory Board. In addition I provided the editorial guidance in this effort. The ODG 2003 board is consulting on establishing scientific standards for healthcare practices for a number of Best Practice Guideline projects. I serve on the Work-Loss Data Editorial Advisory Board for *Official Disability Guidelines* in Treatment in Workers' Comp 2003. This text is establishing national standards for Chiropractic, Medical, and Physical Therapy "Best Practice" and disability duration.

Chief Chiropractic Editor: The Work Loss Data Institute (WLDI) is a for-profit corporation incorporated in the state of Texas engaged in the publication of health care guidelines. The Council of Chiropractic Guidelines for Practice Parameters (CCGPP) is a non-profit organization incorporated in the state of Florida, created by the Congress of Chiropractic State Associates and engaged in the review and dissemination of practice guidelines for the chiropractic profession of the United States. CCGPP and WLDI have commenced this cooperative venture to enable the CCGPP to produce a document which will assist its stakeholders in providing and/or assessing efficacious chiropractic health care. While simultaneously enabling the WLDI to have viable and contemporary product in regard to chiropractic health care guidelines.

I am Board Certified in Chiropractic Forensics, Founding Director of the National Board of Forensic Chiropractors, and the Commission on Independent Forensic Chiropractic Medical Examiner Certification, a Certified Independent Chiropractic Examiner, Certified Disability Examiner, Category I, and completed a 300-hour postgraduate program in Chiropractic Orthopedics.

**The Work Loss Data Institute's <u>Official Disability Guidelines</u>™ Seventh Edition, 2003**
**ODG covers Return-To-Work "Best Practice" Guidelines for Activity Modifications.**

## ACTIVITY MODIFICATIONS:

Manual work: Lifting with knees (with a straight back) not more than 25 lbs up to 15 times/hr; squatting up to 16 times/hr; standing or walking with a 10-minute break at least every 1-2 hours; sitting with a 10-minute break every 1-2 hours; extremes of flexion or extension allowed up to 12 times/hr; extremes of twisting allowed up to 16 times/hr; climbing ladders allowed up to 25 rungs 6 times/hr; driving car or light truck up to a full work day; driving heavy truck up to 4hrs/day.

**(Given the significant degree of work restriction a functional work capacity evaluation is indicated to more accurately determine the examinee's work capacity.)**

### Appropriateness of Care

The client has asked that I specifically address the issue of appropriateness of medical care. Based on the specifics of this care, it is my professional opinion that care has been consistent with the usual standards of care for this problem.

### Recommendations

### Diagnostic/Consultation/Therapeutic Recommendations

I recommend that future therapeutic and diagnostic health care needs will be required for Mr. Babitsky's maintenance and stability of his pathology:

a) Implantable pain device for lumbar spine pain as his condition progresses or deteriorates.

b) Pharmacological pain management approaches with possible injections for lumbar spine pain as his condition progresses or deteriorates.

c) He will require orthopedic surgical evaluations on an as-needed basis or for flares of the lumbar spine as his condition progresses or deteriorates.

d) He will require a drug supply depending on the provider's recommendations and his progressive pathologies as his condition progresses or deteriorates.

e) He will require a psychiatric evaluation and pharmacological intervention to address the chronic behavioral impairments that he has been unable to manage on his own.

f) Given the significant degree of work restriction, a functional work capacity evaluation is indicated to more accurately determine the examinee's work capacity.

**Disclosure Statement**

The above analysis is based upon the available information at this time, including the history given by the examinee, the medical records and tests provided, the results of pain status inventories, and the physical findings. It is assumed that the information provided to me is correct. If more information becomes available at a later date, an additional report may be requested. Such information may or may not change the opinions rendered in this evaluation.

The examiner's opinions are based upon reasonable chiropractic orthopedic certainty and are impartial. Independent Medical Examination is both an art and a science, and although an individual may appear to be fit for work activity, there is no guarantee that the person will not be re-injured or suffer additional injury. If applicable, employers should follow the processes established in the Americans with Disabilities Act, Title I. The opinions on work capacity are to facilitate job placement and do not necessarily reflect an in-depth direct threat analysis. Comments on appropriateness of care are professional opinions based upon the specifics of the case and should not be generalized, nor necessarily be considered supportive or critical of, the involved providers or disciplines.

Any medical recommendations offered are provided as guidance and not as medical orders. The opinions expressed do not constitute a recommendation that specific claims or administrative action be made or enforced.

Thank you for asking me to see this examinee in consultation. If you have any further questions, please do not hesitate to contact me.

Respectfully submitted,

Preston B. Fitzgerald, Sr., D.C., CDE I, CICE, CIFCME
Chiropractic Orthopedist
Certified Disability Examiner, Category I
Certified Independent Chiropractic Examiner
Certified Independent Forensic Chiropractic Medical Examiner

PBF:dc

## Report #6: Motor Vehicle Accident—Neck, Upper Back, and Anterior Knee

This report is most notable for the following.

- It is extremely detailed and extensive.
- It is well written.
- Abbreviations, drugs, and other medical terms are explained.
- Very detailed and well-documented physical examination.
- Diagnoses are listed in a numbered list.
- Objective, non-inflammatory language is used. For example, "there was evidence of symptom magnification and were some nonorganic findings during today's history and examination, respectively. However, neither was flagrant."
- Pain chart timeline effectively presents information.

While this is an excellent report, all reports can be improved. Areas of possible improvement include the following.

- More frequent headnotes would make this extensive report easier to read and use.
- An executive summary on such a lengthy and detailed report would be very helpful.
- If photos of the damaged vehicle were available, the author should have considered putting these in the report. A picture says a thousand words.
- The history of the motor vehicle accident should be broken out from the medical history.
- The examiner may have been getting a little out of his true area of expertise when he commented on the biomechanics of motor vehicle accidents.

---

August 10, 2002

Les Milkum, Attorney at Law
Dewey Cheatum & Howe
1000 First Avenue
Seattle, WA 98104

| Re: | Plaintiff: | Clay Mant |
|---|---|---|
| | Case: | *Mant v. Summe* |
| | Claim Number: | 12-345-678 |

Dear Mr. Milkum:

Thank you for allowing me to perform an independent medical examination (IME) on Ms. Mant. She was informed today's examination was to evaluate specific conditions pertinent to the accident in question and to answer your questions in a report; hence information provided would not be confidential. The history provided and symptoms reported by the examinee were dictated in her presence so additions or corrections could be made as indicated. Ms. Mant was further informed the IME would not constitute a comprehensive medical examination, provide advice or treatment, substitute for evaluation and treatment by her own physician(s), or establish a patient-physician relationship. Prior to the physical examination she was instructed not to perform any maneuver that might cause injury or exacerbation of symptoms, and to advise the examiner to avoid or immediately abort any such test.

The diagnoses and conclusions herein are the opinions of the examiner, based on the history provided, records reviewed, and today's examination findings. These opinions do not constitute per se recommendations for a specific claim or other administrative action, and may be modified if further information becomes available later.

## CHIEF COMPLAINT(S):

Neck-upper back and bilateral anterior knee pain.

### History of Relevant Illnesses-Injuries and Record Review:

This 50-year-old right-handed female has a long history of musculoskeletal complaints. The first relevant record provided is a January 25, 1995, chart note from orthopedic surgeon Mark C. Stars, MD, PhD, documenting a complaint of "pain [radiating] into her right shoulder," apparently from neck, noted upon awakening that morning without known precipitant. Remarkable exam findings included recurrence or worsening of the discomfort with cervical extension and rightward rotation but relief "...with elevation of her arm [presumably shoulder]." Impression was "...acute cervical radiculopathy...likely due to a disk problem." Plan was a soft cervical collar and unspecified nonsteroidal anti-inflammatory drug (NSAID).

On January 31, 1995, Dr. Stars referred the plaintiff to Swedish Medical Center Physical Therapy (SMCPT) for thrice weekly treatments over two weeks including "Local Modalities → ROM/Isometrics."

At SMCPT the plaintiff was evaluated by Brenda J. Mortens, PT on February 1, 1995. Current complaints including aching pain in left posterior neck and interscapular area as well as stabbing pain with pins-and-needles in posterior right shoulder girdle. The pains were worse after "sitting w/no head support," looking up or down, and in the evening; better in the morning, and relieved by heat, cold, a shower, and lying down. Ms. Mant reported she slept "flat on back with C-collar all night." The therapist also noted, "just moved with much lifting (~3 mo) plus shoving furniture. Lifts heavy grandson." Additional complaints included headache, blurred vision, and dizziness. Exam revealed limited and in some cases painful neck motions.

Ms. Mortens rendered three treatments between February 3 and 9, 1995, and noted on the former date "'Felt the best it has in a while' for past 2 days; a little tense today." Abnormal exam findings apparently included diminished grip strength on right, absent C6 (brachioradialis) reflex, tenderness along paraspinal and intervertebral muscles, and limited mobility of C3-4, C5-6, and C6-7 interspaces. Treatment on this and two subsequent occasions included intervertebral mobilization with gentle muscle augmentation, soft tissue mobilization (STM) of neck and upper back, hot packs (HP), gentle manual traction, ultrasound (US), electrical stimulation (ES), and various exercises (cervical isometric and upper extremity strengthening).

On February 8, 1995, Dr. Stars authorized four more physical therapy sessions, twice a week for two weeks, including continuation of current treatment and "work to home program."

A February 14, 1995, progress summary from Ms. Mortens reveals the "significant pain" of neck and right upper extremity (RUE) reported originally was now diminished, and paresthesias resolved. While initially "unable to use" RUE, Ms. Mant was now "using [it] with care." The initially "much ↓" neck motions and 3+/5 weakness of C5 myotome had now normalized, with 5/5 strength. While improved a great deal, the plaintiff still had intermittent RUE pain, and absent right brachioradialis and triceps (C6+7) reflexes. Ms. Mortens found it interesting the weakest muscle was innervated by C5, not C6 or 7. "She still gets muscle spasms in R cerv[ical] area with mild activity + needs cerv. collar in eves." Plan was progressive exercises "…to ↑ tolerance to activity without sx [symptoms]." Sometime thereafter Dr. Stars signed the summary, recommending continued semiweekly therapy visits for three weeks.

An undated Discharge Summary from Ms. Mortens indicates the plaintiff "…was seen in PT 7x + returned 3x after…[Dr. Stars's] prescription renewal…. She was noting some progress, ~85% improved in RUE Sx by 2/16/95. She was given a home ex[ercise] program + home management…discussed…last seen on 2/23/95 and canceled the last 2 appts."

On August 15, 1995, Ms. Mant returned to Dr. Stars complaining of increasing neck pain without distal radiation. Exam revealed "minimal pain with extension and rotation," and decreased right brachioradialis reflex, but normal strength and sensation. Plan was "a step-wise plan," beginning with a cervical collar and Daypro (anti-inflammatory analgesic oxaprozin), with further evaluation and treatment if her symptoms increased.

On December 9, 1996, another orthopedic surgeon, David A. Albertson, MD, obtained a brief history of the plaintiff's prior neck pain and treatment, adding that in October (presumably 1996), without precipitating trauma, she "...developed [recurrent] pain in the back of her neck and up into her head [but]...had no radicular symptoms such as...before." The intermittent but daily pain was "...worse with almost any strenuous activity. She also...is under a huge amount of stress at home and at work..." but "If...in certain positions she can relax." Exam was normal apart from mild tenderness throughout cervical spine. Neck x-rays were normal. Assessments were "Flare-up of her cervical strain," and "...under a lot of stress." Dr. Albertson recommended "physical therapy to work on the soft tissues" and "...counseling to...deal with some of the stress issues."

Ms. Mant reports, however, she did not see a counselor thereafter.

On December 10, 1996, Lori Rogers, PT, evaluated the plaintiff at Theracare Nordstrom and obtained a history of increasing "...neck tightness and discomfort since [insidious onset in] September or October. ...At this point she is afraid to move [for fear]...of increasing her symptoms." The discomfort, characterized as stiffness and pressure, was located primarily at base of right neck and associated with "...an abnormal amount of headaches." Abnormal exam findings included a "slightly forward head and rounded shoulder posture...small...dowager's hump," 25% restricted neck motions, and "very tight and tender throughout bilateral cervical paraspinals and interscapular musculature." Impression was cervical strain, the plan being treatment once or twice a week for four to six weeks including modalities, soft tissue work, range of motion (ROM), stretching, posture, and strengthening exercises, as well as patient education in posture, body mechanics, and a home program.

A February 13, 1997, Progress Summary from Ms. Rogers indicates eight treatments had been rendered thus far, with diminution in pain from 6-7 to 0-3/10 at present, and improvement in function from 50 to 90%. Although "doing much better" now, Ms. Mant was still having "problems getting comfortable at the end of the day," "with increased neck pain and tightness" while sitting, riding the ferry home in the evenings. Exam findings included somewhat improved posture, normal neck motions and upper extremity strength, and "resolving" tightness and tenderness in neck and upper back.

The therapist thought it "appropriate to continue [treatment] once a week or…every other week to progress to a full independent program."

Asked to describe her neck pain just prior to the first MVA (see below), Ms. Mant reports, "I was feeling pretty good because I just finished a round of physical therapy." The plaintiff's cervicalgia at this time was reportedly intermittent and 0-3/10 in severity as documented by Ms. Rogers.

Based on information provided by Ms. Mant and the Police Traffic Collision Report (PTCR), on February 14, 1997, she was driving a 1993 Honda Accord, restrained by shoulder and lap belts on a bucket seat equipped with a head restraint in the down position, and going 45 to 50 miles per hour on a highway when a 1994 Mitsubishi Galant traveling in the opposite direction slowed or stopped, intending to make a left turn. The Mitsubishi was rearended by a 1987 Toyota Camry traveling 60 miles per hour, and pushed forward and leftward such that its front struck the left front corner of the Honda. This caused Ms. Mant's car to veer rightward, while continuing forward, and travel off the road, onto the shoulder, and then down an embankment into brush and trees. The driver's side air bag deployed upon impact.

Multiple color photocopies of photographs of the Honda Accord were provided, including views from all four corners, a few close-ups of left front corner, and two views of the vehicle's interior. There is extensive crush of left front fender extending into the engine compartment. The left third of the hood has been peeled upward. The left third of the bumper cover is abraded and at least partially detached. Left front wheel is angled outward as if making a left turn. The windshield is intact but a plastic drape covers the presumably broken driver's door window. There is no apparent deformation of the steering wheel, although its lower half is obscured by the deflated air bag. The Honda was reportedly totaled due to the damage. Ms. Mant adds she was unable to exit the vehicle since the electrical door locks and windows were inoperable post collision.

Views of all four corners of the Mitsubishi and a single picture of its interior taken from the driver's door reveal moderate crush of both rear and front ends, both the driver and passenger air bags having inflated.

Five views of the exterior of the Toyota Camry, including shots from each corner, and a single view of the interior taken from the driver's door were also provided. There is extensive crush of left front fender, actually crumpled into a mass of sheet metal just rearward of the wheel well. The hood is deformed and buckled upward. The crush extends into engine compartment. The left half of front bumper cover is only minimally deformed. A single view of the interior reveals no obvious deformation of components therein, although there appears to be a broken portion of the plastic grill sitting on the front passenger seat.

At the time of impact Ms. Mant was reportedly "sitting up/driving" looking straight ahead. Upon impact she was "thrust forward/then backward/both knees jammed/whiplash." The plaintiff did not lose consciousness and does not recall striking anything inside the vehicle, but adds, "I didn't know what happened. I was trying to stop the car with the emergency brake [the examinee reaching downward with her right hand to pull on an imaginary brake handle]."

Immediate symptoms consisted of "shock/neck & leg." When asked whether she meant pain, the plaintiff states, "I was not feeling anything at that point." "I just remember looking down and saying, "Oh, that's the air bag. I'd never seen one like that before."

"The car was making clicking noises. My first reaction was, 'I've got to get out, it's going to blow.' That's when I was trying to fiddle with the doors and everything. I was just grasping for anything to get out, so I jumped into the back seat and then…didn't know what to do [plaintiff becoming tearful]. I'm trying to grab at anything to open these doors and windows. I'm trying to pull up the door handle and [push on the door but] just panicked…I got the door open but the brush was holding it closed, so I'm still freaking out. I'm pushing on the door with my shoulder and…still couldn't get it open…so I laid on my back and I'm pushing it with my feet and there's brush in the way and I can't get it open, so I push in the car door and I'm crawling through the brush on my hands and knees…up to the side of the road and there's a woman standing there. I'm trying to reach for her…can't get her and she's telling me it's okay, so I got up there and…just collapsed on the side of the road on the gravel. I asked her what happened and she said you were in a car accident."

The plaintiff's memory is not entirely clear for subsequent events. "There were so many people around asking me questions." Apparently Ms. Mant was interviewed by the investigating police officer and then fire department personnel, who placed her in an aid car, and after "duct taping me to the board," transported the plaintiff to the fire station, where they met an ambulance, which then transported her to and onto the Winslow to Seattle ferry. After arriving in Seattle she was transported to Swedish Medical Center-First Hill (SMC-FH).

A report from Bainbridge Island Ambulance reiterates some of the above information, adding Ms. Mant was complaining of pain in right shoulder, apparently radiating to posterior neck, and bilateral knees. Exam was unremarkable apart from apparent tenderness in these areas, the assessment being "Minor injury to left + rt knee pain in rt shoulder 2° to MVA." She was transported in a cervical collar and on a backboard to SMC-FH with "No changes enroute."

In the emergency room (ER) at SMC-FH, Robert C. George, MD, obtained a brief history of the collision and noted complaints of right neck, right shoulder, and right worse than left anterior knee pain, as well as nausea. Abnormal exam findings included tenderness of "neck following…removal [of] her Philadelphia collar," and "a small laceration over her right knee" which was "distinctly tender." X-rays of cervical spine were read as normal by the ER physician, and normal apart from loss of lordosis by the radiologist. Both physicians read x-rays of right knee as normal. Dr. George's impressions were cervical strain and right knee contusion with a small superficial laceration. The knee wound "was anesthetized with topical lidocaine gel, cleansed and then steri-stripped," followed by a dressing and elastic bandage. A cervical collar was applied and Ms. Mant discharged with prescriptions for Tylox (narcotic analgesic oxycodone with acetaminophen), Motrin (anti-inflammatory analgesic ibuprofen), and Flexeril (muscle relaxant cyclobenzaprine).

When asked today about results of the three medications, the plaintiff reports they helped. "I was feeling no pain as long as I was on the schedule that they said you had to take these medications."

On February 20, 1997, Dr. Albertson obtained a brief, similar history of the collision and ER evaluation. Current complaints included "pain in the base of her neck going into…right trapezius," relieved by wearing a cervical collar and lying down, as well as right knee pain, particularly about "an abrasion that was butterflied over." A pain drawing suggests aching along left and right cervical paraspinal muscles, over C7, right scapula, medial clavicle and pectoral areas bilaterally, and from anterior right knee distally along the shin into dorsal foot. Although "improved somewhat," the plaintiff reported the problem was still "severe," with "Disability function…23 out of 24. She no longer can drive, walk on the ferry…to the upstairs bedroom, or work [and]…rates herself as 4 or 5 on anxiety and 7 or 8 on irritability due to the pain."

Abnormal findings on Dr. Albertson's examination included diffuse tenderness of neck, a "quite sore" right trapezius, limited cervical extension and apparent discomfort on all neck motions, and right knee motion of 0 to 90 degrees with accompanying pain in medial femoral condyle. Assessments were cervical strain and "…contusion of her knee with laceration." Plan was physical therapy, continuation of the Motrin, hydrocodone (sic), and Flexeril, and "…remove the steri-strips on Monday."

On February 20, 1997, Ms. Rogers obtained a brief history of the collision six days earlier and subsequent evaluation and treatment. Current complaints included continuous aching in neck, clavicular area, and interscapular region, as well as "little if any movement and need…to move very slowly." Abnormal exam findings included "extremely guarded" neck motions "less than 25%" of normal; tenderness throughout cervical, upper trapezius, and interscapular muscles as well as clavicular region; and "limping with right knee pain." Impression was cervical strain, the plan being modalities; soft tissue work (STW); ROM, stretching, and cervical stabilization exercises; plus "education and instruction in a home program," with semiweekly visits for four to six weeks.

No subsequent records from Theracare were provided until four months later. Ms. Mant recalls she did continue physical therapy treatments there twice a week for four to six weeks. Treatment reportedly included heat, ice, massage, ultrasound, electrical stimulation, and later on exercises. She also saw a female massage therapist there, possibly Sandy. The treatments reportedly helped. "After I was more mobile they would introduce me to exercises that would help me increase the mobility and be a little more comfortable."

On March 14, 1997, Dr. Albertson noted the neck pain was "markedly better," and not really limiting at this time. Ms. Mant, however, reported "…pain over…bilateral patellar tendons, especially when she goes up and down stairs." The orthopedist "told her…the neck and knees still may take months to calm down," recommended she "get on an exercise bicycle," and planned to "…see her back…on an as-needed basis."

On June 13, 1997, Dr. Albertson noted "…episodes over the last three weeks of a sharp, shooting pain in the right [upper?]…back…if she gets into certain positions, either sitting or twisting. Between episodes, she has no pain…Her neck is overall better. She is still having problems with…bilateral knees [and]…cannot kneel on either one…and the right is much worse than…left." Abnormal exam findings included mild tenderness over right thoracolumbar junction and patellar tendons and "positive patellar apprehension…bilaterally but mostly in the distal poles of the patellae." Assessments were neck pain doing well, mild soft tissue pain in thoracolumbar junction, and bilateral patellar tendonitis. Plan was "physical therapy to work on her knees," the orthopedist adding "…this could be a long-term problem. The key will be her program afterwards. I will see her back prn [as needed]."

On June 20, 1997, Ms. Rogers noted the plaintiff's report that "…on 02/14/97…she hit the dashboard with both knees…has been using ice periodically on the right knee [and]…is not taking any medications." Current complaints included right worse than left knee pain of 4-5/10 in severity and accompanying most activities, especially descending stairs, and with "any pressure on her knee." Additional complaints included knee stiffness and numbness, a feeling "like they could give out on her" with activity, and numerous functional limitations including inability "to sit on the floor and get up…run, or walk fast." Abnormal exam findings included a slow gait with small steps, "decreased superior and inferior patellar glide," pain with resisted knee extension, complaints of "numbness and hypersensitivity in the infrapatellar region," and tenderness of patellar tendon and fat pad on right worse than left. Impressions were bilateral patellar tendonitis and fat pad irritation. Plan was again modalities, soft tissue work, stretching and strengthening exercises, plus "education and instruction in a home program," with visits two to three times per week for two weeks.

A June 30, 1997, Progress Summary from Ms. Rogers indicates the plaintiff had had four treatments consisting of US; soft tissue work including friction massage to patellar tendons; quadriceps strengthening, ROM, and stretching exercises; ice; electrical stimulation (ES); and education and instruction thus far, with some relief of symptoms from modalities, although exercises had been "occasionally irritating," and "…overall no significant change." Exam revealed a slightly improved gait, improved patellar mobility especially superior and inferior glide, and diminished tenderness but persistent pain with resisted knee extension and a squat. Plan was to recheck with Dr. Albertson.

Regarding results of this course of physical therapy Ms. Mant states today it was also helpful. "Same type of thing. They would start introducing me to exercises again."
On July 31, 1997, Dr. Albertson noted, "Her neck [was]…doing…fine over the last couple…weeks [but] for some reason…flared up again…right… cervicothoracic junction." "She…actually did quite well with her knees." Exam revealed a trigger point on right around T1-2 spinous processes. Assessment was "…a localized myofascial type pain syndrome." Plan was "some myofascial type work in the area," and return as needed.

Ms. Mant returned to Theracare Nordstrom on August 5, 1997, and was evaluated by Carrie Mason, PT, who recorded a very brief history of the MVA and subsequent treatment, adding "She continues to complain of patellar tendinitis…" presently 4/10 in severity, and "…is not up to speed with her life, although she is working full time and participating in a 4 hour commute including catching the ferry and buses." Abnormal exam findings included a forward head, dowager's hump, rounded shoulders, flattened thoracic kyphosis, normal to mildly limited neck motions apart from right side bending "20% with stretch on left," and tenderness over lower cervical and upper thoracic vertebrae with "…a quite marked palpable increased curve beginning at the base of the cervical spine extending into the upper thoracic vertebrae." Impressions were "Slight decreased range in cervical spine primarily on right side bending. Postural dysfunction. Overall deconditioned." Plan was postural instruction, cervical flexibility exercises, total body conditioning, aerobic activity, and upper extremity strengthening, with semiweekly treatments for three to four weeks.

A September 3, 1997, Progress Summary from Theracare and Tracey A. Robertson, PT, indicates the plaintiff had had six treatments thus far, including US, STW, various exercises, postural education, and cold packs, in addition to HEP instruction. Her function had increased from 75 to 80%, but pain was unchanged at 4/10 with "...fairly constant ache in the upper thoracic region [and]...numbness/tingling in the interscapular area. She states she has been trying to increase her activity level as tolerated. We have been trying to increase her exercise...but...found that her pain is easily flared." Plan was to gradually progress exercises as tolerated. Dr. Albertson was asked if he "...would like us to continue...physical therapy or...discharge her to an independent home program at this time."

A September 19, 1997, Discharge Summary from Ms. Robertson reveals she had not heard from Ms. Mant or Dr. Albertson since September 3rd, and was "...therefore, discharging her from physical therapy."

The plaintiff reports today this course of PT was also beneficial. In response to a question about whether she had any further treatment for the February 1997 MVA, Ms. Mant states, "That was pretty much the end of it. They had introduced me to all the exercises and I had handouts and sheets of everything. I was on my own to do all the exercises they gave me."

On October 16, 1997, orthopedic surgeon Ray Garrett, MD, performed an IME at Medical Consultants Network, Inc., in Seattle, and obtained a brief, similar history. Current complaints included headaches lasting one or two days, a "very achy [neck] with some numbness and...burning, depending on...her activities, such as yard work, woodworking, or sewing," and "a numb area and achy feeling in her right knee," with similar symptoms on left, although it was "not as numb as the right, but...more pins-and-needles." The plaintiff claimed it was "difficult to descend stairs," with cold sensitivity as well. Examination was for the most part normal. Ms. Mant, however, reported right patellofemoral pain on gait and heel and toe walking. The examiner also noted a "one-quarter inch incision [sic]...in relationship to the inferior medial pole of the right patella," positive apprehension on right, "an area of skin thickening...6 cm above the flare of the medial malleolus [reportedly]...the area of contusion from the car accident," and hypesthesia in a 5 x 2 cm area over inferior right patella. Dr. Garrett "requested" x-rays of neck and both knees. Diagnoses were cervical strain, resolved; contusion and laceration medial inferior pole of right patella, healed; and contusion distal right tibia. The examiner concluded the treatment to date had been "reasonable and necessary over…the initial three to six weeks," but that Ms. Mant had "not reached maximum benefit from treatment." He recommended she continue home isometric quadriceps exercises and be re-evaluated in "…two or three months…for a final examination of her right knee." Dr. Garrett considered the prognosis excellent "in regard to the neck, knee, and distal right tibia," and anticipated the knee complaints would resolve over "the next two to three months."

Just prior to the next MVA (see below), Ms. Mant reports her neck pain was intermittent and of lesser severity, 2/10. "They told me I would carry stress in my shoulders. I was doing the exercises they had given me." She was also reportedly having intermittent bilateral anterior knee pain, 4-6/10 in severity. "When you're doing a four-hour commute every day [on]…public transportation, ferry and bus, and walking up and down hills, it's a lot to carry and try and do your physical therapy and keep your stress level down."

On May 21, 1998, Ms. Mant was the unrestrained left rear seat passenger on a Metro bus traveling about 20 miles per hour uphill on a city street when the vehicle stopped suddenly. More specifically, she was sitting in the left rear corner, at the end of the row of rear seats extending the entire width of the bus, and thrown forward into the end of shorter bench seat facing the center of the bus (see last page of this report containing a diagram drawn by the plaintiff). The end of that bench seat had an arm rest above the padded seat bottom, and another transversely-oriented metal bar, reportedly used as a footrest by passengers, connecting its front and rear legs. Ms. Mant grabbed the armrest with her hands while her anterior knees struck the transverse metal bar. She reports having "been so protective" of her knees for so long it was "like a shock." With the assistance of two other passengers she walked to the front of the bus and "got a card to make a report. When I got off the bus I went and stood in front of a store I was so shook up and leaned against the wall there. I walked to work which is a block down the street very shakily." After arriving at work she "…made an appointment [with a physician] and went to that appointment within an hour."

About 1 hour and 15 minutes following this incident aboard the bus, Ms. Mant presented to internist Omri Tamrind, MD, who recorded a brief similar history of the injuries to "…bilateral knees and inferior legs anteriorly. Has been having more pain, mostly…the left knee and inferior leg." Exam was for the most part normal. Abnormal findings included minimal edema of inferior left knee, tenderness of left worse than right tibial tuberosity, and of "mid anterior distal legs," and gait "…favoring the left side." Impression was contusions bilateral knees and anterior inferior legs. Plan was Aleve and "stay off work for a couple of days so she may work on ice packing the areas…injured." Dr. Tamrind expected "increased pain over the next couple of days," but "…recovery within 1-2 weeks."

However, Ms. Mant reports today "The [knee] pain didn't start until the following day." She did take Aleve and ice her knees, learning that gel-filled plastic packs held on with elastic bandages worked well. The plaintiff had no subsequent formal treatment for effects of this bus accident, but continued to apply cold to both knees, as she reportedly did not recover completely from this bus accident. "I still continue to have problems with my knees."

Just prior to the second bus accident, "I was having [intermittent, 5-6/10, bilateral, anterior] knee pain. When it comes, it's like boom, all of a sudden it's achy, achy, achy from the inside. The stress, tense, but nothing like what I'm feeling now. Still carrying the stress in my neck." More specifically, she was experiencing intermittent neck pain of 2/10 in severity.

On April 30, 2002, Ms. Mant was reportedly on an articulated Community Transit bus traveling along a downtown Seattle street. When the driver announced hers as the next stop she arose from her seat and stood adjacent to the rear door (again see diagram on last page). Being unable to adequately grasp the large diameter padded pole, the plaintiff encircled it with her upper limb, pinching the pole between her arm and forearm. She demonstrates this today by abducting shoulder and flexing elbow with her hand across her chest. Ms. Mant was facing rearward and located just forward of the steps leading down to the rear door, when a pedestrian reportedly ran in front of the bus, prompting the driver to brake hard and stop suddenly. The plaintiff fell backward (towards the front of bus). She unsure exactly what transpired, having "lost consciousness for a short while," after which "all I could see was white," but reportedly struck her head five times, possibly on vertically oriented poles, armrests of seats in front of her, or other objects. Ms. Mant ended up 14 feet forward from where she had been standing, lying on the floor with her head and neck "wedged" against the platform for a longitudinally-oriented bench seat. Upon awakening she saw "several fire department people and police standing over me."

In response to a question about immediate symptoms she states, "I hit my head so hard on the top I couldn't even talk to them when they were asking me questions. I was outside for awhile on a gurney or something as I was waiting to get into an ambulance. Everybody's asking me my name and what hospital I want to go to, what insurance, all that kind of stuff. The firemen duct taped me to a board." She was again transported to the ER at SMC-FH.

In the ER Bruce A. Wilson, MD obtained a briefer history, similar except there was no loss of consciousness. Complaints included severe headache and apparent left shoulder pain. Abnormal exam findings included moderate distress, "abrasion @ apex head," apparent left cervical paraspinal tenderness, and anxious mood. A CT scan of head revealed no acute intracranial hemorrhage and mild chronic right ethmoid sinusitis. Impressions were head contusion and trauma from ground level fall. Treatment consisted of cleansing the wound, tetanus immunization, and Tylenol (acetaminophen). Ms. Mant was advised to followup with Dr. Rogers as needed and take acetaminophen for pain.

The plaintiff reports today, "They said I had a concussion and severe whiplash. They gave me Vicodin [narcotic analgesic hydrocodone with acetaminophen] and [a cervical] collar, and told me to take ibuprofen [sic]."

"I was off work for three weeks in a lot of pain, on medication, and sick, nauseated a lot of the time, real sensitive to light."

On May 2, 2002, the plaintiff returned to her primary care physician, internist Embra Rogers, MD. He obtained a brief history of the fall on the bus, similar except "She may have had some transient loss of consciousness [and] had an abrasion on her scalp that did not require suturing." Current complaints included persistent headache, feeling "somewhat groggy…like it is difficult to carry on a conversation," severe neck pain apparently increased with any motion thereof, difficulty opening and closing her mouth due to the cervicalgia, and weakness of hands.

Abnormal findings on Dr. Rogers's examination included diffuse paracervical tenderness and grade 4.5/5 weakness of upper limbs, limited by neck discomfort. X-rays of cervical spine revealed straightening of lordosis suggestive of muscle spasm per Dr. Rogers. A radiologist interpreted the films as "Right-convexity torticollis with straightening of the normal cervical lordosis."

Dr. Rogers's assessments were status post MVA with blunt head trauma and post-concussive syndrome, but without evidence of significant injury by CT scan, and "Lots of musculoskeletal aches and pains with paracervical muscle spasm." Plan was remain off "work until morning when she will call…to assess her current level of discomfort," "physical therapy when the acute injury has improved," Skelaxin (muscle relaxant metaxalone), and refill the Vicodin.

Upon referral from Dr. Rogers, the plaintiff was evaluated by neurologist Raymond Pick, MD, on May 8, 2002. He obtained a brief history of the fall eight days earlier and subsequent evaluation, similar to Dr. Rogers, noting the plaintiff had "been wearing a soft neck collar…the past eight days," with minimal improvement in ROM, although it was now "…easier to get out of bed." Additional complaints included feeling "dazed and medicated," intermittent dizziness, nausea, and "tenderness in her tailbone." In addition to the Vicodin, which seemed "to be helping," and the Skelaxin which was not, Ms. Mant was taking ibuprofen.

Abnormal findings on Dr. Pick's examination included diminished temperature sensation in feet, moderately to severely limited cervical ROM and bilateral "…severe paracervical spasm." Impression was "Post-concussive syndrome [with]…inattention as well." Plan was nortriptyline (tricyclic antidepressant), discontinuation of the Skelaxin, increased dosage of ibuprofen, warm pads to neck thrice daily, and physical therapy starting next week. Dr. Pick considered the prognosis good, as "Most of her pain is likely due to ligamentous injury." However, the neurologist recommended she "take next week off work," and anticipated driving would be a major issue for the next several weeks.

On May 13, 2002, the plaintiff presented to Leon Victor, LMP, who obtained a brief, similar history of the injury two weeks earlier. The massage therapist added, "HA [headaches] are getting better (subsiding); neck is still very stiff + sensitive. Limited ROM. Unable to drive; using neck brace a few hours every day." Regarding aggravating factors, Mr. Victor recorded, "looking down to table; lifting—unable w/left arm." Heat, sitting still, and a hot shower reportedly provided relief.

Mr. Victor's examination revealed hypertonicity of neck and shoulders with diminished ROM of neck, evidently left worse than right rotation. Treatment consisted of Swedish massage and myofascial release (MFR) of head, neck, and shoulders, which reportedly resulted in diminished hypertonicity and "feeling better." Ms. Mant was advised to "drink lots of water" and continue massage therapy twice a weekly.

Mr. Victor rendered massages on another three occasions between May 16 and 28, 2002, for ongoing similar symptoms. On the 20$^{th}$ he noted, "First day back at work—had difficulty walking down hill back to bus [in] PM.

Mr. Victor performed another five massages between June 1 and 26, 2002. Complaints reported on the former date included "HA last 2 days from the morning—continued throughout the day—also affecting the work." The plaintiff also reported "neck feels really tight—makes it harder to deal w/stress @ work 2° P[ain]." By the latter date the headaches were diminished in severity and frequency, but Ms. Mant was still experiencing stiffness of neck and shoulder, with intermittent pain and limited motions thereof. Treatment again consisted of Swedish massage and MFR, which reportedly resulted in diminished hypertonicity, increased relaxation, and decreased stress.

The plaintiff's most recent visit to Dr. Rogers was reportedly on August 5, 2002, at which time "he said it was okay to start the physical therapy." He also recommended continuation of ibuprofen.

On August 5, 2002, Dr. Rogers noted "...she has been undergoing massage therapy with significant benefit, marked decrease in her muscle tightness, and improvement with relaxation." Ms. Mant, however, was still having left-sided pain and limited ROM of neck, and decreased motions of left shoulder, especially elevation, with "...minor weakness in her grip." Abnormal exam findings included left paracervical and suprascapular tenderness with minimally (4.5/5) diminished grip on left. Dr. Rogers prescribed "physical therapy evaluation and treatment" for neck and left shoulder.

Later that day, August 5, 2002, Ms. Mant began treatment at Stanwood-Camano Physical Therapy, under Joe Beaton, PT. He obtained a history of the fall on April 30th similar to, if briefer than, that reported today, adding, "...she was pretty much out of it for about 3 weeks [thereafter]." The plaintiff was presently taking ibuprofen but no longer using Vicodin. Current complaints included neck pain with associated sleep disturbance, possibly headaches, difficulty with left shoulder elevation, and numbness and tingling in palmar wrist and tips of second and third digits (presumably on left). Ms. Mant reported fear of "...lifting heavy objects such as an ice chest, cartons of forms...at work and kids [at the]...pediatric clinic."

Abnormal exam findings included elevation of left shoulder which was "rounded anteriorly"; limited and apparently painful cervical side bending bilaterally, and apparent discomfort on leftward neck rotation plus "restricted right rotation with symptoms reported on the left;" "left scapula significantly restricted through retraction and elevation both actively and passively," resulting in diminished shoulder ROM; tightness of posterior shoulder capsule; and 4-/5 scapular elevation strength. Functional assessment was "...decreased scapular mobility and muscle guarding in the left scapular region." Plan was "...functional rehabilitation training to decrease guarding and improve scapular mobility...and [progression] to ROM for the left shoulder to establish full functional return." The plaintiff was instructed in a home exercise program.

Mr. Beaton rendered another pair of treatments on August 8 and 12, 2002, including review of therapeutic exercises, scapular circles and clocks with heat, manual scapular mobilization, proprioceptive neuromuscular facilitation (PNF), relaxation techniques with breathing, use of an Aerodyne bicycle, shoulder blade pinches and shrugs, and shoulder ROM exercises.

Assessment on the latter date was "Improved scapular mobility particularly in elevation. Shoulder abduction appears guarded in minimal change." Plan was to continue treatment.

Ms. Mant adds today the physical therapy included "a lot of different exercises to loosen the [left] shoulder area," as well as instruction in various do's and don'ts. Plan is a total of eight semiweekly treatments "to start with. He also wants me in conjunction to have massage therapy with Leon."

She has continued to see Mr. Victor up to the present, apart from "one week when I wasn't able to go." The massages of neck and upper back typically provide partial pain relief for an hour.

Ms. Mant can recall no other evaluation or treatment for musculoskeletal problems over the last several years, but wrote on the questionnaire, "As time goes on the pain continues."

**RECORD SOURCE LIST:**

Following is a list of healthcare providers and the examiner whose records were reviewed, categorized by specialty. Those whose records were not submitted but referenced as rendering evaluation and/or treatment for Ms. Mant are identified by an asterisk. The sources of nonmedical records reviewed are next identified.

| | |
|---|---|
| Allergy-Immunology: | Michael F. Milltowns, MD (1/20/00—7/11/00) |
| Anesthesiology: | Kevin T. Kerns, MD (6/19/01) |
| Dermatology: | Kim G. Abbot, MD (10/15/99—11/14/00) |
| Emergency Medicine: | Robert C. George, MD (2/14/97) |
| | Bruce A. Wilson, MD (4/30/02) |
| Gastroenterology: | Aaron C. Stars, MD (11/9/89—11/28/89) |
| Internal Medicine: | Nancy J. Bakerman, MD (12/1/95) |
| | Marti H. Lighter, MD (12/29/93—3/23/99) |
| | Susannah I. Tyler, MD (6/10/91—12/29/93) |
| | Omri H. Tamrind, MD (5/21/98) |
| Massage Therapy: | Leon Victor, LMP (5/13/02—6/26/02) |

| | |
|---|---|
| | " " " * (after 6/26/02) |
| Neurology: | Raymond Pick, MD (5/8/02) |
| Obstetrics-Gynecology: | Steven G. Beck, MD (6/19/01) |
| | Theresa A. Babcock, MD (6/18/01—6/22/01)<br>" " " "* (before 6/18/01 and after 6/22/01) |
| Orthopedic Surgery: | Ray H. Garrett, MD (10/16/97) |
| | David A. Albertson, MD (3/4/96—7/31/97) |
| | Mark C. Stars, MD, PhD, (1/25/95—8/15/95) |
| Pathology: | Donald R. Hansen, MD (6/19/01) |
| Physical Therapy: | Stanwood-Camano Physical Therapy (8/5/02—8/12/02)<br>Joe Beaton, PT |
| | Swedish Medical Center Physical Therapy (2/1/95—after 2/23/95)<br>Brenda J. Mortens, PT |
| | Theracare Physical Therapy (3/12/96—9/19/97)<br>Lori Gibson, PT |
| | Carrie Mason, PT |
| | Lori Rogers, PT |
| | Tracey A. Robertson, PT |
| Pulmonary Medicine: | Embra A. Rogers, MD (7/13/00—8/5/02) |
| Radiology: | Jay Clark, MD (7/11/00) |
| | Thomas J. Kopple, MD (2/14/97) |
| | Christopher L. Kotsam, MD (1/20/00—7/11/00) |
| | William M. Mack, MD (7/3/91) |
| | John C. McMichael, MD (11/28/89—9/24/92) |

| | |
|---|---|
| | David Riga, MD (5/2/02) |
| | Carlton F. Root, MD (10/15/99) |
| | Janice C. Stacey, , MD (4/30/02) |
| | Thomas P. Sultan, MD (4/13/00) |
| Miscellaneous Records: | Bainbridge Island Ambulance (2/14/97) |
| | Photocopies of photos of vehicles in 2/14/97 MVA |
| | Police Traffic Collision Report (2/14/97) |

## CURRENT SYMPTOMS:

Presently Ms. Mant complains of constant aching, burning, and tightness in cervical paraspinals, and extending distally into medial superior border of trapezius and medial scapular region bilaterally. On the left, the symptoms extend further distally and leftward into posterior, superior, and anterior shoulder. On a scale of 0 (no discomfort) to 10 (the worst pain imaginable), the plaintiff reports her neck pain was a 10 immediately after the February 1997 MVA, and presently is 6-7, having varied from 4 to 8 over the past month with an average of 5. The cervicalgia is worse when driving or "riding on a bus where you constantly have to hold your head." It is diminished by massage and sitting in a hot tub.

Ms. Mant also complains of intermittent bilateral anterior knee pain variously characterized as aching, stabbing, and/or throbbing, with accompanying weakness. The knee pain was reportedly also 10 in severity just after the February 1997 MVA, and is presently 2-4, having varied from 3 to 7 over the past month, with an average of 4 to 5. It is worse with cold weather, sometimes "happens on its own," and is relieved by positional changes and sitting in a hot tub. "In the wintertime when it's colder it can be up to 20, 30 times a day when it's the low-grade pain, then it really hurts and it's gotten worse each year." She denies giving out, locking, swelling, or sensation of loose body in either knee.

Ms. Mant denies any weakness of upper or lower limbs apart from the knees. Last night when doing exercises in physical therapy she noted onset of numbness and tingling in the palmar tips of left index, middle, and ring fingers. Otherwise, the plaintiff has no sensory complaints in upper or lower extremities or any pain in limbs apart from that in left shoulder and bilateral knees.

When graphically describing her current symptoms on the questionnaire completed on April 9, 2002, she wrote, "Neck = stiff & tight sometime burning. Knees = achey pain & weak/sometimes light throb to more intense throb." Today Ms. Mant wrote, "L shoulder/L side of neck now injured still very weak/achey."

In response to a question about any other complaints, the plaintiff adds her knee can be fine and then for no apparent reason while walking down the street she will have "immediate severe pain" in "both [knees] but more the right. My right knee is aching right now."

Ms. Mant believes she is getting worse with time and is concerned about "developing arthritis."

**Activity tolerance:**

On April 9, 2002, Ms. Mant described her typical day as "@ 4:30 am/take Community Transit from Stanwood to downtown Seattle/catch a Metro from 2nd Ave to 1st Hill/standing room only/work in med. office 9 hrs/walk down Madison to 4th Ave catch CT for commute home. Sometime up to 3 hrs 1-way on C.T. is tough if I get an inside seat & am unable to move to get comfortable."

Ms. Mant also reported spending about 40% of waking hours sitting or lying and being limited in all 13 activities listed on the History Questionnaire, including sitting restricted to 30 minutes, as well as driving and standing, adding in each case, "I have to change positions for comfort." Regarding walking, lifting, carrying, bending, reaching, pushing, pulling, and climbing, she stated, "I can do these activities until I feel the slightest knee pain & then I quit. I have learned not to push because the pain will be greater afterwards. Sometimes in the morning after heavy activity it is very painful if I have not p[ai]d attention to pain level." She reported performing no squatting or kneeling due to accompanying knee pain.

Today (August 13, 2002), the plaintiff added with respect to lifting and carrying, "I have not been lifting w/my L side/arm/shoulder." She also reported inability "to reach out w/L arm."

Regarding any other limitations Ms. Mant previously reported difficulty "getting up & down from sitting on the ground or floor. Gardening is limited to staying w[ith]in a comfort level/cold weather. My commute is more difficult/use rakes/chairs etc when bending to the floor/ground reputedly [sic]. Activities w/my 10 yr old grandson are mild." She adds today, "I can't do the games that he would like me to play with him."

With respect to exercise she wrote previously, "Started the swimming 6 mo ago/about 4 x per month right now."

Regarding hobbies, Ms. Mant previously wrote, "I have a complete wood shop & love to make/do wood crafts." By wood crafts she means "small furniture, decorative items for the home, in particular a lot of Christmas decorations."

## REVIEW OF SYSTEMS:

Ms. Mant has no other current complaints.

## PAST AND/OR UNRELATED MEDICAL HISTORY:

In response to a question about any similar symptoms prior to the February 1997 MVA Ms. Mant wrote, "I had neck pain prior to the accident possibly from lifting something heavy."

**Injuries:** None known apart from the above.

**Illnesses:**

*Musculoskeletal:* Ms. Mant developed right lateral epicondylitis in or about February 1996.

In October 1999 she sought treatment for what turned out to be a foreign body (wood fragment) extending from nail fold of left thumb into the nail plate, with a surrounding pyogenic granuloma. The wood and granuloma were excised by a dermatologist.

*Neurological:* No known problems apart from the aforementioned headaches.

*HEENT:* Ms. Mant has had recurrent upper respiratory infections including sinusitis and laryngitis, with presumed eosinophilic nonallergic rhinitis.

She has also had recurrent otitis media, either unilateral or bilateral.

*Respiratory:* Remarkable for recurrent bronchitis and reactive airway disease (asthma).

*Cardiovascular:* The plaintiff has increased cholesterol and triglycerides.

*Gastrointestinal:* She has been diagnosed with possible irritable bowel syndrome due to abdominal pain and constipation, and has gastric reflux and internal hemorrhoids.

*Genitourinary:* Ms. Mant has had pyelonephritis, a ruptured ovarian cyst, and multiple small leiomyomata.

*Dermatological:* She has had dermatitis of hands and onychomycosis.

*Endocrine:* No known problems.

*Psychiatric:* As indicated, the plaintiff's records contain repeated references to stress.

**Surgeries:** The foreign body and pyogenic granuloma were excised from left thumb in October 1999. The plaintiff underwent a total abdominal hysterectomy in June 2001.

**Hospitalizations:** In addition to the latter surgery Ms. Mant was hospitalized for childbirth in September 1972.

## WORK HISTORY:

The plaintiff is employed as the office manager of Polyclinic Pediatrics, and has been worked there for over nine years.

This job reportedly requires sitting three to four hours per day, standing two to three hours, and walking for one hour. Additional duties include frequent bending and twisting, and occasional lifting up to 15 to 20 pounds.

Ms. Mant was reportedly off work for 3½ weeks following the February 1997 MVA, 1 day following the first bus accident, and 3 weeks after the fall on the bus in April 2002. She is presently working full time in her regular occupation.

The plaintiff reportedly enjoys her job, gets along well with her supervisor and coworkers, and has a lot of control in her position as office manager.

## FAMILY HISTORY:

Her father had "three different kinds of cancer," including the spine, and diabetes mellitus.

## SOCIAL HISTORY:

**Marital Status and Dependents:** Ms. Mant has been married, divorced, remarried, and divorced a second time. As implied, she now uses her first married name, Mant.

The plaintiff has one nondependent daughter and presently lives alone.

**Education:** Ms. Mant is a high school graduate, had two years of vocational training in cosmetology and medical office billing, and two years of college.

## MILITARY HISTORY:

None.

## MEDICATIONS AND ALLERGIES:

**Medications:** She currently takes Prilosec daily and Motrin on an as-needed basis.

**Allergies:** None known.

## SUBSTANCE USAGE:

Ms. Mant denies use of tobacco or illicit drugs, either currently or in the past, and drinks alcohol "socially."

When asked if there is anything else she wishes to add the plaintiff states, "I don't think so."

## PHYSICAL APPEARANCE

**General Appearance:** This woman who appears her stated age walked into the conference room with a normal gait and sat without apparent physical distress during today's 2½ hour interview.

However, she did become briefly tearful when describing her difficulty getting out of the Honda Accord following the February 1997 collision, and the accompanying fear and anxiety.

The plaintiff was cooperative in completing the History Questionnaire and a fairly good historian.

Ms. Mant's stated height is 64 inches and weight 170 pounds. Her weight has reportedly increased since the February 1997 motor vehicle collision.

She is right-handed.

Present during the interview and acting as chaperone during the physical examination was Judy Stevens, a paralegal from the office of the plaintiff's attorney.

## ORTHOPEDIC EXAMINATION:

Ms. Mant stood with equal height of shoulders and iliac crests, bearing weight equally on both lower limbs. No abnormal spinal curvatures were visible from behind. From the side, a forward head posture was evident, with shoulders slouched forward and a protuberant abdomen. General muscular development appeared fair.

There was tenderness on superficial palpation over proximal half of left cervical paraspinals and left supraspinatus fossa, but nowhere else about neck, back or shoulder girdles. No additional areas of tenderness were noted upon firm palpation. No muscle spasm was evident.

Active motions of cervical spine were flexion 40 degrees, extension 50 degrees, lateral bending of 30 degrees to left and right, and rotation of 60 degrees to left and 50 degrees to right. Active thoracolumbar motions were flexion 110 degrees, extension 15 degrees, lateral bending of 40 degrees to both left and right, and rotation of 10 degrees bilaterally. She performed the spinal motions more slowly than average, taking a few extra seconds to reach the limit in most cases, but reported no accompanying discomfort or other symptoms.

Gentle axial loading with pressure applied at vertex of the skull, gentle downward pressure on superior shoulders, and gentle en bloc rotation of torso were asymptomatic. Cervical distraction caused "pressure" just inferior to left ear. Foraminal compression tests were not completed on either side as gentle passive extension and leftward or rightward rotation reportedly caused discomfort in proximal sternocleidomastoid bilaterally, before any axial loading was applied.

Active motions of left/right shoulders were abduction 55/160 degrees, adduction 30/30 degrees, extension 35/40 degrees, flexion 125/150 degrees, external rotation 80/80 degrees, and internal rotation 75/75 degrees. The degree of effort put forth on some motions of left shoulder was questionable. For example, during subsequent manual muscle testing the examinee readily mimicked the examiner's demonstration of 90 degrees of shoulder abduction with elbows flexed bilaterally as the position to adopt and maintain while resisting downward force on lateral arms. She demonstrated full motions of elbows, forearms, wrists, and digits in distal upper extremities.

Gentle passive circumduction of left shoulder revealed mild, fairly constant crepitus versus minimal crepitus on the right. Left shoulder was stable anteriorly, inferiorly, and posteriorly.

Gait, heel and toe walking, and tandem gait were normal. Manual muscle testing revealed grade 4/5 weakness upon resisted left shoulder external rotation, flexion, and abduction, with normal strength on resisted motions of right shoulder and both elbows, forearms, and wrists. Finger abduction was initially weak bilaterally, and normal strength achieved only after repeated encouragement. Measured with a Jamar dynamometer in three temporally separate trials, grip strength on left was 10, 6, and 4 kg versus 25, 16, and 14 kg on right. Normal strength was noted throughout both lower limbs.

Deep tendon reflexes were 1+ and symmetrical at biceps, triceps, brachioradialis. Knee and ankle reflexes were 2+ bilaterally. Sensation was intact in all four extremities, including tips of left index, middle, and ring fingers.

Measured 10 cm proximal and distal to flexion crease of elbow respectively, arm circumferences were 32.5 cm on left versus 33 cm on right; while forearm circumferences were 21 cm on left versus 23 cm on right.

Percussion over ulnar notch, pronator teres, radial tunnel, and Guyon's canal was asymptomatic bilaterally. Percussion over left carpal tunnel caused a localized shock sensation. On the right this caused a much more apparent "shocky thing" to radiate from carpal tunnel proximally to anterior shoulder. Phalen test was negative bilaterally.

Knees were normal on inspection apart from a barely perceptible 14 mm long, longitudinal scar over medial portion of medial tibial condyle. No soft tissue swelling or effusion was evident on either side. There was tenderness on firm palpation of anterior portion of medial joint line bilaterally, more so on right than left. Otherwise, both knees were nontender.

Observing patellae on knee extension in the sitting position revealed mild lateral tilting on both sides, but no inverted J sign. Patellar inhibition, apprehension, medial displacement, and grind were all negative, apart from notation of asymptomatic crepitus on the latter. Patellar compression caused pain bilaterally.

Lachman, anterior and posterior drawer, and varus and valgus stress tests in 30 degrees of flexion were negative bilaterally. McMurray test was also negative on both sides. Ms. Mant had full extension and flexion of both knees.

Measured 15 cm superior and inferior to medial joint line of knee respectively, thigh circumferences were 52.5 cm on left versus 53 cm on right, knee circumferences 38 cm on left versus 39 cm on right, and leg circumferences 35 cm on left versus 35.5 cm on right. Lower extremity lengths were equal.

## DIAGNOSES:

1. Chronic intermittent headaches, possibly tension and/or cervicogenic in type, onset in or before January 1995.

2. Probable right posterolateral cervical disc herniation in January 1995, if present probably due to degenerative disc disease, and resultant right C5, C6, and/or C7 radiculopathy.

3. Recurrent neck pain with associated headaches in October 1996, possibly due to recurrence or worsening of the aforementioned disc herniation.

4. Multiple injuries due to the February 1997 motor vehicle collision (left frontal impact), including:
    a) cervical sprain/strain
    b) contusion anterior right and probably left knees
    c) laceration medial right knee.

5. Contusions bilateral knees and anterior legs (shins), due to the May 1998 injury (slid forward striking end of bench seat when bus stopped suddenly).

6. Multiple injuries due to the April 2002 injury (fell backward when bus stopped suddenly) including:
    a) scalp contusions and abrasion
    b) recurrence or worsening of headaches
    c) possible cerebral concussion and post-concussive syndrome
    d) cervical sprain/strain.

7. Possible bilateral carpal tunnel syndrome, probably due to a combination of avocational and occupational activities, and excess weight, if present.

8. Mild lateral tilting of patellae, a congenital-developmental anomaly.

9. Overweight, probably exogenous.

10. Anxiety, definitive diagnosis and causal determination beyond the scope of this examination.

## DISCUSSION:

**Overview of Examinee's History and Exam Findings:** Ms. Mant was a pleasant and cooperative historian. In some cases her characterizations of injuries appeared hyperbolic. For example, she provided an emotionally charged description of her attempts to get out of the Honda Accord on February 14, 1997. Since the examiner originally did not have the ER records following the April 30, 2002, bus accident, the plaintiff was asked to describe what happened at Swedish Medical Center-First Hill. "They said I had a concussion and severe whiplash. They gave me Vicodin [narcotic analgesic hydrocodone with acetaminophen] and [a cervical] collar, and told me to take ibuprofen." The records from Dr. Wilson and the nurse and SMC-FH suggest none of this is true. There was no diagnosis of concussion, presumably because Ms. Mant denied loss of consciousness and was alert and oriented. Dr. Wilson apparently noted left cervical paraspinal tenderness, but did not diagnose whiplash, severe or otherwise. She was given and advised to take Tylenol as needed for pain, which is plausible since it would be inadvisable to prescribe a narcotic such as Vicodin for someone with a possible head injury. No cervical collar was dispensed in the ER, or recommended by Dr. Wilson, although the plaintiff may have kept that applied during ambulance transportation to SMC-FH.

There were some indications of symptom magnification, and the plaintiff's claimed and demonstrated physical restrictions are probably exaggerated. However, her complaints seemed plausible in distribution (see below).

Objective abnormalities on today's examination included the protuberant abdomen, small scar about medial right knee, and mild lateral tilting of patellae. The smaller left arm and forearm are probably due to the plaintiff's right-hand dominance. The examiner is uncertain of an explanation for the smaller circumferences of left thigh, knee, and leg; but the discrepancies were minimal.

Subjective findings included limited neck and back motions, discomfort in sternocleidomastoid with gentle passive extension and leftward or rightward rotation of neck, weakness on resisted motions of left shoulder, shock-like sensations with percussion over carpal tunnel bilaterally (with radiation proximally to shoulder on right), tenderness on firm palpation of anterior portion of medial joint line of knee bilaterally, and pain on patellar compression on both sides.

Nonorganic findings during the examination included the superficial tenderness over left neck and upper back, poor and inconsistent effort upon active motions of left shoulder and grip strength bilaterally, and possibly poor effort during strength testing of left shoulder.

**Causation:** The above diagnoses and causes are stated on a more probable than not basis where possible. However, the diagnoses must be qualified by noting that most are based primarily, if not exclusively, upon subjective complaints and/or physical findings which can neither be confirmed nor denied. Also, it is often difficult, if not impossible, to corroborate or disprove statements of attribution based solely on history.

Independent neurologic evaluation is suggested if a more definitive opinion is desired regarding the cause of Ms. Mant's chronic intermittent headaches, However, they are probably tension and/or cervicogenic in type, and began in or before January 1995.

It is not known with certainty whether Ms. Mant had a right posterolateral cervical disc herniation in January 1995 because no imaging study was performed. However, her symptoms and physical findings suggestive of right C5, C6, and/or C7 radiculopathy indicate something was causing neural impingement. At her age a disc herniation would be more likely than spinal stenosis. Other potential causes such as tumor or infection are relatively rare and likely would have become evident long ago. Absent any known precipitating trauma, the presumed disc herniation was likely caused by progressive disc degeneration, due in turn to genetics and aging.

Many factors determine the likelihood, type, and severity of injury after a collision, which in turn influence the need for treatment, disability, and likelihood of permanent residuals. These include the strength and elasticity of the occupant's tissues (muscle, tendon, ligament, bone, etc.) and hence their ability to resist externally applied direct or indirect stresses. A football player or infant is understandably less likely to be injured in a frontal collision than a frail, elderly woman. Obviously most individuals, including Ms. Mant, fall between these extremes. However, given her pre-existing headaches, neck problems, and anxiety she may have been a physical and psychological "eggshell."

Another factor is body position at the time of impact. An individual in a frontal collision tends to continue traveling forward due to inertia, while the vehicle decelerates. Upon reaching the limit of stretch of shoulder and lap belts (if worn), there tends to be cervical and lesser thoracolumbar flexion, followed by rebound extension. A person whose cervical and thoracolumbar spine are in a neutral position (looking forward) at impact is less likely to be injured than one rotated leftward or rightward, as the facet joints are designed to accommodate flexion and extension in neutral, but to a much lesser extent when rotated. Hence Ms. Mant was less likely to be injured than someone, for instance, looking sideways at impact.

Awareness of the impending collision has a protective effect, tending to prevent or minimize trauma, presumably given the ability of a vehicular occupant to brace, guard, or otherwise contract muscles in preparation for impact. Conversely, individuals with no forewarning of an impact are more likely symptomatic afterward. Ms. Mant apparently was unaware of the impending collision.

Perhaps the most important determinants of bodily injury are the accelerations (g forces) to which an occupant is subjected, and their duration. The higher the acceleration, and longer it is sustained, the greater the likelihood of injury. Since $\Delta v$, the change in velocity of a vehicle, is the area under the acceleration vs. time curve, it combines both factors, and is a useful way to quantify impact severity. In fact, studies have repeatedly shown the crash parameter most closely related to occupant injury potential is $\Delta v$.[20][21][22][23] The change in velocity dictates the speed with which an occupant will strike, or be struck by, its interior, e.g., seat belts, steering wheel, and/or dashboard in a frontal impact such as this. Whatever the interior structure, the faster the speed of interaction with an occupant, the higher the forces on his body, and greater the probability of injury.

$\Delta v$ is dependent in large part upon kinetic energy of the vehicle(s) (KE = ½ mass x velocity$^2$). Understandably, one would be less likely to be injured when striking, or being struck by, a motorcycle than a high mass vehicle such as a semi tractor-trailer. Obviously the Mitsubishi falls between these extremes of mass. Velocity is also an important factor, and since it is squared, assumes greater relative importance at higher speeds. Not surprisingly, collisions occurring at highway speeds such as in this case are more likely injurious than those on city streets or in parking lots.

Characteristics of the vehicle(s), particularly ability to absorb kinetic energy, are also important determinants of bodily injury. Energy-absorbing bumpers and vehicle crush (if any) to some extent dissipate energy that would otherwise be available to accelerate (or in this case decelerate) the subject

---

[20] Kornhauser M: Delta v thresholds for cervical spine injury. *Society of Automotive Engineers* SP-1174, SAE No. 960093:1-13, 1996.

[21] Nahum AM and Gomez MA: Injury reconstruction: the biomechanical analysis of accidental injury. *Society of Automotive Engineers* SP-1030, SAE No. 940568:69-79, 1994.

[22] Rogers VL and Compton CP: The relationship between delta v and injury. *Proceedings of the 37th Stapp Car Crash Conference*, SAE No. 933111:35-41, 1993.

[23] Robinette RD, Fay RJ, Paulsen RE: Delta v: basic concepts, computational methods, and misunderstandings. *Society of Automotive Engineers* SP-1030, SAE No. 940915:309-332, 1994.

vehicle and occupant. Interior features of the vehicle are also important. The presence or absence of an airbag(s), energy-absorbing steering column, padded dashboard, etc., may all influence the nature and extent of occupant trauma. Fortunately, a fair amount of energy was dissipated in crushing all three vehicles involved; and the Honda's air bag deployed.

While the plaintiff was involved in a relatively high $\Delta v$ collision, and one that would cause injury in virtually any occupant, one must recognize that reports of symptoms following an accident do not necessarily reflect the severity of tissue damage. Pain and other complaints are not simply pathophysiologic phenomena, but must be understood in the larger context of the whole person. Whether and how an individual perceives and reports pain, for example, depends on many factors including cultural background, personality, emotional status, level of arousal, past experience, the current situation, and reinforcement contingencies. In cases where there is anger and/or potential compensation, the severity, distribution, and duration of complaints often correlate poorly with the mechanism and magnitude of the real or alleged trauma.

As implied, following a collision occupants having pre-existing psychosocial problems are much more likely to manifest complaints of disproportionate severity and/or distribution, and respond poorly to treatment directed towards physical pathology, resulting in symptoms of unexpectedly prolonged duration as well. Individuals with antecedent neuromusculoskeletal pathology, in particular pre-existing degenerative disease of or trauma to their spine, with or without immediately preceding symptoms, are also more likely to be symptomatic afterward.

There is some question as to whether the plaintiff's left knee pain is attributable to the February 1997 collision. Noticeably absent from the earlier records, including those from Bainbridge Island Ambulance, Dr. George, Dr. Albertson, and Ms. Rogers is any reference to left knee pain. In fact, it appears the first mention of bilateral knee pain was a month after the subject collision, on March 14, 1997, when Dr. Albertson noted "pain over her bilateral patellar tendons." The temporal disparity between the collision and initial symptom onset (or at least report) on left suggests a cause-and-effect relationship is unlikely.

On the other hand, given the principal direction of force, the Honda Accord was decelerated with respect to its forward travel and accelerated rightward. Due to inertia the plaintiff would have continued traveling forward in a straight line to the extent permitted by her shoulder and lap belts. Relative to her vehicle, she would have gone forward and leftward, and may very well have struck her anterior left knee on the door panel, dashboard or some other interior object. Determining factors would include her height, where the seat bottom was adjusted along its tracks, the "snugness" with which the lap belt was applied, and amount of stretch in the belt fabric. Ultimately, given the absence of any other more probable cause for the left knee pain beginning sometime between February 14 and March 14, 1997, the examiner concludes that it, like the discomfort on the right, probably is causally related to the collision on the former date.

Regarding the May 1998 bus accident, there were subjective and objective findings suggesting Ms. Mant sustained contusions of bilateral knees and anterior legs (shins).

There were also subjective and objective findings indicating the plaintiff sustained an abrasion and contusions of scalp in the April 2002 bus accident. At least historically there was also recurrence or worsening of her headaches and neck pain thereafter. This is plausible based on the evidence of scalp injury and the plaintiff's "eggshell" status. Given the conflicting evidence regarding loss of consciousness the examiner cannot state with certainty or even probability whether there was a cerebral concussion at the time of injury and post-concussive syndrome thereafter. Independent neurologic evaluation is again recommended if a more definitive opinion is desired.

Independent psychiatric evaluation is suggested if a better-educated opinion is desired as to precise diagnosis and cause of the anxiety, or to use the plaintiff's term, "stress." However, it pre-existed the February 1997 MVA. The anxiety may be "work-related" as Ms. Mant implied on page 5 of the Personal Health History completed on February 20, 1997. Regardless, various life stressors probably have contributed to her headaches and neck pain, and perhaps other physical complaints as well. Anxiety often causes increased resting muscular tension, and discomfort accompanying same (tension myalgia). Corroborating this conclusion is Dr. Albertson's December 9, 1996, notation "she is...under a lot of stress," and explanation "...to her how chronic stress can...exacerbate muscular tension.

The numbness and tingling in the palmar tips of left index, middle, and ring fingers (median nerve distribution) which Ms. Mant reportedly experienced when doing exercises in physical therapy yesterday, and the shock-like sensations with percussion over carpal tunnel bilaterally (with radiation proximally to shoulder on right) during today's examination suggest she may have mild bilateral carpal tunnel syndrome. If present, the median nerve entrapment is probably due to a combination of avocational and occupational activities and excess weight, but unrelated to any of the aforementioned injuries.

The symmetrical nature of the mild lateral tilting of Ms. Mant's patellae suggests this is the way she was born and/or grew. In other words it is probably a congenital-developmental anomaly. Patellar malalignment can cause anterior knee pain and crepitus. Hence the lateral tilting may be contributing to Ms. Mant's knee discomfort, but it could also be incidental given its mild severity.

Overweight is defined as a body mass index (weight in kilograms divided by height in meters$^2$) greater than or equal to 25. A BMI greater than or equal to 30 constitutes obesity, and 40 or more morbid obesity. Given her reported height of 64 inches and weight of 170 lbs., Ms. Mant's body mass index is 29, which meets the criterion for overweight and approaches that for obesity. As indicated, the excess weight is probably exogenous, due to caloric intake via food and beverages in excess of the body's demands.

As implied by Dr. Milltowns, Ms. Mant probably has "eosinophilic non-allergic rhinitis with mild reactive airway disease," and accompanying sinusitis. These conditions probably have nothing to do with the February 1997 collision or any of her other accidents, although evaluation by an allergist and/or ear, nose, and throat specialist is suggested if a more definitive opinion is desired.

Symptom magnification (SM) is exaggeration of pain or other complaints, often precipitated by an injury or illness. While physical effects of the trauma or disease improve and perhaps resolve, the symptoms persist, and may increase in severity and/or distribution over time. The magnification may be conscious or unconscious.

The severity of pain is commonly exaggerated in SM, e.g. 9, 10 or even greater on a 0-10 scale. Ms. Mant was asked today to quantify her discomfort from 0 (none) to 10 (the worst pain imaginable). While the reader may have another mental picture, the examiner envisions an individual with discomfort of 10 in severity writhing in agony on the ground, floor, or bed while awaiting ambulance transportation to an emergency room. In other words, someone with 10/10 pain is, or should be, hospitalized.[24] Whether the plaintiff was actually having pain of 10 in severity after the February 1997 collision as claimed cannot be confirmed or denied, but she was not hospitalized. A rating of 7 implies moderately severe pain for which one needs to see a doctor now. Notwithstanding her comfortable appearance during the interview, Ms. Mant reported having neck pain of 6-7 in severity at present.

---

[24] Dorto, AJ. Symptom Magnification and the Role of the Disability Evaluating Physician. *ABIME Perspective* Summer 1999, 1-13.

While few musculoskeletal conditions produce constant pain, the most notable examples being infection and tumor, symptom magnifiers often claim omnipresent discomfort. Pain due to physical injuries or degenerative disease is usually mechanical, precipitated by activity or prolonged maintenance of one position, persists for a period of time thereafter, then resolves with cessation of the offending activity and rest, or a change in position. Today Ms. Mant claimed to have constant neck pain.

Sometimes discomfort is hyperbolically characterized, e.g., horrible, unbearable, or devastating. The plaintiff did not use these emotionally laden descriptors. Persons exaggerating their pain or other complaints may also employ "polycharacterization." For example, Ms. Mant characterized her neck pain as aching, burning, and tightness; and bilateral anterior knee pain as aching, stabbing, and/or throbbing.

Symptoms may also be magnified into implausibly widespread or nonanatomical distributions, for example, "everything hurts," numbness "from the elbow down" or weakness "of the whole leg." Sometimes complaints migrate from one side or area to another, or "metastasize," involving progressively more body parts over time. By contrast, Ms. Mant's complaints have been fairly well localized and reasonably consistent in distribution.

Physical examination findings (signs) that do not fit known patterns of injury or illness are labeled nonorganic. In contradistinction to objective findings such as scars, masses, reflexes, or limb circumferences that can be observed, felt, tested, or measured respectively, most signs are subjective, dependent upon the behavior or responses of the patient or examinee. As implied, nonorganic physical findings are not consistent with anatomical or physiological derangement due to trauma or disease. Related terms, sometimes used interchangeably with NPF, are abnormal pain behavior, illness behavior, or functional overlay. However, the latter may be a confusing misnomer, since these signs are almost always associated with some degree of (at least claimed) dysfunction.

Ms. Mant did not put forth good effort upon some left shoulder motions. For instance, abduction was initially limited to 55°. However, shortly thereafter, when beginning upper extremity strength testing, the examiner demonstrated 90° of shoulder abduction bilaterally, with elbows flexed, as the position to maintain while he pushed down on her lateral arms to assess strength of shoulder abductor muscles. Ms. Mant easily adopted the position, nearly doubling her allegedly maximum active shoulder abduction.

The examiner cannot definitively confirm or deny validity of the grade 4/5 weakness demonstrated on left shoulder external rotation, flexion, and abduction. However, suboptimal effort thereon seems probable, perhaps due to the plaintiff's concern about possibly causing pain.

The examiner is unaware of any plausible explanation for the initial weakness of finger abduction bilaterally apart from suboptimal effort. Normal strength was eventually achieved, but only after repeated encouragement.

The instructions regarding grip strength assessment on page 508 of the AMA *Guides to the Evaluation of Permanent Impairment*, Fifth Edition state, "Tests repeated at intervals during an examination are considered…reliable if there is less than 20% variation in the readings. If there is more than 20% variation…one may assume the individual is not exerting full effort." As indicated, Ms. Mant's grip strength was measured with a Jamar dynamometer in three temporally separate trials. The measurements of 10, 6, and 4 kg on left and 25, 16, and 14 kg on right far exceed the 20% variation cutoff for reliability.

SM and NPF are 3 to 4 times more common in the setting of a compensable injury or illness[25]; suggesting claimants or plaintiffs believe they will derive greater monetary or other benefit by inflating the duration, distribution, and/or severity of their complaints and findings. Indeed the most obvious external incentives for these behaviors are tangible. While often financial, e.g., an impairment award, time loss compensation, reimbursement for treatment costs, or judgment for pain and suffering; the tangible motive may be non-pecuniary, e.g., obtaining vocational retraining or drugs such as narcotics. Secondary gain may also be intangible. e.g., avoidance of undesirable occupational or home duties, sympathy from friends and relatives, nuturing from caregivers, etc.

However, because SM and NPF can occur unconsciously, and the individual exaggerating or fabricating the complaints and subjective findings may be unaware of the motivation, one should not necessarily equate their presence with malingering. Nonanatomical-nonphysiological symptoms and signs commonly reflect an individual's psychosocial makeup, including upbringing, cultural background, educational level, family situation, employment or lack thereof, etc.

Persons with pre-existing mental health problems, particularly a prior history of physical, emotional, and/or sexual abuse are prone to develop disproportionate somatic complaints subsequently. However, Ms. Mant did not report any prior or current abuse on today's questionnaire.

---

[25] Snider, RK, editor. *Essentials of Musculoskeletal Care*. Rosemont, IL: American Academy of Orthopaedic Surgeons, 1997, 43-45.

Rather than conscious magnification or fabrication of symptoms and signs for external gain (malingering), SM and NPF are commonly a means to communicate distress: "See how bad I am" or "I'm not getting the help I need." Furthermore, the presence of nonorganic complaints and findings does not rule out organic (physical) pathology. There may be significant underlying injury or illness, masked by the "functional overlay."

SM and NPF are often noted by independent medical examiners, but rarely by treating doctors, therapists, etc. There several possible reasons for the discrepancy. Health care providers often fail to identify SM or NPF because they have not been trained to recognize same. On the other hand, assessment of the validity of symptoms and signs is an integral part of any quality independent medical examination (IME).

The discrepancy in notation may also reflect bias. The attending physician may be a patient and/or personal advocate, perhaps recognizing "there's something wrong with this picture," but fail to report the suspicion fearing it would diminish their patient's credibility and the value of their claim or lawsuit. Notation of SM or NPF might also prompt a third party to conclude diagnostic studies and/or treatment were unnecessary, and deny payment for services rendered, thereby diminishing the provider's income. The examiner may also become an advocate, but for their client, inflating the importance of nonorganic symptoms or signs which are few in number or marginal in significance.

Lastly, patients often behave differently than examinees. To please, and avoid offending, their treating doctor, therapist, etc., patients frequently report more favorable treatment outcomes (lesser symptoms) than they would to an examiner or new health care provider.

By virtue of prior experience or conversation with a coworker, union steward, or attorney, claimants and plaintiffs may also view an IME in an adversarial light, and exaggerate or fabricate complaints and findings in an attempt to avoid cessation of time loss compensation, denial of further treatment, diminution in an impairment award or settlement for pain and suffering, etc.

In summary, there was evidence of symptom magnification and were some nonorganic findings during today's history and examination, respectively. However, neither was flagrant.

**Evaluation and Treatment:**

*Past:* The evaluation and treatment rendered in the ER at Swedish Medical Center-First Hill, by Dr. Albertson, and at Theracare Nordstrom through

September 3, 1997, probably were necessary for injuries sustained in the February 1997 collision. However, no further diagnostic or therapeutic endeavors were necessary for effects of that collision.

*Future:* No further formal treatment appears warranted at present for the plaintiff's neck-upper back-left shoulder or bilateral anterior knee pains. However, as repeatedly advised by others, she would be well advised to continue a self-directed program of stretching, strengthening, and aerobic conditioning exercises. Weight reduction is also recommended. Ms. Mant may also wish to take an over-the-counter analgesic on an as-needed basis provided no untoward side effect results.

**Apportionment:** The plaintiff's current condition is obviously multifactorial, being due in part to whatever was causing her head, neck and radicular pains prior to the February 1997 collision, presumably a cervical disc herniation, or perhaps more than one. It is also due in part to the February 1997 collision which likely caused temporary worsening of her pre-existing neck pain with new onset of bilateral anterior knee pain. Additionally her present condition is due in part to the May 1998 and April 2002 bus accidents. While the first of these appears to be the least severe of all her traumas, Ms. Mant reported today she did not recover completely therefrom. "I still continue to have problems with my knees." Lastly, her physical symptoms are likely due in part to psychosocial factors, probably including anxiety manifested in increased muscular tension and tension myalgia.

It is difficult to provide a precise percentage apportionment. However, in anticipation of such a question, the examiner asked Ms. Mant to quantify her pain levels on a scale of 0 (no discomfort) to 10 (the worst pain imaginable) before the February 1997, May 1998, and April 2002 accidents, and at present, to enable at least a subjective numerical basis for apportionment. The table below summarizes her responses.

| Symptom | Pre-2/97 MVA | Pre-5/98 Bus | Pre-4/02 Bus | Now |
|---|---|---|---|---|
| Neck pain | 0-3 intermittent | 2 intermittent | 2 intermittent | 6-7 constant |
| Knee pain | 0 | 4-6 intermittent | 5-6 intermittent | 2-4 intermittent |

Her current head and neck pain are probably due to two factors, whatever was causing them before the February 1997 MVA, and the April 2002 bus accident. Supporting the collision as a primary cause are the "abnormal amount of headaches," and neck pain for which she began another course of physical therapy on December 10, 1996, which continued up to and including the day prior to the MVA. On February 20, 1997, Ms. Mant reported on page 4 of the Personal Health History at Dr. Albertson's office she "had just finished" therapy prior to the collision six days earlier. However, this is not corroborated by Ms. Rogers's February 13th Progress Summary. The therapist thought it "appropriate to continue [treatment] once a week or...every other week."

While there was increased neck pain after February 1997 MVA, the table reveals it was an exacerbation (temporary worsening) rather than aggravation (permanent worsening). In other words, Ms. Mant's neck pain had returned to its baseline by the time of the May 1998 bus accident. It remained at that level (reportedly 2 but actually 0-2 since it was intermittent) until the April 2002 bus accident, with another spike upwards in head and neck pain thereafter. At least historically Ms. Mant has not recovered to her pre-fall baseline, the previously intermittent cervicalgia now being constant, and increased in severity from 0-2 to 6-7, with new onset of left shoulder pain. Whether she will completely recover from the 2nd bus accident remains to be seen. Hence the fall on the bus would be considered the most proximate and another primary contributor to her current cervicalgia. At present her neck pain is probably due 50% to each, the pre-existing pathology and the April 2002 accident.

By contrast, statements from the plaintiff suggest her bilateral knee pain is due to the February 1997 and May 1998 accidents. She reportedly did not have knee pain before the subject MVA, and stated that discomfort was permanently worsened by striking her knees on the bus seat. However, the table indicates her current knee pain is less than it was both before and after the 1st bus accident, suggesting it was an exacerbation. Given the latter, and the greater magnitude of collision, the examiner would apportion her knee conditions 75% to the February 1997 MVA and 25% to the May 1998 bus accident.

**Disability:**

*Prior:* The periods of time loss reported today by Ms. Mant following her three vehicular accidents appear to have been warranted.

*Current:* While the plaintiff claimed multiple different activity restrictions, and limitation in some avocational pursuits, which the examiner can neither confirm nor deny, there appears to be no occupational disability, as she is now and has been for some time employed full time in her regular occupation.

**Medical Stability:** Ms. Mant probably reached the point of maximum medical improvement with respect to the February 1997 collision by

September 3rd of that year, seven months later, when she discontinued treatment.

**Prognosis:** It is difficult to understand the plaintiff's claim she is presently getting worse, which is inconsistent with the natural history of the vast majority of trauma. In other words, injuries tend to gradually improve, if not resolve, over time as a result of the body's natural healing processes, even in the absence of treatment. The examiner suspects her current neck-left shoulder and bilateral knee pain will improve (but not resolve completely) over the subsequent months and years barring recurrent injury. The improvement will likely be expedited if she exercises regularly, including performance of short-arc and isometric quadriceps strengthening. Weight reduction will likely also improve her general well-being, and diminish the loads on her knees.

The examiner has been asked whether he agrees or disagrees with the diagnoses and recommendations of Dr. Garrett. Based on the history reported and records reviewed today, there is no indication apart from his report of a contusion of distal right tibia in the February 1997 MVA. Hence, no such diagnosis was listed. The other two diagnoses recorded by Dr. Garrett, the cervical strain and contusion-laceration of right patella, appear justified for the most part, although based on today's examination the laceration was not over the patella, but rather medial tibial condyle. Dr. Garrett's diagnoses are also incomplete, likely due in part to the fact he was not provided with records prior to the February 1997 collision, nor could he have been aware of the May 1998 and April 2002 incidents as they had not yet occurred. I agree with the preceding orthopedic examiner that there is "no disability at the present time," but am more pessimistic than Dr. Garrett who anticipated an excellent prognosis. Specifically, if the plaintiff's knee pain was going to resolve, it probably would have done so by now. This suggests she will be left with mild but continued intermittent knee pain. I agree with Dr. Garrett the treatment to date was necessary, and regarding the advisability of performing isometric quadriceps exercises on a home basis, but disagree with his conclusion that she had "not reached maximum benefit from [formal] treatment" by the time of his IME.

Charles N. Brooks

Charles N. Brooks, MD, PC

**Report #7: Brain Injury**

This report is most notable for the following.

- It is well organized. Good use of headnotes and numbered lists.
- Good presentation of introductory information.
- Records and other documents reviewed are clearly documented.
- Precision of examination time (e.g., terminated at 12:08 P.M.).
- Detailed, well-documented examination.
- Examiner stays within his area of expertise (e.g., by not commenting on the etiology of cardiac tamponade).
- Report is objective and balanced.
- Disagreements with other experts (e.g., concerning the life care plan) are made objectively and without inflammatory language.

While this is an excellent report, all reports can be improved. Areas of possible improvement include the following.

- An executive summary would have been a helpful addition to this complex, lengthy evaluation.
- Some superfluous information is included (e.g., comments about do-not-resuscitate orders in brain-injured individuals).
- Literature cited should be cited with more specificity (e.g., a more specific cite than "several recent papers").
- Somewhat excessive boilerplate language at the end of the report.

---

## INDEPENDENT MEDICAL EVALUATION

| | |
|---|---|
| **EXAMINEE:** | Cate Warren |
| **DATE OF BIRTH:** | 8/2/1953 |
| **CHRONOLOGICAL AGE:** | 47 years |
| **SOCIAL SECURITY NUMBER:** | 123-45-6789 |
| **DATE OF IME:** | 3/2/01 |
| **EXAM TIME:** | 10:30 A.M. to 12:08 P.M. |
| **DATE OF INJURY:** | 5/5/97 |

| | |
|---|---|
| **PARTY REQUESTING IME:** | Jarret Schweighart<br>Geiser & Willey, P.A.,<br>Attorneys-at-Law<br>900 N. Glencoe Ave.<br>Torrence, FL 30000<br><br>Tel: 555-555-1111<br>Fax: 555-555-2222 |
| **PARTY RESPONSIBLE FOR PAYMENT:** | Same as above |
| **REASON FOR IME:** | Assessment of current impairment and disability-related issues as germane to history of hypoxic-ischemic brain insult. |

**BASIS OF REPORT:**

1. IME of March 2, 2001

2. Review of records provided through Attorney Schweighart's office including:

   St. Hilary's Hospital records 6/92 through 7/92

   Records of Glen Caudwell, PA-C, 8/96 through 6/97

   Terrace Medical Center records, 3/14/97 through 4/10/97

   Lincoln Medical Center, 4/10/97 through 5/1/97

   Trustworthy Home Health Care, 5/2/97 through 5/4/97 (certified through 7/2/97)

   Records from Ocean View Medical Center, emergency room, 5/3/97

   Records from Lincoln Medical Center emergency department, 5/3/97

   Records from Lincoln Medical Center 5/4/97 through 6/3/97

   Records from Alliance Health Care Company 6/97 through 7/97

Records from Terrace Medical Center 8/22/97 (emergency department)

Hospital admission records from Terrace Medical Center, 8/26/97 through 9/4/97

Miscellaneous emergency room visits 8/97 through 6/00, Terrace Medical Center

Records from Alliance Health Care Company, Subacute Unit, 6/1/97 through 9/19/97

Records from Valencia Hospital 9/19/97 through 12/12/97

Records of Blaine Gryce, 1997 through 1998

Video tape 3/23/98 of Cate Warren at Windsor Rehabilitation Center - 31 minutes duration

Records from Windsor Rehabilitation & Health Care Center, 1998

Record from Alexander Scully, M.D., 1998
Records of Jordan Mullens, Jr., M.D., 2/22/99

Records from Union HealthCare Plaza - Outpatient records of Louis Branda, M.D., 3/22/99 through 9/00

Records of Stewart Kaplan, M.D., 9/10/99

Richard Grant, DMD, Terrace Surgery Center, 10/4/99

Records from Union Hospital, miscellaneous, from year 2000

"Comprehensive Rehabilitation Evaluation", prepared by Colin King, M.D., on Cate Warren, 10/20/00

Form letter form Daniel Arzbecker, M.D., State University, regarding neuronal cell implantation for the treatment of stroke

Depositions:

A. Jack Warren, 1/11/00 and 10/18/00

B. Colin King, M.D., 2/22/01

## HISTORY OF PRESENT ILLNESS, BASED ON RECORD REVIEW:

The examinee's medical history pre-dating her cerebral hypoxic ischemic insult secondary to cardiac tamponade on 5/5/97 is quite complex. Based on available information, she had been in and out of various hospitals and medical care practitioners' offices from the latter part of 1996 through the time of her unfortunate turn of events in May of 1997.

When seen in the latter part of 1996 through her primary care physicians office, Dr. Harold Walsh (although I would note it appears that she was often seen by other persons in the office, including a physician's assistant). It was noted that she had mid-epigastric pain for several months' duration. She was initially thought to have a hiatal hernia versus peptic ulcer disease. Her symptoms progressed over time to the point where she was admitted in early 1997 (1/97) to the emergency room at Torrence Hospital with a presumptive diagnosis of "strep throat." A subsequent upper endoscopy (esophagogastroduodenoscopy) was unremarkable. She continued to have continued somatic symptoms, complaints consistent with dysphagia (difficulty swallowing), as well as thoracic pain.

On 3/14/97, she was again admitted to the hospital with a diagnosis of fever, leukocytosis associated with chest pain, which they felt, at that time, was possibly related to some type of gastrointestinal tract pathology. She was also concurrently diagnosed with H.pylori positive gastritis. She underwent a number of different tests including tests to rule out pericarditis. She was noted to have a small posterior pericardial effusion in addition to moderate tricuspid regurgitation. Chest x-ray demonstrated perihilar vascular prominence with focal consolidation overlying the left hilum and bilateral lung based pleural densities.

A colonoscopy was done on 3/23/97 and noted problems leading from the sigmoid and/or descending area. The discharge summary from this hospitalization notes the following "discharge diagnoses..." (1) fever of unknown origin; (2) leukocytosis; (3) status post gastrointestinal bleed and anemia.

On the 4/10/97 admission at the Lincoln Medical Center, due to her persistent blood loss, she was transfused 8 units of packed bed blood cells and received fresh frozen plasma as well. Her chest x-ray continued to worsen. Multiple cultures were done, all of which were negative except for one positive coagulase negative staphylococcus epidermidis, which was felt to likely be a contaminate. She was started on multiple antibiotics. Eventually, her leukocytosis reached a peak level of 69,000 which is extremely elevated. All cultures were negative. Biopsy revealed non-specific acute and chronic interstitial pneumonitis which was felt to be consistent with a chemical pneumonitis. Due to her leukocytosis, a bone marrow aspirate was performed and showed increased white blood cells but otherwise was within normal limits. She was "shot-gunned" relative to the antibiotic approach and received a multi-drug regimen including a four-drug anti-TB regimen, anti-pseudomonal Penicillin, and steroids, the latter being non-antibiotic/fungal medication. During this time, her lactate dehydrogenase level (LDH) was noted to be quite elevated at 1173. HIV testing was also done which was negative.

On 4/10/97, the patient was transferred to The Lincoln Medical Center for evaluation of her fever of unknown origin. During this hospitalization, the treating physicians concluded that her fevers might actually be related to a drug reaction. The agent which was felt to be the culprit in this reaction was an H2 blocker that is known to cause febrile leukemoid reactions. With discontinuation of H2 blocker, her leukocytosis apparently started to resolve over a 4-day period but then on the 4th day of admission, she spiked a fever to 105 with an elevated white count over 20,000. She was also started on Diflucan for oral candidiasis. She received a high dose antibiotic and was begun on empiric therapy for a number of etiologic infectious agents that might be responsible for her fever. Hepatitis profile was negative. Multiple imaging studies were done including scans of the head, neck, chest, abdomen and pelvis which revealed no abscess or hidden source of infection. Bone marrow biopsies were negative. A white blood cell scan only showed increased uptake in the base of the lung. Complete work ups by gynecology and ophthalmology were also performed and were unremarkable.

An echocardiogram done on 4/17/97, one month after the prior of 3/17/97, was somewhat limited but noted mild mitral and tricuspid regurgitation with mild concentric hypertrophy with grossly normal left ventricular systolic function and esophagogastroduodenoscopy (EGD) was done on 3/20/97 with impression of "duodenal ulcer, active GI bleed and status post injection therapy."

At the time of his discharge on 5/1, it was the treating physician's opinion that there was no known etiology for what was believed to have been an infectious cause to her clinical presentation. The possibilities that were considered included non-pulmonary or disseminated tuberculosis. A lung biopsy was recommended as a method to establish such a diagnosis but apparently was refused by Ms. Warren. Other possibilities that her treating doctor considered at that time included disseminated fungal infection. The possibility of this condition was addressed in treatment with high dose, long term antifungals in the form of Fluconazole. Other possibilities considered included atypical Zoonosis and atypical manifestation of CMV (cytomegalovirus). Although Mrs. Warren tested positive for both IgG and IgM titers, suggesting the possibility of a convalescent stage for cytomegalovirus, her IgM titers were not elevated enough to make this a likely possibility. I would note that serum and urine protein electrophoresis studies were also performed and revealed no evidence of malignancy. Ultimately, her treating doctors concluded that her pulmonary infiltrates might, indeed, have been secondary to a chemical pneumonitis from aspiration related to a procedure such as an esophagogastroduodenoscopy.

Connective tissue work up was done, all of which was negative. She was felt to have a hemolytic anemia secondary to infection or medication. At the time of discharge on 5/1/97, Mrs. Warren continued to spike fevers to 102 degrees while maintaining a leukocytosis of approximately 20,000 with 90% polymorphonuclear leukocytes and a left shift, including 15-20 band. Mrs. Warren apparently expressed her wishes.... "to return home and continue any further work up of this syndrome as an outpatient." The procedures that were not performed but were recommended to be considered in the future include a lumbar puncture, pleural biopsy and perhaps, a repeat analysis of her pleural effusion.

Mrs. Warren was apparently re-admitted to the Lincoln Medical Center on 5/4/97, presenting with continued fevers and shortness of breath. At the time of her admission, she was described as over-weight but in no acute distress. She had a 2/6 systolic ejection murmur without associated gallop. Lungs were noted to have diffuse crackles half-way up and were dull at the bases. She had 1+ edema bilaterally in the lower extremities. She was started on anti-fungal, Diflucan, as well as, an antibiotic, Doxycycline for presumptive infection. An echocardiogram and transesophageal echocardiography were ordered to rule out endocarditis. A cardiothoracic surgery consult was requested to evaluate for pleural biopsy to rule out granulomatous disease. The echocardiogram revealed impending tamponade. Cardiology was asked to see this patient.

She apparently collapsed in the latter part of the day at approximately 6 p.m. on 5/5/97 en-route to the bathroom. When the cardiology service arrived, she was tachycardic, tachypneic and cyanotic and was bagged with 100% oxygen. She was transferred immediately to the CCU for bedside pericardiocentesis. On arrival to the CCU she apparently became unresponsive, pulseless and cyanotic. Her cardiac rhythm was noted to be electromechanical dissociation (EMD) and an ACLS (Advanced Cardiac Life Support) protocol was initiated. Emergent pericardiocentesis was performed with removal of approximately 100 ccs of serosanguineous fluid being removed from the pericardial space. A second pericardiocentesis was performed later that night and drew off 280 ccs of fluid, concurrent with an increase in her systolic blood pressure from the 70s to 110. Following the second procedure, Mrs. Warren apparently had some seizure activity and went into status epilepticus (examiner's note: generally defined as a seizure lasting longer than 30 minutes). She was treated with IV Ativan and Dilantin. It was at this point that an apparent diagnosis of anoxic brain injury was made. Based on available records, the patient's anoxic event occurred following the pericardiocentesis and associated with her cardiac arrest and presumed lack during this time of adequate cerebral perfusion. She was apparently noted to have been "down" without adequate cerebral perfusion for about 6 minutes.

After her seizures were controlled and she was neurologically stabilized, there was not noted to be any change in her neurological status. She developed acute renal failure which was felt to probably be secondary to low perfusion injury from her cardiac arrest resulting in acute tubular necrosis. Due to her renal complications, she was placed on dialysis. She also developed secondary elevations in her liver transaminase levels which were also felt to be related to anoxic/hypoxic-ischemic perfusion injury. Although the feeling was that her overall presentation was consistent with a bacterial infection, no positive cultures could be established. She had no re-accumulation of her pericardial effusion. She subsequently completed a full course of multi-antibiotic therapy. Sputum cultures did grow out positive for Klebsiella pneumoniae. Due to respiratory failure, Mrs. Warren required being placed on a ventilator. No cardiothoracic procedures were performed due to the patient's neurologic status and the families desire to hold off on surgery, given her overall neurological condition.

Follow up electroencephalogram performed later during her hospitalization at the Lincoln Medical Center noted in the conclusion that she had sustained a severe anoxic brain injury with severe cortical anoxic damage and very poor prognosis for recovery. Neurologically, she remained relatively stable. Myoclonic jerks were noted, consistent with her diagnosis of anoxic brain injury. A Tussio catheter was placed on 5/22/97 for hemodialysis. A subsequent percutaneous tracheostomy, as well as, gastrostomy tube were placed prior to her discharge on 6/1/97. At that time, she was discharged to Alliance Health Care, subacute unit.

She was apparently hospitalized at the Alliance skilled nursing facility from 6/1/97 through 9/19/97. Based on available documentation, it appears that she remained in a vegetative state. Based on the information garnered elsewhere, it appears that during her hospitalization at the subacute facility, she remained on renal dialysis until it was discontinued some time in July when her kidneys started to apparently function again. Venous access was apparently maintained, due to the historical difficulties in intravenous accessibility. Due to medical complications, Mrs. Warren was transferred to Terrace Medical Center on 8/22/97 for fevers where she was diagnosed with sepsis and acute pyrexia in the emergency room. She was apparently sent back to the nursing home on that day and then readmitted on 8/26/97 in septic shock to the same institution. She was discharged again on 9/4/97 after being medically stabilized.

On 9/12/97, the examinee was apparently admitted to Terrace Medical Center after she "sat up in bed, had tremors, and her eyes rolled back into her head." She was diagnosed with apparently seizure activity and apparently not admitted to the hospital for this, but was just seen in the emergency room and released.

Following her discharge from Alliance skilled nursing facility in September, she was admitted to Valencia Hospital in Garden Springs, Florida, on 9/19/97. At this facility, non-successful attempts were made to wean her off her respirator. I am not sure I have all the notes from this facility as everything is computer generated and I have no written notes or orders for review. She did have problems due to multiple loose teeth and tongue biting, per available documentation.

Mrs. Warren was subsequently transferred to Windsor Rehabilitation facility in Weston, Virginia on 12/12/97. She stayed at this institution through 5/28/98 at which time she was apparently discharged to her home in Florida to her husband's care. There are very scanty notes from this institution. I am not sure if the chart is incomplete. Based on review of the available notes, it appears that Mrs. Warren remained vegetative during this hospitalization. Interestingly, a chest x-ray done on 5/19/98 was unremarkable without any active evidence of pleural or parenchymal change from 12/13/97. During this hospitalization, she was weaned from her ventilator.

Since returning home to her husband's care in May of 1998, she has been relatively medically stable. I would note that based upon review of available records, she has undergone a bone densitometry study in 3/00 which showed apparent normal bone density in the lumbar spine with osteopenia of the femoral neck. Thyroid function testing including TSH was within normal limits in August of '99, as was an endocrine work up including LH (leuteining hormone) and FSH (follicles stimulating hormone). This work up was apparently done due to the fact that Mrs. Warren has not had any menstrual periods in 2 years.

There were apparently efforts made in the latter part of 2000 to get Mrs. Warren admitted into Bradley Rehab in June of 2000, but this was apparently denied by the insurance carrier. Mrs. Warren subsequently incurred a left leg femur fracture just above the knee from a fall during a transfer. This was apparently incurred during a commode transfer that Mr. Warren was doing with his wife.

Efforts were made since her discharge home to decannulate her. However, this has been unsuccessful, although her tracheostomy has been downsized and she is now apparently using it most of the time in a "capped" manner. There is also a notation in the history of hyperparathyroidism but with apparently normal calcium and phosphorus levels, based on available laboratory data (although she did suffer from hypercalcemia later in her post-injury course).

In October of 2000, she apparently had a broken G-tube and underwent replacement for it at the time this was done on 10/6/00. There were no apparent complications. G-tube replacement was also performed on 5/3/00.

Records of Dr. Alexander Scully were also reviewed. These document care provided by the family practitioner during the year of 1998. I would note that on review of laboratory testing, I noted that her triglyceride level was 235 with normal being less than 200. As of the date of assessment, 9/98, I would also note that glucose level was very low at 27. There is also documentation in Dr. Scully's records relative to an article entitled, "The Physiological Response to the Procedure of Masking." This technique apparently involved increased carbon monoxide exposure in the air administered to the patient in question without exposing the individual to hypoxic conditions. This technique has apparently been used predominately in children, as per the protocol described.

Mrs. Warren did apparently undergo a mammogram which was normal with the exception of what was probably a small benign lymph node in the right breast in September of 1998.

Records of Dr. Richard Grant were also reviewed, dating from 1997 to 1998. These records document late 1997 dental extractions. Dr. Grant appears to have been the attending physician at Windsor Rehabilitation and Health Care Center. Based on his report of 12/97 to Dr. Hooper, Dr. Grant felt that Mrs. Warren had sustained hypoxic encephalopathy related to cardiac arrest after pericardiocentesis. Based on his neurologic exam, the patient was most likely in a vegetative state at that time. Based on the discharge summary from Windsor, it appears that during her hospitalization at that institution, she developed hypercalcemia when her calcitonin was discontinued, as related to her apparent diagnosis of hyperparathyroidism. Calcitonin was reinstated and her serum Calcium came down to "reasonably minimally elevated levels."

Records from Dr. Jordan Mullens were also reviewed. These records were limited to an evaluation conducted on 2/22/99. Of note is the fact that he felt that Mrs. Warren was at a Rancho Los Amigos level of II when he examined her, yet for some reason in his diagnostic impression/assessment, he noted that she was "low functioning, Rancho Los Amigos level II/III." Among other assessments, he also noted that she had muscle and joint contractures. In his plan, Dr. Mullens felt that Mrs. Warren would be a good candidate for the response enhancement program on the inpatient service and then went on to detail areas that needed to be addressed during such a hospitalization. He noted that the estimated length of stay would be 10 days for the evaluation.

In September of 1999, Mrs. Warren underwent an evaluation by Dr. Stewart Kaplan. This was a limited assessment with the only diagnostic impression being "status post encephalopathy." A PET-scan was ordered to "ascertain the functional part of her brain." A PET-scan demonstrated "unusual FDG PET that shows global hypometabolism in the cerebral cortex with the most intense area of activity center primarily in the brain stem. This study was performed at Union Hospital. In 10/99, Mrs. Warren underwent extraction of all her remaining teeth by Dr. Grant.

I would note that there is also a letter in the records from Dr. Daniel Arzbecker from the State University, Department of Neurological Surgery regarding their research protocol on "Study of Neuronal Cell Implantation for the Treatment of Stroke." I do not have adequate records to know whether this was pursued.

**<u>CURRENT EQUIPMENT:</u>**

1. Single hospital bed, manual crank bed with bilateral non-split rails. The rails run the length of the bed.

2. Rotating transfer disk.

3. InvaCare Jeri-chair with tilt feature, but no recline feature; back tilts to 30 degrees; foot rests elevate 90 degrees to 180 degrees

4. Kangaroo pump; on IV pole; used intermittently for feedings

5. InvaCare pneumatic lift

6. Electric suction machine used p.r.n.

7. Lasko humidifier

8. Air cleaner with Ionizer-Holmes brand

9. InvaCare 9000-XT wheelchair with recline but no tilt feature, solid wheels without rims and elevating foot rests with a gel cushion, as well as, an InvaCare head rest

10. Mat in adjacent room for range of motion and "patterning"

11. Bilateral wrist finger orthoses - Helix Plus extended with thumb abductor feature

12. Bilateral Multipodus boots

**ARCHITECTURAL ISSUES:**

The residence that Mrs. Warren resides in with her husband is a modest home in a residential neighborhood. The only access she uses is the front door. At this entrance, there is a small 5" step going up to a landing of about 4 by 6 and then a 1' step into the front door. There is no ramping currently to the front entrance. The home is not wheelchair accessible nor are the doorways going from her bedroom to the adjoining bathroom.

Per Mr. Warren, his wife spends most her time in her bedroom, which is approximately 13 by 15 feet. There is an adjoining bathroom which is not wheelchair accessible. The toilet is not raised but has elevated support bars bilaterally. He has to transfer her into the bathroom to use the toilet. There is also a walk-in shower in the bathroom which is approximately 2 1/2 feet by 5 feet with a step-up of approximately 6".

**PERSONS PRESENT DURING EVALUATION:**

1. James Coolidge, Esq. - plaintiff's attorney
2. Gregory Stanish, Esq. - Attorney representing retaining firm
3. Mark Pye, MSH, CRC, CDMS, CCM, Disability Analyst
4. Jack Warren

**EXAMINER'S NOTE:**

This examiner would note that the entire assessment, aside from the time spent looking at architectural issues and accessibility was videotaped by the legal representative of Mrs. Warren, Mr. Coolidge. Additionally, for the record, I had requested an opportunity to interview Mr. Warren related to my normal IME methodology of attempting to acquire as much information as possible from corroboratory sources. This request, however, was denied by the attorneys representing Mrs. Warren.

I would also note that on my entry into the Warren home, Mr. Warren was apparently taken somewhat by surprise when I introduced myself as Dr. Zasler, he shared with me that he had wanted to contact me to get my input regarding his wife's status, given my affiliation with the Brain Injury Clinic and my knowledge in this area of brain injury care but had, instead, contacted Dr. Gene Foley.

## FAMILY HISTORY:

Positive for cancer in father.

## ALLERGIES:

Allergic to Tetracycline with sequela of venous sclerosis. Sensitive versus allergy to Biaxin with nausea and vomiting.

## MEDICATIONS:

Based upon available information garnered from Dr. King's evaluation, the Mrs. Warren was on the following medications at the time of his evaluation in 10/00:

1. Baclofen 10 milligrams 1 p.o. three times a day

As per Mr. Schweighart's office, the examinee is currently on:

1) Calcet (dose unspecified)
2) Zantac (dose unspecified)
3) Calcium supplement
4) Liquid lortab for pain

## PAST MEDICAL HISTORY:

1. Status post surgery in 1992 involving left L5-S1 hemilaminectomy and diskectomy under microscopic control and diagnosis of L5-S1 herniated disk on the left side with left S1 hyperesthesia and radiculopathy.

## SOCIAL HISTORY:

Based on available information, Ms. Warren was neither a smoker nor a drinker. There is no history of illicit drug use. She works in a local book store. She was married without children.

## PHYSICAL EXAMINATION:

**General:** The patient is arousable/alert but not aware. She demonstrates decerebrate posturing spontaneously with positive spontaneous bruxing and snout reflex.

**Skin:** Slight excoriation, bilateral undersides of breasts; lumbar scar from prior back surgery; and bilateral groin irritation without breakdown. No evidence, whatsoever, of skin breakdown or maceration/excoriation in the buttocks or perineal area. No skin problems otherwise noted.

**HEENT:** Normocephalic, atraumatic. Edentulous. TMs are well visualized with clear ear canals. Nasal mucosa are well hydrated. I did not visualize the examinee's mouth well due to clinching and strong bite reflex. Examination reveals head forward posture with increased cervical tone. There was no palpable thyromegaly, lymphadenopathy or observable jugular venous distention. The examinee was noted to have a capped, #4, cuffless, Shiley tracheostomy in place.

**Lung Examination** revealed scattered bronchi with decreased breath sounds, left lower lobe and decreased inspiratory "effort."

**Cardiovascular Examination** reveals regular rate and rhythm without audible murmur, rubs, or gallops. There were no bruits noted (carotid, temporal, ocular or mastoid).

**Abdominal Examination** reveals bowel sounds to be hyperactive. There was a vertical scar, transabdominally, presumptively related to prior laparotomy. No palpable hepatosplenomegaly or masses. In the left upper quadrant, a gastrostomy tube "button" was in place.

**Extremity Examination** revealed on passive range of motion testing of the right upper extremity shoulder abduction 90 degrees and flexion 120 degrees. Elbow range of motion, functional with both extension and flexion (the latter with increased triceps tone noted). Wrists and fingers with increased flexor tone but without gross contracture. In the left upper extremity, shoulder abduction was approximately 130 degrees and flexion was approximately 150 degrees. Elbow range of motion was functional with less triceps tone than on the right side. Wrist and fingers demonstrated increased flexor tone without gross contracture. Lower extremity exam revealed left tibial external rotation posturing. Hip range of motion was full with increased adductor tone noted. Knee range of motion was full. Ankle to approximately 90 degrees without significant toe range of motion restrictions or contractures. In the right lower extremity, hip range of motion was functional with increased adductor tone. Knee range of motion was functional with positive patellar crepitation noted on passive range of motion. Ankle range of motion to 90 degrees in dorsiflexion. Toe range of motion is intact passively without evidence of contracture. Finger and toenails are all well trimmed without evidence of significant pathology otherwise noted.

**Neurological Examination** revealed **cranial nerve** assessment to be limited by patient's neurological state of function. A strong bite reflex was noted which made it impossible for this examiner to evaluate gag reflex. The examinee blinked to finger snap and demonstrated a generalized response to loud clap. No visual or auditory tracking was noted. Pupils were slightly reactive to light with questionable bilateral cataracts. Fundi were poorly visualized. Left gaze preference was noted. No response to visual threat or any visual stimulus in either hemifield. Examinee demonstrated bilateral corneal reflexes and positive doll's eyes. **Deep tendon reflexes** exam revealed generalized hyperreflexia with bilateral extensor plantar responses with associated bilateral ankle clonus. Positive crossed adductor responses were noted. On assessment of pathologic reflexes, the examinee demonstrated bilateral Babinski's, Chaddock's and Stransky reflexes, as well as, bilateral Tromner's, Hoffmann's, and palmomental reflexes. Additionally, positive snout and jaw jerk were elicited with an equivocal glabellar reflex. **Sensory examination** revealed no sustained orienting response to any stimuli including visual, auditory or olfactory. No vocalization was noted, although the examinee did make sounds intermittently; e.g. vocalized (albeit no verbalizations). On sensory stimulation, including nociceptive stimulation, withdrawal was noted in the arms and legs without evidence of localization anywhere else on the body including chest and abdomen, bilaterally, as well as, ears and extremities, bilaterally. The examinee alerted/aroused slightly to sternal rub. **Cerebellar examination** demonstrated no spontaneous nystagmus. **Motor examination** revealed spastic quadriparesis without spontaneous movement that could be interpreted to be volitional in nature. **Mental Status Examination:** There was no command following. The examinee was asked to stick out her tongue by verbal commands, as well as, move each extremity by verbal commands without response. I also placed a mirror in front of her and tracked it across both hemifields without any visual orienting response noted.

**<u>OBSERVATION OF MR. WARREN WITH HIS WIFE:</u>**

After a long discussion, there was final agreement to allow me to observe Mr. Warren interact with his wife in an attempt to elicit behavior. I specifically requested that he try and interact with her in a way that demonstrated responses that he thought were consistent with awareness and/or volitional behavior on her part. Based on my observations, which were also recorded on videotape by a legal representative of the examinee, there was no command following observed. It appears that tactile triggers, such as touching her forehead, prompted reflexive responses that are being misinterpreted as "volitional responses." I saw nothing during the time that Mr. Warren interacted with his wife that would suggest that he was eliciting any type of awareness and/or volitional cognitive, behavioral or motor responses.

## OTHER ASSESSMENTS:

1. **Functional Independence Measure**

   All scores were noted to be 1 (e.g., total assist).

2. **Disability Rating Scale (DRS)**

   0,4,2,3,3,3,5,3 = 23. This score is consistent with a disability category of vegetative state.

3. **Rancho Los Amigos Cognitive Behavioral Rating Scale - II**

   This score is consistent with a vegetative state level of function.

## MMI (MAXIMAL MEDICAL IMPROVEMENT):

Based on the examinee's time post injury, it is this examiner's opinion with a degree of medical probability, that she has reached neurologic MMI, as well as functional MMI due to the fact that she can be stated, based upon current diagnostic and prognostic criteria, to be in a "permanent" or chronic vegetative state secondary to her initial hypoxic ischemic insult to the brain. Based on the 1994 physician paper published in the "New England Journal of Medicine," by the Multi-Society Task Force, permanency can be established at three months, post insult, for hypoxic ischemic brain injury.

Given her time post insult, and the current accepted diagnostic criteria for "permanency," following hypoxic ischemic brain insult, Mrs. Warren has reached MMI (maximal medical improvement). MMI is defined by the Guides for Evaluation of Permanent Impairment published by the AMA (5th Edition) as that point in time at which an individual's total body impairment can be stated to be likely not to change more than 3% over the ensuing year. I would also note here that the issue of permanency remains debatable. This examiner has some reservations on the use of the term "permanent" given the fact that there are several reported cases in the literature where individuals following traumatic brain injury or hypoxic ischemic brain injury have emerged from otherwise "permanent" states of unconscious after the so-called cut-off period; e.g. 1 year after trauma and 3 months after hypoxic ischemic insult. This terminology remains somewhat in debate and this fact must be acknowledged in the context of any responsible discussion of Mrs. Warren's condition. Nonetheless, the general consensus opinion in the neuroscience community is that any aggressive medical and/or rehabilitative efforts in an individual who is otherwise in a permanent vegetative state, would be medically futile. As per various physician papers, assignment of a "DNR (Do Not Resuscitate)" order should be considered, both by family and treating clinicians, in such a context.

## APPORTIONMENT AND CAUSALITY:

This is a very complex case as related to the medical course pre-dating her acquired brain injury. I will defer the etiology of her cardiac tamponade to those appropriately qualified to make this determination. Clearly, the examinee's hypoxic ischemic brain injury resulted from her cardiac arrest which was secondary to her cardiac tamponade. Her current permanent vegetative state is 100% apportionable to the sequela of her hypoxic ischemic brain injury, based upon information available to this examiner at the time of this report.

## RESTRICTIONS AND RISKS:

Mrs. Warren is at increased risk for a variety of morbidity conditions associated with relative immobility including skin breakdown, pneumonia, and urinary tract infections. Other potential complications include contractures, GI complications, cardiopulmonary compromise and peripheral vascular morbidity associated with venous thrombosis, although the latter is very uncommon in the chronic phase of care in these types of patients in my experience.

Given the kind of care that she has been receiving, her morbidity risk is significantly decreased, based on not only the high attention level that her husband provides to her daily care but also the fact that he regularly mobilizes his wife. Based on this clinician's experience, such mobilization is a significant positive factor in decreasing long-term medical morbidity associated with any low level neurologic state.

## LIFE EXPECTANCY PROGNOSTICATION:

Based on my assessment of Mrs. Warren and review of the available records, I would note the following with regard to her life expectancy prognostication. Firstly, Mrs. Warren has multiple ongoing risk factors for medical morbidity and mortality. Nonetheless, she has remained more medically stable with time than less medically stable which, in and of itself, is a positive prognostic indicator for a longer than shorter life expectancy. Given her current level of neurological functioning, she remains at risk for recurrent infections including pneumonia and urinary tract infections. These types of infections, as well as, other complications such as skin infections due to pressure sores, seizures and aspiration risk, can lead to complications in and of themselves, as well as, secondary complications such as systemic bacteremia (e.g. sepsis). Mrs. Warren also remains at risk for progression of contractures due to her hypertonicity. Such contractures can further limit mobility and increase risk for skin breakdown and associated complications. Certain risk factors such as the presence or absence of a protective cough and gag reflex were unable to be fully evaluated due to the patient's strong bite reflex.

Mr. Warren seems to be providing a very high level of attention to his wife's maintenance care, a level which would be hard to duplicate in most care settings in this examiner's experience. Clearly, the level of care and attention being provided is a significant prophylactic in and of itself to potential consequential medical morbidity. If such care were to continued, it certainly would seem to provide a further argument for endorsing a longer than shorter life expectancy. If all current morbidity risk factors were optimally addressed, realizing that no risk factors can be negated fully by even the best of care, it is this examiner's opinion that Mrs. Warren's life expectancy would be anticipated to be 10-15 years from now with the understanding that actuarial norms for a black female at the time she was injured need to be used to predict her life expectancy had it not been for her acquired brain injury. Any determination of life expectancy must consider any other medical morbidity that may have shortened her projected actuarially based life expectancy. This examiner makes the aforementioned probability predictions and statements:

1) Having been involved with national and international guideline development in the area of vegetative state and minimally consciousness state assessment and management.

2) Being familiar with the literature relating to life expectancy in persons with severe neurologic impairment due to acquired brain injury.

3) Having examined and followed well over 300 vegetative and minimally conscious patients over the last 16 years.

It is also this examiner's opinion that life expectancy determinations are best made on an individual basis. There is some data on life expectancy determination in severely disabled persons following acquired brain injury as well as other conditions; e.g. developmental disabilities where the major common factor is severe immobility as the major morbidity/mortality factor in this group of patients. The literature on vegetative state patient life expectancy must be interpreted cautiously due to methodological concerns and small sample size issues. The most current, widely accepted treatise on this topic was published in the New England Journal of Medicine in 1994 and authored by the Multi-Society Task Force on the vegetative state. In that document, the consensus panel concluded that the average life expectancy for a patient in a vegetative state was 3-5 years and that a life expectancy beyond 10 years was rare. There is also a significant amount of population-based literature on life expectancy in severely disabled, immobile patients that demonstrates an overall trend to early demise in these individuals; the work by Eyman et al is probably the most well quoted in this area.

There is no literature that this examiner is aware of that has prospectively examined, in a methodologically sound fashion, specific morbidity risk factors and/or quality of care after severe brain injury in either vegetative or minimally conscious individuals as related to acquired brain injury. There have been several recent papers, one published in the "Archives of Physical Medicine and Rehabilitation" and the other, published in the journal, "Brain Injury," dealing with life expectancy issues after severe TBI. Certainly, one can draw some parallels with population-based studies when trying to assess particular individual's life expectancies such as Mrs. Warren. However, use of population-based studies as the only means to determine one specific person's life expectancy is, in this examiner's opinion, faulty logic. Such a practice goes against appropriate use of population-based prognostic data in this examiner's extensive clinical experience in this area. Therefore, one must delineate person-specific risk factors and historical events of significance to arrive at a medically probable life expectancy.

This examiner has not included any decrease in life expectancy related to pre-injury medical conditions which, at the time of this report, are still somewhat of a puzzlement to this clinician due to the fact that the examinee's complex pre-ABI history is outside the domain of my expertise. If she persists with any chronic condition that increases her morbidity and/or mortality risks, this will need to be determined by a clinician so trained and qualified to make such a determination.

It is important to recognize that appropriately conducted life expectancy determination in a case such as Mrs. Warren's involves examining historical records for past and current risk factors for medical morbidity as well as prior infections and complications documented post-injury and for that matter, pre-injury as relevant. Risk factors for medical morbidity such as immobility, recurrent pulmonary or urinary tract infections and/or poorly controlled epilepsy and/or spasticity all have the potential to decrease life expectancy in and of themselves as related to their correlation with morbidity and therefore mortality.

Another factor to analyze is the temporal relationship of illness to injury. That is, the examinee who remains more stable over time than less stable, tends to live longer than shorter. The examinee who seems to get worse over time and less medically stable tends to live a shorter life than a longer one. Given the relative stability of Mrs. Warren's medical condition over the last two years, even considering her compromised neurological and functional status, one would have to conclude that her chance of living longer was higher than had she been persistently medically unstable and in and out of the hospital over the referenced period of time. Clinical observations have clearly demonstrated that the duration of survival in a person in a vegetative state or, for that matter, minimally conscious state, seems to be positively correlated with longer life span; that is, the longer one lives, the longer one lives. The fact that Mrs. Warren is approaching 3 years post injury with the latter half of these 3 years demonstrating a fairly solid level of medical stability. Based on available information, one would have to conclude that her chance of living longer was fairly high and certainly her chance of living longer than the anticipated average of 3-5 years predicted by the Multi-Society Task Force seems a strong probability (aside from the fact that there are methodologic concerns with the MSTF mean life expectancy determination).

An additional fact is that the apparent aggressiveness that Mr. Warren is taking with regard to his wife's care, particularly with regard to her mobilization. A recent study published by Strauss, et. al., in "Archives of Physical Medicine and Rehabilitation" in 1998, expounded on the benefits of mobilizing patients relative to the impact on life expectancy.

## **PAIN AND SUFFERING:**

It is important to acknowledge that based on exam and the diagnostic conclusion that Mrs. Warren is in a "chronic" or "permanent" vegetative state, it can be stated with a degree of medical probability that she does not consciously appreciate pain, nor does she suffer as a result of her current condition. Clearly, as with any individual in a vegetative state, there is always a question of observed response to painful stimuli and their implications on conscious pain experiences. It is important for all involved parties to understand that even patients in vegetative states respond to pain but that these responses which may include limb withdrawal, sweating, tachycardia and even primitive motor responses may occur but do so at a subcortical level without conscious awareness. Additionally, based on our understanding of vegetative state, Mrs. Warren does not, in all medical probability, have any appreciation for any aspect of her condition and/or predicament. Inherent in this absence of awareness is the inherent implication that she is not able to suffer from an emotional standpoint due to her own lack of internal perception and/or awareness of her condition.

## VOCATIONAL PROGNOSIS:

Clearly, Mrs. Warren is totally and permanently disabled from any type of employment, competitive or otherwise, as a result of her May 1997 hypoxic ischemic brain insult.

## FUTURE CARE NEEDS:

As an examiner who is also a practicing clinician who has been involved in both national and international efforts and guideline development for assessment and care of persons in a vegetative, as well as minimal conscious state, I would recommend that as with any other examinee who is vegetative that Mrs. Warren's care be structured in accordance with the recommendations made by the Dordt work group, as published in the "Journal of Head Trauma Rehabilitation" (article enclosed).

## COMMENTS REGARDING LIFE CARE PLAN OF DR. COLIN KING:

This report is an extremely comprehensive report, including extensive record review and accompanying documentation including a life care plan. I would note the following regarding the report:

1. Dr. King, the examiner, had an opportunity to interview Mr. Warren.

2. The following are subcategorizations of where opinions were provided. Generic IME with diagnostic impressions (albeit no impression that the examinee was in a vegetative state), vocational position statement, AMA Impairment Rating, "Functional Impairment Rating," continuation of care summary report, photographs and documentation.

3. Dr. King's impairment rating demonstrates an unfamiliarity with the use of the *Guides to Evaluation of Permanent Impairment,* published by the AMA, either 4th or 5th Edition. Given the examinee's/patient's vegetative state, it would be much easier and certainly more logical to rate her using Chapter 13, section 3A (Disturbances in levels of consciousness and/or awareness), where she would receive a 90% impairment rating based on being in a chronic or permanent vegetative state and requiring total support). I would note that his rating of her station and gait is inaccurate, as she cannot rise to a standing position and maintain it with difficulty on her own, and therefore would actually fall, if one was even using this criteria to rate impairment, in Class 4, which gives an impairment rating of the whole person of 40-60%. The impairment rating for

respiration really is irrelevant in the context of rating someone in a chronic/persistent vegetative state, as is the use of upper extremities, given the existing ratings for consciousness and awareness. One could certainly add sexual functioning; however, it would seem to be implicit, although there are no specific directions in the Guides to note this. Other areas rated would also seemingly be subsumed under the recommended category of 13A for rating this examinee including aphasia, mental status impairment and emotional disturbances. Additionally, and maybe most importantly, as noted by Dr. King, on the last paragraph of page 4, the largest value or greatest percentage of the seven categories of impairment is used to represent the impairment of all types." In this case, he should have certainly utilized the altered awareness and/or "disturbances in level of consciousness and/or awareness" e.g. table 13-2, on page 309, in the 5th Edition of the Guides.

4. There is no scientific methodology to justify the science, evidence based or otherwise, to support the manner in which Dr. King calculated Mrs. Warren's "permanent functional impairment." The methodology used has no basis aside from a list of diagnostic impressions. It seems to this examiner that what Dr. King is really defining is the degree of disability that Mrs. Warren has sustained as a result of her hypoxic ischemic brain injury. My greater concern is the use of a percentage to express her degree of disability rather than simply saying that she is totally and permanently disabled as the result of her acquired brain injury. Once again, there is no scientific methodology to justify a percent disability rating and/or percent "functional impairment rating," whether specific to this case or not. Additionally, neither proposed rating would meet Daubert criteria from a medicolegal standard.

5. Life Care Plan Comments

   a. The medical follow up is excessive, as the examinee, by my evaluation, has no current needs for neurosurgical, neurological, neuro-ophthalmological, ENT or infectious disease follow up at the current time. It cannot be stated, with a degree of medical probability, that she will require such services in the future. It is not unreasonable to have a certain number of orthopedic evaluations calculated into the life care plan, however, I think that an up-front conclusion that she will require a one time per year orthopedic evaluation for the rest of her life is unreasonable. GI follow up, given continued PEG feedings is reasonable on a once a year basis with some prn visits calculated in over her lifetime, as is follow up for her tracheostomy and pulmonary problems which can be done either by a pulmonologist or a good family practitioner. Regular medical care which typically occurs on a one time per year frequency for general medical maintenance, should not be calculated into the life care plan. Urological follow up in a patient who is not otherwise having urological complications and who is in a vegetative state is certainly reasonable, on a one time per year basis. In an otherwise vegetative patient/examinee, who is not having any significant morbidity, physiatric follow up at 4 times per year would seem excessive. Reasonable follow up would be 2x/per year given the examinee's historical medical stability and the current level of care being provided.

b. There is no medical justification for any of the tests noted on page 3 of the life care plan at this point in time, given the patient's history and current neurological status. With regard to the tests on page 4, there is no justification or rationale for an MRI of the hips. Urological follow up should include a yearly KUB and probably renal ultrasound; however, an IVP does not need to be done yearly in someone who is otherwise medically stable. From a urological standpoint, it can be done every 3-5 years in a patient with the examinee's degree of immobility. X-rays are not unreasonable if there is progression of functional/neuromuscular scoliosis; however, at the current time, there is no evidence that this is the case and stating that such x-rays are necessary one time per year for life is unreasonable and not supported by either medical experience or literature. Urinalysis should be conducted at the time of general medical follow up, based upon need, not based upon frequency, set at two times per year, in an otherwise urologically/medically stable patient/examinee. There is no justification for the frequency of laboratory studies being recommended on page 5 including anticonvulsant levels, which need only be checked one time per year, assuming the patient is otherwise medically stable and not having seizures. General laboratory tests should be checked one time per year unless there is some indication otherwise to do so more frequently… which, at the current time, this examiner cannot justify. I would note, however, that based on available information, Mrs. Warren is not on any seizure medicine and the likelihood that she will need to take this is certainly not able to be stated with a degree of medical probability.

c. The medical procedures on pages 6-7 are all stated as "possible procedures" and should not therefore be included as costs in the life care plan, aside from the fact that their likelihood is low. As an example of this, the likelihood of Mrs. Warren developing hydrocehalus or complications thereof is pretty much nil given the mechanism of her brain injury, her time post injury and the absence of any evidence that she has had a hydrocephalic disorder. At the current time, there is no evidence that there is any potential benefit to be derived from either ocular or contracture surgery. Additionally, there is no evidence to suggest Mrs. Warren is having significant cardiopulmonary compromise from neuromuscular scoliosis to even justify in an otherwise vegetative-state patient surgery for neuromuscular scoliosis.

d. With regard to housing, it is this examiner's opinion that the current house is not appropriate architecturally for Mrs. Warren and that a wheelchair accessible home and/or architectural modifications to make the current residence as wheelchair accessible as possible would be medically and rehabilitatively appropriate if the examinee is to continue to be cared for by her husband and/or ancillary staff in the home environment.

e. With regard to medications, it is this examiner's opinion that additional medications may want to be considered as being more likely than not, medically appropriate for Mrs. Warren, including potentially, higher doses of Baclofen, as well as a stool softener and/or rectal suppository.

There are discrepancies in Dr. King's reporting of medications relative to present reported drug regimen as per the retaining party's office which need to be clarified. Medications for hyperparathyroidism are unrelated to the injury and would not be compensable.

f. Although I have no problem with a re-evaluation by physical therapy or occupational therapy one time per year, I see no medical justification for yearly speech/cognitive re-evaluation, unless there is some, albeit unexpected, change in her status (which is not medically anticipated with a degree of probability). Outpatient therapy 5 hours per week, 50 weeks per year, as recommended on pages 8 and 9, is not medically indicated and suggests a poor understanding on the part of the physician making these recommendations of current accepted treatment standards for an individual in a chronic/permanent vegetative state. I do agree, however, with the treatment recommendations for family counseling which are reasonable, and could benefit Mr. Warren and/or other involved family members.

g. It would be my recommendation that if Mrs. Warren is to be cared for at home, that she should have trained aide care, not necessarily CNA level care, although the latter would certainly be acceptable. Her current care would be considered custodial and the level of training necessary for taking care of an individual in such as state could be provided by trained lay persons in a much more cost-effective manner than care rendered by licensed personnel. Clearly, as state regulations require, certain types of activities will need to be done by skilled/licensed personnel such as tracheostomy changes or G-tube changes, if not also medication administration which might also be performed by Mr. Warren, as he so desires to be involved, once additional ancillary care might be provided.

h. Depending upon who was normally doing housekeeping prior to Mrs. Warren's acquired brain injury, provision of a housekeeper may be reasonable; however, the current recommended hours of 4 per day certainly seems excessive for a house as small as the Warren's and one that is as sparsely furnished.

i. The recommended equipment for activities of daily living are all unreasonable in an otherwise vegetative state patient.

j. Certainly adaptive equipment for bathing and mobility need to be considered and the recommendations made seem reasonable, as do the replacement rates. I am not sure why so many different bathing/toileting DME items are required, however (as noted on page 12).

k. I have no problem with the recommendations for an electric hospital bed, Hoyer lift, feeding pump or reclinable Geri-chair; however, the Geri-chair may be duplicative if the examinee has an appropriate tilt-and-recline wheelchair. The rehabilitation equipment recommended is not medically necessary or indicated, given the patient's chronic/permanent vegetative state.

l. I have no problems with the recommendations made on page 14.

m. I have no problems with the recommendations made on page 15.

n. With regard to the Model 2 life care plan, which denotes care in an extended care facility, I would note that for an otherwise vegetative state individual, the rate being quoted seems to be excessive, given my own knowledge of national rates for these types of facilities. It is unclear what other comparisons were done to establish whether the rate of $450 per day is reasonable, as the only facility quoted was the Florida Institute for Neurologic Rehabilitation.

   I took the liberty of calling the FINER program and was told that they do not even accept patients who are below a Rancho level of IV. Additionally, I contacted a couple of Florida nursing homes and found out that rates normally range from $130/day to $150 per day for in house care of any otherwise vegetative state examinee/patient.

o. All of the therapy services/additionally billed services are not medically indicated and not supported by current neuroscience consensus opinion regarding the long term care of an individual in a vegetative state.

**IMPRESSIONS – Injury-Related:**

1. Status post hypoxic ischemic brain injury 5/5/97 secondary to cardiac arrest as a result of cardiac tamponade.

2. Permanent/chronic vegetative state secondary to #1.

3. Spastic quadriparesis secondary to #1.

4. Limb contractures–secondary to #1 and #2.

5. Bowel and bladder incontinence secondary to #1 and #2.

6. Inadequate support resources for examinee's care in home environment.

7. Major concerns regarding potential for caretaker (e.g., Mr. Warren) to "burnout" due to being primary/sole caretaker for his wife.

8. Functional dependent state secondary to #1 and #2.

9. History of post-anoxic seizures (last in 9/97)–currently no active problem with epilepsy based on available information.

10. History of amenorrhea–likely secondary to #1.

11. History of prolonged ventilatory support (> than 6 months) status post anoxic event of 5/97.

12. Status post left femur fracture secondary to fall during transfer by husband–2000.

13. Status post various early (within first 6 months post insult) hospitalizations for medical complications.

14. Status post tracheostomy–chronic indwelling tracheostomy by history.

15. Status post gastrostomy–now with gastric "button."

16. Status post renal failure due to hypoxic/shock related renal insult requiring long term dialysis.

17. Status post placement of Tussio catheter for #16.

18. Status post bronchoscopy.

**IMPRESSIONS - Non-Injury-Related:**

1. Status post lumbar spine surgery for L5-S1 herniated disc in 1992.

2. Hyperparathyroidism.

3. Hypertriglyceridemia.

4. Complex medical course predating 5/97 hypoxic ischemic brain injury which appears to have been initiated during an EGD procedure.

5. History of gastritis (heliobacter pylori) and duodenal ulcer.

6. Status post diaphragmatic hernia.

## RECOMMENDATIONS:

1. Establish code status if not already done–as per current guidelines, strongly consider DNR.

2. Provision of basic interventions essential to daily care including range of motion exercises (passive), positioning protocols, dietary/nutritional management and modulation of hypertonicity with main treatment endpoint of morbidity prophylaxis.

3. Optional interventions, such as sensory stimulation or pharmacologic trials to enhance potential from emergence from the vegetative state should be considered unjustified in this examinee given the time post injury and lack of any intercurrent issue suggesting that such treatment would have any scientific rationale.

4. Provision of an adequate plan of care as noted and critiqued on pages 17 through 20 of this report.

5. Family education and counseling regarding the examinee's condition and prognosis.

6. Provide Mr. Warren with information regarding withdrawal of care; although I fully suspect that he would not want to pursue such a measure given my perceptions of his level of commitment to his wife and her care. I am unclear, however, as to how much he fully understands her current condition and its associated prognosis and ramifications.

7. Attempt to wean tracheostomy as it is a potential morbidity risk factor–assuming it is not medically necessary, which is unclear based on available information.

8. Nurse case manager 1 to 2 hours per month to oversee medical and custodial care issues.

***NOTE:*** *Any comments on appropriateness of care are professional opinions based upon the specifics of the case and should not be generalized, nor necessarily be considered supportive or critical of the involved providers or disciplines. Any medical recommendations offered are provided as guidance and not as medical orders.* ***I always request that the examinees' treating physician(s) receive a copy of my IME****. I am also willing to discuss my opinions with the examinee's treating doctors with permission from the retaining party. The opinions expressed do not constitute a recommendation that specific claims or administrative action be made or enforced. Medicine is both an art and a science and although an individual may appear to be fit* *for work activity, there is no guarantee that the person will not be re-injured or suffer additional injury. If applicable, employers should follow the processes established in the Americans with Disabilities Act, Title I. The opinions on work capacity are to facilitate job placement and do not necessarily reflect an in-depth direct threat analysis.*

*This independent medical evaluation is based upon the available history provided by the examinee, IME of 2/16/01, and medical record review. This examiner's expertise as a board certified physiatrist, Fellow of the American Academy of Physical Medicine and Rehabilitation, Fellow of the American Academy of Disability Evaluating Physicians, diplomate of the American Academy of Pain Management and certification as an Independent Medical Examiner were also contributory to the opinions generated in this case. I am a physician duly licensed to practice medicine in the state of Virginia. All opinions are based upon a reasonable degree of medical probability unless otherwise stated. If further information is required, please contact the undersigned.*

*The opinions rendered in this case are the opinions of this evaluator based on his training, experience and expertise in the field of physiatry (Physical Medicine and Rehabilitation) - please refer to attached C.V. in Appendix 1. The conclusions of this report are based in part on the assumption that the materials provided for review are true and correct. I declare that the information contained within this document was prepared by this examiner and is true to the best of my knowledge at the time of issuance of this report. If more information becomes available at a later date, opinions are subject to change. I am being reimbursed at a rate of $400/hour for my time in this case as per my contractual agreement, which is also enclosed as an appendix.*

Should there be additional questions, please feel free to call this examiner at (555) 555-1234.

Sincerely,

____________________________________

Nathan D. Zasler, MD

Fellow, American Academy of Physical Medicine and Rehabilitation
Fellow, American Academy of Disability Evaluating Physicians
Diplomate, American Academy of Pain Management
Certified Independent Medical Examiner
Medical Director, Concussion Care Centre of Virginia, Ltd.
Medical Consultant, Pinnacle Rehabilitation, Inc.
Medical Director, Tree of Life, LLC

**Report #8: Workers' Compensation—Lower Back**

This report is most notable for the following.

- It is thorough, yet concise.
- It is well organized.
- The examiner personally reviewed the diagnostic studies.
- The examiner answers the specific questions asked by the client.
- The report is objective and balanced.

While this is an excellent report, all reports can be improved. Areas of possible improvement include the following.

- More identifying and introductory information at the beginning of the report.
- An executive summary at the beginning of the report would have been helpful.
- The medical records reviewed should have been more specifically identified (e.g., by providing the name of the treating provider).
- The examinee should be referred to as "the examinee" and not "the patient."

---

April 19, 2002

Ms. X is a 39-year-old woman referred for evaluation of low back and right lower extremity discomfort.

**HISTORY OF PRESENT INJURY:**

The patient indicates that her history of low back problems dates back to June of 1998, when she injured her low back in the course of her work as a preloader at ACME Shipping. She recalls twisting while trying to catch a computer that was falling to the floor. She apparently had abrupt onset of pain in her low back.

She reports that following this injury she remained off work until about December of 1998. She went through a work hardening program as she attempted to return to her job.

She indicates that between December of 1998, and August of 2001, she was able to keep up with her work responsibilities at ACME, although she had ongoing problems with her low back.

She indicates that her situation deteriorated substantially in August of 2001. She recalls that she was loading a 40-pound box onto a truck. She advanced her right leg and felt a jolt of pain in the lumbosacral region with radiation over the right buttock. She says that she lost control of her bowels.

She says that she reported the event to her supervisor and was referred to "a company doctor." This physician apparently ordered an MRI scan. He then indicated that she could return to her ACME job, although she should have light duty restrictions. She says that her supervisor told her that she needed to continue working on the conveyor belt where she had worked before, although she was given the opportunity of sitting down and resting if she needed to do this. She indicates that she continued working (apparently for a couple of weeks), but then went off work sometime in September. She has been consistently out of the workforce since then except for one day in about December of 2001, when she tried to return to work. She says that when she made this attempt, she was told that she needed to be able to function 100% before she could go back to ACME. She went off work again and says that she is currently receiving time loss benefits through a workers' compensation claim.

She indicates that she has been seeing Dr. A since September of 2001. He referred her to physical therapy, but the patient says that this made her symptoms worse, so that therapy was discontinued in about January. She does have a self-directed exercise program that she learned as she went through her 1998 injury. She recalls undergoing several injection procedures. An epidural injection done shortly after onset of her symptoms in August provided no benefit. She recalls undergoing three nerve root blocks (right S1 selective nerve root blocks) performed by Dr. A. She says that these helped for about three or four hours. She reports that she has recently undergone a three level discography. She indicates that she experienced severe pain during injections of two of the three discs and at least moderate pain during injection of the third disc. She says that she had a marked flare-up of pain that lasted for days after the discography. She indicates that a physician (presumably Dr. A) has now recommended either an IDET procedure or a spinal fusion.

## CURRENT COMPLAINTS:

Currently, Ms. X reports pain that seems to start in the right lumbosacral junction region. It spreads over the right buttock. It then seems to jump to the anterior aspect of her right knee. As far as sensory dysfunction in the right lower extremity is concerned, she says that she gets paresthesias affecting the little toe of the right foot and the lateral border of the right foot. She cannot identify focal weakness in the right lower extremity, but does note that her knee hurts when she tries to use it so that it is hard for her to do certain right lower extremity activities. She denies any problems with her left lower extremity. She has no problems with bowel or bladder control at this time (although she did have fecal incontinence in the late summer of 2001). Overall, she makes it clear that her most severe pain is at the lumbosacral junction. She rates her average pain at 7/10.

As far as routine activities are concerned, the patient initially reported that she was able to be up all day long. She qualified this to say that she has to lie down a few times a day and do a knee/chest exercise. She experiences increased pain with bending activities such as mopping a floor. Walking can also be painful for her. The effect of sitting is variable. Sometimes she gets cramping and paresthesias in the right lower extremity when she sits for a long period of time. She has a lot of difficulty with heavy lifting. For example, she says that she has to make several trips from the grocery store to her car because she can't manage heavy bags of groceries. Coughing tends to aggravate pain in her back. Sexual activities are painful. At night she gets significant discomfort that interferes with sleep. She describes her pain and activity limitations as "mentally exhausting." She indicates that her social activities have been significantly restricted because of her pain.

**MEDICAL HISTORY:**

CURRENT MEDICAL PROBLEMS: As far as her general health is concerned, she indicates that she has undergone a hysterectomy and ovariectomy. She is taking Estratest for this. She reports that she has had pneumonia on several occasions.

CURRENT MEDICATIONS: Currently, her medications consist of Vicodin, 4-6 tablets per day, and Estratest.

ALLERGIES: She describes herself as allergic to Penicillin, Codeine, Morphine, and aspirin.

PREVIOUS INJURIES: The patient denies any significant problems with her low back prior to 1998.

PRIOR HOSPITALIZATIONS/SURGERIES: She has also undergone a Mumford procedure on her right shoulder and some procedure on her right knee. She can't give any details.

HABITS: She smokes about a pack and a half of cigarettes per day. She describes herself as an occasional drinker and denies a history of drug or alcohol abuse.

## SOCIOECONOMIC:

The patient indicates that she has worked as a preloader for Acme Shipping for more than four years. She indicates that she is divorced and has two dependent children. She has a tenth-grade education. (She indicates that she subsequently got a GED.)

## PHYSICAL EXAMINATION:

General: The patient did not demonstrate any dramatic pain behaviors during the interview. Mood and affect were noteworthy in that she seemed somewhat distressed and slightly irritable at the outset of the evaluation, but seemed to warm up and relax as the evaluation went on.

The patient is 6'0" in height. Her weight is 235 pounds. Inspection reveals a large, somewhat overweight woman. She intermittently unloads her right lower extremity, although this is not dramatic. The pelvis is level, and she has a good lumbar lordotic curve. There is a gentle C-shaped scoliosis running much of the length of her back with convexity to the left. Her head tilted to the right.

The patient transfers slowly getting on and off the examination table. She walks slowly and demonstrates a distinct limp favoring her right lower extremity. She complains of pain at the lumbosacral junction on the right side during a short walk.

Palpation in the lumbosacral region reveals soft tissue hypersensitivity off-center to the right at the level of the lumbosacral junction and to a lesser extent over the right gluteal muscles. The patient does not demonstrate any midline tenderness over the lumbar spine or sacrum.

Range of motion of the lumbar spine is measured with the two inclinometer system. The patient flexes 26 degrees and extends 14 degrees. She reports lumbosacral junction pain with both maneuvers. She does not report any radicular symptoms. Lateral bending is 14 degrees to the right and 24 degrees to the left. Straight leg raising is negative bilaterally when the patient is sitting. When she lies supine she reports pain on left straight leg raising when her hip is flexed 50 degrees. On the right side she reports pain when her hip is flexed 24 degrees. She describes this pain as being in the low back and in the hamstring region of the right lower extremity. It appears to be somewhat aggravated by dorsiflexion and plantar flexion of the ankle.

Her responses are difficult to interpret because she also reports significant pain when her right lower extremity is held in a 90/90 position and when the right hip is flexed or rotated. Passive motions of the left hip are tolerated well and appear to be normal in extent.

The patient reports increased discomfort when she lies supine with her hips and knees extended. She is able to do one crunch, but reports that this aggravates her back pain. She reports increased pain when she tries to lie prone. She is, however, able to hyperextend her spine and demonstrate fairly good lumbar paraspinal muscle tone.

Inspection of the distal lower extremities does not reveal any abnormalities. Peripheral pulses are intact.

Neurologic: Knee jerks are trace positive bilaterally. Ankle jerks are 2+ bilaterally with facilitation. Thigh circumference (4 inches above the knee) is 21-1/8 inches on the left and 21-1/4 inches on the right. Calf circumference is 17-3/4 inches on the left and 17-1/2 inches on the right. On pinprick examination the patient reports some diminution of sensation over the lateral border of the right foot. She does not report any sensory disturbance in the right calf. On manual muscle testing the patient demonstrates mild weakness in plantar flexion, inversion, and eversion of the right ankle and more definite weakness in dorsiflexion of the ankle. Pain inhibition seemed to be playing a role in this weakness. Flexion and extension of the toes is normal in strength, although she does report some sense of cramping when she flexes the toes of the right foot. She demonstrates significant pain inhibited weakness in right knee extension and in activation of all muscle groups around the right hip. Strength is 5/5 on the left side.

Overall, the patient demonstrated very significant functional limitations on examination and significant non-organic signs. Her Waddell score was 3/5.

**X-RAYS:**

I reviewed her lumbar MRI scan from 08/17/01. Sagittal images demonstrate some desiccation of the L4-5 and L5-S1 discs and perhaps the L2-3 and L3-4 discs in comparison to the ones above. Disc height is maintained at all levels. There are slight bulges at L4-5 and L5-S1. Axial images do not reveal evidence of compromise of neural elements. (The radiology report mentions a small lateral L3-4 disc protrusion. I did not see this.)

There is a contrast enhanced lumbar CT scan dated 03/12/02. This is a post-discogram CT scan. There appears to be central spinal stenosis at L3-4. I did not see evidence of leakage of contrast material. Similarly, I did not see evidence of major disc pathology or leakage of contrast material at L4-5. (The radiology report mentions subtle annular tears to the left at both levels.) At L5-S1 there is a central posterior protrusion of contrast material consistent with an annular tear or bulge. There is some evidence of bilateral facet arthropathy at this level and the L4-5 level.

## MEDICAL RECORDS:

There is a physician's report dated 08/16/01. In the patient's portion of the report, the text says: "Have had continued discomfort from injury in 1998. Pain increasing is overwhelming." I cannot read the signature of the physician who filled out the medical portion of the form. The physician notes that the patient has had pain for several years and is now getting pain with radiation into the right thigh. She was noted to have some rectal incontinence. The plan was to have her undergo an MRI scan and to give her Ultram and Robaxin.

There is a report of plain x-rays of the lumbar spine from 08/16/01. The impression was some early osteoarthritis.

There is report of a lumbar MRI scan from 08/17/01. The impression was 1) small lateral L3-4 does not appear to be compressing nerve root, 2) degenerative joint disease at L4-5 and L5-S1, 3) small annular bulges at these two levels, but no thecal sac or nerve root compression.

There is a physician's report from 08/21/01. The physician noted the MRI scan findings and indicated a plan of having the patient undergo an epidural steroid injection. There is report of a lumbar epidural steroid injection performed by Dr. B on 08/22/01.

There is a report by Dr. Milton Greene dated 09/05/01. Dr. A noted that the patient had a history of a back injury in June of 1998, and that he had seen her in January of 1999, when she was doing quite well. His impressions were 1) sensory radiculopathy of the right S1 distribution, 2) MRI reportedly shows disc protrusion at two levels. His plan was to start the patient on Vicodin, Flexeril and Naprosyn. He referred her to Physical Therapy program #1. He raised the possibility of electrodiagnostic studies and epidural injections.

On 09/27/01 Dr. A noted that the patient was returning on a semi-emergent basis. She reported loss of bowel control during the previous two weeks. He expressed the view that her stool incontinence was caused by her low back problem.

In a follow-up note of 10/09/01 Dr. A indicated that the patient had undergone evaluation regarding her rectal incontinence. He stated, "She was evaluated by Dr. C, who felt that the transient incontinence was caused by Valsalva maneuver or a vagal response due to significant pain reflex. She was not concerned about a gastrointestinal problem." Dr. A's plan was to do a selective nerve root block of the right S1 nerve root.

There is a procedure note from 10/12/01. This is described as a right S1 transforaminal epidural steroid injection.

In a follow-up note of 11/28/01 Dr. A indicated that the patient had reported substantial relief of her symptoms following the right S1 and caudal epidural steroid injection he had done in October. He indicated that she had returned to work, but had experienced a marked exacerbation of her pain. His impression was chronic right S1 radiculopathy.

On 12/04/01 Dr. A performed a selective right S1 nerve root injection followed by caudal epidural steroid injection.

On 12/12/01 Dr. A indicated that the patient reported 15% improvement since his last injection and requested another one. On 12/18/01 Dr. A performed a caudal epidural steroid injection and selective nerve root block at S1 on the right side.

On 12/27/01 Dr. A noted that the patient did not report benefit from the last injections. He noted that she had completed a set of three steroid injections and that further interventional therapy would not be helpful for her. He suggested that she resume physical therapy.

On 01/16/02 Dr. A indicated that the patient's physical therapist noted that she had responded only minimally to weight control and aerobic conditioning. The therapist expressed the view that she had evidence of a "persisting facet component." His plan was to schedule her for a median branch block. He noted that if there was no response he would place her at medical stability.

There is a procedure note from 01/22/02. Dr. A performed median branch blocks on the right side at L3-4, L4-5 and L5-S1.

In a follow-up note of 02/06/02 Dr. A noted that the patient had not gotten any benefit from the median branch blocks. His plan was to have her undergo a functional capacities evaluation and then determine permanent partial impairment.

On 02/28/02 Dr. A summarized the results of a physical capacities evaluation that had been done on 02/12/02. He indicated that this concluded that she was not able to return to her usual and customary job, but would need to seek work that falls into the light/medium work category. He noted that her preloader job at ACME required her to lift up to 70 pounds.

On 03/12/02 the patient underwent discography at L3-4, L4-5 and L5-S1. The procedure was performed by Dr. D. The patient was noted to get concordant pain at all three levels, although it was apparently most pronounced at L5-S1.

There is report of a CT scan from 03/12/02. This was done following the discograms. The impression is 1) there are findings consistent with annular tears left laterally at both L3-4 and L4-5. 2) There appears to be a small midline annular tear at L5-S1 with an associated small protrusion that does not cause significant mass effect upon adjacent neural elements. 3) There is moderate central spinal stenosis at L4-5 and mild central spinal stenosis at L3-4. No severe central or foraminal spinal stenoses are defined. 4) There is bilateral facet arthropathy at L4-5 and L5-S1.

**DIAGNOSIS:**

1. **Ms. X presents with low back pain associated with some right lower extremity symptoms. Her symptoms raise the possibility of mild irritation of the right S1 nerve root. However, her most severe pain is clearly in the lumbosacral region by her report, and she does not have anatomic evidence of compromise of the right S1 nerve root or focal neurologic signs that indicate a right S1 radiculopathy. My overall impression is that she has an axial lumbar spine pain syndrome. This may be a reflection of discogenic pain, although, as usual, it is difficult to identify a precise pain generator when a patient has largely axial pain.**

2. **It is worth noting that the patient has undergone three level discography. The interpretation of this is somewhat elusive to me. The patient has a clear recall that she had severe pain during the injections of two of the three discs and some pain during injection of the third disc. This is consistent with the procedure report by Dr. A dated 03/12/02. Also of note is the fact that anatomic abnormalities on post-discography CT scan were rather subtle. All in all, it does not appear to me that the three level discography procedure identified a precise generator of Ms. X's pain.**

3. **Of note is the fact that the patient reports very significant activity restrictions that she relates to her back pain and demonstrates substantial functional limitations and non-organic signs on physical examination. Overall she appears to present with more disability than one would expect in a patient with multi-level degenerative disc disease.**

**DISCUSSION AND RECOMMENDATIONS:**

In response to the questions posed in the cover letter of April 15, 2002:

1. What is your current diagnosis and prognosis for Ms. X? Please list any preexisting factors.
**Ms. X most probably has symptomatic multi-level lumbar degenerative disc disease. Her prognosis is guarded. That is, she is at significant risk to remain symptomatic or to have an aggravation of symptoms if she engages in heavy physical labor. She has preexisting factors in that she injured her back in June of 1998, and gives the impression that she never fully recovered from this.**

2. Are Ms. X's subjective complaints supported by objective findings? How do the findings relate to the injury of 08/13/01?
**The patient appears to have more disability than one usually sees in an individual with multi-level degenerative disc disease. I have no explanation for this. She reports a marked aggravation of her symptoms on 08/13/01. There is no medical basis on which I can either confirm or disconfirm this report. It is worth noting though that many individuals with vulnerable low backs will report marked aggravations of their symptoms in response to relatively modest trauma.**

3. Have her work duties been a substantial factor in the cause of her current symptoms, claimed disability and/or reason for continued medical treatment?
**The patient gives a history of a dramatic deterioration in her back condition while she was carrying an object for ACME. I have no independent basis for confirming or disconfirming this history. If it is true, I would conclude that her work activities have been a substantial factor in her current symptoms.**

4. If not, please provide an alternative explanation which would exclude work-related factors as a substantial cause of the current disability and need for treatment.
**Please see #3 above.**

5. Do you think the work duties have been a temporary aggravation of a preexisting condition? If so, do you feel that she has now reached pre-aggravation status?
**It appears that the patient's work duties in August of 2001, aggravated her underlying lumbar degenerative disc disease. She reports that her symptoms have not yet returned to pre-aggravation status. This statement is somewhat difficult to assess since she has some elements of a chronic pain syndrome. Overall though, the information available to me indicates that the patient's symptoms have not yet reached pre--aggravation status.**

6. Do you agree with the recommended course of treatment, to include the possible IDET procedure?
**I do not believe that an IDET procedure is appropriate for her. Her discography seems to indicate three level disc problems. In my opinion, surgical intervention has a very low yield when a person has multi-level disc problems.**

7. What are your recommendations for future medical care? Please be specific with regard to the frequency and duration of this care. Is this care needed as a direct result of the accident of 08/13/01?
**There are certainly no curative therapies for her condition. She has a chronic multi-level lumbar degenerative disc condition. She needs to understand that self-care will be the key to management of this problem. Since there has been some uncertainty about future options for her, I think it would be reasonable for her to have one additional brief trial of physical therapy that focuses on teaching her a self-directed exercise program. Additional pharmacologic management might also be appropriate as long as her response is carefully monitored and it is clear that the pharmacologic interventions are helping. One possibility would be to modify her opiate regimen. More importantly, I think that she could benefit from anti-depressant medication to help her deal with emotional distress related to her ongoing back pain and disability. This care would be appropriate to help her return to the functional status that she had prior to 08/13/01. Her need for treatment appears to be a direct result of her injury of 8/13/01, as noted above.**

8. Do you feel that she has reached medical stability as defined under the terms of Alaska Workers' Compensation Act in relation to the injury of 08/13/01?
**The patient meets the statutory definition of medical stability.**

9. Do you feel that she has sustained permanent partial impairment? If so, kindly provide your rating based on AMA Guidelines, 5th Edition.
**The patient warrants a DRE Category II impairment of the lumbar spine. This is associated with 5% permanent partial impairment.**

Sincerely,

James Robinson, M.D., Ph.D.
Physiatrist, Psychologist

JR/jrs

**Report #9: Personal Injury—Multiple Injuries**

This report is most notable for the following.

- Objectively documented presence of examinee's attorney during history-taking and introduction.
- Economy of words and an absence of superfluous language.
- Thorough and well-documented musculoskeletal examination.
- Examiner resists commenting on areas outside of the scope of the evaluation (e.g., he does not comment on the possible effect of cannabinoids on the cause of the accident precipitating the injury).
- The report does not overuse boilerplate language.
- Crisp, well-supported conclusions.

While this is an excellent report, all reports can be improved. Areas of possible improvement include the following.

- More headnotes in the beginning of the report, such as "Introduction," "History of Injury," and "Current Status."
- Include an executive summary.
- The record and study review might be more valuable if it were organized chronologically and not by provider. Specific dates on each record summary would add value as would more specificity in the number of records reviewed (e.g., stating "14 x-rays of teeth" as opposed to "numerous x-rays of teeth").
- Better proofreading after dictation to eliminate dictation errors (e.g., "Marshall Arts").
- Avoid self-serving, subjective language (e.g., "Comprehensive" musculoskeletal evaluation. Stating that the evaluation was "comprehensive" will open the examiner to cross-examination highlighting each and every test that was not done.).

---

Dear Mr. ____

The above person was seen by me at your request on 11/04/02 for the purpose of an Independent Medical Evaluation (IME). Mr. _____ understands I will be evaluating him and not offering any treatment. He has his own treating physicians. No doctor/patient relationship is established. Present for the history taking and introduction part of this evaluation is Mr. _____'s attorney, _____. Mr. _____ left prior to the physical examination.

Mr. __ is a 30-year-old right-handed Hispanic male who complains of the following: 1. low back pain with radiation into the right buttock, 2. headaches radiating from the right side to the back of his head, 3. neck pain/stiffness, and 4. the left eye tends to close.

Mr. __ states that his right lower extremity is shorter than the left. He rates his low back at the present time as 8/10. The least amount of pain is 4-5/10 and the and worst amount of pain is 10/10.

Mr. __ states that on 12/18/99 he was putting his Christmas lights on the sliding door out by his balcony on the third floor when he leaned back on the balcony railing, it collapsed, and he fell from the third story onto the concrete parking lot below. Emergency medical rescue arrived at the scene and reported there was no loss of consciousness. However, Mr. __ states he did not remember anything until he woke up in the emergency room. He was taken to Baptist Hospital Medical Center, evaluated and admitted. He experienced multiple trauma including fracture of the right wrist, fracture of the right leg/ankle, fracture of the right femur/hip, facial bone fractures, fracture of the base of the skull, left carpal tunnel syndrome, fracture of the orbits, and fracture of the right fifth metatarsal. He has seen numerous physicians and has had numerous procedures done, as will be enumerated below.

He denies any bladder or bowel dysfunction. He states he does not have a sense of taste or smell. He states nothing in particular reduces his pain. He feels worse during and after exercises, prolonged sitting more than one hour, standing more than thirty to forty minutes, he is able to walk one mile with rest periods. He also feels worse with bending backwards and forwards. He states he is able to drive an automatic shift car. He is independent with all activities of daily living. He states he applied for Social Security Disability and was denied several times. He states on the most recent attempt he was given Social Security Disability, however, it has not been finalized yet.

He states that due to the accident of 12/18/99 he is not able to cook, participate in sports (baseball, Marshall arts, and run). He has difficulty reading, the left eye tends to close, difficulty concentrating and remembering. He states he wakes up at 7:30 am, has coffee for breakfast and makes his bed. He plays with his one-year, seven-month-old child. He reads a book. He also does his home exercise program. Mr. __ states he had three molars (teeth) removed due to this accident.

CURRENT CARE: 1. Dr. __ (orthopedic surgeon), every other month. He states Dr. __ is going to remove the hardware from the right lower extremity in the future. His next appointment is December 2002. 2. Dr. __ (neurologist), every other month for nervousness, decreased memory, and hand swelling. He is not involved in any formal exercise or therapy program. He was admitted into Baptist Hospital on 12/18/99 and discharged home on 01/04/00. He went for therapy as an outpatient for a period of time thereafter.

PAST MEDICAL HISTORY: 1. Tonsillectomy (prior). 2. Right ankle ORIF (current). 3. Right wrist ORIF (current). 4. Right femur/hip ORIF – intramedullary nail (current).

SOCIAL HISTORY: He smokes one pack of cigarettes every three days. He denies consumption of alcohol. He is involved in a home exercise program three times per week. He consumes one cup of coffee per day. He lives with his common-law wife, who is currently pregnant, and with their one-year, seven-month-old son.

CURRENT MEDICATIONS: 1. Vioxx 25 mg q.d. 2. Paxil 20 mg q.d.

DRUG ALLERGIES: NKA

EDUCATIONAL HISTORY: High School Graduate. Certificate in office machine repair (six month course), Cannon Company.

FAMILY HISTORY: Father alive, age 66, healthy. Mother alive, age 64, healthy. Sisters: two, both alive, ages 34 and 36, healthy. Brothers: one alive, age 38, healthy.

WORK HISTORY: At the time of his injury he was employed as a chef for __ restaurant for two years. He learned how to be a chef by "on-the-job training." He has not worked since the date of injury, 12/18/99.

REVIEW OF RECORDS:

1. BAPTIST HOSPITAL – 12/18/99 – 01/04/00

Diagnostic Studies:

- Lateral cervical spine x-ray – negative for fracture, muscle spasm present.
- Facial and nasal bones: fracture right inferior orbital wall and possible lateral wall.
- Increased density of right ethmoid sinus, unable to visualize well. Nasal bones are negative.
- Chest x-ray: no evidence of pneumothorax
- Thoracic spine: minimal compression fracture of T8 (subtle irregularity only).

- Lumbosacral spine: fracture right superior and inferior pubic rami near the synphysis pubis. No lumbar spine fractures are noted
- Right wrist x-rays: fracture of distal radius with extension into the joint. There is also a chip fracture of the ulnar styloid process.
- Right hip x-rays: comminuted fracture of the proximal shaft of the right femur, avulsion of the right lesser trochanter with the fracture extending into the intertrochanteric part of the femur. Also, pubic rami fractures as noted.
- Right femur: comminuted fracture of right femoral shaft, avulsion of lesser trochanter.
- Right knee: negative
- Right tibia and fibula: comminuted fracture of the distal tibia with extension through the posterior, medial, and inferior rip of the lateral malleolus (ankle).
- Right foot/ankle: comminuted fracture of the distal tibia into the malleolus. Also fracture of the head of the fifth metatarsal.
- CT scan of the brain: right-sided facial fractures. Right orbital floor fracture, comminuted anterior wall and right maxillary antral floor fracture. Comminuted, depressed right anterior/lateral maxillary antral wall fracture. Displaced and depressed right zygomatic arch fracture with mild impingement of the temporalis muscle. Mild comminuted fracture of the right lateral orbit with a small amount of intraorbital air present. Linear nondisplaced fracture along the right middle cranial fossa in the greater wing of the sphenoid bone. There is a small intracranial tear located at this site. Associated soft tissue swelling in the right facial and periorbital region. Question of mild hemorrhagic contusion of the right frontal base. Ventricles are normal in midline, no edema or midline shift. Small amount of air adjacent to the left TMJ and this is usually associated with a basilar skull fracture. There is a basilar skull fracture on the right, but it is difficult to see on the left, may need CT scan of the skull base. Small amount of fluid in the spenoid and ethmoid sinuses.
- CT scan of the brain: prior extensive fractures previously noted of the facial bones. No intracranial hematoma, no definite contusion seen at this time. There are tiny dots of intracranial air and air along the left TMJ suggesting left-sided basilar skull fracture.
- Right wrist x-rays (postoperative): external fixation device in place for stabilization of the comminuted fracture of the right distal radius.
- Pelvis: intramedullary rod into the right hip, comminuted proximal third femoral fracture with some displacement of the bone fragments. Comminuted fracture of the inferior and superior right pubic ramus.
- Right femur: status post hip pinning with an intramedullary rod through the femoral shaft to transfix a markedly comminuted fracture of the

subtrochanteric femur and lesser trochanter. Fracture fragments are 1-2 cm displaced and angulated.

- Right femur: mid and proximal third femoral fracture, with rod through femoral shaft and screw through femoral neck. Proximal femoral fracture is displaced laterally and lesser trochanter is more medial.
- Right tibia and fibular (during surgery): plastic cast obscuring detail of tibia and fibula. Also external device through proximal tibial shaft, talus and calcaneuus. Comminuted fractures of the medial, posterior, and possibly lateral malleolus (ankle) with widening of the ankle mortise.
- Right ankle x-rays: external fixation device over the comminuted distal tibial fracture.
- CT scan of the right ankle (12/21/99): comminuted displaced fractures of the right distal tibia with disruption of the ankle mortise. Also displaced avulsion type fraction of the distal fibula. External fixation device in place.
- Follow-up diagnostic studies – 12/22/99.
- X-rays of the orbits: comminuted fracture of the right orbital floor with opacification of the right maxillary sinus, fracture of greater wing of the spenoid bone, questionable fracture of the lateral wall of the right orbit.
- CT scan of the orbits: multiple facial and skull fractures with air fluid levels in the maxillary, ethmoid, and sphenoid sinuses with diffuse subcutaneous soft tissue swelling. Fracture of the right zygomatic arch, comminuted fracture of the orbital rim to the posterior lateral wall of the maxillary sinus. Comminuted fracture of the lateral wall of the orbit anteriorly. Comminuted and depressed fracture of the wing of the sphenoid bone, extends to the orbital plate of the frontal bone on the right laterally. Associated nondisplaced fracture of the right nasal bone.
- Follow-up diagnostic studies 01/03/00 – right wrist x-rays: external fixation device over a fracture of the distal radius in satisfactory alignment and position. Small avulsion chip fracture of ulnar styloid process in satisfactory position.
- Pelvis: fracture of right superior and inferior pubic rami with fracture extending into the pubis superiorly. There is also a previously noted fracture of the proximal right femur with satisfactory alignment.
- Right femur: fractures previously described, transfixed by rod and screws, satisfactory position and alignment.
- Right tibia and fibular: external fixation device remains in place with satisfactory alignment of the fracture. Fracture of distal tibia, chip fracture of the inferior aspect of the lateral malleolus (ankle).
- EEG: abnormal EEG with evidence of diffuse slowing of the dominant background rhythm. No epileptiform activity, asymmetries, focal pathology or paroxysmal events noted.

X-rays from the office of Dr. (Orthopedic Surgeon)

- Right wrist: healing intraarticular distal radius fracture, satisfactory alignment.
- Right femur: minimal callus formation a very comminuted subtrochanetric femoral fracture with intake locked rod. The patient is strictly non-weightbearing.
- Right tibia and fibula: satisfactory alignment of the intraarticular distal tibial fracture and hardware.
- 3/01/00 – Right wrist: progressive healing, good alignment.
- Right femur good rod positioning, early callus formation with parts of the communited fracture.
- Right tibia and fibular: satisfactory alignment with external fixator in place with intraosseous screw fixation.
- 3/22/00 – Right ankle: x-rays of the right ankle with the external fixator removed.

Progressive fracture healing but still able to see the fracture lines.
05/24/00 – Right wrist: satisfactory alignment and remodeling around the fixator pin sites.
05/24/00 – Right femur: early remodeling around severely comminuted fracture with satisfactory position of hardware.
05/24/00 – Right ankle: well aligned with no mortise subluxation but mild arthrosis about the tibia – talar joint but no ossesous spurs that would block motion.
05/11/00 – MRI of the brain: maxillary sinus mucosal thickening, no intracranial abnormality.

Lawrence __, DDS
Numerous x-rays of the teeth.

2. __, MD (Orthopedic Surgeon)
02/02/00 – It is now six weeks after his multiple trauma. He is not taking any significant amount of pain medication. X-rays of the right wrist reveal evidence of healing of the intra-articular distal radius fracture in satisfactory alignment. X-rays of the right femur revealed minimal callus formation at that point of a very comminuted subtrochanteric femur fracture with an intact locked rod. X-rays of the right tibia and fibula reveal maintenance of satisfactory alignment of the intraarticular distal tibia fracture and hardware. Impression: 1. Status post multiple trauma.

03/01/00 – Follow-up. It is now two months after his pilon fracture fixation and one month out of the fracture of right wrist. X-rays of the right wrist, right femur, and right tibia and fibula reveal progressive healing. Impression: 1. Stable, status post multiple trauma.

03/22/00 – Follow-up. X-rays of the right ankle reveal satisfactory alignment and progressive healing. Impression: 1. The overall impression is stable, status post multiple trauma.

03/29/00 – Follow-up. He now complains of right-sided facial numbness and continued numbness in his left index and long fingers. He is non-weight bearing with crutches, in an air cast. Right lower extremity wounds are clear. The external fixator is intact. He is referred to a neurologist for reassessment of his possible neurological sequelae from his multiple trauma.

05/24/00 – Follow-up. It is now five months from his date of injury (12/18/99). He has discomfort in the right thigh and ankle. He still has persistence of left index finger and left middle finger numbness, posttraumatic. X-rays of the right wrist reveal satisfactory alignment and remodeling about the fixator pin sites. The right femur x-rays reveal early remodeling about a very comminuted subtrochanteric fracture with the intact nail with satisfactory position of the screws, without any hardware breakage. X-rays of the right ankle reveal well aligned tibial plafond surface with no mortise subluxation but some mild arthrosis about the tibio-talar joint, no evidence of any osseous spurs that might be blocking motion. Impression: 1. Persistent ankle and thigh tendinitis and tenosynovitis with mold ankle arthrosis, posttraumatic, status post right wrist, right femur, and right tibia pilon fractures.
01/12/00 – Impression: orthopedically stable, status post multiple trauma.

02/04/00 – Follow-up

3. MIAMI-DADE FIRE RESCUE REPORT 12/18/99
The patient states he fell off of a 20 foot height balcony onto concrete pavement. There is no loss of consciousness, no neck or back injury, no abdominal pain. He is alert and oriented x 3, in no acute distress. He has primarily right-sided pain and swelling. The patient will not elaborate about the fall/jump.

4. BAPTIST HOSPITAL TRAUMA ADMISSION 12/18/99 – 01/04/00
Discharge Summary – 01/04/00 – Admitting/discharge diagnosis: 1. Closed head injury concussion with post-concussive syndrome. 2. Possible basilar skull fracture. 3. Right-sided superior, inferior pubic ramus fractures. 4. Right femur subtrochanteric fracture. 5. Right distal tibia intraarticular pilon fracture. 6. Right distal radius fracture. 7. Right fifth metatarsal neck fracture. 8. Left upper extremity head probably neuropraxic, etiology unclear. 9. Orbital fractures for which no intervention was opted for.

History: This is a 27-year-old male with multiple trauma who states he fell off a third floor balcony after hanging some Christmas lights. He states the balcony gave way as he leaned against it. There was probable loss of consciousness and head injury. He was slightly confused but communicating verbally in the emergency room. He had obvious facial injuries and facial fractures. He was in significant pain.

During this admission he underwent numerous orthopedic procedures. He was placed on prophylactic antibiotics. He was able to ambulate with a platform walker. He was not considered a candidate for the inpatient rehabilitation program since financial arrangements were not made. He will follow-up as an outpatient for therapy. He was advised of the possibility of right ankle arthrosis, arthritis and possibly an ultimate ankle fusion and the need for extensive therapy. He will follow-up on an outpatient basis with physical therapy and orthopedic follow-up care. He will also have follow-up dental care. Dental service had recommended tooth extraction on a follow-up basis. There is no acute infection but he had multiple broken teeth from the accident and some chronic decay in teeth numbers 19 and 30.

- Numerous handwritten follow-up physician progress notes.
- Steven A. __, MD (Neurologist) – consultation 12/18/99. This patient sustained multiple trauma following a fall from a third floor balcony. A review of laboratory studies reveals the toxicology to be positive for cannabinoids. It was otherwise negative for other agents. Impression: 1. Closed head injury, currently alert and oriented x 3. 2. Multiple trauma secondary to fall from third story balcony with orbital fractures, right femoral fracture, pubic fracture, wrist fracture, tibial fracture, all on the right side.
- ___, MD (PM&R) - 01/04/00 Impression 1. Multiple trauma secondary to fall with orthopedic injuries, closed head trauma, orbital fractures and basilar skull fractures. 2. Left carpal tunnel syndrome, rule out median nerve injury. 3. History of right orbital injuries and blunt facial trauma. Plan: Outpatient therapy to include physical therapy and occupational therapy. He will need a left carpal tunnel syndrome splint for nigh-time use, as well as, outpatient EMG study with myself or neurology.
- Operative report – 12/19/99 – Procedure: 1. Right femur manipulation with intramedullary locked rod fixation. 2. Right distal tibial closed manipulation with external fixation. 3. Right distal radius closed manipulation with external fixation.
- Operative report 12/28/99 – Surgical procedure: 1. Numerous orthopedic procedures to the right lower extremity.
- 12/18/99 – Toxicology drug screen: positive for cannabinoid (urine). All others were negative.
- 12/18/99 – Drug screen positive for tricyclic antidepressant (NG/ML); 24.
- 12/21/99 – Physical upper initial evaluation

5. BAPTIST HOSPITAL
PHYSICAL THERAPY/REHABILITATION RECORDS
- Dates of service: 01/17/00 – 06/16/00 Numerous handwritten therapy notes.

6. __, MD 04/26/00 – Initial neurology consultation
- Impression: 1. Post-concussive syndrome.
- Numerous follow-up notes.
- 09/06/00 – Final neurology consultation. Impression: 1. Post-concussive-syndrome. 2. Orbital fractures. 3. Right pubic ramus fracture. 4. Right femur fracture. 5. Right tibia fracture. 6. Right radius fracture. 7. Right fifth metatarsal fracture. 8. Probable right distal hand neuropraxia. He is at MMI as of this time (09/06/00). Permanent impairment rating is ten percent whole person according the AMA Guides. This is pertaining to his head and right hand nerve damage. Any impairment rating regarding the orthopedic part of it is deferred to Dr. ___.

7. ___, PhD, AHPP (Neuropsychologist)
04/225/00 – Neuropsychological evaluation – Diagnosis: DSMIV (Axis 1) Major Depression, Recurrent, Moderate. Axis II – No diagnosis. Axis III: closed fracture of pubis, fracture of femur, closed fracture of neck femur, postconcussion syndrome, fracture of right ankle, fracture of distal end of right radius, fracture of metatarsal bone, closed fracture of orbital floor (blowout), fracture facial bones, disorder of teeth and supporting structures, open wound of internal structures of mouth uncomplicated, open wound of face without complication, forehead, carpal tunnel syndrome.

## *COMPREHENSIVE MUSCULOSKELETAL EVALUATION*

Mr. ___ is 5'8" tall and weights 190 pounds. The blood pressure is 120/74. The pulse is 94 and regular. The heart has an S1/S2 rhythm, the lungs are clear. No rales or wheezes are heard. Positive bowel sounds are heard.

Evaluation of the cranial nerves reveals the left eyelid tends to droop, however, the muscle tone is good for opening and closure. The pupils are round, equal, and reactive to light and accommodation. He has loss of smell and taste to alcohol. The tongue is midline. The gag reflex is intact. Speech is functional. All other cranial nerves are within normal limits bilaterally.

The range of motion of the cervical spine is as follows: flexion 70 degrees (60 degrees), extension 35 degrees (75 degrees), right and left rotation 80 degrees (80 degrees), right lateral bending 30 degrees (45 degrees), left lateral bending 35 degrees (45 degrees). There is restricted active cervical range of motion. Postural examination reveals the right shoulder to be approximately one-half inch to one inch lower than the left. There are no gross spinal deformities noted. Forward flexion brings the fingertips lacking 8" from the floor, extension is 20 degrees, right side bending brings the fingertips 3" below the popliteal crease, left side bending brings the fingertips 3" below the popliteal crease. He has difficulty toe and heel walking on the right side, left side is normal. He ambulates independently with a straight cane with a mild limp as he bears weight on the right lower extremity. He uses a cane in the right hand.

The muscle stretch reflexes are one plus in both upper extremities, the right knee jerk and ankle jerk is two plus. The left knee jerk is one plus, the left ankle jerk is two plus, the plantar responses are down-going bilaterally. Sensation is intact to sharp sensation, vibration and cold sensation in both upper and lower extremities.

Measurement of the right lower extremity from the ASIS to the internal malleolus is 33-1/8" left 34-1/4". Measurement of the lower extremity from the umbilicus to the internal malleolus on the right side is 36-7/8", left 38". There is an anatomical short right lower extremity of 1-1/8". This is due to the fracture of the right femur, more likely than not. The pulses in both upper extremities are intact.

Measurement of the right arm/forearm 4" above and below the distal elbow crease is 12-3/4"/12" left 12-3/4"/11-3/4" no appreciable difference. Measurement of the right thigh/calf measured 5" above and below the medial tibial plateau is as follows: 18-1/2"/14-3/4" left 19"/15-1/4" mild reduction in the right quad/calf which may be related to the fracture of the right femur/ankle. Measurement of the right ankle in the bi-malleolar region on the right side is 10-3/4" left 10-1/8" swelling is noted about the right ankle.

The straight leg raising test was negative at 90 degrees in the seated position bilaterally. In the supine position he complained of right hip pain at approximately 80-90 degrees, negative on the left. Patrick's test was positive for hip pain on the right, negative on the left. Flexion of the thighs onto the abdomen reproduced right hip pain on the right, negative on the left. Tinel's test was negative at the wrists and elbows. The arm drop test was negative bilaterally. The cervical compression and distraction tests and Phalan's test was negative bilaterally. Manual muscle testing of both upper and lower extremities was 5/5 (normal). Manual muscle testing of the abdominals and back extensors revealed good strength. Palpation did not reveal any muscle spasm or trigger points in the posterior cervical region or trapezii. There was tenderness to palpation in the midline at L5/S1. There is also tenderness in the right posterior buttock region. There was no sciatic notch tenderness. There was no tenderness in the popliteal spaces with deep pressure over the sciatic nerves.

Mr. __has tight hamstrings with a popliteal angle on the right of 25 degrees and on the left 40 degrees. Active range of motion of the wrists is as follows:

| | Right Wrist | Left Wrist | Normal |
|---|---|---|---|
| Extension | 70 degrees | 70 degrees | 60 degrees |
| Flexion | 60 degrees | 90 degrees | 70 degrees |
| Radial Deviation | 30 degrees | 50 degrees | 20 degrees |
| Ulnar deviation | 20 degrees | 40 degrees | 30 degrees |

There is mild limitation of active ROM of the right wrist.

The active range of motion of the right ankle is as follows: dorsiflexion 0 degrees (20 degrees), plantar flexion 25 degrees (40 degrees), inversion 15 degrees (30 degrees) eversion 0 degrees (20) degrees. There is reduced active range of motion. Manual muscle testing of the right ankle within the available range overall was 4+/5. The active range of motion of the hips is as follows:

| | Right | Left | Normal |
|---|---|---|---|
| Flexion | 90 degrees | 110 degrees | 100 degrees |
| Extension | 0 degrees | 10 degrees | 30 degrees |
| Abduction | 45 degrees | 50 degrees | 40 degrees |
| Adduction | 25 degrees | 30 degrees | 20 degrees |

There is restricted active range of motion (ROM) of the right hip.

Hand grip strength testing using the Jamar Dynamometer in five separate positions on the right side reveals the following: 0 pounds, 0 pounds, 0 pounds, 0 pounds, 0 pounds. On the left side the readings are as follows: 3 pounds, 12 pounds, 21 pounds, 20 pounds, 3 pounds. Using the Jamar Dynamometer in the #2 position with three consecutive trials on the right side is as follows: 0 pounds, 0 pounds, 0 pounds, on the left the readings are as follows: 18 pounds, 14 pounds, 15 pounds. Using the Bulb Dynamometer the reading on the right side was 9 pounds and on the left 20 pounds. These findings indicate lack of effort on the right side. The left side reveals consistent effort. I was able to put my two fingers in his palm and not pull them out.

The range of motion of both knees is 0-150 degrees. Orthopedic testing of the right knee reveals good medial and lateral stability. The patella moves freely. No effusion is noted. Orthopedic testing for meniscus injury was negative.

Body Scars:
Right forearm: There is a one inch vertical scar on the lateral aspect of the right midforearm.
Right lower extremity: There is a 4-1/2" curved scar on the right posterior/lateral aspect of the right pelvis. There is also a 2 –1/4" vertical scar along the mid lateral thigh region. There are two small posterior right distal thigh scars present.
Right ankle: There is a 3" curved scar on the anterior aspect of the right ankle. On the medial aspect of the right ankle there is a 1 – ½" scar.

IMPRESSION: 30-year-old right-handed Hispanic male status post fall injury from a third floor balcony, 12/18/99 with the following:

Status-post multiple trauma as described above with ORIF of right femur with good results and ORIF of right ankle with anatomical short right lower extremity of 1 – 1/8".
Mechanical low back pain secondary to short right lower extremity with resultant gait dysfunction.
Subjective complaints of headaches, probably secondary to cervical sprain/strain.
Loss of taste and smell sensation most probably secondary to basilar skull fracture with cranial nerve involvement.
Droopy left eyelid secondary to facial/head injury.
Other multiple trauma, i.e. fractures of right wrist, right 5th metatarsal, and pelvis.
Closed head injury.
Left carpal tunnel syndrome by documentation, negative clinical examination.
Other medical data as enumerated above.

**COMMENTS:**

1. Mr. __ gave an incomplete effort with the hand grip strength testing on the right side. In essence, he has normal strength in both upper and lower extremities, including the abdominals and back extensors. There was some discomfort with strength testing of the right hip and ankle.
2. During the course of an eight hour day at the present time he is able to do the following: sit 8 hours, stand 4 hours, and walk 4 hours. He is able to occasionally left/carry 11-20 pounds, bend, squat, stoop, kneel, and crouch. He should never crawl, climb, balance, work at unprotected heights, be exposed to extreme cold or whole-body vibration. He can use his hands on a frequent basis for fingering, feeling, grasping, and reaching while seated. While standing, he can use the left upper extremity on a frequent basis, (presently using the

cane in the right hand). He can operate foot controls while seated, right occasionally, left frequently.

3. He is not at MMI at this time. Pending removal of hardware in the near future and also pending possible lengthening procedure of the right lower extremity. His future functional ability will increase due to the future surgeries which will eliminate the need for the cane, balance his spine, improve his gait, and increase his functional ability of both upper extremities. After the above surgeries are done, he should be able to frequently lift/carry at least 30-40pounds, bend, squat, stoop, and push/pull while standing. Occasionally kneel, and crouch. He should never crawl, climb, or balance. He will most probably be at MMI within one year from the date of the right femur lengthening procedure, if no complications arise.
4. According to Mr. __ he has been awarded Social Security Disability, effective date is to be determined. This has not been finalized.
5. I discussed the future medical care issues at length with Dr. __ Vocational/Rehabilitation/and Life Care Planning expert. Please refer to his report for full details.

The opinions rendered in this case are the opinions of this evaluator. This evaluation has been conducted on the basis of the medical examination and documentation as provided, with the assumption that the material is true and correct. If more information becomes available at a later date, an additional service/report/reconsideration may be requested. Such information may or may not change the opinions rendered in this evaluation. This opinion is based on a clinical assessment, examination, and documentation. This opinion does not constitute per se a recommendation for specific claims or administrative functions to be made or enforced.

I hope this report addresses all of your concerns. Should you require additional information, please do not hesitate to contact me.

Sincerely,

Anthony J. Dorto, MD, FAAPMR, FAADEP

**Report #10: Workers' Compensation—Arm Injury**

This report is most notable for the following.

- It is concise.
- The report appears to be balanced and objective.
- Absence of superfluous or subjective language.
- Client's questions are answered in an easy-to-understand fashion.
- Respectful treatment in the report of the examinee, other providers, and the workers' compensation system. No "pot shots" were taken at anyone.
- The detailed physical examination is documented.

While this is an excellent report, all reports can be improved. Areas of possible improvement include the following.

- Avoid use of medical abbreviations. (For example, state "History" instead of "HX" and "Physical Examination" instead of "PE.") This report was written for an administrative law judge, not other healthcare providers.
- Inapplicable boilerplate language. (For example, multiple use of the word "they" to refer to this single examinee.)
- Excessive boilerplate language. The last three full paragraphs are all boilerplate. This excessive use of boilerplate language takes away from the report.
- Obtain more of the medical records for review prior to generating the report.

---

May 28, 2002

The Honorable
Administrative Law Judge
Wichita, KS

**RE:** Charles Smith

**DOO:** 12/1/00
**CC:** Painful left arm
**MEDS:** One aspirin per day
**ALLERGIES:** NKMA
**CO MORBID:** Two herniated discs in neck

**HX:** Charles Smith is a 53-year-old right-handed Caucasian male who confirmed his identity with the picture on his driver's license. He states that on 12/1/00 he noted symptoms of pain and numbness in his left arm extending up into his left shoulder and neck that occurred after a fall. He was working on a step-up platform that was 12 inches above the floor. He stepped back and fell onto the floor using his left hand to catch himself. He does not remember if there was any swelling or bruising of the left upper extremity. Over the next two weeks, the pain moved down his arm into his fingers. He is uncertain which fingers were affected. He states that he believes that his pain became worse because he does repetitive work. He shared his concerns with his supervisor the next day who suggested that he see ___ medical. The company physician examined Mr. Smith and obtained X-rays. His treatment included Motrin and heat. Mr. Smith states that he had no improvement over the next 4 weeks and was referred to Dr. Watts for an NCT/EMG which was completed on 03/30/01. The NCT/EMG was reported electrophysiologic evidence for cervical polyradiculoneuropathy (roots C6 through T1), sensory and motor, predominantly axonal with some demyelinating features, chronic with evidence of active denervation. Over the next 4 weeks, little improvement was experienced. He says he was frustrated by Workers' Comp. and elected to get an attorney. He says his attorney referred him to Dr. Mission for a disability rating and work restrictions so he could be off work.

The employer wanted a second opinion and he was sent to Dr. Lawance. Dr. Lawance told him that he had a pinched nerve in his elbow but suggested a cervical MRI. The cervical MRI was completed on 05/03/01 with a report of degenerative change greatest at C5-6 with central and lateral stenosis, marrow changes along the end-plates of C5-6 are probably related to degenerative change, and left posterolateral disc bulge at C6-7. On return to Dr. Watts, he was started on a 6-week physical therapy program for his neck.

At the suggestion of his attorney, he saw Dr. Mission again. Dr. Mission's diagnosis was neck pain secondary to polyradiculopathy and left carpal tunnel syndrome. Mr. Smith was provided an impairment rating of 25% based on cervical DRE category IV page 104 and was given light-work-only guides.

He was then referred to a neurosurgeon for possible surgery. Treatment included 3 epidural injections for the cervical spine without improvement. Surgery with diskectomy and fusion was discussed.

The company physician suggested medium-level work and limit hand-over-shoulder activities on the left. He has continued in this work pattern with persistent but not progressive symptoms. His current work activities are outlined below.

**RECORDS AVAILABLE FOR REVIEW:**
05-03-01 - The cervical MRI was completed on 05/03/01 with a report of degenerative change greatest at C5-6 with central and lateral stenosis, marrow changes along the end-plates of C5-6 are probably related to degenerative change, and left posterolateral disc bulge at C6-7.

**ROS:** Mr. Smith describes himself to be in good health with his last general medical history and physical to have been 4 years ago. He feels there has been no change in his mental status and he is able to get adequate sleep each night. Tobacco-2 ppd, Alcohol-12 ppw, Drugs-negative, Sports-negative

**HEENT:** Glasses

**RESP**: Negative

**CV**: HBP

**GI**: Negative

**GU:** Negative

**MS**: Negative except for current complaints. No history of previous trauma or injury. No symptoms of arm weakness, pain, or abnormal feeling before current trauma event.

**CNS/PNS:** Negative

**PSYCH**: Negative

**REF:** Referred by administrative law judge

**FMD:** None

**LMD:** Dr.

**ATTORNEY:** His attorney is David Jones, Esq.

**PRESENT EMPLOYMENT:** He is a sheet metal assembler for Airplane Company, having started on 1/31/89 to present. He describes his job as working 8-10 hours per day, 5 days per week, standing, sitting, drilling holes, and shooting rivets. His work activities have changed due to the restrictions of limited hand-over-shoulder. On average, he does about 10 parts per hour.

**EDUCATION:** High School

**HOBBIES:** Golf and music. He does his normal daily activities, leisure activities, and driving a car. He enjoys playing a guitar, but he cannot do so at this time. He used to play golf a few times per month.

**FH:** His son, Jamie, is 24 and in good health. His parents, Robert and Wilma, are 84 and in good health.

**PE:** Today, the physical examination is consistent with a 53-year-old Caucasian male with an appropriate musculoskeletal build for his stated age, height of 5'11", weight of 210 lb., and heart rate of 78. His ambulatory skills were appropriate for his age and current health condition. The physical examination for the fingers, thumbs, hands, wrists, elbows, shoulders, cervical and thoracic spine were considered age-appropriate for the multiple systems of skin, muscle, bone, nerve, vascular, and lymphatic except as follows.

Mr. Smith was in no acute distress and he cooperated with the examination. His stationary and Romberg were negative. Intrinsic muscle loss on the left hand was present but absent on the right. Grip strength by Jamar was 20, 21, 22 kg left and 55, 54, 53 kg right. Grips in five left 16, 18, 22, 18, 14 and right 50, 50, 54, 50, 49.

On the right, the examination demonstrated a positive percussion, Phalen's, negative reverse, negative direct, pronator and plus/minus Finkelstein's. On the left, there was a positive percussion, Phalen's, negative reverse, direct, pronator, and plus/minus Finkelstein's. Percussion of the ulnar nerve wrist and elbow was negative right. Percussion of the ulnar nerve wrist was negative on the left but on the left elbow caused increasing symptomatology and flexion testing was positive. Medial and lateral epicondylar signs were negative for both the right and left.

Range of motion of the fingers, wrist and elbow were equal but he complained of decreased strength on the left. Range of motion of the shoulders caused discomfort on the left compared to the right, although apprehension, impingement, thoracic outlet, and crepitus were negative for right and left. The cervical and thoracic spine appeared appropriate for stated age and musculoskeletal build. Cervical distraction and compression increased complaints on the left with radicular signs left present.

Sensory was intact for two point, light touch, and vibratory on the right. On the left, altered sensory for two point, light touch, and vibratory in the C5-6 dermatome was present. Deep tendon reflexes were decreased on the brachioradialis. Forearm circumference was 2 cm smaller on the left than the right.

**X-RAYS:** Seven views of the cervical spine were consistent with the MRI degenerative changes at C5-6. Three views of the left shoulder appeared to demonstrate normal bone structure.

**DX:**
1. 12/01/00 – History of fall on left upper extremity
2. 12/01/00 – Painful left upper extremity with altered sensory and muscle weakness
3. 12/01/00 – Possible ulnar nerve entrapment elbow left
4. 12/01/00 – History of CTS but not present on current examination
5. 12/01/00 – Cervical spine degenerative changes at C5-6 with radiculopathy and muscle loss
6. 12/01/00 – MRI with left posteriolateral disc bulge
7. 12/01/00 – Post-epidural injections

**TX:**
Based on the information contained in the report, I believe that this individual is a reasonable candidate for continued treatment. I would agree with Dr.___'s recommendation that the NCT/EMG should be repeated to better understand the possible ulnar nerve elbow entrapment from the C5-6 cervical radiculopathy. At the same time, the test can be used to address the history of CTS that was not supported on the current examination.

I agree with the neurosurgeon that cervical surgery with diskectomy and/or fusion is appropriate. I would proceed with the cervical surgery before considering surgery for the ulnar nerve elbow if conservative treatment fails and most current NCT/EMG is positive.

**WORK GUIDES:**
Before the surgery, this individual may continue with the company physician's suggested work guides of medium-level work and limited hand-over-shoulder activities on the left since his symptoms have not progressed. Additional restrictions will be appropriate in the post-operative period.

In response to questions outlined in your letter:

1. Objective versus subjective complaints: As outlined above, this individual does have objective findings for cervical radiculopathy and possibly left ulnar nerve elbow entrapment.

2. Current diagnosis: Cervical radiculopathy at C5-6 left, painful left upper extremity, weakness left upper extremity, and possible left ulnar nerve entrapment elbow.

3. Causation: Most likely, this individual had a cervical radiculopathy

before the trauma event (fall) as described. Since the fall occurred on the job, the current symptoms represent a permanent aggravation to a preexisting condition.

4. Underlying medical conditions: I am unaware of any additional underlying medical conditions that contribute to this individual's current symptomatology except for the risk factor of alcohol use.

5. Treatment options: Outlined above.

6. Work guides: Outlined above.

7. Maximum Medical Improvement and Impairment Rating: MMI has not been reached.

Today, the medical records (chief complaint, history of present illness, review of systems, past family and social history, work activity history, and comorbidities) and supporting materials were reviewed and a physical examination commensurate with the current medical condition and previous medical conditions that may be influencing the current medical condition was completed. Furthermore, the individual was told and they indicated they understood that they were undergoing a medical examination and/or evaluation at the request of an attorney, an employer, a physician, or an insurance company. They understand that no doctor-patient relationship will be established. They authorize and release Dr. Melhorn to discuss information concerning the results of the medical examination and/or evaluation to any third party, and to testify without limitation, as to all findings of said medical examination and/or evaluation, in any legal action, judicial or administrative proceedings to which they are, or may become, a party or in which they have, or may have, any interest. They waive on behalf of themselves and any persons who may have an interest in the matter, all provisions of law, if any, relating to the disclosure of information acquired through such examination.

An assessment of function was completed and a discussion held, which reviewed their activity levels for home and work. In addition, the activity and/or work guides provided today were provided with the understanding that this individual may appear to be fit to return to activities and/or work duties under the guides provided, however, there is no guarantee that the individual will not report a re-injury or additional injury once they return to activities and or work. Each individual experiences physical activity, including work, differently and the individual should take responsibility to notify their employer or their physician of any change in symptoms. These activities and/or work guides have been provided to the individual and they have indicated their understanding and agreement.

If appropriate, a treatment plan was formulated after medical decision-making was used to develop a diagnosis of the injury/illness using the medical records, materials provided today, the physical examination, and supporting studies. Medicine is both an art and a science. The opinions rendered for this examination are the opinions of this evaluator based on a clinical history, examination, and documentation. These opinions are based upon reasonable medical probability. This evaluation has been conducted based on the medical examination and documentation as provided, with the assumption that the material is true and correct. If more information becomes available later, an additional service, report, or reconsideration may be appropriate. Such information may, or may not, change the opinions rendered in this evaluation. This opinion does not constitute per se a recommendation for specific claims or administrative functions to be made or enforced.

Sincerely,

*J Mark Melhorn, MD*

# Appendix

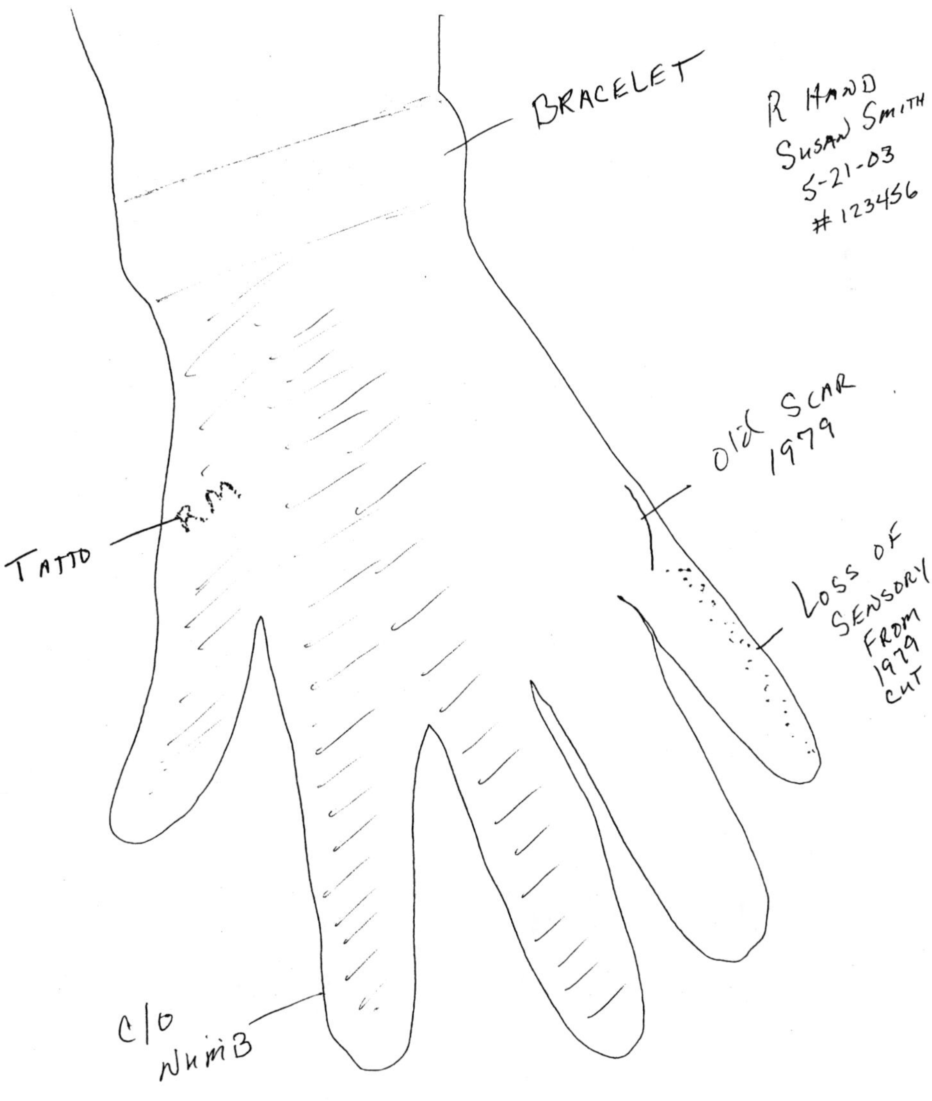
BRACELET
R HAND
SUSAN SMITH
5-21-03
#123456
OLD SCAR
1979
TATTO
R.M.
LOSS OF
SENSORY
FROM
1979
CUT
C/O
NUMB

The Hand Center

ORTHOPAEDICS OF THE HAND & UPPER EXTREMITY

Please circle the level of your pain today

| 0 | 1 | 2 | 3 | 4 | 5 | 6 | 7 | 8 | 9 | 10 |
|---|---|---|---|---|---|---|---|---|---|---|
| No pain | | | | | Moderate pain | | | | | Worst possible pain |

In general, are your symptoms (circle one) same, better or worse?

Please mark the areas on your body where you feel the following described sensations. Use the symbols as provided. Mark all affected areas.

| numbness | pins & needles | burning | stabbing | aching |
|---|---|---|---|---|
| = = = = | o o o o | x x x x | I I I I | • • • • |
| = = = = | o o o o | x x x x | I I I I | • • • • |

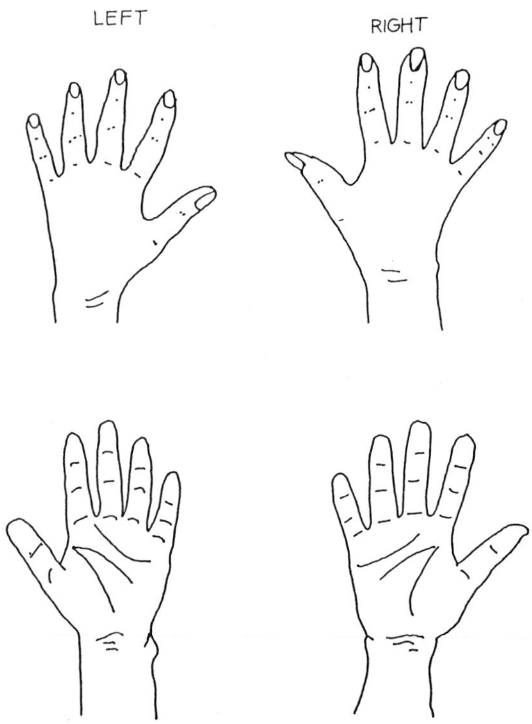


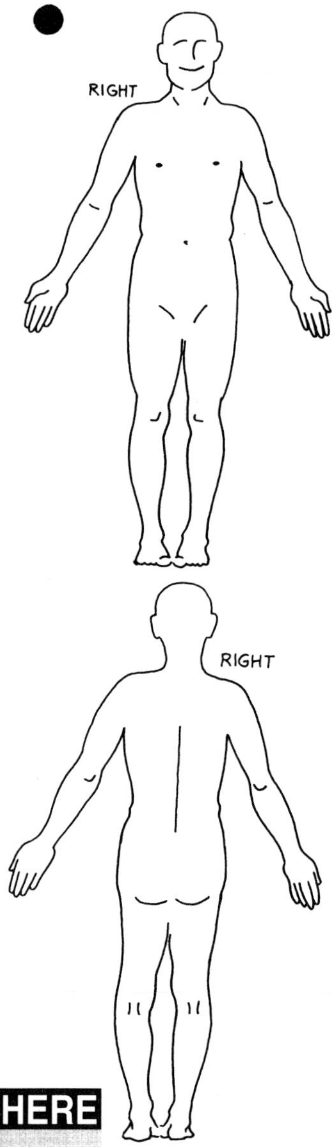


**PLEASE SIGN HERE** — PATIENT SIGNATURE REQUIRED

**DATE HERE** — TODAY'S DATE

THC-6

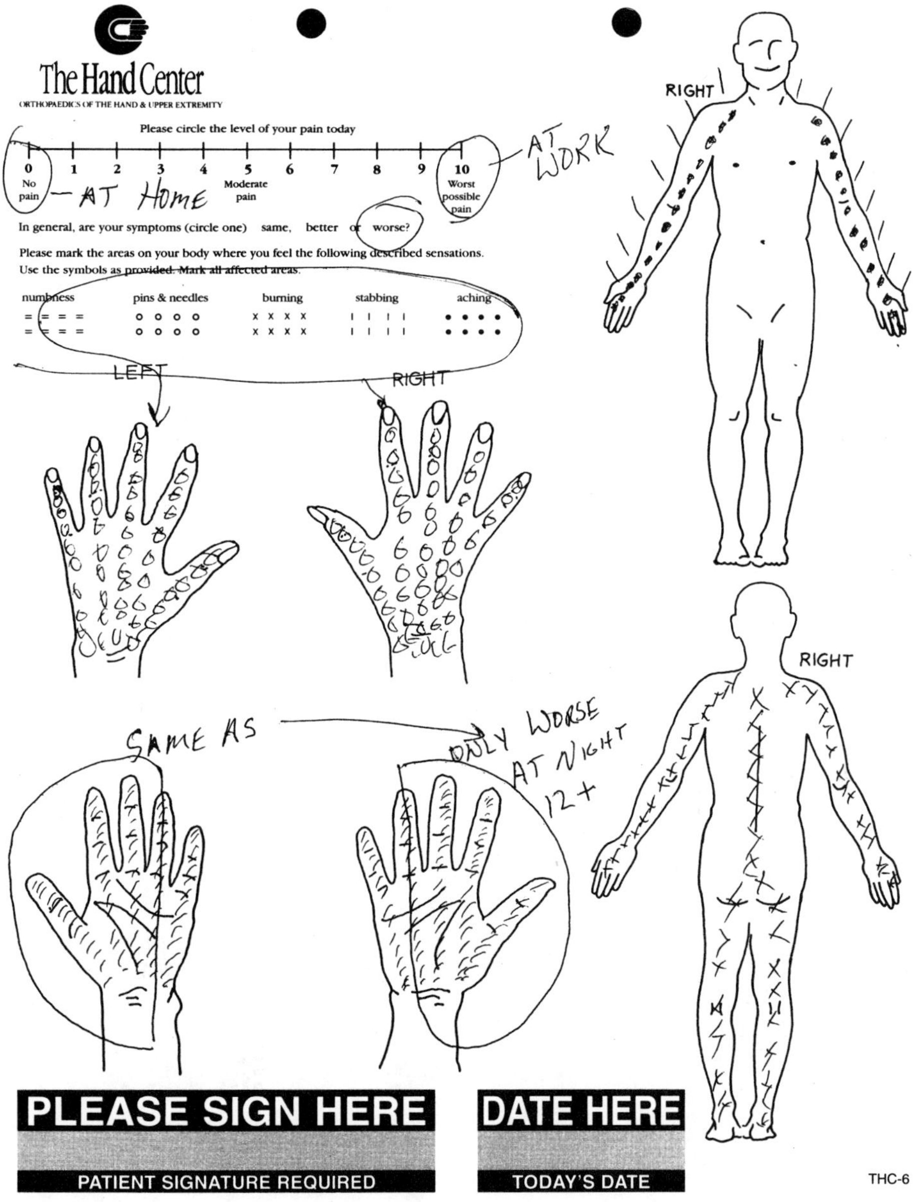

The Hand Center
ORTHOPAEDICS OF THE HAND & UPPER EXTREMITY

Please circle the level of your pain today

0 No pain — AT HOME | 1 | 2 | 3 | 4 | 5 Moderate pain | 6 | 7 | 8 | 9 | 10 Worst possible pain — AT WORK

In general, are your symptoms (circle one) same, better or worse?

Please mark the areas on your body where you feel the following described sensations.
Use the symbols as provided. Mark all affected areas.

| numbness | pins & needles | burning | stabbing | aching |
|---|---|---|---|---|
| = = = = | o o o o | x x x x | I I I I | • • • • |
| = = = = | o o o o | x x x x | I I I I | • • • • |



PLEASE SIGN HERE

PATIENT SIGNATURE REQUIRED

DATE HERE

TODAY'S DATE

THC-6

# INDEX